Revisiting Cardiac Anatomy

Revisiting Cardiac Anatomy

A Computed-Tomography-Based Atlas and Reference

EDITED BY

Farhood Saremi, MD
Professor of Radiology and Medicine
Department of Radiological Sciences
University of California
Irvine
CA, USA

Stephan Achenbach, MD
Professor of Medicine
Department of Cardiology
University of Erlangen
Erlangen
Germany

Eloisa Arbustini, MD, FESC
Prof.ssa Specialista in Cardiologia, Anatomia Patologica, Genetica
Direttore Centro Malattie Genetiche Cardiovascolari
Area Trapiantologica
IRCCS Fondazione Policlinico San Matteo
Pavia
Italy

Jagat Narula, MD, PhD, FACC, FRCP
Professor of Medicine, School of Medicine
Chief, Division of Cardiology & Director, Cardiovascular Center
UC Irvine Douglas Hospital
Director, Memorial Heart & Vascular Institute, Long Beach Memorial Hospital
Medical Director, Edwards Lifesciences Center for Advanced CV Technology, School of Engineering
University of California
Irvine
CA, USA

WILEY-BLACKWELL
A John Wiley & Sons, Ltd., Publication

Blackwell Publishing was acquired by John Wiley & Sons in February 2007. Blackwell's publishing program has been merged with Wiley's global Scientific, Technical and Medical business to form Wiley-Blackwell.

Registered office: John Wiley & Sons Ltd, The Atrium, Southern Gate, Chichester, West Sussex, PO19 8SQ, UK

Editorial offices: 9600 Garsington Road, Oxford, OX4 2DQ, UK
The Atrium, Southern Gate, Chichester, West Sussex, PO19 8SQ, UK
111 River Street, Hoboken, NJ 07030-5774, USA

For details of our global editorial offices, for customer services and for information about how to apply for permission to reuse the copyright material in this book please see our website at www.wiley.com/wiley-blackwell

Library of Congress Cataloging-in-Publication Data
Revisiting cardiac anatomy : a computed-tomography-based reference and atlas / edited by Farhood Saremi . . . [et al.].
p. ; cm.
Includes bibliographical references.
ISBN 978-1-4051-9469-3 (hardback)
1. Heart–Anatomy–Atlases 2. Heart–Tomography–Atlases I. Saremi, Farhood.
[DNLM: 1. Heart–anatomy & histology. 2. Tomography, X-Ray Computed. WG 201 R454 2011]
QM181.R48 2011
611′.12–dc22

2010023428

A catalogue record for this book is available from the British Library.

This book is published in the following electronic formats: ePDF 9781444323207; Wiley Online Library 9781444323191

Set in 9.5/12pt Palatino by Aptara® Inc., New Delhi, India
Printed and bound in Singapore by Markono Print Media Pte Ltd

1 2011

Contents

List of Contributors

Amir Abolhoda, MD
Associate Professor of Surgery
Division of Cardiothoracic Surgery
Department of Surgery
University of California
Irvine, CA, USA

Gustavo Abuin, MD
Chief, Cardiovascular Surgery
Instituto Cardiovascular Rawson;
Director of the Cardioanatomy Research Laboratory
Instituto de Neurobiologìa
Buenos Aires, Argentina

David H. Adams, MD
Professor and Chairman
Department of Cardiothoracic Surgery
The Mount Sinai School of Medicine
Los Angeles, CA, USA

Hatem Alkadhi, MD
Associate Professor
Institute of Diagnostic Radiology
University Hospital Zurich
Zurich, Switzerland

Daniel S. Berman, MD
Professor of Medicine
Director, Cardiac Imaging
Cedars-Sinai Medical Center
Los Angeles, CA, USA

Emanuela V. Büchel, MD
Division of Pediatric Cardiology
University Children's Hospital
Zurich, Switzerland

Javier G. Castillo, MD
Research Fellow
Department of Cardiothoracic Surgery
The Mount Sinai School of Medicine
Los Angeles, CA, USA

Lotus Desbiolles, MD
Institute of Diagnostic Radiology
University Hospital Zurich
Zurich, Switzerland

Niraj Doctor, MBBS
Research Fellow
Cedars-Sinai Medical Center
Los Angeles, CA, USA

Roberto Dore, MD
Chief, Chest Radiology Section Radiology Department
IRCCS Foundation Policlinico San Matteo
Pavia, Italy

Valentina Favalli, BME
Research Fellow
Telethon Centre for Inherited Cardiovascular Diseases
IRCCS Foundation, Policlinico San Matteo
Pavia, Italy

Gregory P. Fontana, MD
Vice Chairman of Surgery
Attending Cardiac Surgeon
Cedars-Sinai Medical Center
Los Angeles, CA, USA

Carla Frescura, MD
Department of Medico-Diagnostic Sciences
University of Padua Medical School
Padua, Italy

Mario J. Garcia, MD
Professor and Director of Noninvasive Cardiology
The Zena and Michael A. Wiener Cardiovascular Institute
The Mount Sinai School of Medicine
Los Angeles, CA, USA

Fabiana Isabella Gambarin, MD
Cardiologist, Echo-Lab Centre for Inherited Cardiovascular Diseases
IRCCS Foundation Policlinico San Matteo
Pavia, Italy

Siew Yen Ho, PhD
Royal Brompton Hospital and Imperial College London
London, UK

Sebastian Leschka, MD
Institute of Diagnostic Radiology
University Hospital Zurich
Zurich, Switzerland

Raj R. Makkar, MD
Director, Interventional Cardiology and Cardiac Catheterization Laboratory
Cedars-Sinai Medical Center;
Associate Professor
UCLA School of Medicine
Los Angeles, CA, USA

Massimo Massetti, MD
Professor of Thoracic and Cardiovascular Surgery
Chief, Division of Cardiac Surgery
University Hospital of Caen
Caen, France

James K. Min, MD
Assistant Professor of Medicine
The Department of Medicine and Radiology
Weill Medical College of Cornell University
The New York Presbyterian Hospital
New York, NY, USA

Horia Muresian, MD, PhD
San Donato Milan
Italy
and
The University Hospital of Bucharest
Bucharest, Romania

Hursh Naik, MD
Interventional Cardiologist
Cardiovascular Intervention Center
Cedars-Sinai Medical Center
Los Angeles, CA, USA

Eric Saloux, MD
Chief, Echo-Lab Division of Cardiology
University Hospital of Caen
Caen, France

Damián Sánchez-Quintana, MD
Professor of Anatomy and Human Embryology
Department of Anatomy and Cell Biology
School of Medicine of Badajoz
University of Extremadura
Badajoz, Spain

Leslee J. Shaw, PhD
Professor of Medicine
Emory University School of Medicine
Atlanta, GA, USA

Gaetano Thiene, MD, FRCP
Professor
Department of Medical-Diagnostic Sciences and Special Therapies
University of Padua Medical School
Padua, Italy

Hyun Woo Goo, MD
Associate Professor
Department of Radiology
Asan Medical Center
University of Ulsan
Seoul, Korea

Preface

The past two decades have witnessed a revolution not only in management but also in the diagnostic approach to cardiovascular disease. Modern imaging tools provide invasive and noninvasive strategies that allow increasingly accurate characterization of morphology and function of the heart. Nuclear medicine, echocardiography (including transesophageal, intravascular, and intracardiac imaging) as well as cardiac magnetic resonance have all immensely contributed to the ability to provide accurate diagnostic and prognostic information. At the same time, modern surgical and interventional treatment requires accurate anatomic information and guidance. The success of increasingly complex coronary and noncoronary structural interventions as well as electrophysiological procedures depends on ever more detailed imaging support. The interface between imaging, diagnosis, and treatment is of tremendous importance and at the same time needs to face increasingly challenging requirements.

In addition to the more established techniques, high-resolution multidetector CT imaging of the heart and cardiovascular system has recently entered the stage. Modern hardware allows truly isotropic imaging with high temporal resolution and a spatial resolution of 0.5 mm or better. Two-dimensional and three-dimensional reconstructions allow to perform "virtual dissection" of complex cardiac anatomy with phenomenal image quality. In fact, in vivo imaging will often provide a more realistic depiction of true anatomic relationships than postmortem analysis.

However, while modern imaging provides new possibilities, it also creates new needs and challenges. To fully realize the potential inherent to the large, detailed datasets, a new type of "imager," needs to fulfill many roles—from teaching medical students and residents to helping the cardiologist better define and the interventionalist or surgeon better correct cardiovascular defects by fully understanding the underlying anatomy.

Hence, as we embarked on this atlas, we set ambitious goals for our project. We resolved to provide a valuable resource and useful companion to a broad spectrum of readership, from medical students starting their career in a dissection hall to cardiologists and cardiothoracic surgeons who rely on ever more accurate imaging for diagnosis and treatment. This atlas is a fresh approach to cardiac anatomy that provides high-quality in vivo anatomy through carefully rendered images with explanatory texts of the clinically relevant underlying anatomic concepts. In spite of amazing proliferation of information on the Internet and multiple Web sites filled with up-to-date information, there is no similarly detailed and systematic compilation of morphological imaging with CT to demonstrate normal in vivo anatomy of the heart and its variants. For good understanding of health and disease, a good anatomy book is irreplaceable and will allow both for systematic learning and as a quick, yet detailed reference for specific clinical questions.

The fantastic imaging quality that can be achieved with state-of-the-art CT imaging hardware and protocols in the hands of experts has deeply impressed and convinced us. We are confident that it will also convince our readership: imaging is a virtual reality.

1 Anatomy of the Heart for a Dissector

Farhood Saremi[1] & Damián Sánchez-Quintana[2]

[1] *University of California Irvine, CA, USA*
[2] *University of Extremadura, Badajoz, Spain*

Introduction

This chapter provides a general description of the heart anatomy and offers an outline of the relevant clinical information. Images are produced using state of the art multidetector scanner on living subjects and by meticulous dissection techniques on cadaveric specimens. Detailed discussions on specific anatomic locations are presented in the subsequent chapters.

Heart Orientation within the Thorax

Generally, cross-sectional imaging study of the heart requires reconstruction of two groups of imaging planes including body and heart planes. Standard body planes include three orthogonal cuts in axial (transverse), coronal, and sagittal orientations. Heart planes also include three orthogonal planes in relation to the heart axes [1,2]. Short-axis images, which correspond to the plane of the atrioventricular (AV) groove, are oblique and are oriented closer to the vertical than to the horizontal plane. Horizontal long-axis (four-chamber) views are double oblique planes perpendicular to both the interventricular septum and the AV plane of the heart. Vertical long-axis (two-chamber) views of the heart are parallel to the interventricular septum (Figure 1.1).

Everyone must be familiar with radiographic borders of the heart in different projections (Figure 1.2). On anterior projection, the right cardiac border is formed by the right atrium (RA), while the left cardiac border is formed by the left ventricle (LV). The right ventricle (RV) and the left atrium (LA) are superimposed structures and are not border-forming, and additional projections are required to review them. Diaphragmatic surface is formed by the RV. On the lateral projection, the anterior cardiac border is the RV, while the posterior cardiac border is composed of both the LV and the LA.

Anteriorly, the heart is covered by the sternum and the costal cartilages. The heart has an extensive diaphragmatic surface inferiorly (Figure 1.3). Posteriorly, the heart lies on the esophagus and the tracheal bifurcation, and bronchi that extend into the lung. The sternum lies anteriorly and provides rigid protection to the heart during blunt trauma.

The true posterior surface of the heart is commonly termed the base of the heart, which is formed largely by the LA. The term "base of the heart" is not frequently used and is restricted to the "origin of the great vessels." The inferior surface of the heart is also closely related to the diaphragm and should not be entirely called posterior. In supine position, along with elevation of the diaphragm, the lower surface of the heart largely faces inferiorly; however, in upright position, with full inspiration, the heart stands vertically and these walls face posteroinferiorly [1]. Because of the obliquity of the surfaces of the ventricles, the diaphragmatic surface of the RV is truly inferior and the diaphragmatic wall of the LV faces posteroinferiorly (Figures 1.3–1.5).

The heart is a three-sided pyramid located in the middle mediastinum. When viewed from its apex, the three sides of the ventricular mass are readily seen (Figure 1.5). Two of the edges are named. The acute margin lies inferiorly and describes a sharp angle between the sternocostal and diaphragmatic surfaces. The obtuse margin lies superiorly and is much more diffuse. The posterior margin is unnamed but is also diffuse in its transition.

The Right Atrium

The RA is the chamber of the heart that receives systemic venous blood return from the superior vena cava (SVC)

Revisiting Cardiac Anatomy: A Computed-Tomography-Based Atlas and Reference, 1st edition. Edited by Farhood Saremi, Eloisa Arbustini, Stephen Achenbach and Jagat Narula.

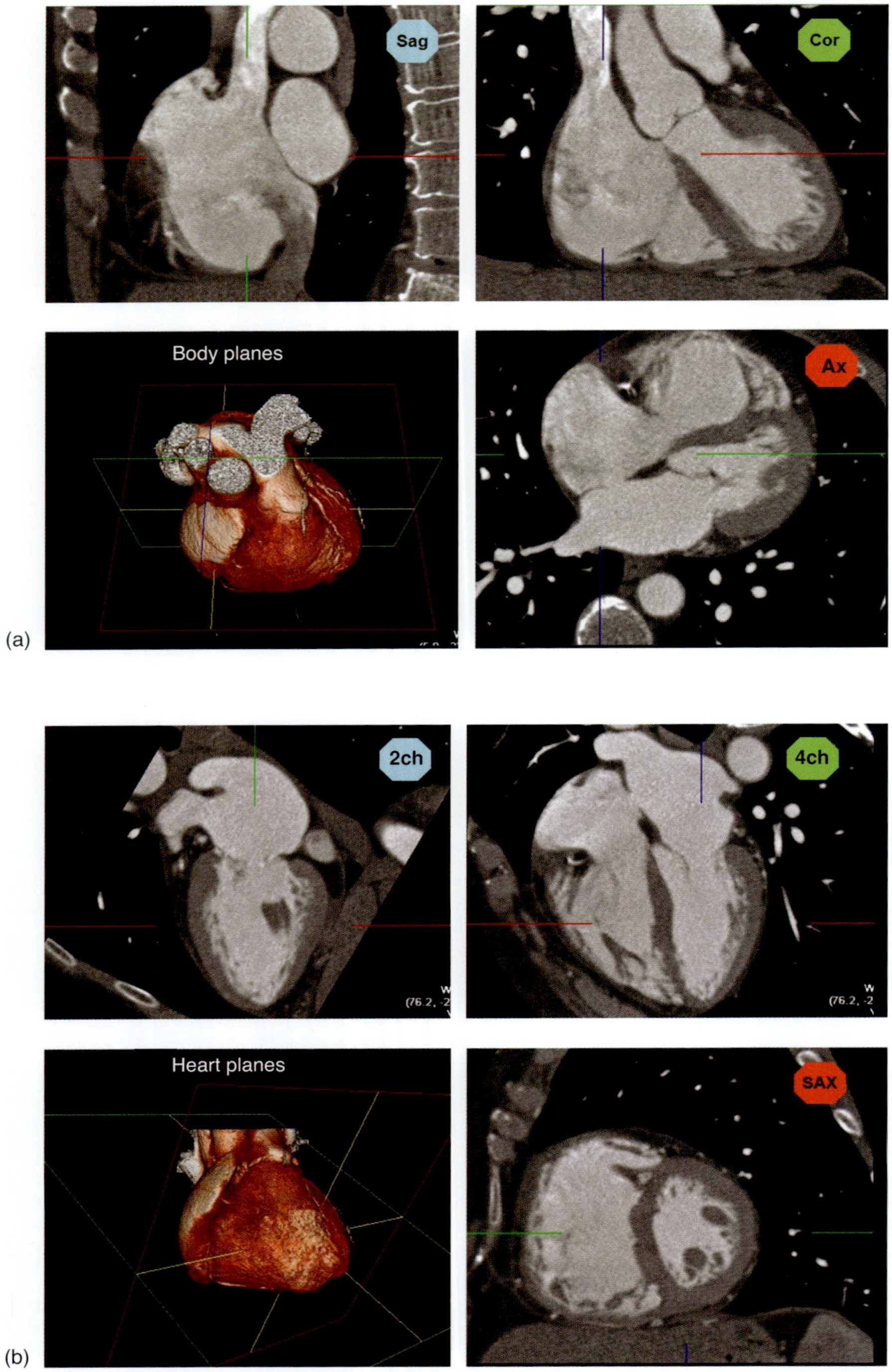

Figure 1.1 Standard body (a) versus heart planes (b). The heart may be viewed in three standard anatomic planes: transaxial (Ax), coronal (Cor), and sagittal (Sag). The three major planes of the heart include short axis (SAX), horizontal long axis (four chamber, 4ch), and vertical long axis (two chamber, 2ch). Although these planes are perpendicular to one another, the body planes transect the heart obliquely, while the heart planes transect the body obliquely.

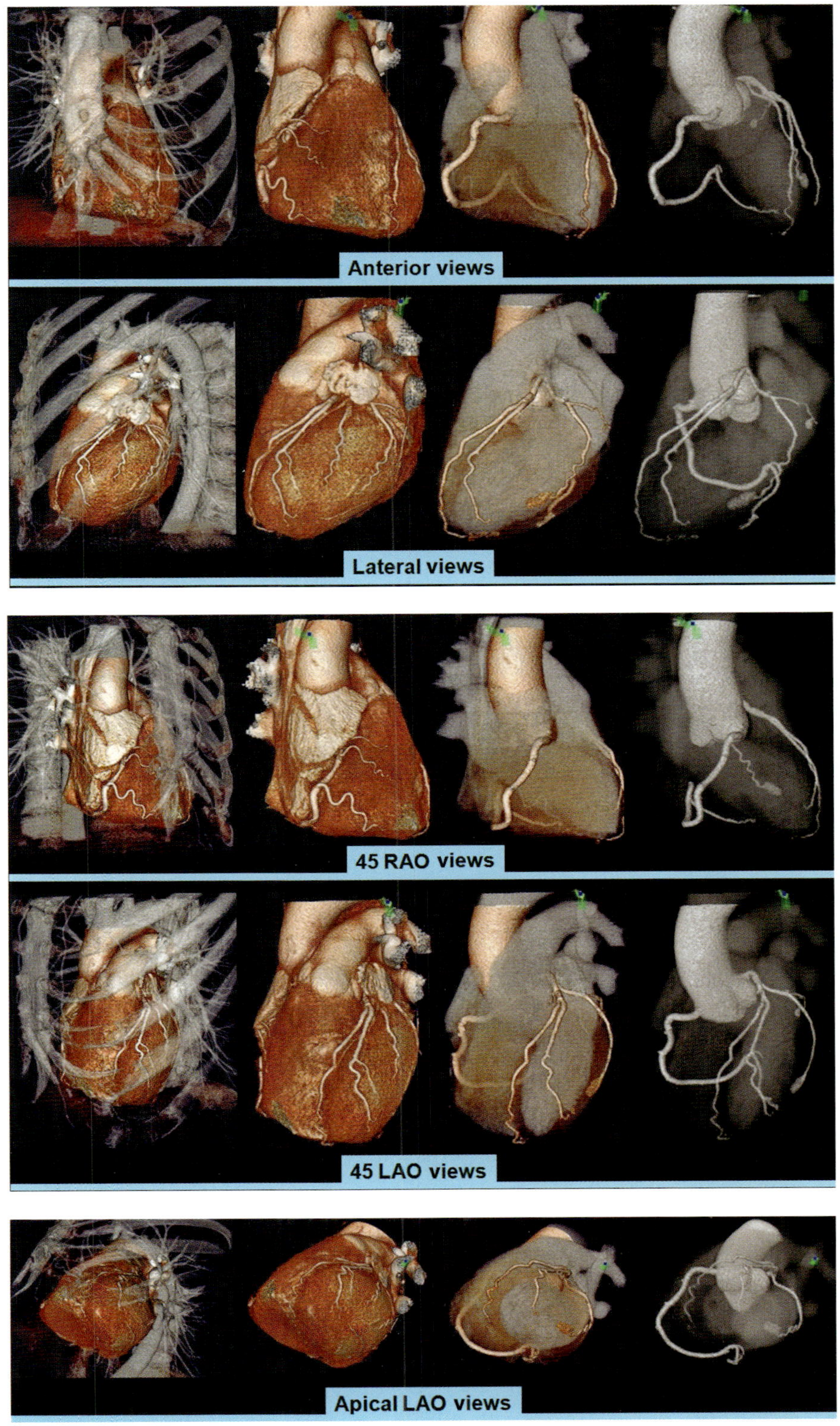

Figure 1.2 Radiographic projections are shown. All images are obtained with a 64-slice MDCT with three-dimensional reconstruction. Postprocessing is performed to show the relationship of the heart to the thoracic cage. Angiographic projections show the relation of the coronary arteries to the cardiac chambers. LAO, left anterior oblique projection; RAO, right anterior oblique projection.

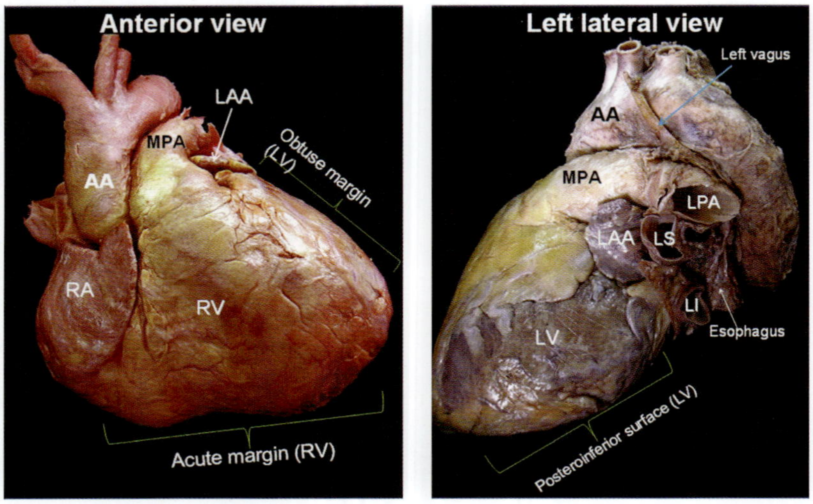

Figure 1.3 Ventricular margins and surfaces of cadaveric heart photographed in attitudinal positions to simulate the views as seen in living condition. (a) Anterior view and (b) Left lateral view of the heart. AA, ascending aorta; LAA, left atrial appendage; LPA, left pulmonary artery; LS and LI, left superior and left inferior pulmonary veins; LV, left ventricle; MPA, main pulmonary artery; RA, right atrium; RV, right ventricle.

and inferior vena cava (IVC) and coronary venous return from the coronary sinus. Looking at three-dimensional images of the heart from the top, RA is positioned to the right and anteriorly, while the LA is situated to the left and mainly posteriorly [3] (Figure 1.6)

From a spatial point of view, the RA may be divided into lateral, medial, inferior, and posterior walls. The RA comprises three components: the appendage, the venous part (sinus venarum), and the vestibule [4,5]. One of morphologic characteristics of the RA is the presence of the crista terminalis. This C-shaped muscular ridge separates the smooth-walled sinus venarum from the trabeculated appendage (the right half of the primitive atrium) [6]. The crista terminalis varies in size and extent in different individuals (Figure 1.7; see also Chapter 9, cardiac anatomy for electrophysiologic interventions). Another indicator of the right atrial morphology is a large, wide-based appendage (Figure 1.6). Some anatomists define the appendage as the anterosuperior protrusion of the body of the RA, an anatomic feature rather than an anatomic subdivision. The vestibule, also known as supravalvular lamina, is a smooth muscular rim surrounding the tricuspid orifice [1] (Figure 1.8). The pectinate muscles do not reach this area (Figure 1.5; see also Chapter 9). The right coronary artery (RCA) runs in the epicardial fat next to the vestibule.

Terminal groove is a fat-filled sulcus on epicardial side, which corresponds internally to crista terminalis (Figure 1.6, the right lateral view). The sinus node and terminal

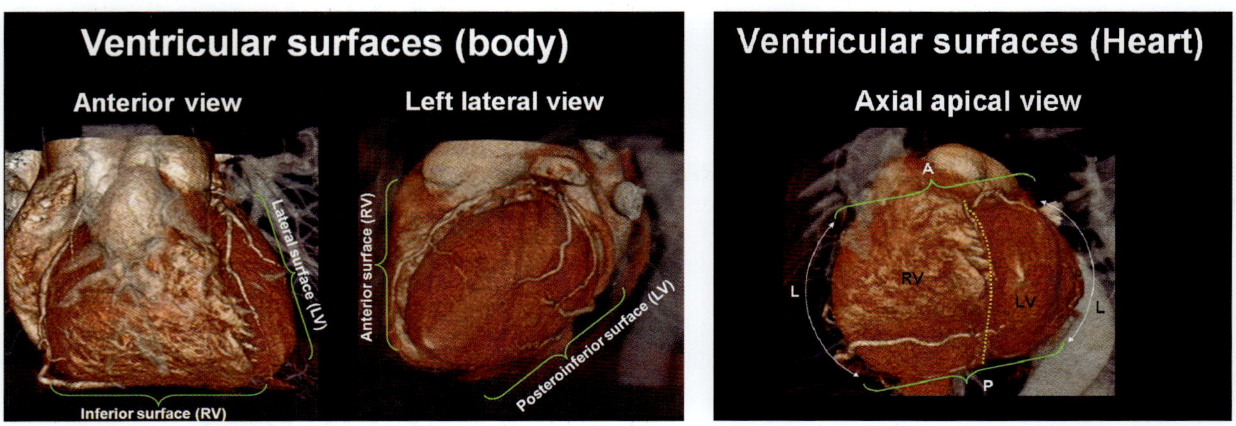

Figure 1.4 CT angiography views. The ventricular surfaces are shown is relation to the thorax (body) and the heart itself. A, anterior; dotted yellow line, interventricular groove; L, lateral; LV, left ventricle; P, posterior; RV, right ventricle.

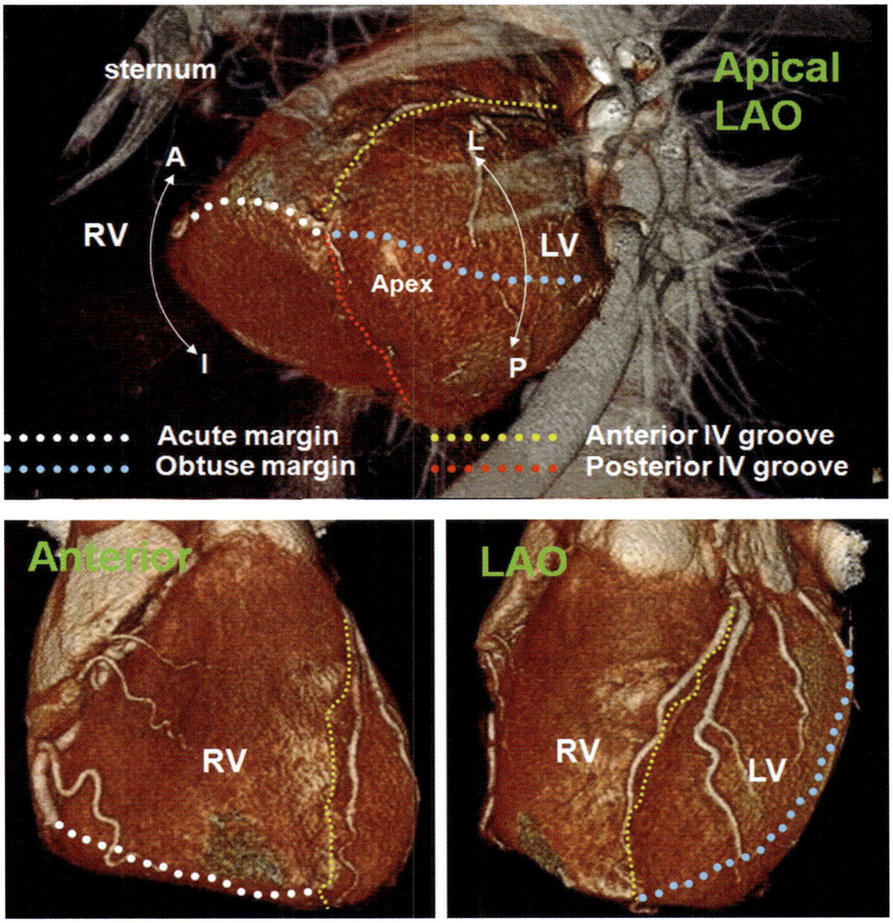

Figure 1.5 The margins of the heart. The acute margin is applied to the right ventricle (RV) only between the sternocostal (A, anterior) and diaphragmatic (I, inferior) surfaces. In an anterior view, the acute margin forms the lower border and the right atrium forms the right lateral border of the heart. The term "obtuse margin" denotes the posterolateral aspect of the left ventricle and atrium. It is defined as the junction between the lateral (L) and posterior (P) walls of the left ventricle (LV). In left anterior oblique (LAO) projection view, it forms the left border of the heart. Obtuse margin is a critical anatomic landmark, and in many instances, an artery (obtuse marginal, a branch of the LCx artery) runs along it.

segment of sinoatrial (SA) node artery are located in this groove, close to the superior cavoatrial junction.

The sinus venarum is mainly located in the posterolateral wall of the RA between the SVC and IVC orifices [7] (Figure 1.6). From the third week after the development of the primitive heart tube, the primitive atria are separated from the sinus venosus by a segmentation termed the SA ring. The sinus venosus has two horns. The right horn gives rise to all the intercaval regions of the RA including the crista terminalis, the Eustachian ridge, and the Thebesian valve (Figure 1.6). The left horn gives rise to the coronary sinus [8]. The interatrial septum is located posteromedially.

The RA is home to important parts of the cardiac conduction system including the SA and the AV nodes (AVNs) [9–11]. The SA node (SAN) is a banana-shaped structure in the subepicardial side of superior cavoatrial junction, composed of cells slightly smaller than normal working cells (Figure 1.11; see also Chapters 9). It is the source of the cardiac impulse. Because of the vicinity of the sinus node to the epicardial surface, it may be damaged in selected cardiac surgeries or extensive pericardial diseases [9]. The SAN is supplied by the SAN artery. The SAN artery is usually, a single branch, arising from the proximal RCA (60%) or the left circumflex (LCx) artery (40%) (see Chapter 4 and 9 for details). In the majority of hearts, the SAN artery passes through the center of SAN [11] (Figure 1.9).

The AVN is located within the boundaries of Koch's triangle near its apex. The triangle of Koch is an important anatomic landmark of the RA, which is commonly used for electrophysiologic studies (Figure 1.17; see also Chapter 9). This triangle is bordered posteriorly by the tendon of Todaro (fibrous extension from the Eustachian valve), anteriorly by the septal leaflet of the tricuspid valve, and inferiorly by the ostium of the coronary sinus (Figure 1.10). The size of Koch's triangle is variable in different

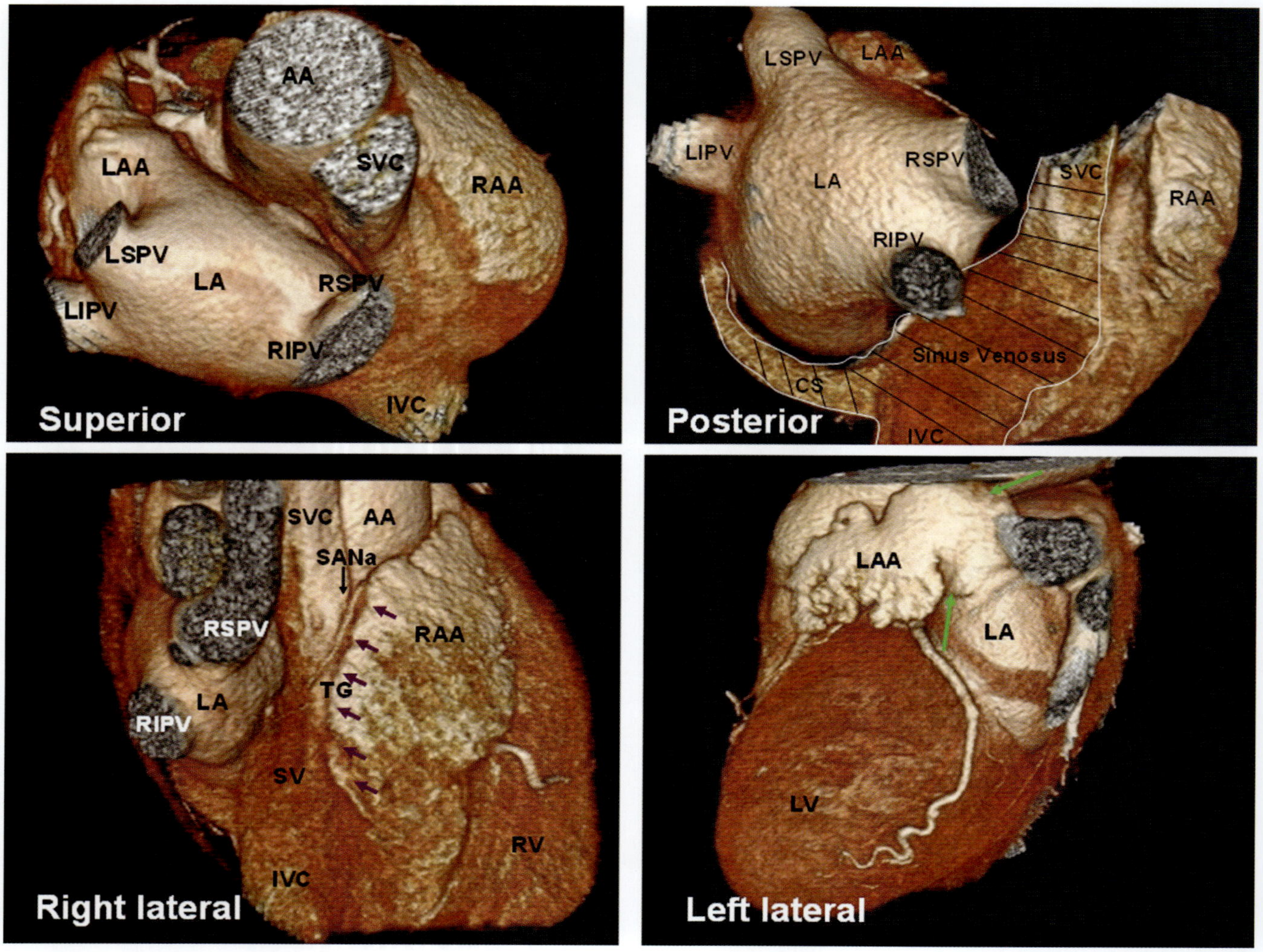

Figure 1.6 Atrial epicardial views. When viewed from the top (superior), the cavity of the right atrium is positioned to the right and anterior, while the left atrium is situated to the left and mainly posteriorly. On the posterior view, the anatomic boundaries of structures arising from the sinus venosus (SV) of the right atrium are shown (shaded area). Lower images are right and left lateral views of the heart. The dominant feature on the right side is a large, triangular shaped, atrial appendage. Terminal groove (TG) is between sinus venosus and RAA (small arrows). Note the sinoatrial node (SAN) artery running in this groove. The left atrial appendage (LAA) is a small lobulated structure. It is a potential site for deposition of thrombus owing to its trabeculated margin and narrow neck (green arrows). AA, ascending aorta; CS, coronary sinus; IVC, inferior vena cava; LA, left atrium; LIPV, left inferior pulmonary vein; LSPV, left superior pulmonary vein; LV, left ventricle; RA, right atrium; RAA, right atrial appendage; RIPV, right inferior pulmonary vein; RSPV, right superior pulmonary vein; SANa, sinoatrial node artery; SVC, superior vena cava. (Reprinted from Saremi and Krishnan [3], with permission.)

individuals. The apex of this triangle corresponds to the central fibrous body of the heart [12].

The AVN consists of a compact portion and an area of transitional cells. The compact portion lies over the central fibrous body [13] (Figure 1.19; see also Chapter 9). The AVN continues distally with the penetrating bundle of His. The AVN artery originates from the distal RCA (80–90%) and penetrates into the base of the posterior interatrial septum (inferior pyramidal space) at the level of crux of the heart in 80–87% of patients (Figure 1.11). In the remaining, it originates from the distal LCx artery [14–16].

The inferior wall of the RA is a complex area with several important anatomic landmarks [7, 17]. The IVC and the coronary sinus connect to this portion of the RA. The Eustachian valve guards the anterior margin of the IVC. It is usually membranous and variably developed (Figure 1.26; see also Chapter 9). It may look fenestrated or contain muscles. Usually it inserts medially to the Eustachian ridge or sinus septum, which is the border between the oval fossa and the coronary sinus. The medial border of the Eustachian valve continues as a tendon of Todaro that runs in the musculature of the Eustachian ridge. Mistakenly,

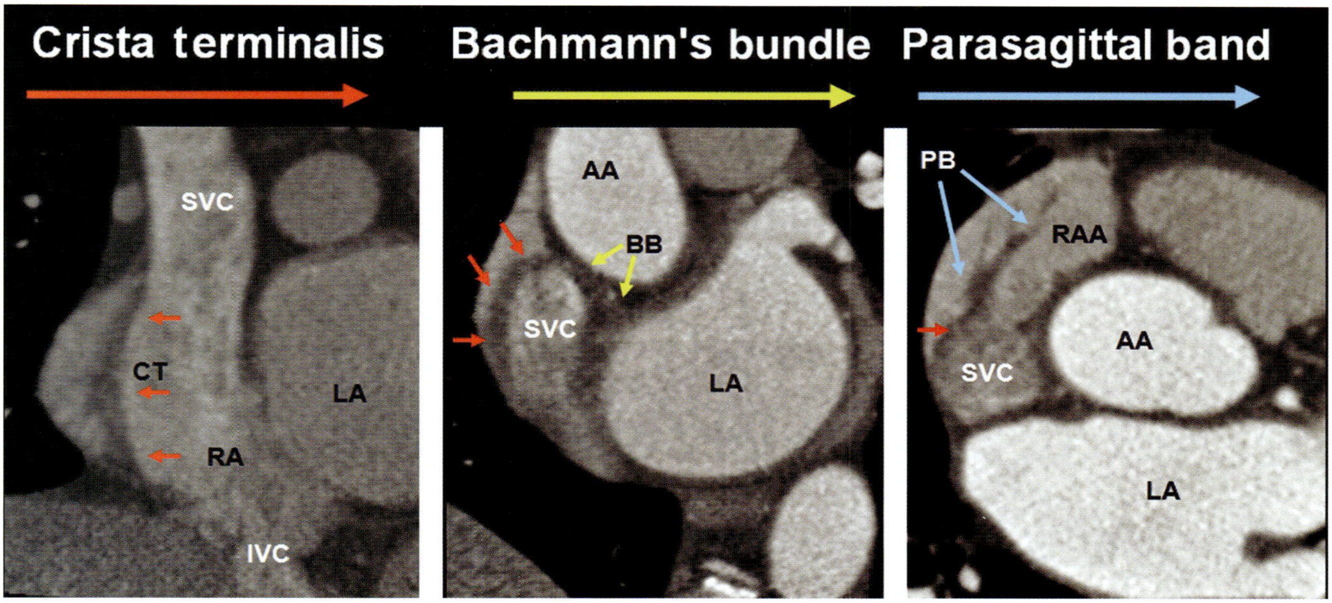

Figure 1.7 Crista terminalis (CT) is a fibromuscular ridge formed by the junction of the sinus venosus and primitive right atrium (red arrows). The entire CT lies between the pectinate muscles and the sinus venarum. The origin of the crest at the interatrial groove is confluent with the origin of another important muscular fascicle, Bachmann bundle (yellow arrows). The crest arches anterior to the orifice of the SVC (precaval band) and extends to the area of the anterior interatrial groove. The parasagittal band (PB, blue arrows) or septum spurium is a large pectinate muscle arising from the precaval portion of the crest. It divides the right atrial appendage into medial and lateral compartments. The inferior border of the CT near the IVC orifice is unclear. It breaks up into a series of trabeculations in the area of the atrial wall known as the cavotricuspid isthmus. AA, ascending aorta; BB, Bachmann bundle; IVC, inferior vena cava; LA, left atrium; RA, right atrium; RAA, right atrial appendage; SVC, superior vena cava.

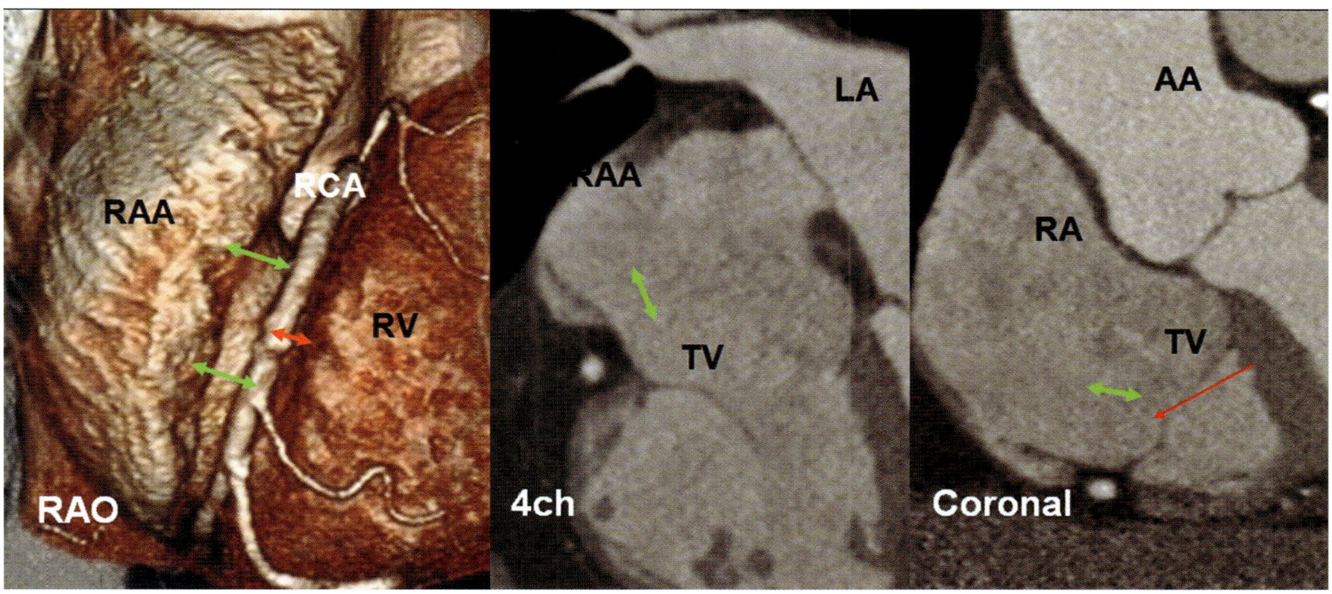

Figure 1.8 The right atrial vestibule, also known as supravalvular lamina, is a smooth muscular rim surrounding the tricuspid orifice (green arrows). The pectinate muscles do not reach this area. The right coronary artery runs in epicardial fat next to the vestibule. A thin fibrous membrane extends between the tricuspid annulus and the ostium of the right ventricle (RV), known as subvalvular membrane (red arrows). The fragile nature of this complex membranous structure should be remembered in tricuspid valve (TV) repair or replacement. 4ch, four chamber; AA, ascending aorta; LA left atrium; RA, right atrium; RAA, right atrial appendage; RAO, right anterior oblique projection; RCA, right coronary artery.

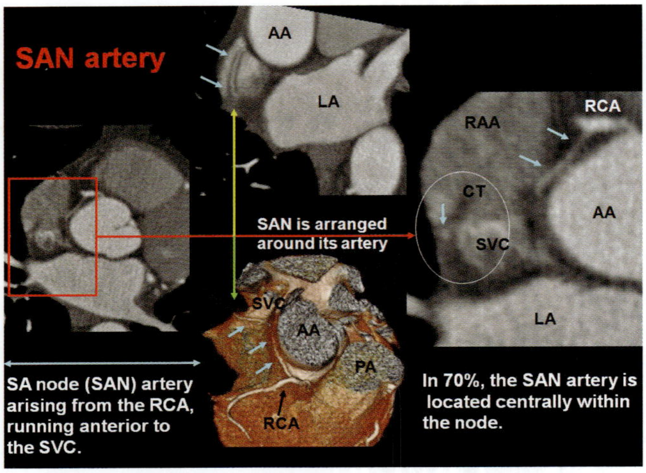

Figure 1.9 Sinoatrial node (SAN) artery arising from the right coronary artery (RCA). Axial and short-axis images at cavoatrial junction show terminal portion of SAN artery running in myocardial tissue of crista terminalis (CT). SAN tissue is arranged around SAN artery in 75% of cases. AA, ascending aorta; LA, left atrium; LV, left ventricle; PA, pulmonary artery; RA, right atrium; RAA, right atrial appendage; SVC, superior vena cava. (Reprinted from Saremi and Krishnan [3], with permission.)

the valve may be sutured to the anterior rim of an atrial septal defect at the time of shunt repair. Laterally, the Eustachian valve merges into the crista terminalis. In some cases, it is large, posing an obstacle to pass a catheter.

The inferior wall of the RA between the IVC and the tricuspid valve is a quadrilateral region known as cavotricuspid isthmus [18]. It is the target of catheter ablation techniques for isthmus-dependent atrial flutter [19]. Autopsies and angiographic findings have shown a highly variable isthmus anatomy that can make ablation difficult. Obstacles such as large Eustachian ridge/valve, aneurysmal pouches, or even a concave deformation of the entire isthmus may lead to more difficult ablation sessions. Therefore, knowledge of anatomic variants of this region is very important. Cardiac multidetector CT (MDCT) provides detailed anatomic information, including the size and anatomic variants of cavotricuspid isthmus, coronary sinus, and Eustachian ridge [20] (Figures 1.10 and 1.12).

It is common to observe outpouchings in the medial and lateral margins of the inferior wall of the RA (Figure 1.13). The medial outpouching inferior to the orifice of the coronary sinus is known as the sub-Eustachian sinus of Keith. When seen in attitudinally correct orientation, it is anterior to the orifice of the IVC and sub-Thebesian rather than sub-Eustachian [4] (Figure 1.14). Because of its special arrangement of muscle fibers, it can be the substrate for reentrant circuit during atrial flutter. This peculiar anatomy is recognized as one of the major procedural difficulties in catheter interventions of the RA (details in Chapter 9).

The RA and the coronary sinus form a unit that wraps around the LA. The coronary sinus is highly variable in morphology and its length varies between 30 and 50 mm

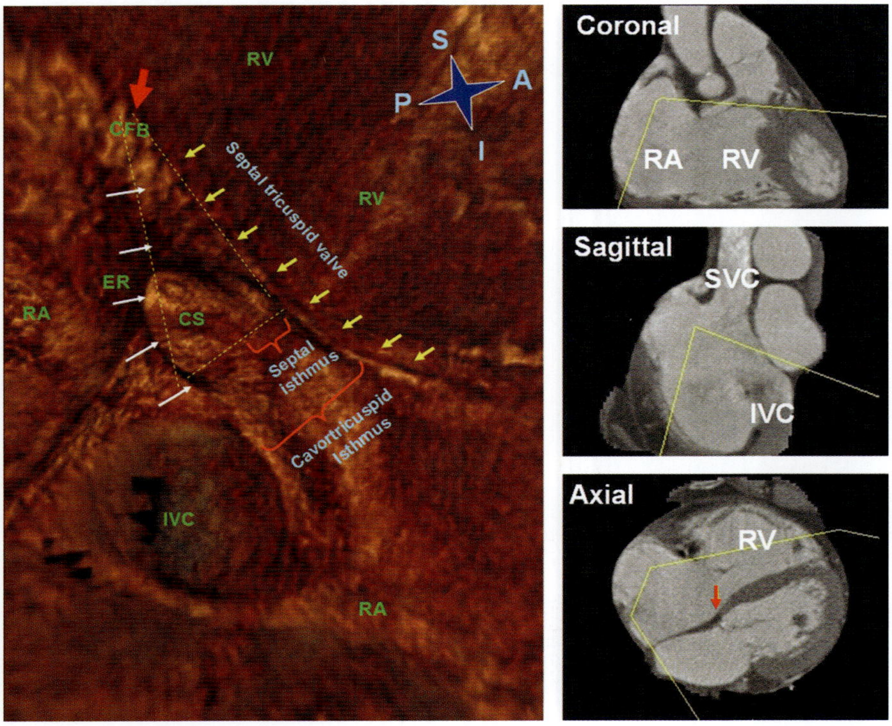

Figure 1.10 The triangle of Koch and related structures. Endocardial view of the right AV junction shows the triangle of Koch and the right atrial isthmus. The triangle of Koch is demarcated by the tendon of Todaro/Eusthasian ridge (ER) posteriorly (white arrows), the attachment of septal tricuspid leaflet (yellow arrows) anteriorly, the coronary sinus inferiorly, and the central fibrous body (CFB) at the apex (red arrows). The septal isthmus (small bracket) is part of the smooth vestibule. The cavotricuspid isthmus lies between the orifice of the IVC and the tricuspid valve (large bracket). Reference CT images on the right show the anatomic position of the Koch triangle (yellow lines) from different perspectives. A, anterior; AVN, atrioventricular node; CS, coronary sinus; I, inferior; IVC, inferior vena cava; P, posterior; RA, right atrium; RV, right ventricle; S, superior; SVC, superior vena cava. (Reprinted from Saremi and Krishnan [3], with permission.)

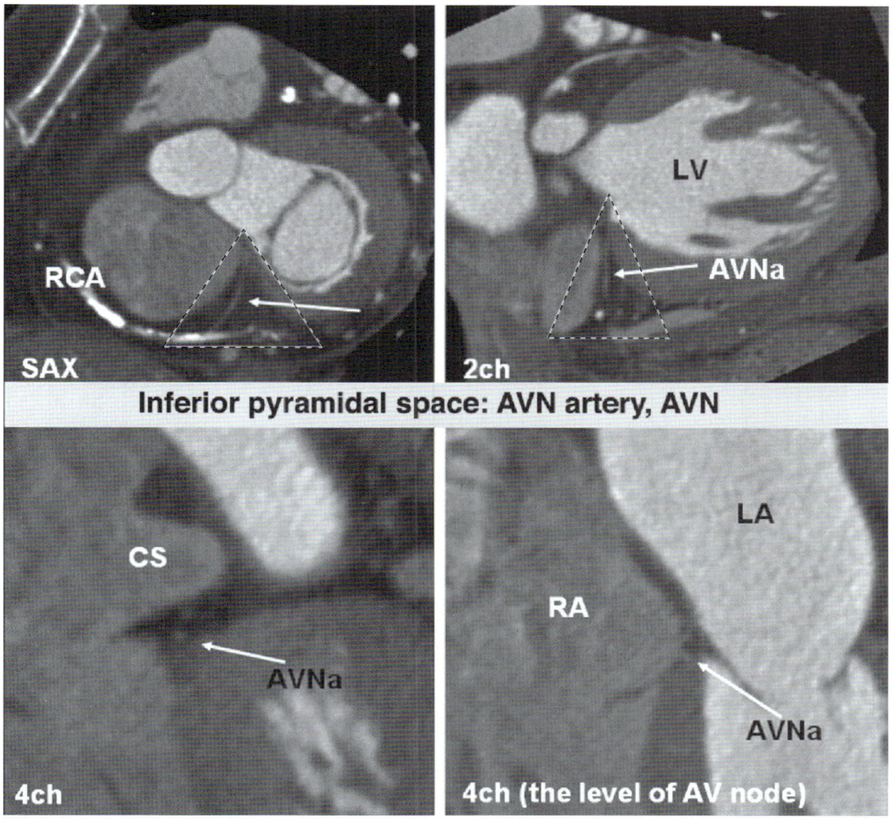

Figure 1.11 Inferior pyramidal space (dotted triangle) is the anatomic location of atrioventricular node artery (AVNa). The AVNa originates from the distal right coronary artery (RCA) and penetrates into the base of the posterior interatrial septum. The AVNa supplies the AVN at the apex of the pyramid in close proximity to the muscular atrioventricular septum. This area is not a true septum, but extracardiac fat sandwiched between the right atrium (RA) and the left atrium (LA). 2ch, two-chamber view; 4ch, four-chamber view; CS, coronary sinus; LV, left ventricle; SAX, short-axis view.

in 75% of cases [21, 22] (Figure 1.64; see also Chapter 9). The coronary sinus ostium is at the inferomedial corner of the RA and posteroinferior to the AVN. It is guarded by the Thebesian valve. The valve is usually a thin semilunar fold in antero-inferior rim of the ostium (Figure 1.15). It is continuous with the Eustachian valve. The coronary sinus collects blood from most of the epicardial coronary veins serving the left heart.

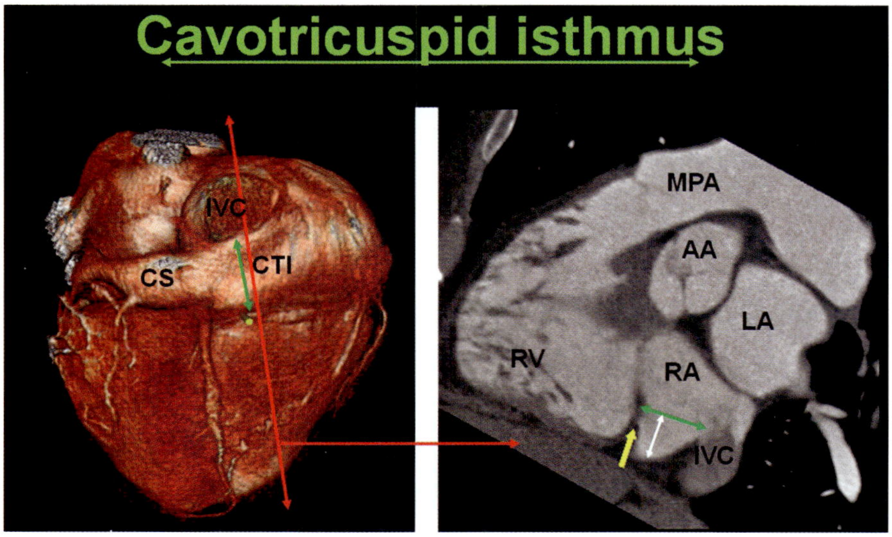

Figure 1.12 Cavotricuspid isthmus is a quadrilateral area in the floor of the RA bounded by the inferior vena cava (IVC) and the Eustachian ridge posteriorly and the septal attachment of tricuspid valve anteriorly (yellow arrows). On a two-chamber view of the right side of the heart through the central portion of the CTI as indicated by the red double-headed arrow in the posterior three-dimensional image, the IVC is closest to the atrioventricular (AV) groove (yellow arrows). The length and depth of the central isthmus (green and white double-headed arrow respectively) can be measured on this view. AA, ascending aorta; CS, coronary sinus; CTI, cavotricuspid isthmus; LA, left atrium; MPA, main pulmonary artery; RA, right atrium; RV, right ventricle.

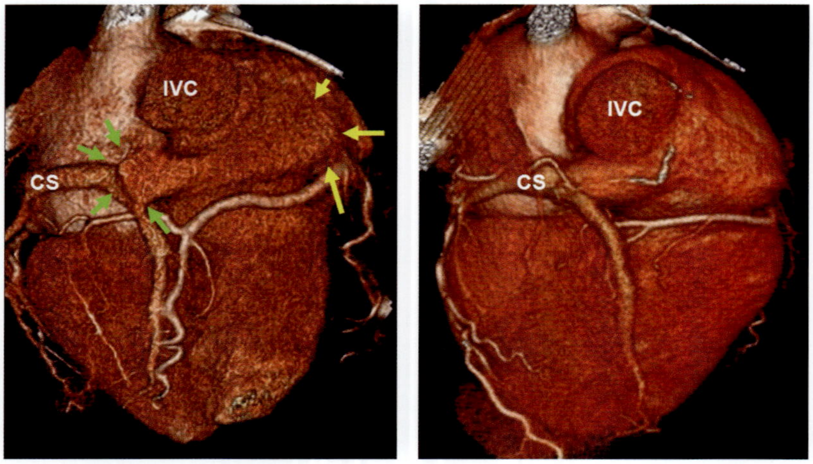

(a) (b)

Figure 1.13 Posterior three-dimensional images of the heart demonstrate the inferior wall of the right atrium in two different patients. (a) It is common to observe two pouches: one medially and one laterally. The inferomedial pouch has been termed sub-Eustachian sinus of Keith (green arrows). It extends below the ostium of the coronary sinus and may interfere with percutaneous catheterization of the coronary sinus. The inferolateral pouch is usually smaller (yellow arrows). (b) Posterior view in a different patient shows smooth contour of the inferior wall with no outpouching. CS, coronary sinus; IVC, inferior vena cava.

The Left Atrium

The LA is the posterior chamber of the heart (the RA is the right lateral, the RV the anterior, and the LV is the left lateral chamber) that receives pulmonary venous drainage from the four pulmonary veins [1]. With the exception of the interatrial muscle bundles (Bachmann bundle), the muscles of each atrium are confined to its wall. The shape of the LA may be compared to an inverted box with a large opening attached to the mitral valve. The relations of the LA to adjacent structures are important (Figure 1.16). The LA is divided into five poorly demarcated walls: anterior, posterior (posteroinferior), superior, lateral, and right medial (septal).

As with the RA, the LA consists of a venous component, an appendage, and a supravalvular vestibule [2,4] (Figure 1.34; see also Chapter 9). Most part of the LA except the appendage is smooth-walled. The superior and posterior walls of the LA form the pulmonary venous component, with the venous orifices at each corner.

The left atrial appendage (LAA) is derived from the primitive atrium and has a rough, trabeculated surface [23]. The orifice of the LAA is anterior to the left superior pulmonary vein. Below this level, the interatrial Bachmann bundle marks the junction of the anterior and superior walls of the LA. The LAA is a potential site for deposition of thrombus owing to its narrow neck with the LA [24]. The proximal portion of the LCx artery runs in contact with the inferior wall of the LAA. A variable relationship

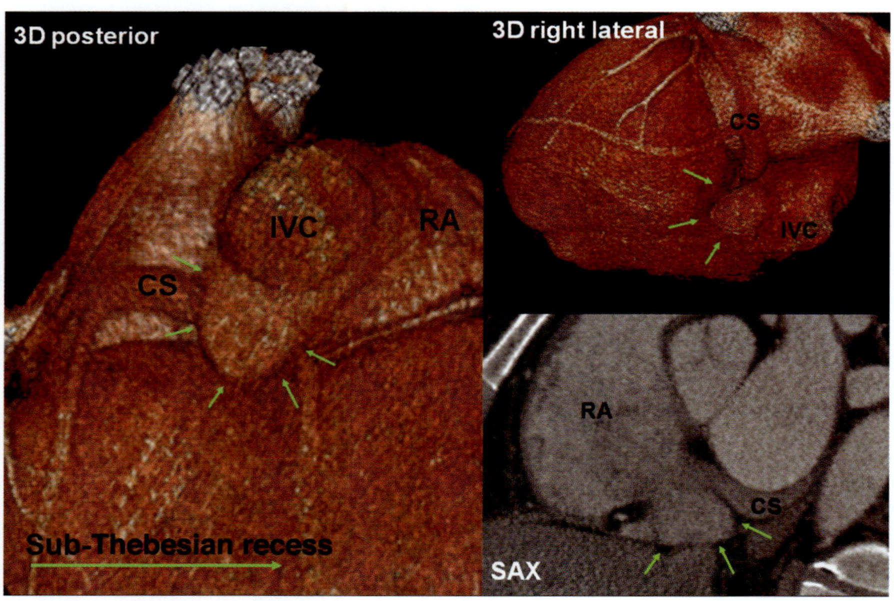

Figure 1.14 Sub-Thebesian pouch is a diverticular extension of cavotricuspid isthmus under coronary sinus. Posterior three-dimensional (3D) view and short-axis (SAX) image at the level of coronary sinus (CS) demonstrate a relatively large sub-Thebesian recess inferior to the Thebesian valve (green arrows). It is anterior to the orifice of the IVC and sub-Thebesian rather than sub-Eustachian. IVC, inferior vena cava; RA, right atrium.

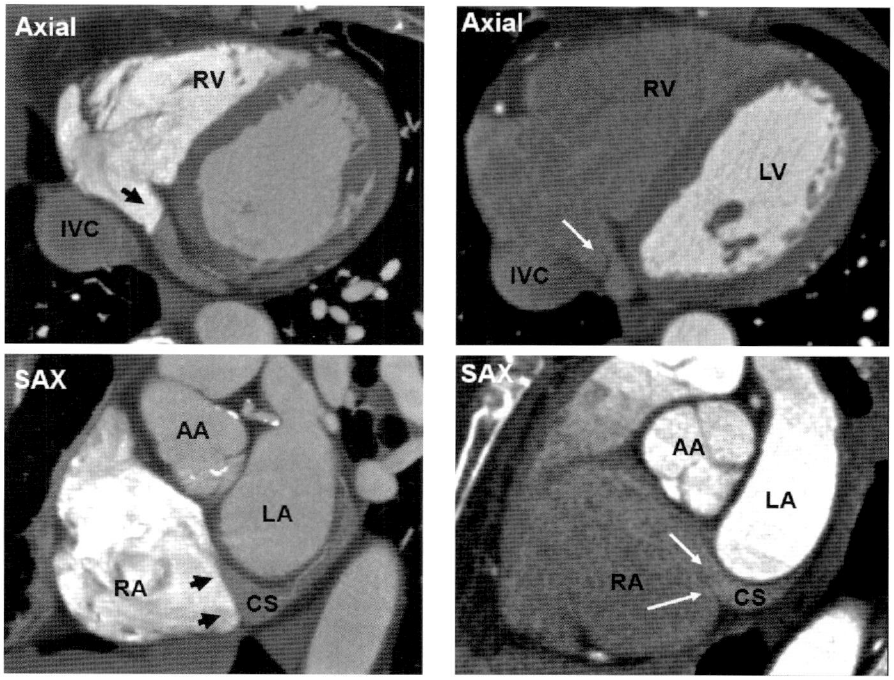

Figure 1.15 Normal anatomy of the ostium of the coronary sinus. Axial and short-axis (SAX) images of two different patients are shown. The Thebesian valve is shown by the arrows. AA, ascending aorta; CS, coronary sinus; IVC, inferior vena cava; LA, left atrium; LV, left ventricle; RA, right atrium; RV, right ventricle.

of the coronary arteries to the LAA exists. There is a wide variation in the configuration of the LAA (Figure 1.17).

The orifice of the LAA is at the junction of the anterior and the lateral wall, anterior to the left superior pulmonary vein. The axis is directed posteriorly, inferiorly, or anteriorly. It may rotate internally into the transverse sinus (Figure 1.18). It should be differentiated from attachment of the LAA to the anterior wall (bridging), a less common variant. Rarely the tip of the LAA may reopen into the anterior wall of the LA (double orifice).

The vestibular component surrounds the mitral orifice. Large branches of the LCx artery extend to the posterior aspect of the LA vestibule usually 10 mm above the ostium of the LV. In a dominant LCx, artery distal branches can reach to the external crux of the heart. However, exceptions occur and large RCA branches may run in contact with the vestibule. An anatomical area of the vestibule located between the left inferior pulmonary vein and the mitral annulus is known as left atrial isthmus [25] (Figure 1.19). It may be the source of recurrence after circumferential pulmonary vein catheter ablation for atrial fibrillation [26] (Figure 1.44; see also Chapter 9).

Components of the Interatrial Septum

Atrial septation is a complex process involving several tissue components [27]. The flap of the foramen ovale (septum primum) closes against the atrial septum (septum secundum), with fusion usually occurring within the first two years of life. Fusion is incomplete in about 25% of people, resulting in probe patent defect, termed a patent foramen ovale [28] (Figure 1.20). The size is usually <5 mm. A septum is best defined as a wall that can be removed without exiting from the cavities of the heart. The floor of the oval fossa represents the embryonic primary atrial septum. The superior and posterior rims of the fossa, often referred to as the septum secundum, is the infolded wall between the SVC and the right pulmonary veins known as interatrial groove and not a true septum [29] (Figures 1.20–1.24). Therefore, inadvertent puncture outside the limited margins of the oval fossa during transseptal interventions will perforate the heart, rather than provide access to the LA via the septum [27] (Figure 1.29; see also Chapter 9).

Anteriorly and inferiorly, the rim and its continuation into the atrial vestibules overlie the muscle masses of the ventricles with the fat-filled inferior pyramidal space intervening (Figures 1.21 and 1.22). The right atrial aspect gives the impression of a larger septal component, mainly because of the expansion of the atrial wall that is described as the aortic mound. This is the anterior wall of the RA just behind the aortic root (Figure 1.21).

Bachmann bundle is a subepicardial muscular bridge at the anterosuperior margin of the interatrial groove [30,31]. On the right, it extends into the anteromedial wall of the RA, anterior to the SVC, where its fibers intermingle with those of the precaval bundle, the superior extension of the crista terminalis. On the left, it blends in with the LAA

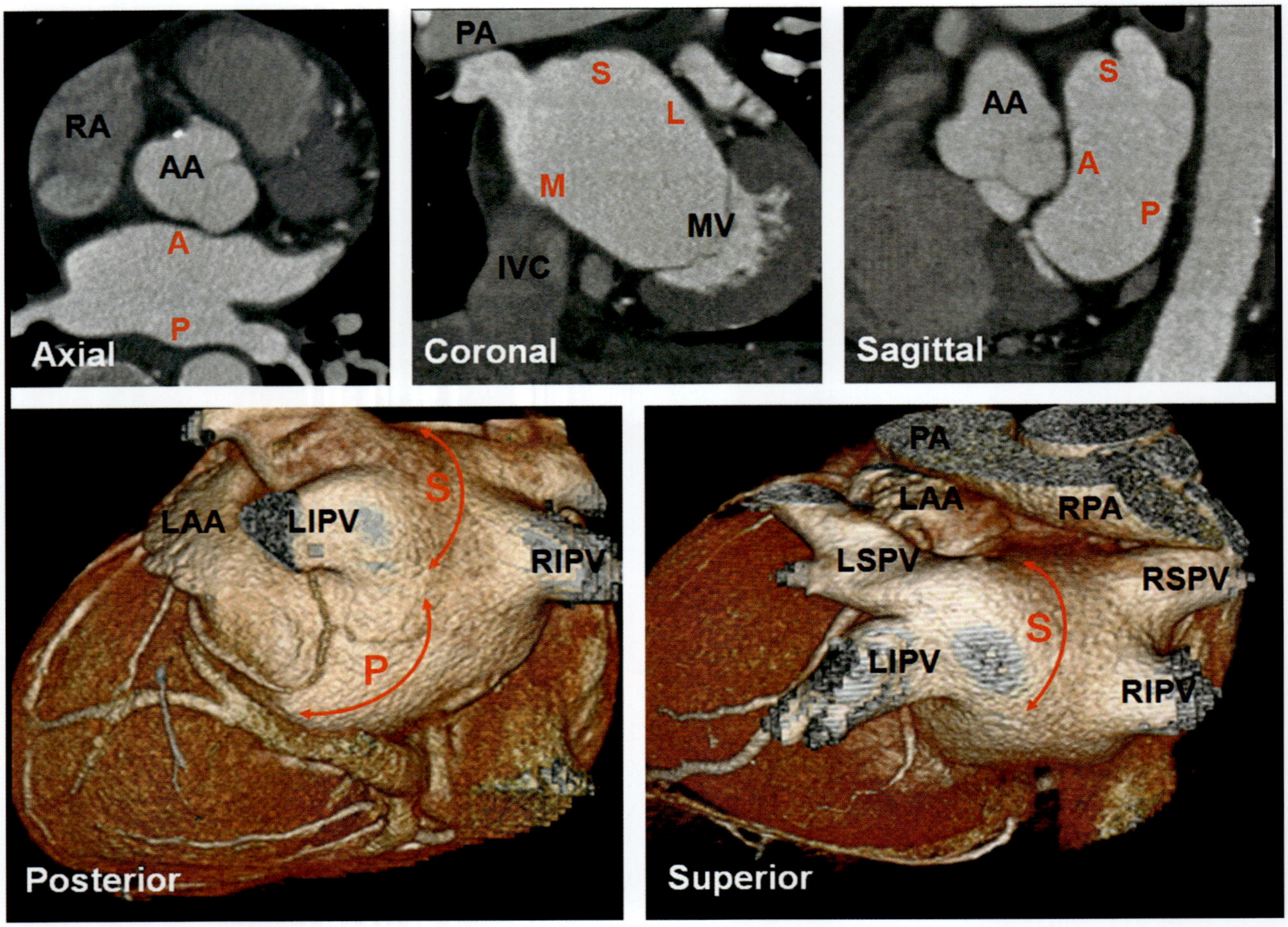

Figure 1.16 The boundaries of the left atrium are shown in different two-dimensional and three-dimensional projections. The left atrium is box-like chamber in the posterior aspect of the heart. The pulmonary artery (PA) and the right pulmonary artery (RPA) are separated from superior wall (S) of the left atrium (LA) by the transverse sinus. The highest portion of the LA is at the ostium of the left superior pulmonary vein. The left pulmonary veins (PVs) are usually higher than the right PVs (see Chapter 9 for further detail). The ascending aorta (AA) is related to the anterior wall (A) of the LA and the anteromedial wall of the right atrium (RA). It is separated inferiorly by adipose tissue of the interatrial groove and superiorly by the transverse sinus of the pericardium. The left sinoatrial node artery travels in the epicardial fat at the junction of the superior and anterior walls of the LA. Behind the middle of the noncoronary (posterior) sinus of the aorta, the anterior wall of the LA meets the anteromedial wall of the RA (fat filled interatrial groove). The anterior wall is usually thin and poorly muscled and vulnerable to being torn. The superior wall, or dome, is the thickest, measuring 3.5–6.5 mm (Anderson RH). The interatrial septum forms the medial wall (M) of the LA. The posteroinferior (P) wall is in close proximity to the esophagus. L, lateral wall; LAA, left atrial appendage; LIPV, left inferior PV; LSPV, left superior PV; MV, mitral valve; RIPV, right inferior PV; RSPV, right superior pulmonary vein.

musculature (Figure 1.24). The principal vascular supply of Bachmann bundle is branches of the SAN artery and its branches [32] (Figure 1.24). The role of this interatrial band is to ensure rapid interatrial conduction, leading to physiological biatrial contraction [33].

Septal Components of the AV Junction

The septal components of the AV junction are important because they conduct the cardiac impulse from the atria to the ventricles [4, 13]. At the crux of the heart, there is an area where tricuspid valve is attached to the septum closer to the ventricular apex than the mitral valve (Figure 1.25). In this region, the cavity of the RA is separated from that of the LV by the AV muscular sandwich, erroneously described as the "muscular AV septum." As stated by Anderson *et al.* [13], this area is not septal because the epicardial fibro-fatty tissue of inferior pyramidal space containing AVN artery is sandwiched between the atrial wall and the ventricular musculature (Figures 1.11, 1.22, 1.23).

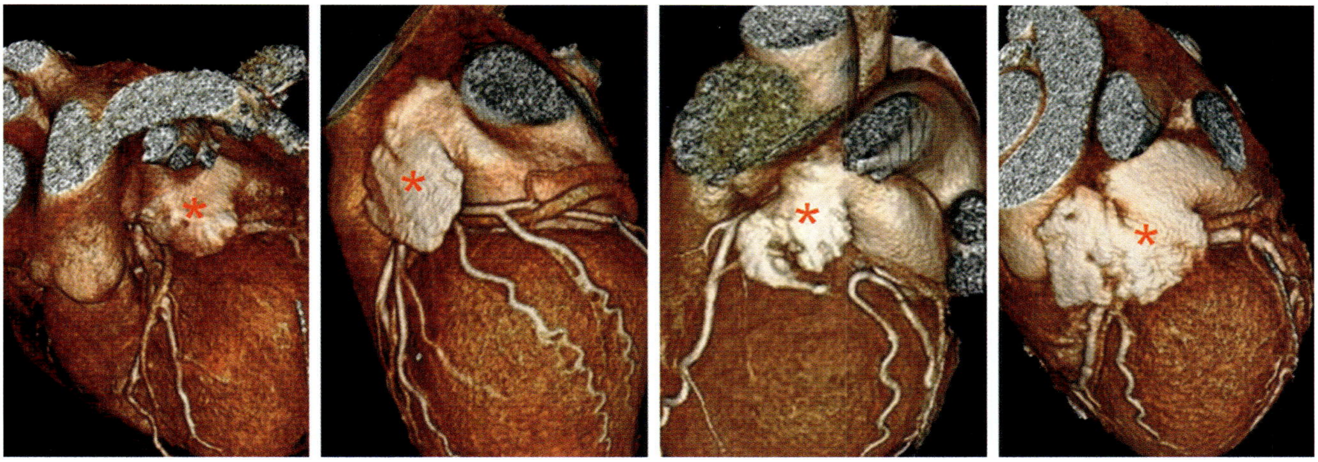

Figure 1.17 The left lateral views of the heart in four different patients demonstrate variation in shape and size of the left atrial appendage (LAA). The size of the neck of the LAA is also variable. The left circumflex (LCx) artery runs very close to the orifice of the LAA. Asterisk denotes left atrial appendage. .

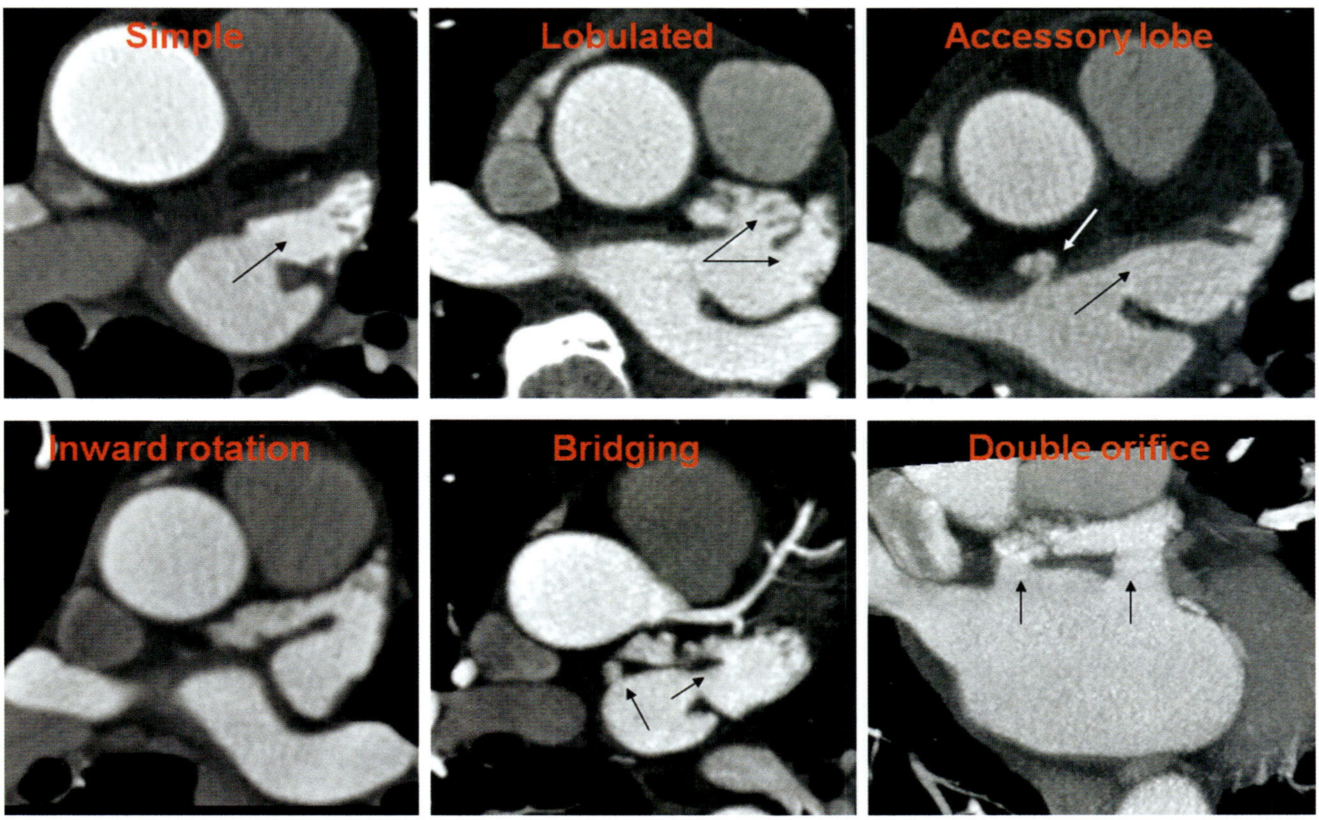

Figure 1.18 Anatomical variations of the left atrial appendage (LAA) (arrows). The LAA may be simple looking with one trabeculated cavity. It may be lobulated with two or three lobules. The axis of the LAA is usually directed anteriorly or inferiorly. Inward rotation is not uncommon. Accessory appendage is also common arising from the roof (anterior wall) of the left atrium (LA). These small outpouchings may connect with an internally rotated LAA giving the bridging or double orifice variants of the LAA.

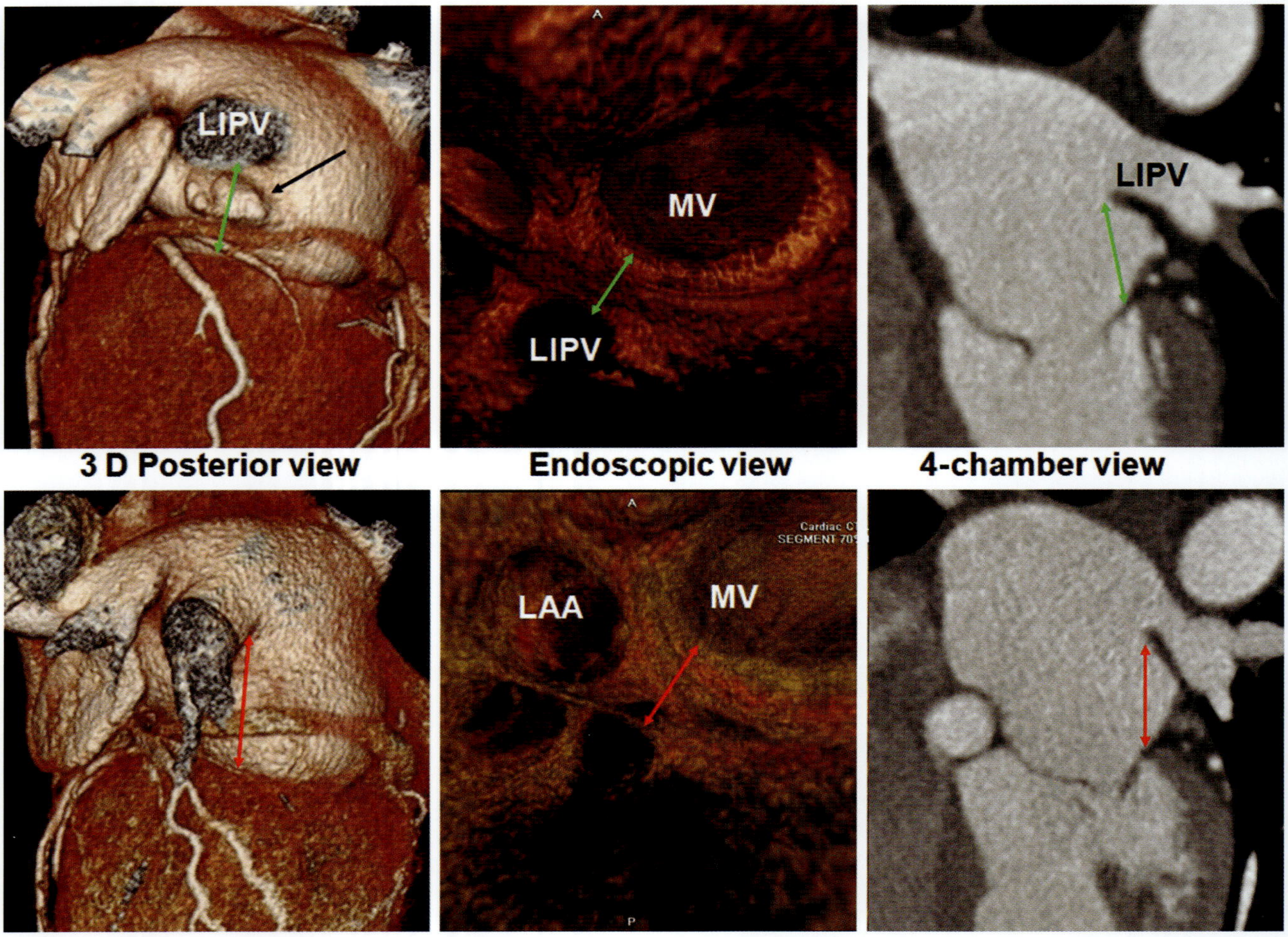

Figure 1.19 The left atrial isthmus is shown in two different patients. The length of isthmus varies in different individual. Upper row demonstrate shorter but deeper left isthmus compared to lower images. The left atrial isthmus is the area between the orifice of the left inferior pulmonary vein (LIPV) and the posteroinferior margin of mitral annulus (arrows). CT can easily evaluate the length, depth, and morphologic variants of this region. Note accessory LAA is common in this anatomic region (black arrow). CT endoscopic views are shown in the middle and four-chamber images on the right. LAA, left atrial appendage; MV, mitral valve.

The central fibrous body lies superior and anterior to the muscular AV septum (Figure 1.26). The central fibrous body is made up, in part, by the right fibrous trigone, and in part by the membranous septum and welds together the aortic, mitral, and tricuspid valves [13,34]. The membranous septum itself is divided into two parts by the septal leaflet of the tricuspid valve: an AV component between the RA and the LV, and an interventricular (IV) component (Figures 1.26 and 1.27). The relative sizes of the two components are variable and determined by the site of attachment of the septal leaflet of the tricuspid valve to the membrane [1]. For example, the AV component can be much larger than the IV component. Additionally, the size of membranous septum varies directly with the height of the posterior aortic sinus. Of surgical importance is the close proximity of the conduction system of the heart to the attachments of septal leaflet to the membranous septum. The bundle of His penetrates the right fibrous trigone and runs along the inferior margin of the IV component of the membranous septum.

The Right Ventricle

The RV is the most anteriorly situated cardiac chamber and lies behind the sternum. The normal RV wraps around the LV and varies in sizes and shapes. Traditionally, the RV is divided into the sinus and conus parts. The lower margin of the moderator band is the border between the conus and the trabeculated sinus (Figures 1.28 and 1.29). Some believe, the morphology of both the right and LVs can be better defined by dividing the ventricles into three components: the inlet, apical trabecular, and outlet

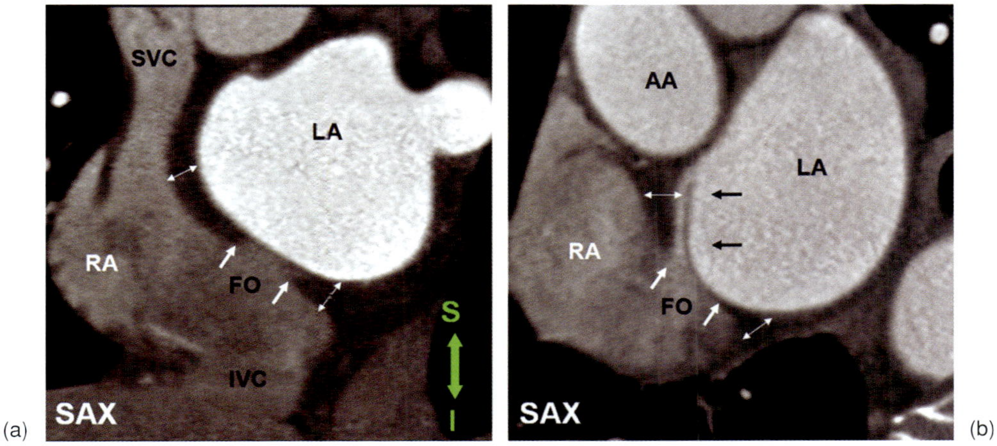

Figure 1.20 Anatomy of the interatrial septum and patent foramen ovale (PFO). Short-axis (SAX) images perpendicular to the interatrial septum show the fossa ovalis (FO) in (a) and a well-structured PFO in (b). The septum primum (black arrows in (b)) is fused to the inferior rim of FO and extends superiorly as a flap. The superior and the inferior rims (white arrows) of the FO are formed by infolding of the right atrial wall [interatrial groove (IAG) or the septum secundum]. IAG (double headed arrows) contains extracardiac fat. The infolding of the right atrial wall overlaps the flap of septum primum, forming a narrow tunnel through which a probe can be passed. AA, ascending aorta; I, inferior; LA, left atrium; RA, right atrium; S, superior; SVC, superior vena cava.

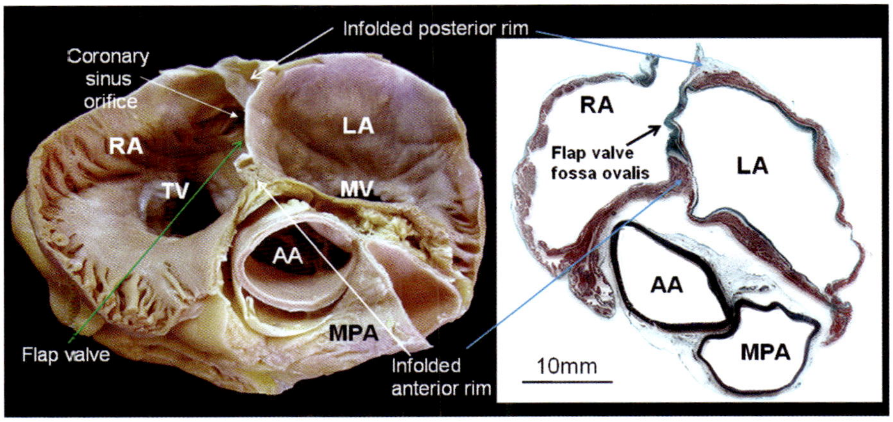

Figure 1.21 Short-axis sections across the atrial chambers through the flap valve of the fossa ovalis showing how the rim is simply the infolded atrial walls. AA, ascending aorta; LA, left atrium; MPA, main pulmonary artery; MV, mitral valve; RA, right atrium; TV, tricuspid valve.

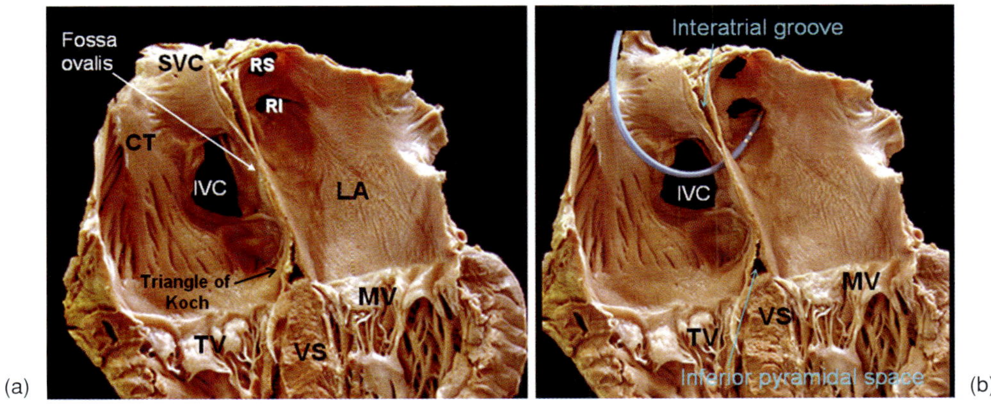

Figure 1.22 Horizontal long-axis (four-chamber) views of dissected human heart are shown (a, b). A probe is passed through the fossa ovalis and its end is placed into the right inferior (RI) pulmonary vein (image b). The superior rim of the fossa is the infolded wall between the SVC and the right pulmonary veins is known as interatrial groove (Waterston's or Sondergaard's groove). Anteriorly and inferiorly, the rim and its continuation into the atrial vestibules overlie the inferior pyramidal space. CT, crista terminalis; IVC, inferior vena cava; LA, left atrium; MV, mitral valve; RS, right superior pulmonary vein; SVC, superior vena cava; TV, tricuspid valve; VS, ventricular septum.

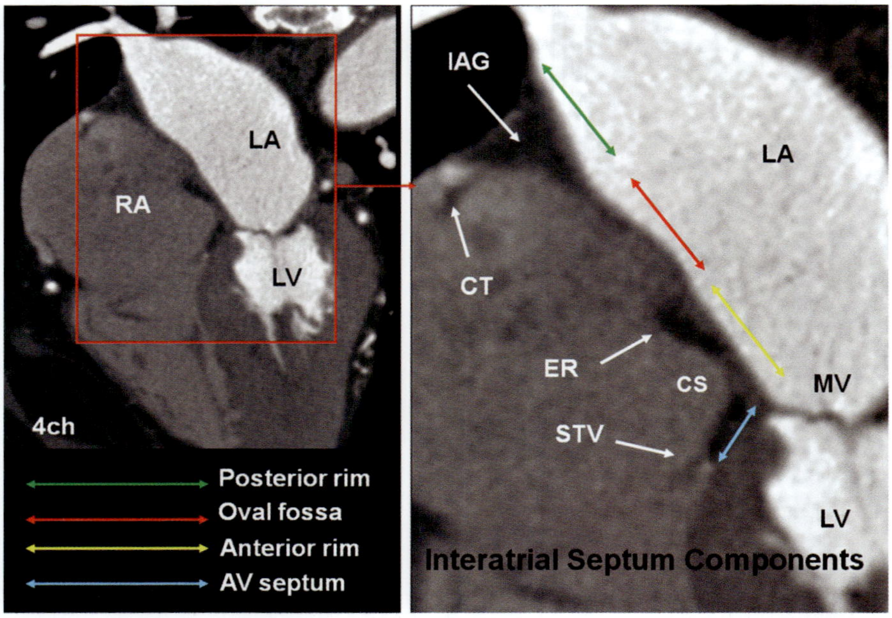

Figure 1.23 Components of the atrial septum on long-axis four-chamber (4ch) view. The right image is a magnified view of the left image. The slice is passed through the orifice of the coronary sinus (CS). The only true septum between the two atria is confined to the area of the fossa ovalis. The anterior rim is directly continuous with the Eustachian ridge (ER) that separates the orifices of the inferior vena cava (IVC) and the coronary sinus. Note separation of the septal attachment of the tricuspid valve (STV) from anterior mitral valve (MV) attachment by the muscular atrioventricular septum (blue arrow). 4ch, four chamber; CT, crista terminalis; IAG, interatrial groove; LA, left atrium; LV, left ventricle; MV, mitral valve; RA, right atrium.

portions [35–37]. The inlet portion of the RV surrounds and supports the tricuspid valve and its tension apparatus. A distinguishing feature of the tricuspid valve is the direct attachment of its septal leaflet to the ventricular septum [36]. The trabecular portion of the RV extends out to the apex and is characterized by coarse trabeculations typical of the RV. At the apex, the wall of the ventricle is quite thin and vulnerable to perforation by cardiac catheters and pacemaker electrodes. The RV can also be divided into basal, mid, and apical sections as well as anterior, lateral, and inferior walls [38].

The apical trabecular portion is continuous with the apparatus of the tricuspid valve. A well-known prominent trabeculation is the septomarginal trabeculation (septal band) that consists of a body and two limbs (Figure 1.29). The anterosuperior limb extends along the infundibulum to the leaflets of the pulmonary valve [4]. The posterior limb runs backward and inferiorly toward

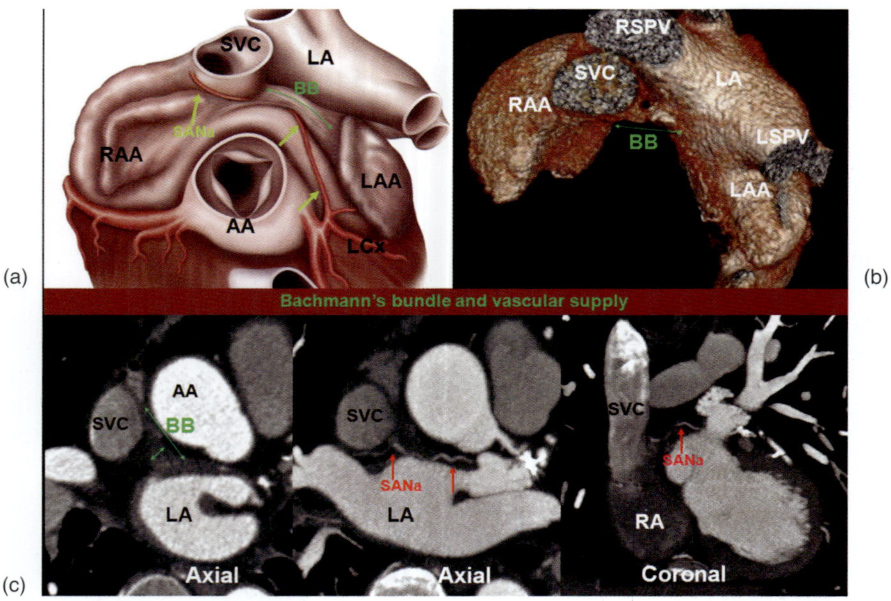

Figure 1.24 Part (a) is an illustrative superior view of the heart showing the anatomic location of Bachmann bundle and supplying left SA node artery (SANa) (from the left circumflex). Part (b) is a sculptured three-dimensional superior image of the atria. Bachmann bundle is shown (green arrows) connecting the two atria anteriorly up to the junction of the superior vena cava (SVC) in the right atrium (RA) and extending to the left atrial appendage (LAA) in the left atrium (LA). In part (c), the SANa (yellow and red arrows) is shown arising from the left circumflex, passing through Bachmann bundle and ending retrocavally. AA, ascending aorta; BB, Bachmann bundle; LCx, left circumflex; LSPV, left superior pulmonary vein; RAA, right atrial appendage; RSPV, right superior pulmonary vein.

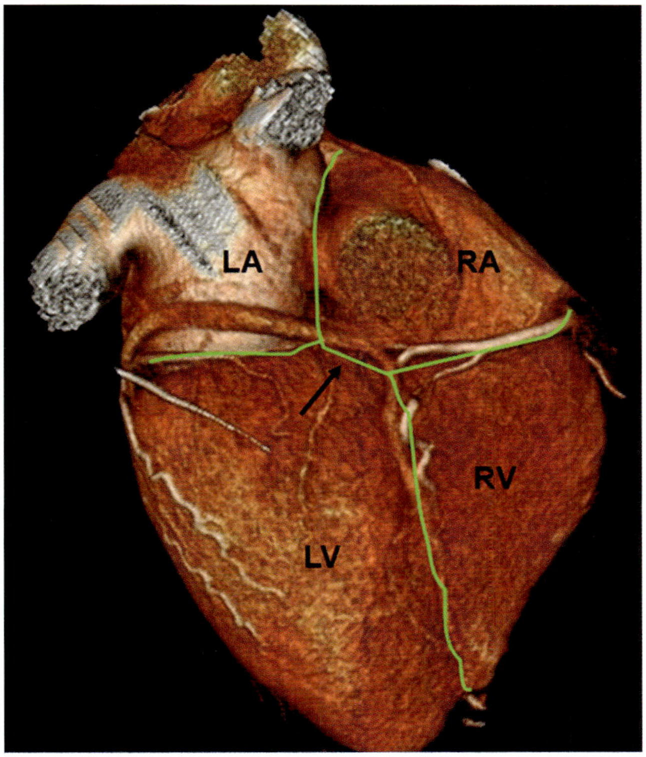

Figure 1.25 External cardiac crux is an area in the posterior aspect of the heart where cardiac chambers show their maximum proximity (arrow). This area is filled with fat. The vertical and horizontal lines in the cardiac crux are not perpendicular (green lines). As seen in this inferior view of the heart, the interatrial groove meets the left atrioventricular groove at right angle, and the interventricular and the right atrioventricular grooves are perpendicular. The right atrioventricular (AV) groove is inferior to the left AV groove due to inferior position of the septal leaflet of tricuspid relative to the mitral valve. LA, left atrium; LV, left ventricle; RA, right atrium; RV, right ventricle.

the right ventricular inlet (Figure 1.29). The body of the septomarginal trabeculation runs to the apex of the ventricle, where it gives rise to the anterior papillary muscle before breaking up into the general apical trabeculations (Figure 1.29). The anterior papillary muscle itself continues as an important muscular strand, the moderator band, to the parietal wall of the RV. When abnormally formed or hypertrophied, the septomarginal band can divide the ventricle into two chambers (double-chambered RV) [36].

Tricuspid Valve

The ostium of the tricuspid valve is elliptical. The tricuspid annulus is almost completely muscular. The three leaflets of the tricuspid valve are named for their anatomic location: septal (medial, conal), anterosuperior, and inferior (posterior) (Figure 1.30). The number of leaflets is variable. The largest is usually anterosuperior. The inferior leaflet may be very small or absent. The septal leaflet attaches to the septal and in part inferior wall of the RV. Septal attachment over the membranous septum divides it into AV and interventricular portions (Figure 1.27). However, presence of a gap in the leaflet at the attachment site to the membranous septum is not infrequent [36]. The commissures form where the leaflets join together at their peripheral ends. However, the three leaflets are not always well separated and their commissures may be poorly developed. There is no well-formed fibrous annulus for the tricuspid valve. Instead, the vestibule of the RA is separated from the ventricular ostium by the fibro-fatty tissue of the AV groove. The entire parietal attachment of the tricuspid valve usually is encircled by the RCA (Figure 1.30) running within the AV groove.

The papillary muscles (PM) of the tricuspid valve are termed septal, anterior, and inferior (posterior) [39]. The anterior (single or bifid) (Figure 1.30) and inferior (one or two) PM (Figure 1.30) are attached to the anterior and inferior walls of the RV, respectively, provide insertion for the chordae from the nonseptal leaflets of the tricuspid valve. A second inferior papillary muscle may be attached to the septum (Figures 1.30 and 1.31). Almost all the chordae from the septal leaflet are attached with or without the intermediation of septal PM to the septal wall; however, some pass to the inferior PM. Septal PM can be single or multiple and may receive chordae from the anterior leaflet. The septal PM usually arises from body or posterior limb of the septomarginal trabeculation. The one arising from the posterior limb is called conal (medial or Luschka) PM [2]. The septal PM is located below the right coronary sinus of the aorta and may fuse to the septal band. It is absent in 20% of the hearts [39]. The right bundle branch of cardiac conduction system runs immediately beneath the septal papillary muscle and then within the body of the septomarginal trabeculation before reaching the moderator band [34].

The Right Ventricular Outflow Tract (Pulmonary Infundibulum)

The pulmonary infundibulum (conus) is a tubular muscular structure that supports the leaflets of the pulmonary valve. The length, size, and angle of the conus vary (Figure 1.31). However, the size of the infundibulum is independent of the general size of the RV [1]. One determinant of the size of the infundibulum is the axis of the pulmonary trunk (Figure 1.32). The infundibulum is less well-developed in the presence of a horizontal axis of the pulmonary trunk (horizontal heart).

The posterior wall of the infundibulum (conus) is formed by a prominent muscular ridge, known as the

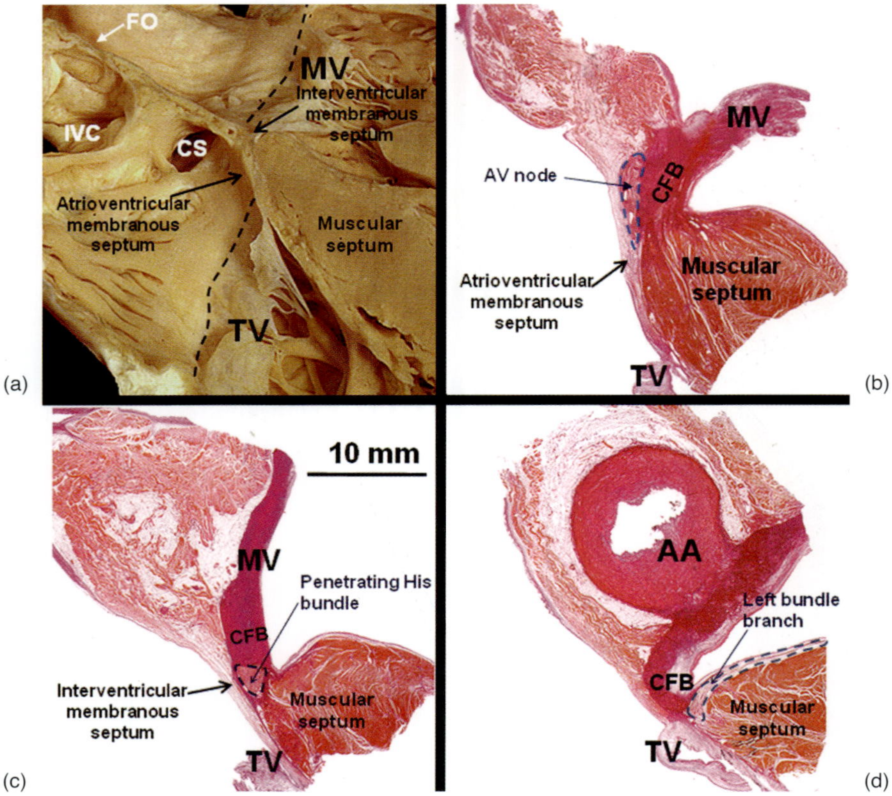

Figure 1.26 (a) Four-chamber section shows the attachment of the septal leaflet and mitral valve to the ventricular septum, and the location of atrioventricular (AV) and interventricular membranous portions of the membranous septum. (b–d) Histological sections corresponding to the location of the specialized AV conduction system (AV node, penetrating His bundle and left bundle branch) between the membranous septum and the muscular ventricular septum. AA, ascending aorta; CS, coronary sinus orifice; CFB, central fibrous body; FO, fossa ovalis; IVC, inferior vena cava; MV, mitral valve; TV, tricuspid valve.

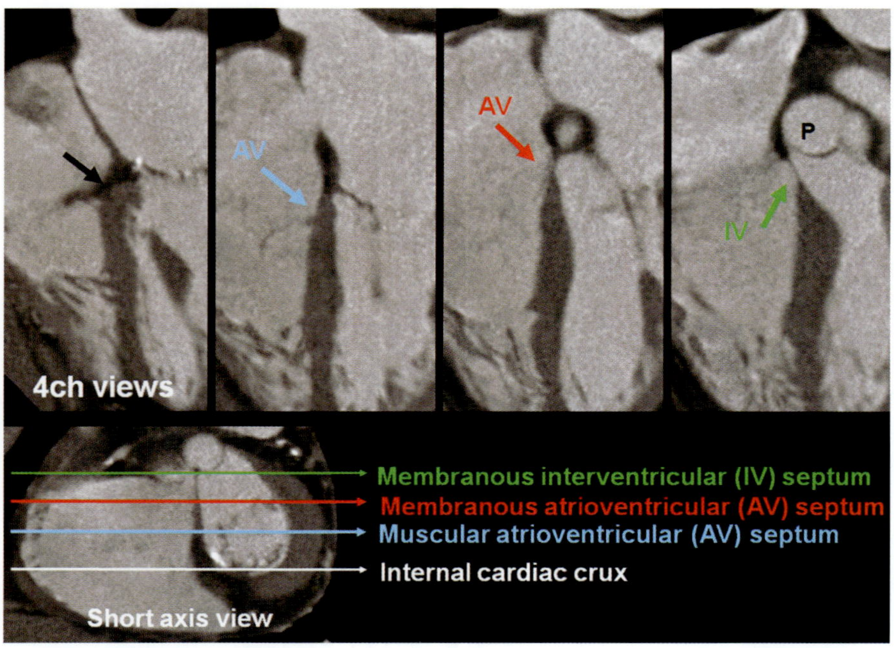

Figure 1.27 The septal components of the atriventricular (AV) junction. Using a short-axis view at the level of membranous septum, four-chamber (4ch) slices are reconstructed at the levels of internal cardiac crux (black arrow), muscular AV septum (blue arrow), membranous AV septum (red arrow), and membranous interventricular (IV) septum (green arrow). Note the offset between septal attachment of tricuspid valve and mitral valve at muscular AV septum. The membranous septum itself is divided into two parts by the septal leaflet of the tricuspid valve. (Reprinted from Saremi and Krishnan [3], with permission.)

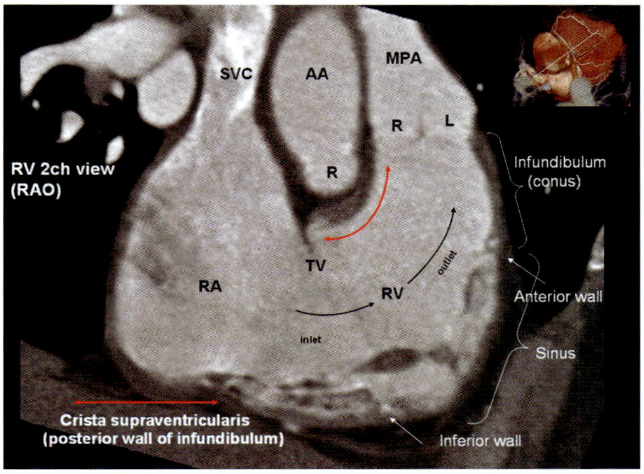

Figure 1.28 The right anterior oblique view (two chamber) of the right heart is shown. The right ventricle (RV) can be divided into inflow and outflow segments. The outflow tract, the infundibulum or conus, separates the inflow and outflow valves. The axis of the orifices of the two segments roughly forms an angle of 60°. The posterior wall of the infundibulum (the infundibular septum) extends between the septal papillary muscle and the right pulmonary sinus (R). It is in contact with the right aortic sinus (R). It is separated from the right aortic sinus by epicardial fat. A thin membranous segment of the posterolateral of the conus may exist. This is a possible cause of an aneurysmal bulge of this region when pressure in the RV is high. 2ch, two chamber; AA, ascending aorta; L, left pulmonary sinus; MPA, main pulmonary artery; RA, right atrium; SVC, superior vena cava; TV, tricuspid valve.

crista supraventricularis (supraventricular crest, infundibular septum) that separates the tricuspid and pulmonary valves (Figures 1.28, 1.31, 1.33). This is in contrast to what is seen in the LV where the aortic and mitral valves are in fibrous continuity. The length of crista supraventricularis varies from patient to patient; however, most of it is separated from the aorta by epicardial fat and can be surgically removed without entering the left ventricular cavity [4]. Only the central portion of its inferior part forms part of the interventricular septum. Incisions through the crista supraventricularis should be made carefully, as it may injure the RCA (Figure 1.33).

The crista supraventricularis is located between the septal and parietal bands of the infundibulum (Figure 1.33). Parietal extension of infundibular musculature (beyond the level of membranous septum) is called parietal band (ventriculoinfundibular fold). The septal band or septomarginal trabeculation is a prominent Y-shaped muscle column that divides into anterosuperior and inferoposterior limbs (Figure 1.34). The body of septomarginal trabeculation extends to the apex of the ventricle, where it divides into smaller trabeculations including the moderator band. The moderator band is variable in size and inserts into the anterior papillary muscle (Figures 1.29 and 1.34). Arterial supply to the moderator band originates from septal branches of the anterior descending artery [40]. Anastomotic vessels with the RCA exist at the level of the anterior papillary muscle.

The Pulmonary Valve

When heart is viewed in attitudinal anatomic position as sitting in the thorax, the pulmonary leaflets and sinuses are seen to be posterior, right anterolateral, and left anterolateral [1] (Figure 1.35). However, in relation to the heart the pulmonary sinuses can be named anterior, left posterior, and right posterior. Because of the semilunar shape of the pulmonary leaflets, this valve does not have a ring-like annulus (similar to the aortic valve). The sinotubular junction of the pulmonary trunk marks the level of the commissures between the annuli (Figure 1.35). A second junction exists at the ventriculoarterial junction. The base of the sinuses within the ventricle crosses the anatomic ventriculoarterial junction [41] (Figure 1.36).

The leaflets of the pulmonary and aortic valves have different levels of attachments, and there is an extracardiac tissue plane between the walls of the aorta and the pulmonary trunk (Figure 1.36). This anatomic feature makes possible the safe separation of the pulmonary valve, including its basal attachments within the infundibulum from the rest of the RV outflow tract for use as a valve autograft (i.e., the Ross procedure) [42,43].

The Left Ventricle

The LV is a conical structure with trabeculated walls that narrow down to a rounded apex (Figures. 1.5, 1.34, 1.38). The boundaries, especially between the septal and posterior walls, are imprecise. The opening of the LV is called the ostium [1]. It provides attachment for the mitral valve, aortic annuli, and aortoventricular membrane. The highest point of the ostium is the interannular trigone between the left and right aortic annuli. The lowest point of the ostium is approximately 1.5 cm posterior to the inferior commissure of the mitral valve. Similar to the RV, the LV cavity can also be subdivided into three components. The inlet component is surrounded by the mitral valve and its tension apparatus, and the outlet supports the aortic valve. The anterior leaflet of the mitral valve separates the inlet from the outlet. The outlet component is incomplete posteriorly so that the leaflets of the aortic and mitral valves are in fibrous continuity (Figure 1.37). The apical trabecular component of the LV extends to the apex. It is characterized by fine trabeculations where the myocardium is surprisingly thin (Figure 1.37). Perforation of the LV apex is surprisingly uncommon in contrast to perforation of the apex of the RV during catheterizations or biopsy

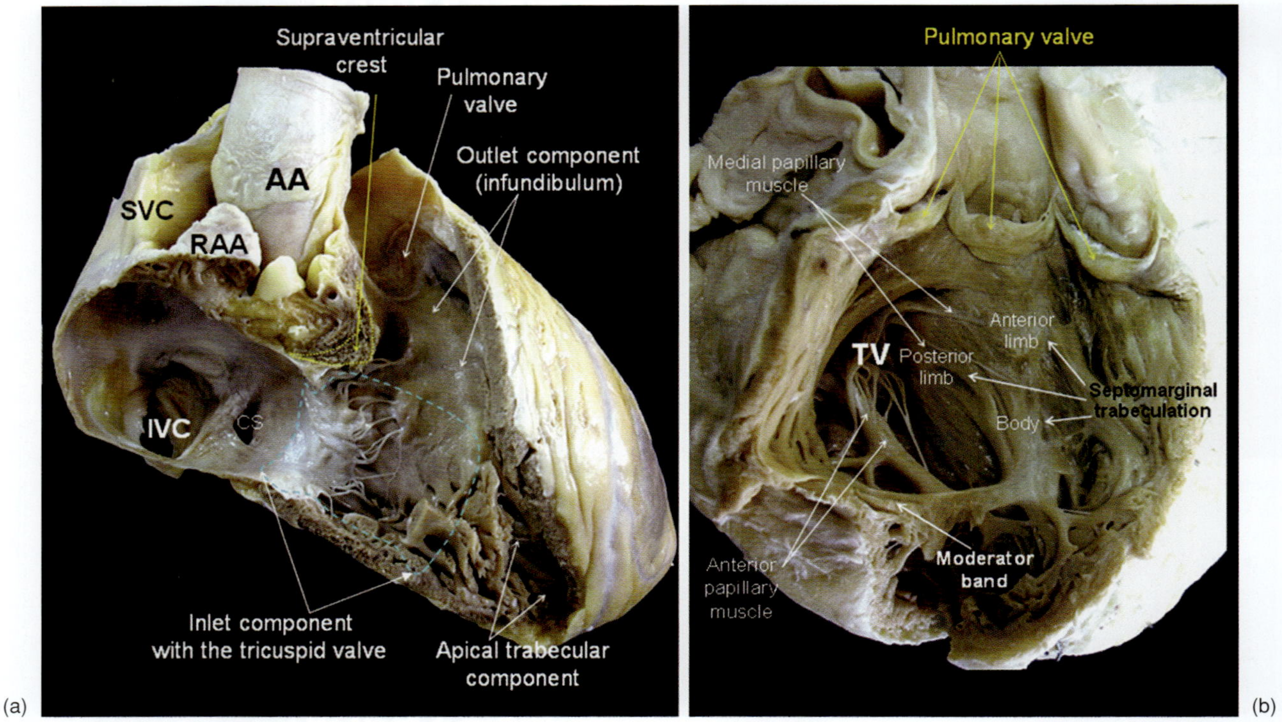

Figure 1.29 (a) Window dissection of a heart prepared by removing the anterior superior wall of the right ventricle. The three components of the right ventricle are revealed. (b) The right ventricle is opened from the front to show the tricuspid valve, the pulmonary valve, and the septomarginal trabeculation. AA, aorta appendage; CS, coronary sinus orifice; IVC, inferior vena cava; RAA, right atrial appendage; SVC, superior vena cava; TV, tricuspid valve.

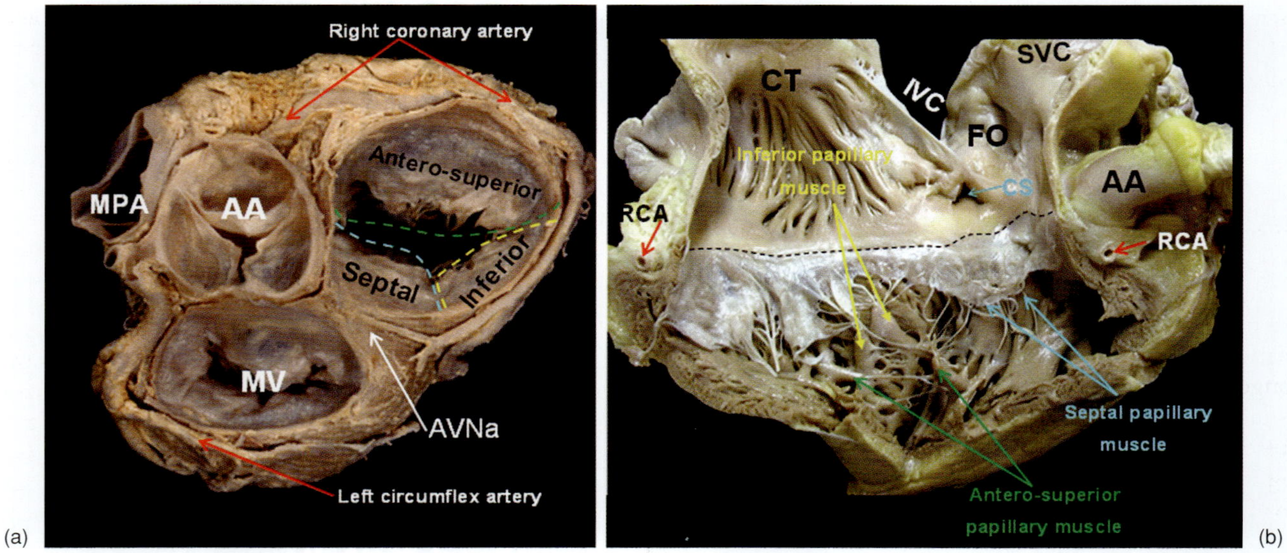

Figure 1.30 (a) The ventricular base of the heart is viewed from the atrial aspect. This figure shows the leaflets of the tricuspid valve. The right coronary artery passes round the atrioventricular groove in the right parietal junction and gives rise to the atrioventricular nodal artery (AVNa). (b) The right side of the heart is opened to show the hinge of the tricuspid valve (dotted line) and the location of the right papillary muscles. AA, ascending aorta; CS, coronary sinus orifice; CT, crista terminalis; FO, Fossa ovalis; IVC, inferior vein cava; MPA, main pulmonary artery; MV, mitral valve; RCA, right coronary artery; SVC, superior vena cava.

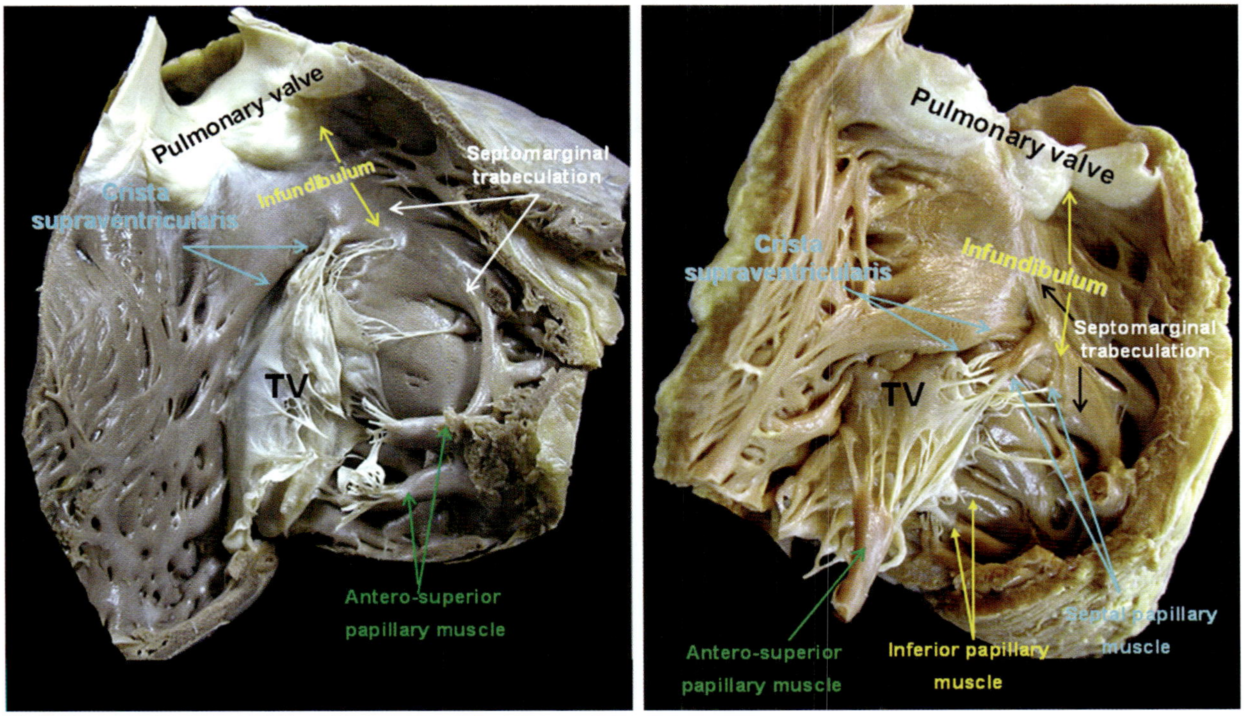

(a) (b)

Figure 1.31 Two different specimens are shown (a, b). The anterior wall of the right ventricle is opened to show the different sizes of infundibulum (yellow arrows) of the right ventricle and the location of the crista supraventricularis and septomarginal trabeculation. In each specimen, the anterior and posterior limbs of the septomarginal trabeculation are shown by arrows. TV, tricuspid valve.

procedures. The relation of the apices of the ventricles to each other is not without clinical significance. The apex of the RV may be demarcated from the left, producing an incisura (Figure 1.38). However, it is the apex of the LV (not the RV), which is readily identified at fluoroscopy. On the basis of recommendation of American Heart Association, a standardized segmental model is proposed for tomographic imaging of the heart [44]. In this model, the muscle and cavity of the LV is divided into a 17 segments that are assigned to coronary arterial territories.

The trabeculations of the LV including its septal wall are quite fine compared with those of the RV, a useful characteristic in diagnosis of ventricular morphology in congenital heart disease. The outlet part of the septum is usually smooth (Figure 1.37b). The two PM are termed posterior (posteromedial) and lateral (anterolateral), arising from the posterior and lateral walls at midventricular level (Figure 1.37 and 1.39). Usually, no papillary muscle attaches to the left side of the interventricular septum. PM are extensions of the ventricular muscle, and their function relate to the integrity of LV function and geometry. Knowledge of the variation in the location and number of PM is useful in mitral valve surgery and reconstruction of the LV wall aneurysm. Accessory, basal, or apical PM may be present (Figure 1.39). The anterolateral PM is supplied by branches of the left anterior descending artery and the posteromedial by branches of the dominant right coronary or the LCx artery. Chordae tendineae (tendinous chords) may originate from the papillary muscle or the wall of LV [45]. Common anatomic variants such as large Thebesian sinusoids, myocardial cleft, or muscle bridges within the LV cavity should not be confused with pathologies [21,46] (Figure 1.40).

The Mitral Valve

AV valve (mitral and tricuspid valves) components include valvular apparatus (annulus, leaflets, and commissures) and tension apparatus (PM and chordae tendineae) [47,48]. The two leaflets of the mitral valve have different appearances. The attachments site of the anterior (aortic) leaflet is shorter than the posterior (mural) leaflet and comprises approximately one third of the circumference of the mitral annulus (Figure 1.41 and 1.42). When the valve is closed, the surface area of the anterior leaflet is larger than the posterior leaflet (3/1 or 2/1). The posterior leaflet has a scalloped appearance with three or more segments separated by clefts [48].

Unlike the tricuspid valve, the mitral valve leaflets are supported by a rather dense collagenous annulus, also

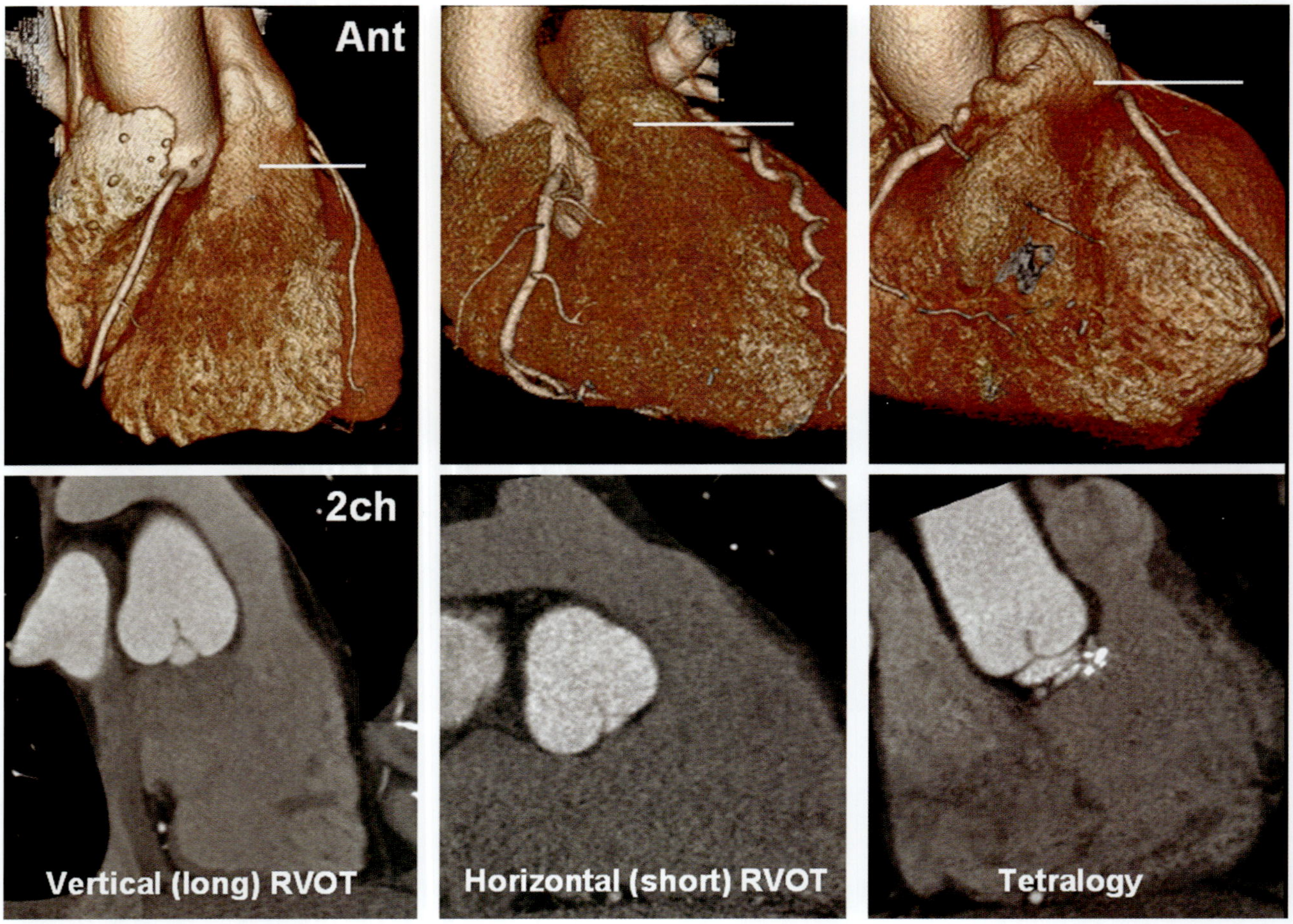

Figure 1.32 Different morphologies of the right ventricular outflow tract (RVOT) are shown. Anterior (Ant) three-dimensional images are presented on the top row with the corresponding two-chamber (2ch) views of the right heart on the lower row. The superior margin of the left ventricle is demarcated by the white lines. The posterior wall of infundibulum (infundibular septum) may be short below the upper surface of the left ventricle (LV) or high above the LV upper margin or rises above the level of the right aortic sinus. Its size is mainly determined by the axis of the plane of the pulmonary ostium. When this plane extends anterosuperiorly, a large infundibulum occurs. When it is almost horizontal, a small infundibulum results (middle images). In tetralogy of Fallot, a short thickened infundibulum is seen causing subvalvular stenosis.

known as subvalvular membrane [1]. The annulus is a sheet-like structure, not a ring or cord-like structure, and extends peripherally from the fibrous trigones (Figure 1.43). It is deficient toward the aorta at the level of mitral-aortic curtain extending between the two trigones (aortic-mitral annulus) [48]. For surgical purposes, the annulus is considered the area of the attachment of the valve leaflets to the atrial muscle.

The mitral valve annulus is a functional component and demonstrates nonplanar saddle morphology [49]. The complex three-dimensional geometry of the mitral annulus may play an important physiological role in the proper and durable function of the valvular complex. The annulus height to commissural width ratio will be increased during systole in normal hearts. This relationship is markedly altered in mitral insufficiency because of acute posterior wall ischemia or cardiomyopathy. It is shown that this ratio is lower in the hearts with posterior wall ischemia [50]. The saddle morphology of the annulus imposes leaflet curvature that—in combination with leaflet bulging—reduces stress on valve components during systole and may contribute to valve competence [51].

Annulus calcification is common and usually involves the posterior mitral ring (Figure 1.44).

In mitral valve replacement, the attached border of the posterior leaflet is of particular interest because of the danger of periprosthetic leak. This complication is less common in relation to the anterior valve as its attachments to the fibrous trigones are stronger and less involved with calcifications. Placement of sutures in the muscle of the ventricle and subvalvular membrane may interfere with durability of the sutures [1]. The circumflex coronary artery and the coronary sinus run close to the posterior mitral annulus (Figures 1.41 and 1.45).

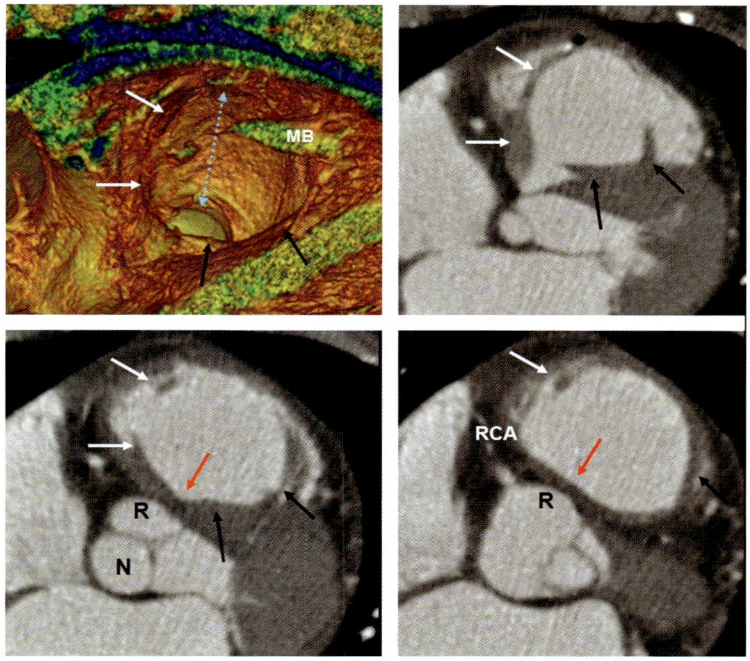

Figure 1.33 Endoscopic view (a) shows the tubular structure of the infundibulum (blue dotted arrow). (b–d) are axial images at three levels through the conus. The muscles of infundibulum are divisible into parietal and septal bands. White arrows demarcate the parietal band and black arrows show the septal band. The parietal band lies anterior to the right aortic sinus. These muscular bands form the posterolateral and posterior walls of the infundibulum, respectively. The junction of these two bands is often indicated by a ridge extending from septal papillary muscle to the right pulmonary annulus known as crista supraventricularis (red arrows). Some anatomists or surgeons have used the term to comprise the entire infundibular musculature. In some normal hearts, the parietal and septal bands are poorly developed. Note close proximity of the RCA to the crista supraventricularis. MB, moderator band; N, noncoronary sinus of the aorta; R, right coronary sinus of the aorta; RCA, right coronary artery.

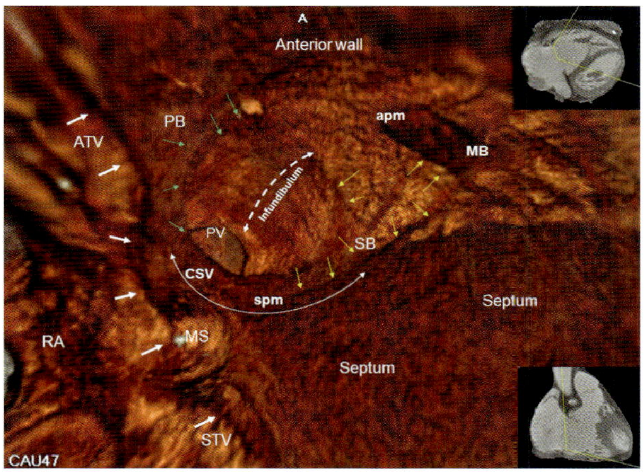

Figure 1.34 The right ventricle outflow tract is shown in this endoscopic view of MDCT study of the heart. The crista supraventricularis (CSV) is located between the septal and parietal bands (SB, PB). The septal band (septomarginal trabeculation) consists of multiple trabeculae (yellow arrows). The extension of the septomarginal trabeculation to the anterior wall of the RV forms the moderator band (MB) and the anterior papillary muscle (apm). The parietal band (green arrows) projects anteriorly (forms posterolateral wall of the right ventricular outflow tract (RVOT)) and fades out above the anterior papillary muscle. The septal (medial) papillary muscle (spm) arises from the junction of the septal and parietal bands. Note septal attachment of the tricuspid valve (STV) passing over the membranous septum (MS). ATV, anterior tricuspid valve; PV, pulmonary vein; RA, right ventricle.

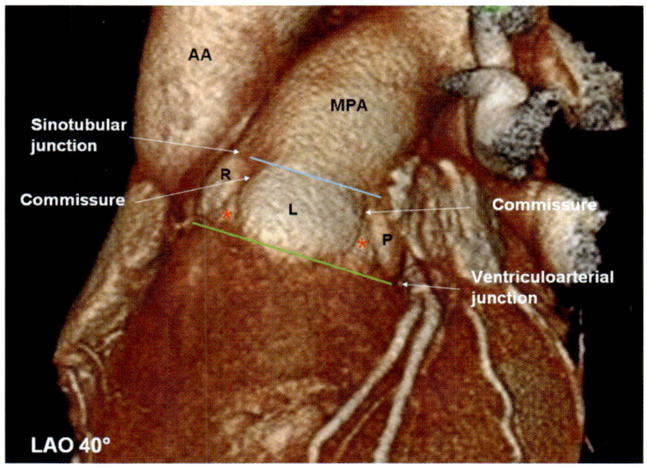

Figure 1.35 Forty degrees left anterior oblique projection (LAO) view of the main pulmonary artery (MPA) is shown. The pulmonary sinuses including the right (R), left (L), and posterior (P) annuli are seen. The term "pulmonary annulus" denotes the semilunar fibrous attachment of each of the pulmonary leaflets that gives the shape of a triradiate crown to the arterial root. The annuli of the pulmonary valve contribute to the fibrous skeleton of the heart; however, they are much less sturdy than the aortic annuli. The ventriculoarterial junction is demarcated by the green line. Interannular fibrous trigones are shown (red stars). The commissures between the annuli are marked by arrows indicating peripheral apposition of the leaflets. The blue line connecting the commissures marks the sinotubular junction. AA, ascending aorta.

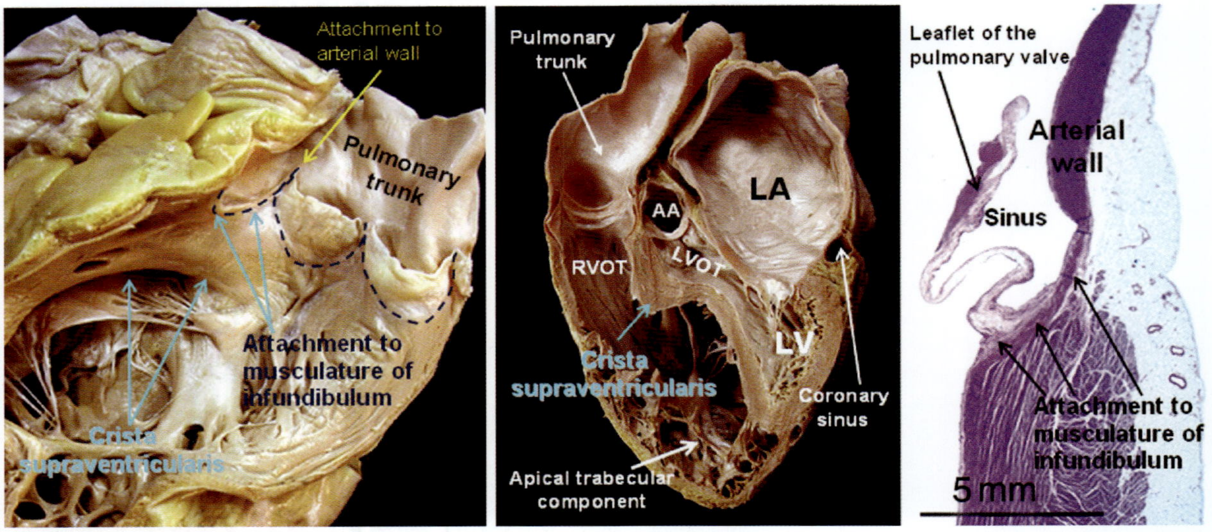

Figure 1.36 (a) The leaflets of the pulmonary valve are mainly supported by the infundibulum of the right ventricle. However, at their commissures the leaflets are attached to the pulmonary artery trunk (sinotubular junction). (b) Longitudinal section of the right ventricle shows that a small portion of the crista supraventricularis (posterior wall of the RVOT) extends beyond the limits of left ventricular outflow tract and separates the leaflets of the pulmonary valve from the left ventricle. (c) Histological section of the pulmonary valve shows how the attachment of the musculature (myocardium) of the infundibulum (arrows) to the pulmonary leaflet extends well proximal to anatomic ventriculo-arterial junction. AA, ascending aorta; LA, left atrium; LV, left ventricle; LVOT, left ventricular outflow tract; RVOT, right ventricular outflow tract.

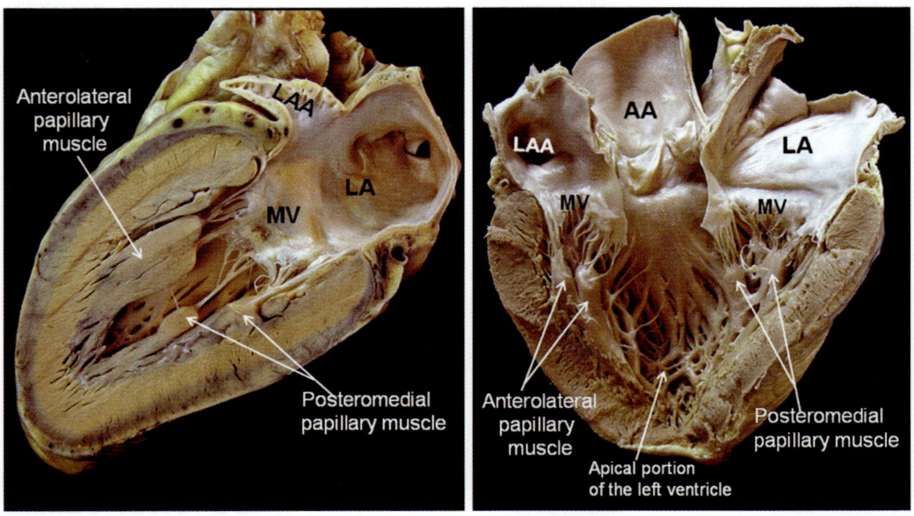

Figure 1.37 (a) Window dissection into the left ventricle shows the inlet portion surrounding the mitral valve (MV), the papillary muscles of the left ventricle, and the fine criss-crossing trabeculations at the apex. (b) Opened view of the ventriculo-aortic junction shows the outlet portion of the left ventricle and the typical semilunar attachments of the leaflets of the aortic valve. Note fine trabeculations in the apical zone. The anterolateral and posteromedial papillary muscles are shown. Each mitral leaflet receives chordae from both papillary muscles. The anterolateral papillary muscle is attached to by chordae tendineae to the left half of the anterior and posterior leaflets, whereas the posteromedial papillary muscle is attached to by chordae tendineae to the right half of the anterior and posterior leaflets. AA, ascending aorta; LA, left atrium; LAA, left atrial appendage; MV, mitral valve.

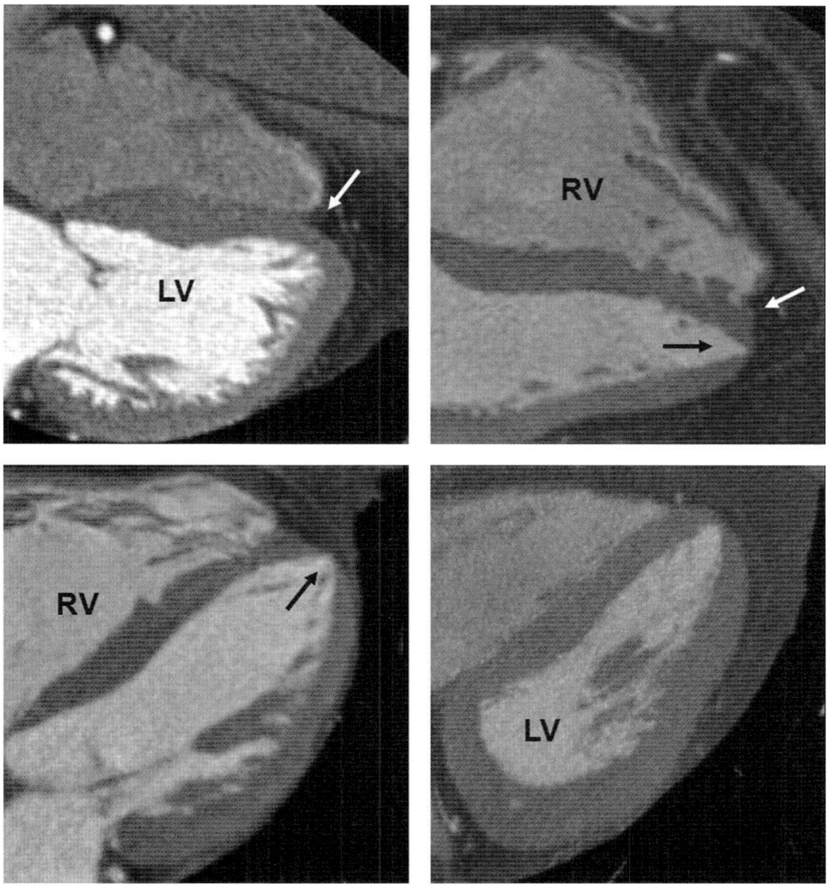

Figure 1.38 Four-chambers views demonstrate varying shapes of the apices in four different examples. The apex of the left ventricle may be sharply angular or smooth and spherical. The location of the right ventricle (RV) apex is important during right heart catheterization. It is anterior to the left apex and can be demarcated from the left apex by an incisura (white arrows). In some cases, the apex of the RV is thin and sharply angulated, which results in vulnerability to perforation. Note the paper thin left ventricle (LV) apex (black arrows). Perforation of the LV apex is surprisingly uncommon in contrast to perforation of the apex of the RV during catheterizations or biopsy procedures.

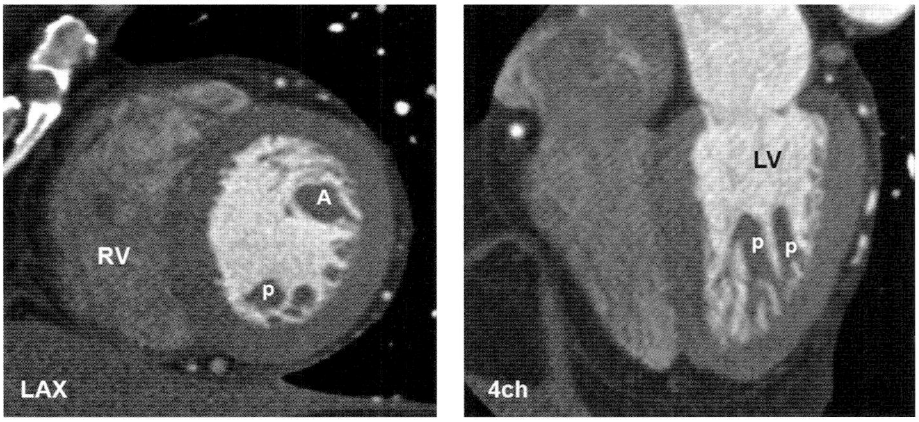

Figure 1.39 The left ventricle (LV) papillary muscles (PM) are shown. Short-axis (LAX) image at midventricular level shows the anterolateral (A) and the posteromedial (P) PM. The anterior PM is larger and less tethered to the LV wall than the posterior. In approximately two thirds of people the anterior PM is a single structure and the posterior consists of one or two based columns with one or two heads. Variants of the papillary muscle exist. The chords arising from a basal PM (arrow) is shown attaching to the basal zone of the posterior leaflet. 4ch, four-chamber view; RV, right ventricle.

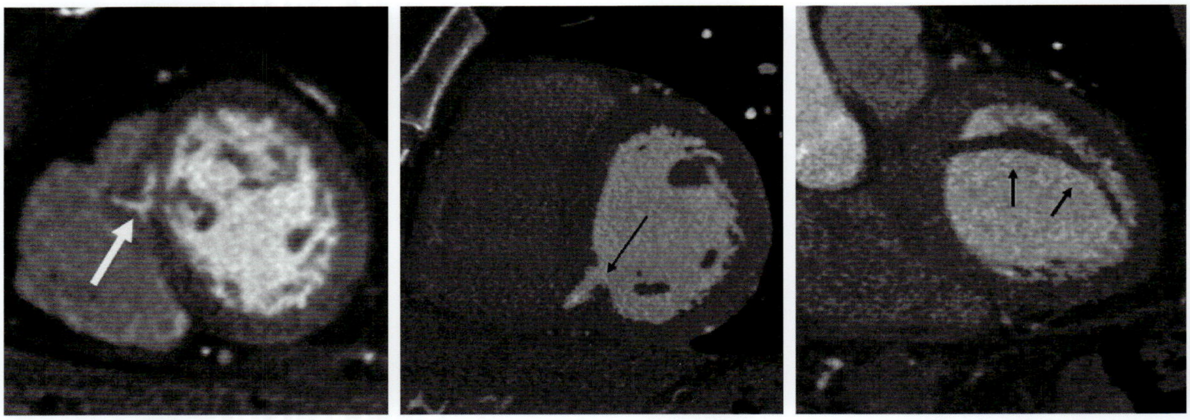

(a), (b) (c)

Figure 1.40 Short-axis images of the left ventricle show common anatomic variants including large (a). Thebesian sinuses (white arrow), (b). myocardial cleft (long arrow), and (c) intraventricular muscular bridge (black arrows) extending between septum and lateral wall of the left ventricle (LV).

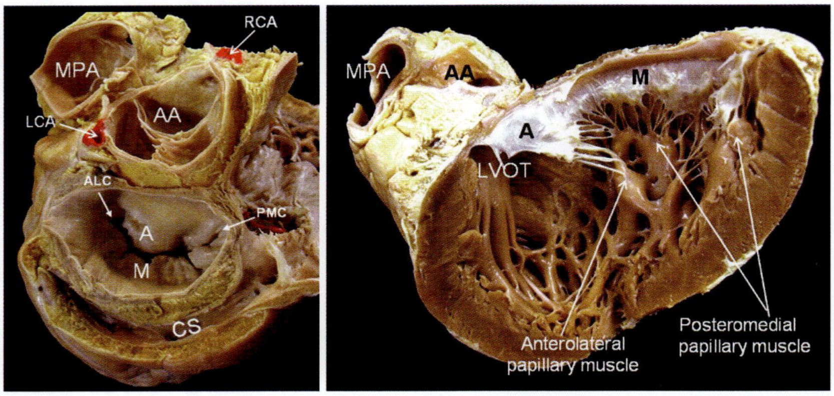

(a) (b)

Figure 1.41 (a) The kidney-shaped vestibule of the mitral valve is shown from the atrial side. The zone of opposition (the commissure) between the leaflets and the fibrous continuity in the ventricular roof between the aortic (b) leaflet of the mitral valve and the aortic sinuses are shown. Note the coronary sinus (CS) in the left atrioventricular groove surrounding the mitral valve from behind. (b) The left ventricle is opened to show the anterior [aortic (A)] leaflet that is shorter than the posterior [mural (M)] leaflet of the mitral valve. AA, ascending aorta; ALC, anterolateral commissure; CS, coronary sinus; LCA, left coronary artery; LVOT, left ventricle outlet tract; MPA, main pulmonary artery; PMC, posteromedial commissure; RCA, right coronary artery.

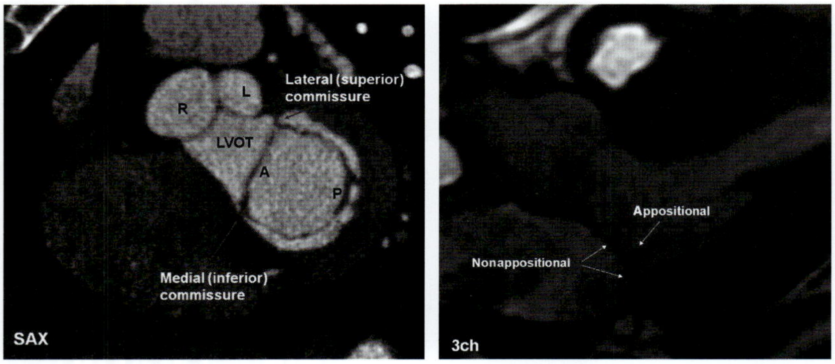

(a) (b)

Figure 1.42 (a) Short-axis view at the level of the mitral valve (mid-diastole). The commissure is defined as the junction of the mitral leaflets. The anterior (A) and posterior (P) leaflets are confluent at the commissures and do not reach the annulus. At the commissures, it is approximately 1 cm in width. In this image, the commissures are named by their attitudinal anatomic position in the thorax. (b) The appositional and nonappositional fractions of the mitral leaflets are shown in this three-chamber view (3ch) obtained by CT during systole. L, left coronary sinus; LVOT, left ventricle outflow tract; R, right coronary sinus; SAX, short axis.

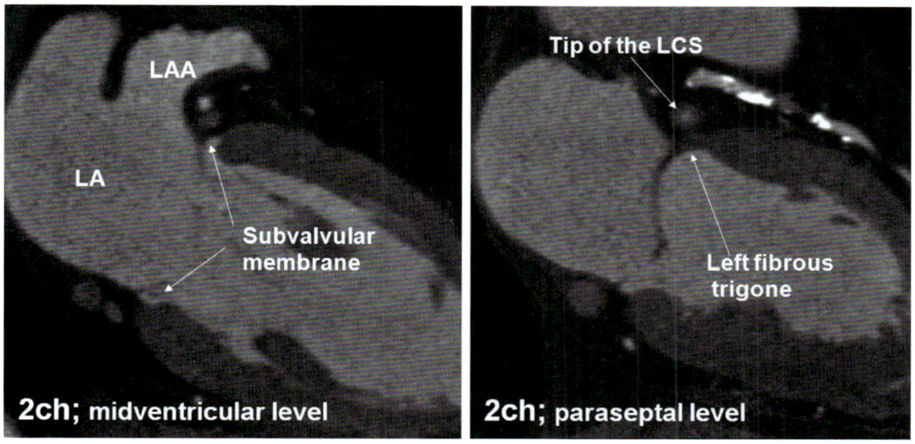

Figure 1.43 Two-chamber (2ch) views of the left ventricle at midventricular and paraseptal levels are shown. Mitral leaflets are attached to the left ventricle (LV) ostium by subvalvular membrane. It is a strip of fibrous tissue (annulus) with only a few millimeters (6–8 mm) in thickness encircling the ostium of the left atrium (LA). It is continuous with the right fibrous trigone on the right and the left fibrous trigone on the left at the aortic valve level. Note close approximation of the left fibrous trigone with the tip of the left coronary sinus (LCS). Annulus is a nonconductive fibrous sheet that electrically isolates the left atrium from the left ventricle. Aneurysmal bulge of the subvalvular membrane may develop. These aneurysm can be developmental or a result infection or surgery. LAA, left atrial appendage.

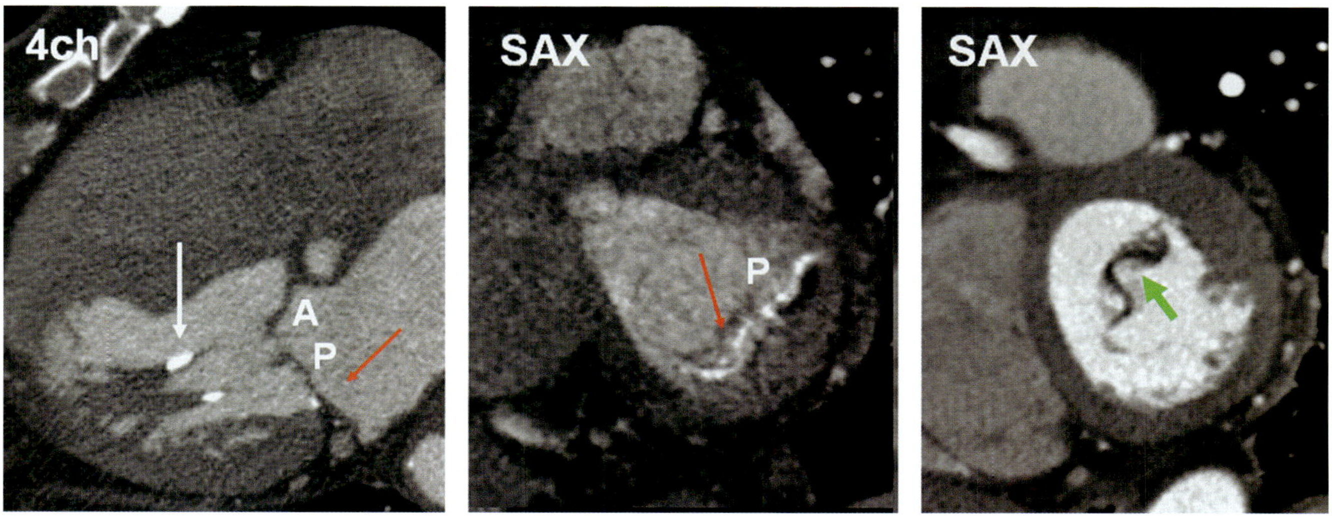

Figure 1.44 Calcification of the mitral annulus is common and usually involves the posterior leaflet, subvalvular membrane, and left ventricle (LV) ostium (red arrows). Papillary muscles may calcify too (white arrow). At the midpoint of the posterior leaflet of the mitral valve, the subvalvular segment of the atrioventricular (AV) membrane narrows and in some cases not visible. This is the region where calcification of the annulus develops the most. Usually, no serious functional abnormality occurs. Thickening and fatty degeneration of free edge of the mitral leaflets may develop with aging (green arrow). 4ch, four-chamber view; A, anterior mitral leaflet; P, posterior mitral leaflet; SAX, short-axis view.

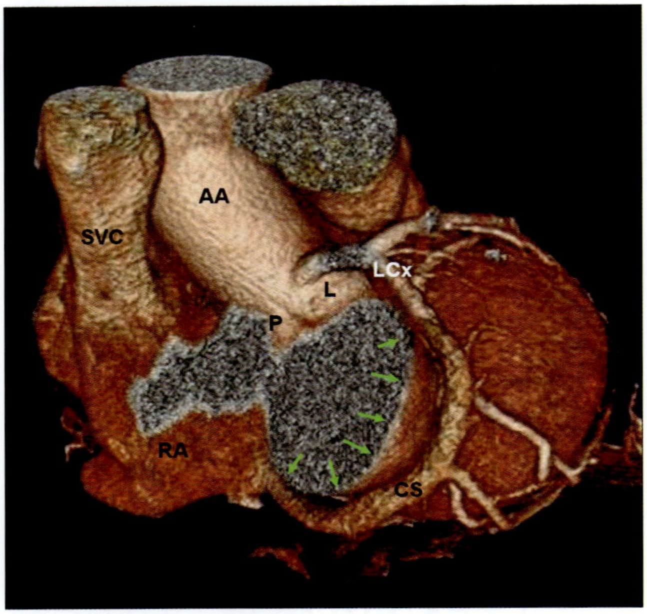

Figure 1.45 The relationship of the posterior mitral ring (green arrows) with coronary vessels is shown in this three-dimensional image of the heart. The left atrium is removed from the image. The left circumflex artery (LCx) runs adjacent to the superior margin of the posterior leaflet, whereas the coronary sinus (CS) is adjacent to the inferior margin of the mitral ring. These structures can be damaged during surgical or percutaneous mitral valve interventions. When the circumflex artery is dominant, the entire attachment of the posterior leaflet may be closely related to this artery. AA, ascending aorta; L, left coronary sinus; P, posterior coronary sinus; RA, right atrium; SVC, superior vena cava.

In contrast to the tricuspid valve, there is no direct attachment of the mitral valve to the ventricular septum, although the PM are frequently connected to the septum or to the right fibrous trigone by false cords [45]. The attached border of the anterior leaflet is divisible into three segments (Figure 1.46). The middle segment is the longest and in fibrous continuity with the aortic valve (posterior and left annuli). This segment extends between the right and left fibrous trigones (LFTs). This relation is important in aortic valve replacement surgery. For example in aortic root enlargement surgery, an incision through the atrial wall in this segment of the anterior leaflet may be extended into the subaortic outflow tract to dilate the aortic valve annulus [1]. The anterior and posterior segments are attached to the ostium of the LV and found between the mitral commissures and the fibrous trigones (Figure 1.46). Variations are seen in the length of ostial attachments of the anterior leaflet beyond the fibrous trigones.

The Left Ventricular Outflow Tract

The left ventricular outflow tract (LVOT) supports the aortic valve (Figures 1.47 and 1.53). In contrast to the RV infundibulum, which is comprised entirely of muscle, the LVOT consists of both muscular and fibrous portions. With the exception of the posterior leaflet of the mitral valve, all components of the aortoventricular membrane are part of the LVOT including the anterior mitral leaflet, fibrous trigones, intervalvular trigone, and membranous interventricular septum [1].

The Aortoventricular Membrane

The aortic annuli and the LV ostium are attached by aortoventricular membrane, part of the fibrous skeleton of the heart (Figure 1.49). This membrane is thicker between the nadir of the posterior (noncoronary) annulus and the ostium of the LV, forming a triangular structure known as the right fibrous trigone (RFT) (the term "central fibrous body" is also applied to this area) (Figure 1.53). The central fibrous body marks the junction of the left and right atrial attachments with the posterior annulus and the ostium of the LV. A similar thickened membrane, the LFT, exists between the left annulus and the LV. Large LFT result in minimal attachment of the left sinus to the LV. In contrast, muscular replacement of the LFT may rarely exist, causing direct attachment of the left sinus to the LV muscle. Between the two trigones, is the fibrous continuity of the anterior mitral leaflet with the aortic valve. Muscular replacement is more common in the right aortic annulus. Particular care is necessary in placing sutures in the muscular portion or paravalvular leak may result. Peripherally, the trigones are continuous with the annulus of the mitral valve (subvalvular membrane).

The Membranous Interventricular Septum

The RFT is continuous with membranous interventricular septum (Figure 1.49). The septal attachment of the tricuspid valve demarcates the AV and interventricular divisions of the membranous septum (Figure 1.27). The left bundle of the cardiac conduction system enters the LVOT posterior to the membranous septum [34] (Figure 1.51).

The Aortic Valve

The aortic valve is a semilunar valve. Behind each leaflet, the aortic wall bulges outward to form the three sinuses of Valsalva designated as right coronary, left coronary, and noncoronary (posterior) sinuses [52] (Figure 1.52). Between the sinuses the commissures are formed [53]. Similar to the pulmonary valve, the aortic valve does not have a discrete annulus. The fibrous annuli conform the shape of sinuses. They provide attachment to both the aortic wall and the leaflets of the aortic valve. Both the aortic and the pulmonary roots have ventricular musculature at the base of their sinuses (ventriculoarterial junction).

(a) 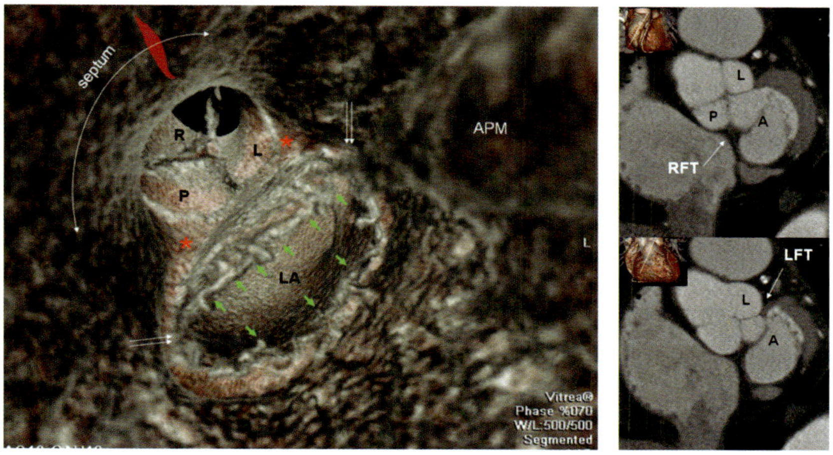 (b)

Figure 1.46 (a) Endoscopic view of the mitral and left ventricular outflow tract (LVOT) at diastole. The view angle is at the apex of the left ventricle. Anterolateral papillary muscle (APM) is seen at the upper right corner of the image. The fan-shaped closed leaflets of the aortic valve are seen anteriorly. Oval shaped mitral ring is seen posteriorly. Mitral valves are widely open during diastole. The anterior leaflet covers the anterior third of the mitral ring. Free margin of mitral leaflets are shown by green arrows. Medial and lateral commissures are marked by double arrows. Middle segment of the anterior leaflet is continuous with the medial aspect of the posterior (P) and left (L) aortic annuli. The right and left fibrous trigones (LFTs) are seen between the lateral attachments of the anterior mitral leaflet and aortic annuli (red stars). The trigones are in continuity with mitral annulus (subvalvular membrane) (pinkish band of tissue around the mitral valve). In surgical repair of the LVOT in obstructive hypertrophic cardiomyopathy, a longitudinal incision in the axis of the left ventricle (LV) is made under the left side of the right aortic sinus (red patch). Both commissures are well posterior to their related fibrous trigones. The lateral mitral commissure is approximately 15 mm behind the LFT and the medial 10 mm from the right fibrous trigone (RFT). The LFT may be large and confluent with the intervalvular membrane or may be very small or absent. (b) Short-axis images at two different levels show the anatomic location of the RFT and the LFT. A, anterior mitral leaflet; LA, left atrium; R, right aortic sinus.

(a) 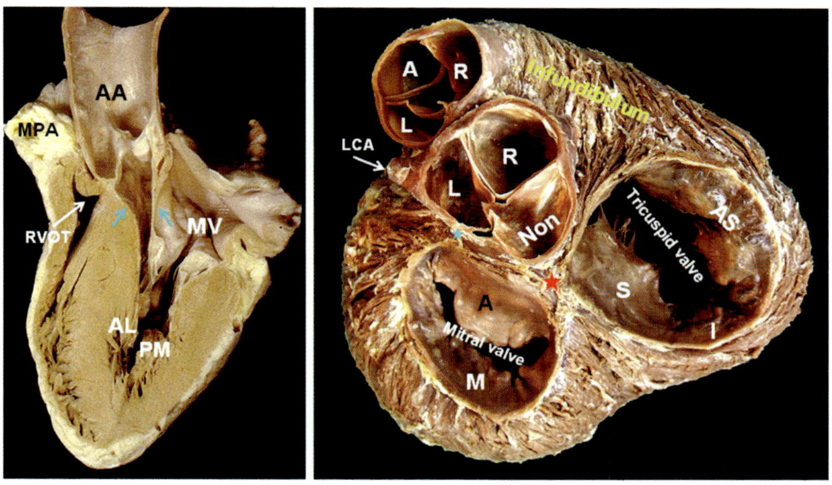 (b)

Figure 1.47 (a) Longitudinal section through the parietal walls of the ventricles shows the subaortic outflow tract and its muscular and fibrous components (blue arrows) and how the papillary muscles of the mitral valve are closely faced each other. (b) Short-axis view from atrial side, after removal of the epicardium and coronary vessels, shows the relationship of the aortic valve and the right (red star) and left (blue star) fibrous trigones. Pulmonary sinuses are named according to their relationship to the heart (nonattitudinal), which include anterior (A), left (L) posterior, and right (R) posterior. The right (R), left (L), and noncoronary sinuses of the aortic valve are shown. Note the origin of the left coronary artery (LCA) from the left coronary sinus. The aortic (A) and mural (M) leaflets of the mitral valve and the septal (S), anterosuperior (AS), and inferior (I) leaflets of the tricuspid valve are seen. AA, ascending aorta; AL, anterolateral papillary muscle; MPA, main pulmonary artery; MV, mitral valve; PM, posteromedial papillary muscle; RVOT, right ventricular outflow tract.

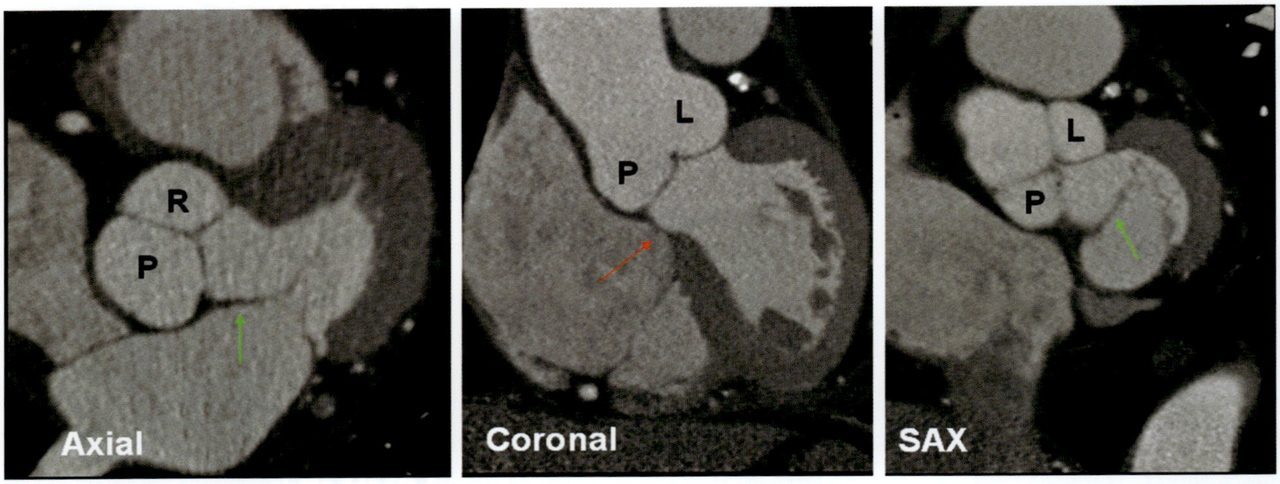

Figure 1.48 The left ventricular outflow tract, three different projections. The septal wall of the left ventricular outflow tract includes the interventricular septum with its membranous portion (red arrow). The posterior quadrant of the outflow tract consists of anterior mitral valve (green arrows) with its fibrous attachment to the wall containing left and right fibrous trigones that also support the posterior and left aortic annuli in the area of aortomitral continuity. The lateral side of the outflow tract is again muscular and consists of the posterolateral margin of the inner curvature of the left ventricle (LV). L, left; P, posterior sinuses; R, right.

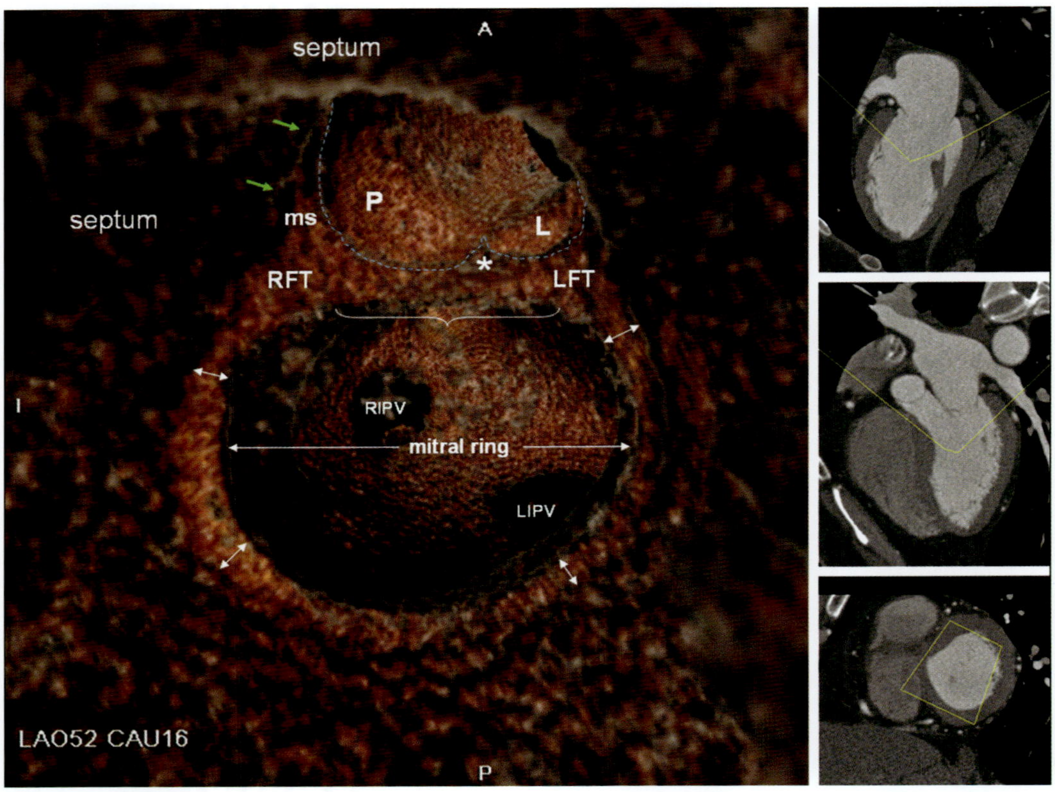

Figure 1.49 Components of the aortoventricular membrane as viewed from the left ventricle (LV) apex, the ostium of the LV, consists of aortic and mitral divisions. The width of junction of the anterior mitral valve and the aortic valve (left and posterior sinuses) is approximately 3 cm extending between the left and right fibrous trigones, also known as fibrous continuity of mitral valve (large bracket). The right fibrous trigone (RFT) is in continuity with membranous septum (ms, green arrows). Intervalvular fibrous trigone (marked by "star") between the aortic annuli is also continuous with the rest of fibrous membrane. Note the subvalvular membrane around the mitral ring (small double headed arrows) meets the left and right fibrous trigones anteriorly. A, anterior; L, left coronary sinus; LFT, left fibrous trigone; LIPV, left inferior pulmonary vein; P, posterior coronary sinus; RIPV, right inferior pulmonary vein.

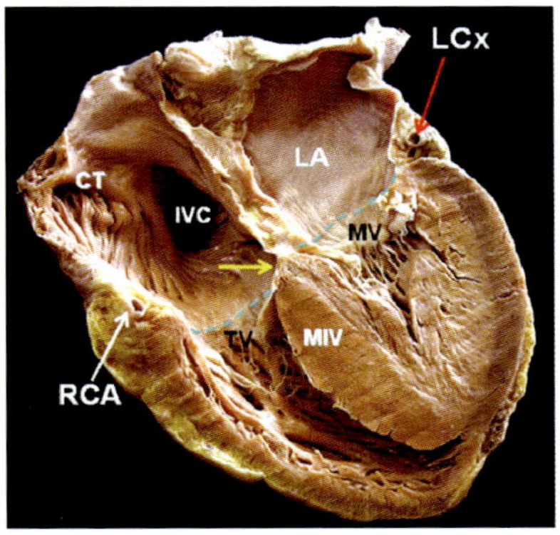

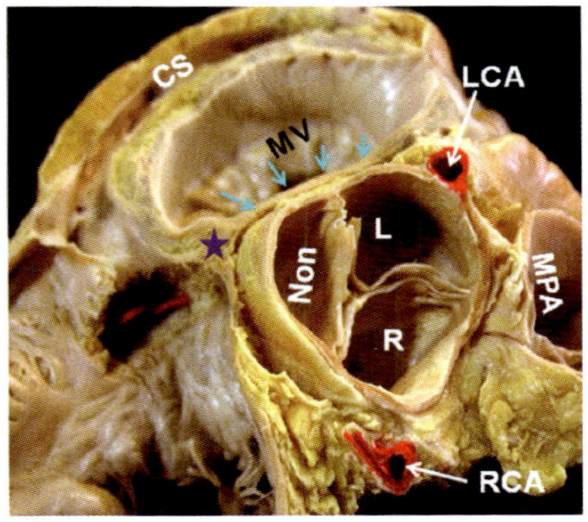

Figure 1.50 (a) Long-axis section (four chamber) shows how the muscular atrioventricular septum (yellow arrow) is formed by the attachment of the atrioventricular valves at different levels. (b). The aortic valve is seen from above with closed leaflets. Note the fibrous continuity of the medial part of the noncoronary (non) and left coronary (L) leaflets with the aortic leaflet of the mitral valve (blue arrows). This important area is also known as the aortomitral curtain. Purple star, right fibrous trigone; CS, coronary sinus; CT, crista terminalis; IVC, inferior vena cava; L, left coronary leaflet; LA, left atrium; LCA, left coronary artery; LCx, left circumflex artery; MIV, muscular interventricular septum; MPA, main pulmonary artery; MV, mitral valve; R, right coronary leaflet; RCA, right coronary artery; TV, tricuspid valve.

Ventricular musculature is circumferential in the pulmonary root. On the other hand, ventricular musculature is incomplete in the aortic root at the level of the noncoronary sinus due to the continuity between the leaflets of the aortic and mitral valves [54]. Extension of ventricular myocardium in to aorta or pulmonary artery beyond the ventriculoarterial junction is not uncommon. The clinical significance of this extension is unknown [54].

The aortic valve is related to each of the cardiac chambers and valves (Figure 1.53). The relationship is very important to understanding aortic valve pathology and many congenital cardiac malformations. The adjoining halves of the posterior and left aortic sinuses are anterior to the LA. The left atrial attachment to the aortoventricular membrane extends between the nadirs of the left and posterior aortic annuli. The relationship is important in aortic valve replacement surgery, since the prosthetic valve may be sutured to the membrane just below the left atrial attachment. The anterior half of the posterior sinus (adjoining to the right sinus) bulges into the medial wall of the RA (Figure 1.53). The midpoint of the posterior sinus faces the interatrial junction (Figure 1.53). However, clockwise or counterclockwise rotation of the aortic annuli may be present [1].

The right aortic sinus is in close relation to the posterior wall of RVOT and the parietal band (Figure 1.33). It is also partially covered by a large epicardial fat pad. The commissure between the posterior and right coronary annuli is located directly above the penetrating AV bundle and the membranous ventricular septum (Figure 1.51B).

Intervalvular trigone between the right and left coronary sinuses of the aorta (Figure 1.52B) is anterior to the LFT and forms the uppermost part of the subaortic LVOT (sagittal body planes, image 18). An incision through this area passes into the space between the aortic root and the pulmonary trunk. Only a small part of this area in the normal heart is a true outlet septum (infundibular septum). Thus, although the outlet components of the right and LV face each other, an incision below the aortic valve enters low into the infundibulum of the RV.

The Pericardium

The pericardium surrounds the heart and extends superiorly to cover part of the SVC, ascending aorta, and main pulmonary artery (Figure 1.54). Normal pericardium can be identified at CT images as a thin line of soft tissue density outlined by mediastinal and epicardial fat (Figure 1.55).

The pericardium consists of an outer fibrous component and an inner double-layered serous sac that surrounds the heart [55]. The outer serous layer that is closely attached to the fibrous layer is the parietal pericardium. The visceral serous pericardium, or epicardium, adheres to the heart and great vessels and forms recesses and sinuses. Normally, the pericardial sac contains 15–50 mL of fluid allowing visualization of the pericardial recesses on CT or MR imaging studies [56]. The fibrous pericardium is fused with the central tendon of the diaphragm inferiorly and with the tunica adventitia of the great vessels superiorly. Anteriorly, it is attached to the sternum by superior and inferior sternopericardial ligaments (Figure 1.55).

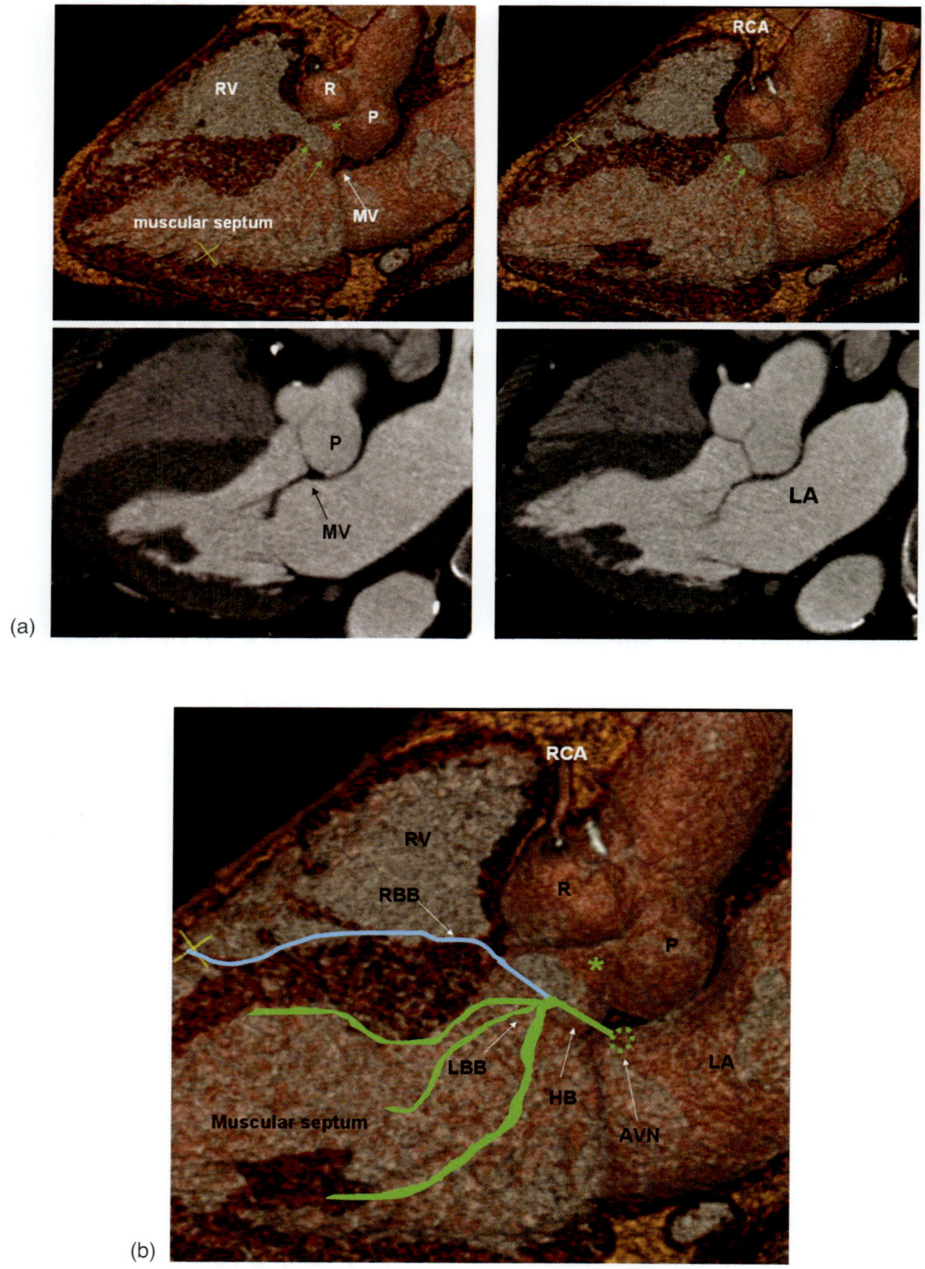

Figure 1.51 (a) Endoscopic views of the left ventricular septal wall with corresponding three-chamber slices show the membranous septum as a bluish area (green arrows) below the intervalvular fibrous trigone (green star) of posterior and right coronary sinuses. Note that the right coronary (R) sinus bulges into the right ventricle (RV) and the posterior (noncoronary) sinus (P) protrudes the left atrium (LA). The attachment of the anterior mitral leaflet (MV) to the nadir of the posterior sinus is seen (black arrow). (b) Close-up view of the septal wall of the LVOT is shown. The left bundle branch (LBB) of the cardiac conduction system enters the left ventricular outflow tract posterior to the membranous septum and immediately beneath the commissure between the right and posterior annuli of the aortic valve. After traveling a short distance down the septum, the left bundle divides into two or three main divisions. The AV node (AVN) is in the Koch's triangle (the right atrium) just beneath the right fibrous trigone, below the nadir of the posterior aortic sinus. The bundle of His (HB) penetrates the right fibrous trigone and travels along the inferior margin of the membranous septum. It divides into the left and right bundles at the level of septal attachment of the tricuspid valve to the membranous septum. RBB, right bundle branch; RCA, right coronary artery.

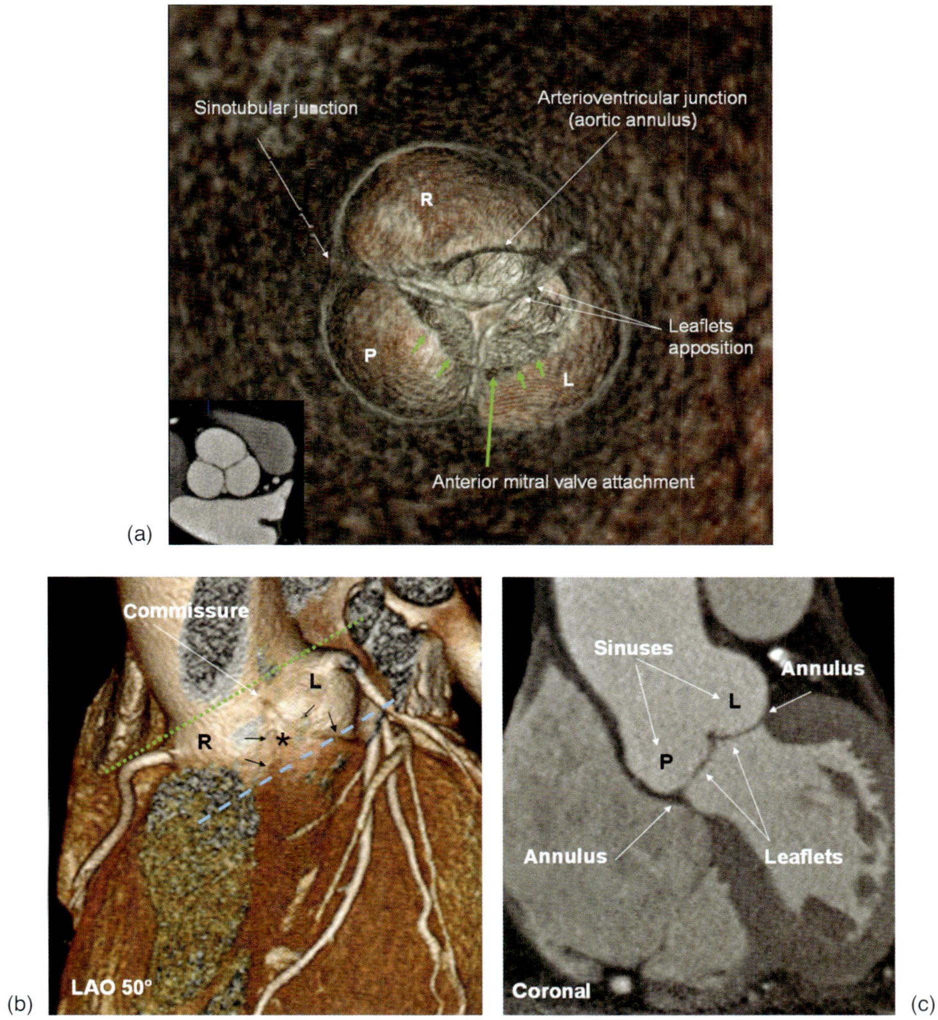

Figure 1.52 (a) Endoscopic view of the aortic side of the aortic valve using MDCT. Corresponding axial image is shown at the left lower corner. The images are obtained during diastole. The semilunar leaflets are in apposition. Three aortic sinuses are shown including posterior (P), left (L), and right (R). A variation in size of the sinuses and leaflets is present; the right is the largest. The site of aortomitral continuity is shown by green arrows. Fenestration is common in the appositional side of the aortic leaflets. (b, c) are three-dimensional and coronal images of the aortic root. Each leaflet forms its U-shaped annulus (small black arrows in (b)). Intervalvular fibrous trigone between the right and left coronary sinuses of the aorta (black star) is anterior to the left fibrous trigone and forms the uppermost part of the ostium of the left ventricle (LV). The sinotubular junction is demarcated by the green line and the ventriculoarterial junction by the blue line. The axis of the aortic annulus is 30° above the horizontal plane. Characteristically, the posterior sinus is the lowest and the left the highest. However, in a small percentage of people the right sinus is at the same level or rarely below the posterior. LAO, left anterior oblique projection.

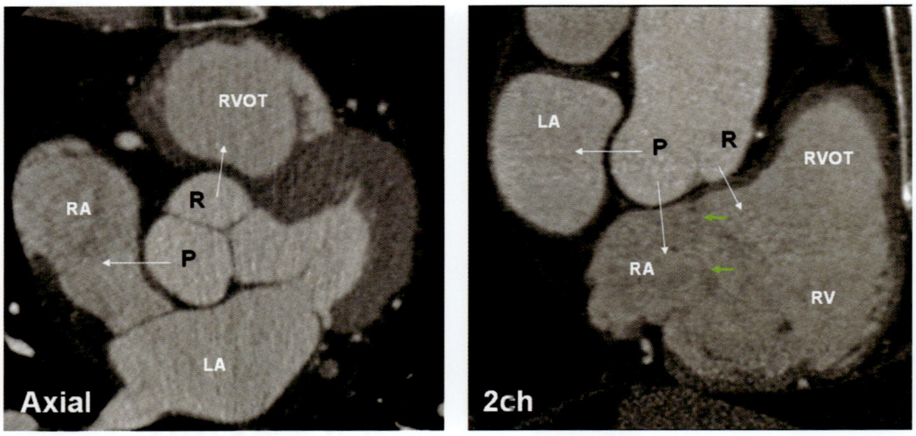

Figure 1.53 Relationship of the aortic sinuses to the cardiac chambers. Because of the central position of the aortic valve relative to the other valves and cardiac chambers, abscess formation can produce fistulas between the aorta and any of the four chambers of the heart. The right aortic sinus (R) is in close relation to the posterior wall of right ventricular outflow tract (RVOT). The most common location for congenital aneurysm of the sinus of Valsalva is the left side of the right coronary sinus bulging into the RVOT. The septal papillary muscle of the tricuspid valve is below the nadir of the right coronary sinus. The anterior half of the posterior sinus (adjoining to the right sinus) bulges into the medial wall of the right atrium (RA). The commissure between the two is close to the atrioventricular (AV) node. Fistula from posterior sinus aneurysm most often communicates with the RA. The attachment of the septal leaflet of the tricuspid valve to the membranous septum is variable. However, it usually underlies the commissure between the two sinuses (green arrow). When it extends beneath the posterior sinus, the fistula may enter the right ventricle (RV). Aneurysm of the left aortic sinus is very rare and anatomically a fistula can develop into the left ventricle (LV) or the left atrium (LA). P, posterior or noncoronary sinus.

(a)

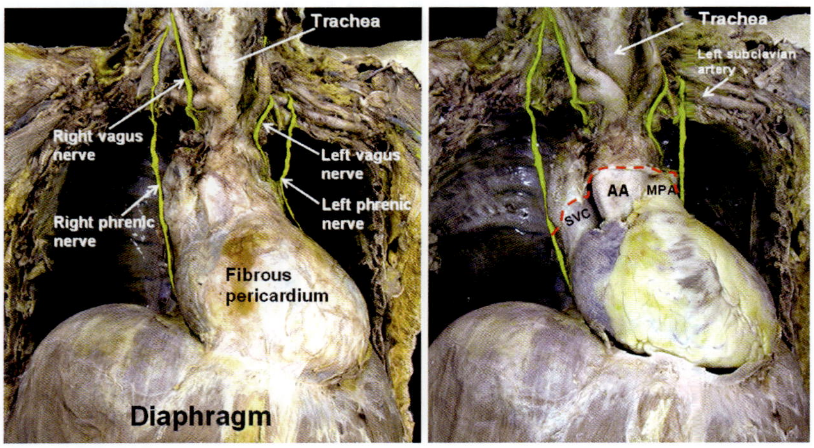

(b)

Figure 1.54 (a) An anterior view of the heart with the fibrous or parietal pericardium around it. The lungs are removed. The phrenic and vagus nerves are painted in yellow. (b) The fibrous pericardium has been removed. The superior reflection of the parietal pericardium on the superior vena cava (SVC), ascending aorta (AA), and main pulmonary artery (MPA) is seen (red line).

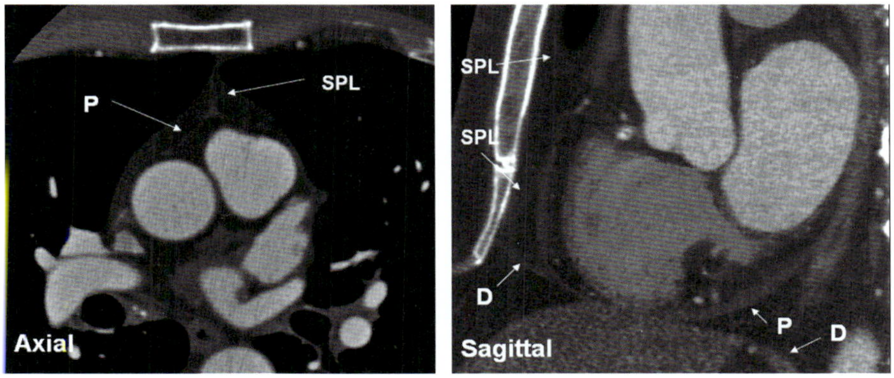

Figure 1.55 Attachments of fibrous pericardium (P) to the sternum by superior and inferior sternopericardial ligaments (SPL) and to the central tendon of the diaphragm (D) are shown.

The reflections of the serosal layers are arranged around two complex tubes. One tube encloses the aorta and pulmonary trunk. The second tube encloses the SVC, the IVC, and the four pulmonary veins [55, 56]. The transverse sinus is the passage between these two pericardial tubes (Figures 1.56–1.57) (Figures 1.59 and 1.60). At the level of transverse sinus, it is possible to pass a finger posterior to the aorta and pulmonary trunk and anterior to the LA and SVC. The oblique sinus is the cul-de-sac located posterior and superior the LA.

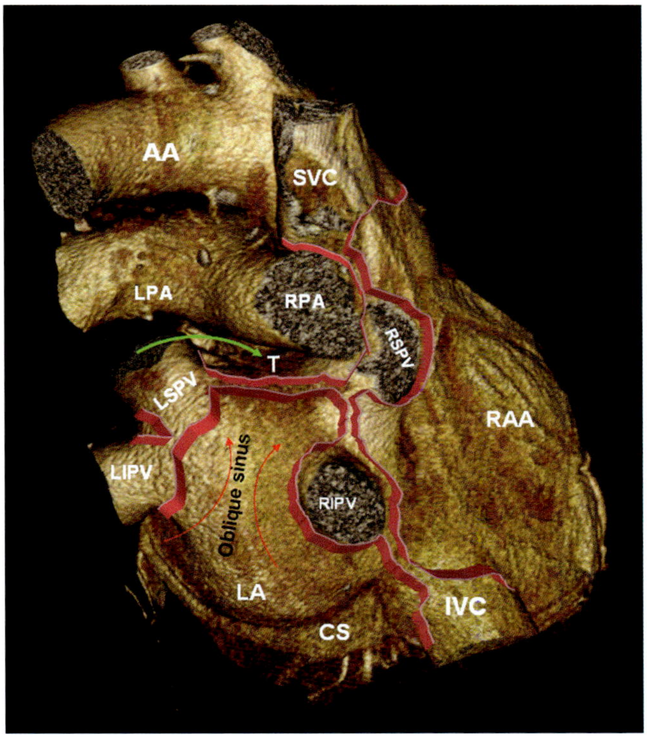

Figure 1.56 The right lateral view of the heart demonstrates the oblique sinus separated from the transverse sinus (T) by two layers of pericardial reflections that run between the left and right superior pulmonary veins. AA, ascending aorta; CS, coronary sinus; IVC, inferior vena cava; LA, left atrium; LIPV, left inferior pulmonary vein; LPA, left pulmonary artery; LSPV, left superior pulmonary vein; RAA, right atrial appendage; RIPV, right inferior pulmonary vein; RPA, right pulmonary artery; RSPV, right superior pulmonary vein; SVC, superior vena cava.

The Transverse Sinus

The transverse sinus is located inferior and posterior to the aorta and the pulmonary trunk, and above the LA. It is subdivided into the superior and inferior aortic recesses and the right and left pulmonic recesses [57] (Figure 1.57). The superior extent of the transverse sinus along the aortocaval space is the superior aortic recess [58]. Some authors further divide this recess, based on its relationship to the aorta, into posterior, lateral, and anterior portions. Cephalad extension of this recess into the high right paratracheal region (high riding recess) can be mistaken for pathologies such as a bronchogenic cyst [59] (Figure 1.58).

The anterior extension of the superior aortic forms a characteristic crescent in front of the aorta and pulmonary artery. Inferior extension of the transverse sinus along posterior wall of the aorta and above the LA is called the inferior aortic recess. Lateral extent of the transverse sinus forms the left and right pulmonic recesses between the pulmonary artery and superior pulmonary vein on each side [60]. The left pulmonic recess is bounded medially by the fold of ligament of Marshall (Figure 1.59).

The Pericardial Fat

Pericardial fat composes of the epicardial fat and the paracardial fat [61, 62] (Figures 1.47 and 1.60). Paracardial (mediastinal) fat is situated on the external surface of the parietal pericardium within the mediastinum. Epicardial (subepicardial) fat is located between the visceral layer of the pericardium and the myocardium. Epicardial adipose tissue is supplied by branches of the coronary arteries, whereas paracardial fat is supplied from different sources including the pericardiacophrenic artery, a branch of the internal mammary artery.

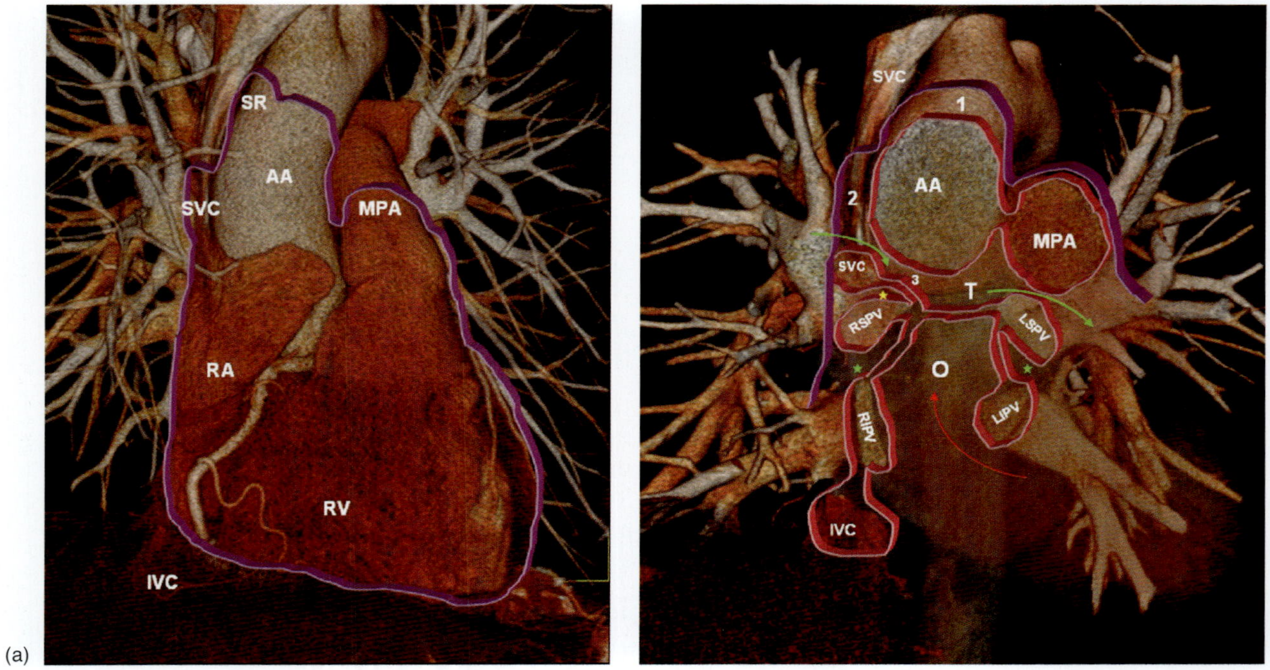

Figure 1.57 (a) The anterior view of the heart with drawing of the fibrous (parietal) pericardium around it (purple). (b) Drawing of the visceral pericardial sac (in red) around large vessels at their cardiac origin after removal of heart. Superior attachment of the parietal pericardium is again shown (in purple). The ascending aorta (AA) and main pulmonary artery (MPA) are enclosed in one tube. The superior vena cava (SVC), inferior vena cava (IVC), and pulmonary veins (PVs) are enclosed in other tube. Transverse sinus (T) is complex interconnecting passage between these two tubes. Double layer of serous pericardium (*arrow*) separates transverse sinus and oblique sinus. Components of the superior aortic recess anterior (1), lateral (2), and posterior (3) to the aorta are shown. The oblique sinus (O) is located behind the left atrium. Retrocaval recess (yellow star) is located between the SVC and the right superior PV (RSPV). The left and right lateral recesses (green stars) are formed between superior and inferior PVs. LIPV, left inferior pulmonary vein; LSPV, left superior pulmonary vein; RA, right atrium; RIPV, right inferior pulmonary vein; RSPV, right superior pulmonary vein; RV, right ventricle.

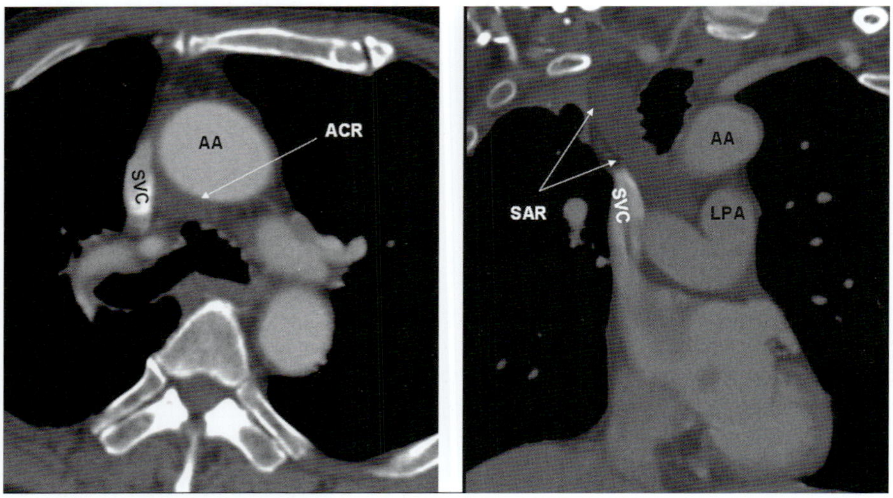

Figure 1.58 High riding aortocaval recess (ACR) with its superior extent rising to the level of the thoracic inlet. AA, ascending aorta; LPA, left pulmonary artery; SAR, superior aortic recess; SVC, superior vena cava.

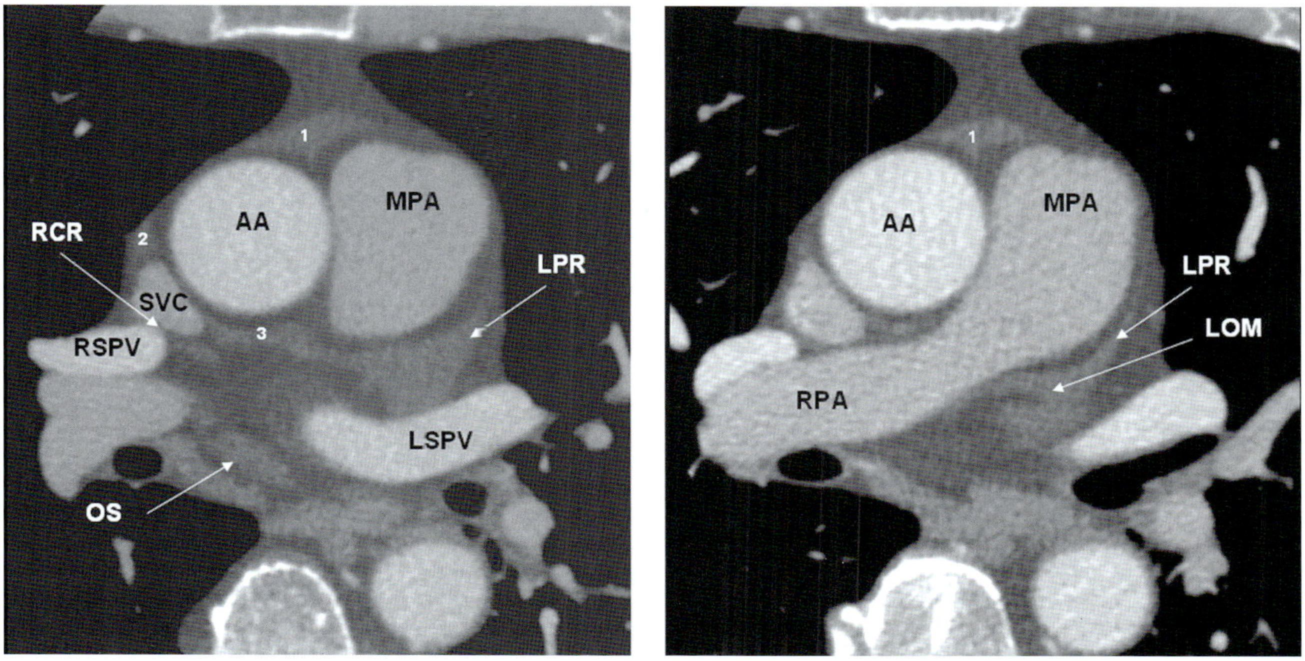

Figure 1.59 Axial images of the heart at the level of the transverse sinus are shown. Components of the superior aortic recess anterior (1), lateral (2), and posterior (3) to the ascending aorta (AA) are evident. The left pulmonic recess (LPR) of the transverse sinus is seen anterior to the left superior pulmonary vein (LSPV). Fold of the ligament of Marshall (LOM) is seen deep in the LPR. A small retrocaval recess (RCR) and the superior portion of oblique sinus (OS) are also seen. MPA, main pulmonary artery; RPA, right pulmonary artery; RSPV, right superior pulmonary vein; SVC, superior vena cava.

(a) (b)

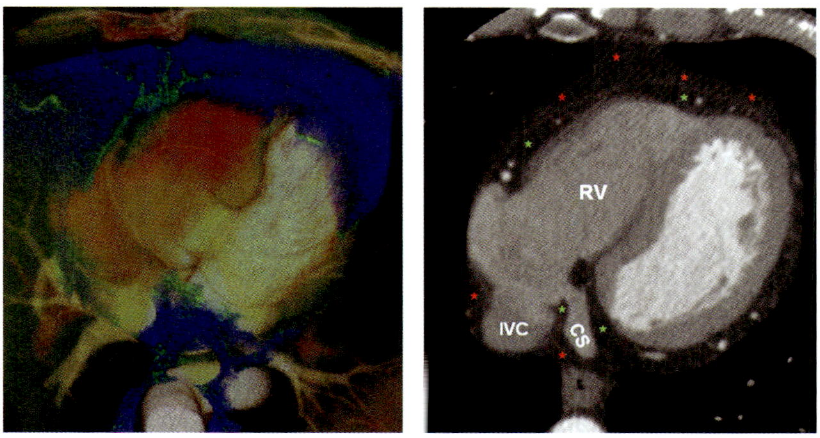

Figure 1.60 (a) Three-dimensional color mapping of the pericardial fat is shown in blue. (b) Axial image of the heart at the level of the coronary sinus (CS) shows different compartments of the pericardial fat including the epicardial (green stars) and the mediastinal (red stars) fat. The pericardial sac is shown as a thin line between the two compartments. Epicardial fat is located between the pericardial sac and the myocardium. The coronary vessels and the coronary sinus are embedded in the epicardial fat. The mediastinal fat covers outside the pericardial sac. IVC, inferior vena cava; RV, right ventricle.

Epicardial fat covers 80% of the heart's surface and is largely concentrated around the anatomic course coronary vessels in the AV or interventricular groove [63,64]. There is three- to fourfold more epicardial fat associated with the right than the LV. Epicardial fat is not limited to the surface of the heart but can penetrate deep in the interatrial septum and septal AV junction (Figure 1.60).

References

1. McAlpine WA. (1975) *Heart and Coronary Arteries: An Anatomical Atlas for Clinical Diagnosis, Radiological Investigation, and Surgical Treatment*. Springer-Verlag, New York, pp. 160–178.
2. Kouchoukos NT, Blackstone EH, Doty DB, Hanley FL, Karp RB. (2003) Anatomy, dimensions, and terminology. In *Kirklin/Barrett-Boyes Cardiac Surgery* (3rd edition). Churchill Livingstone, Philadelphia, pp. 3–22.
3. Saremi F, Krishnan S. (2007) Cardiac conduction system: anatomic landmarks relevant to interventional electrophysiologic techniques demonstrated with 64-detector CT. *Radiographics* 27(6):1539–1565.
4. Anderson RH, Brown NA. (1996) The anatomy of the heart revisited. *Anat Rec* 246:1–7.
5. Wilcox BR, Cook AC, Anderson RH. (2004) *Surgical Anatomy of the Heart*. Cambridge University Press, Cambridge, pp. 11–82.
6. Sanchez-Quintana D, Anderson RH, Cabrera JA *et al.* (2002) The terminal crest: morphological features relevant to electrophysiology. *Heart* 88:406–411.
7. Matsuyama TA, Inoue S, Kobayashi Y *et al.* (2004) Anatomical diversity and age-related histological changes in the human right atrial posterolateral wall. *Europace* 6:307–315.
8. Anderson RH, Webb S, Brown NA. (1999) Clinical anatomy of the atrial septum with reference to its developmental components. *Clin Anat* 12:362–374.
9. James TN. (1977) The sinus node. *Am J Cardiol* 40:965–986.
10. Sow ML, Ndoye JM, Lo EA. (1996) The artery of the sinoatrial node: anatomic considerations based on 45 injection-dissections of the heart. *Surg Radiol Anat* 18:103–109.
11. Sánchez-Quintana D, Cabrera JA, Farré J, Climent V, Anderson RH, Ho SY. (2005) Sinus node revisited in the era of electroanatomical mapping and catheter ablation. *Heart* 91(2):189–194.
12. Ho SY, Anderson RH. (2000) How constant anatomically is the tendon of Todaro as a marker for the triangle of Koch? *J Cardiovasc Electrophysiol* 11:83–89.
13. Anderson RH, Ho HY, Becker AE. (2000) Anatomy of the human atrioventricular junctions revisited. *Anat Rec* 260:81–91.
14. Saremi F, Abolhoda A, Ashikyan O *et al.* (2008) Arterial supply to sinuatrial and atrioventricular nodes: imaging with multidetector CT. *Radiology* 246(1):99–107.
15. Anderson KR, Murphy JG. (1983) The atrio-ventricular node artery in the human heart. *Angiology* 34:711–716.
16. Arid JM, Armstrong O, Rogez JM, Robert R, Lardoux MC, Leborgne J. (2000) Arterial vascularisation of the atrioventricular node. *Surg Radiol Anat* 22:93–96.
17. Sanchez-Quintana D, Ho SY, Cabrera JA *et al.* (2001) Topographic anatomy of the inferior pyramidal space: relevance to radiofrequency catheter ablation. *J Cardiovasc Electrophysiol* 12:210–217.
18. Cabrera JA, Sanchez-Quintana D, Farre J, Rubio JM, Ho SY. (2005) The inferior right atrial isthmus: further architectural insights for current and coming ablation technologies. *J Cardiovasc Electrophysiol* 16(4):409–410.
19. Olgin JE, Kalman JM, Fitzpatrick AP, Lesh MD. (1995) Role of right atrial endocardial structures as barriers to conduction during human type I atrial flutter: activation and entrainment mapping guided by intracardiac echocardiography. *Circulation* 92:1839–1848.
20. Saremi F, Pourzand L, Krishnan S *et al.* (2008) Right atrial cavotricuspid isthmus: anatomic characterization with multidetector row CT. *Radiology* 247(3):658–668.
21. von Lüdinghausen M. (2003) The venous drainage of the human myocardium. *Adv Anat Embryol Cell Biol* 168(I-VIII): 1–104.
22. Silver MA, Rowley NE. (1988) The functional anatomy of the human coronary sinus. *Am Heart J* 115:1080–1084.
23. Ho SY, Sanchez-Quintana D, Cabrera JA *et al.* (1999) Anatomy of the left atrium: implications for radiofrequency ablation of atrial fibrillation. *J Cardiovasc Electrophysiol* 10:1525–1533.
24. Veinot JP, Harrity PJ, Gentile F, Khandheria BK *et al.* (1997) Anatomy of the normal left atrial appendage. A quantitative study of age-related changes in 500 autopsy hearts: implications for echocardiographic examination. *Circulation* 96:3112–3115.
25. Becker AE. (2004) Left atrial isthmus: Anatomic aspects relevant for linear catheter ablation procedures in humans. *J Cardiovasc Electrophysiol* 15:809–812.
26. Jais P, Hocini M, Hsu LF *et al.* (2004) Technique and results of linear ablation at the mitral isthmus. *Circulation* 110:2996–3002.
27. Anderson RH, Brown NA, Webb S. (2002) Development and structure of the atrial septum. *Heart* 88:104–10.
28. Hagen PT, Scholz DG, Edwards WD. (1984) Incidence and size of patent foramen ovale during the first 10 decades of life: an autopsy study of 965 normal hearts. *Mayo Clin Proc* 59:17–20.
29. Saremi F, Channual S, Raney A *et al.* (2008) Imaging of patent foramen ovale with 64-section multidetector CT. *Radiology* 249(2):483–492.
30. Bachmann G. (1916) The inter-auricular time interval. *Am J Physiol* 41:309–320.
31. Lemery R, Guiraudon G, Veinot JP. (2003) Anatomic description of the Bachmann bundle and its relation to the atrial septum. *Am J Cardiol* 91:1482–1485.
32. Saremi F, Channual S, Krishnan S, Gurudevan SV, Narula J, Abolhoda A. (2008) Bachmann Bundle and its arterial supply: imaging with multidetector CT—implications for interatrial conduction abnormalities and arrhythmias. *Radiology* 248(2):447–457.

33. Ariyarajah V, Fernandes J, Apiyasawat S, Spodick DH. (2007) Angiographic localization of potential culprit coronary arteries in patients with interatrial block following a positive exercise tolerance test. *Am J Cardiol* 99(1):58–61
34. Anderson RH, Yanni J, Boyett MR, Chandler NJ, Dobrzynski H. (2009) The anatomy of the cardiac conduction system. *Clin Anat* 22(1):99–113.
35. Haddad F, Hunt SA, Rosenthal DN, Murphy DJ. (2008) Right ventricular function in cardiovascular disease, part I: Anatomy, physiology, aging, and functional assessment of the right ventricle. *Circulation* 117(11):1436–1448.
36. Ho SY, Nihoyannopoulos P. (2006) Anatomy, echocardiography, and normal right ventricular dimensions. *Heart* 92(Suppl 1):i2–i13.
37. Goor DA, Lillehei CW. (1975) Congenital malformations of the heart. In Goor DA, Lillehei CW. (eds) *Congenital Malformations of the Heart: Embryology, Anatomy, and Operative Considerations* (1st edition), pp. 1–37. Grune & Stratton, New York.
38. Jiang L. (1994) Right ventricle. In Weyman AE. (ed.) *Principle and Practice of Echocardiography*, pp. 901–921. Lippincott Williams & Wilkins, Baltimore, MD.
39. Nigri GR, Di Dio LJ, Baptista CA. (2001) Papillary muscles and tendinous cords of the right ventricle of the human heart: morphological characteristics. *Surg Radiol Anat* 23(1):45–49.
40. Reig J, Albertí N, Petit M. (2000) Arterial vascularization of the human moderator band: an analysis of this structure's role as a collateral circulation route. *Clin Anat* 13(4):244–250.
41. Anderson RH, Razavi R, Taylor AM. (2004) Cardiac anatomy revisited. *J Anat* 205:159–177.
42. Ross DN. (1967) Replacement of aortic and mitral valve with a pulmonary autograft. *Lancet* 2:956.
43. Luciani GB, Favaro A, Casali G, Santini F, Mazzucco A. (2005) Ross operation in the young: a ten-year experience. *Ann Thorac Surg* 80(6):2271–2277
44. Cerqueira MD, Weissman NJ, Dilsizian V *et al*. (2002) American Heart Association Writing Group on Myocardial Segmentation and Registration for Cardiac Imaging: Standardized myocardial segmentation and nomenclature for tomographic imaging of the heart. A statement for healthcare professionals from the Cardiac Imaging Committee of the Council on Clinical Cardiology of the American Heart Association. *Circulation* 105(4):539–542.
45. Loukas M, Louis RG Jr, Black B, Pham D, Fudalej M, Sharkees M. (2007) False tendons: an endoscopic and cadaveric approach. *Clin Anat* 20:163–169.
46. Johansson B, Maceira AM, Babu-Narayan SV, Moon JC, Pennell DJ, Kilner PJ. (2007) Clefts can be seen in the basal inferior wall of the left ventricle and the interventricular septum in healthy volunteers as well as patients by cardiovascular magnetic resonance. *J Am Coll Cardiol* 50(13):1294–1295.
47. Anderson RH, Frater RW. (2006) How can we best describe the components of the mitral valve? *J Heart Valve Dis* 15:736–739.
48. Muresian H. (2009) The clinical anatomy of the mitral valve. *Clin Anat* 22(1):85–98.
49. Levine RA, Handschumacher MD, Sanfilippo AJ *et al.* (1989) Three-dimensional echocardiographic reconstruction of the mitral valve, with implications for the diagnosis of mitral valve prolapse. *Circulation* 80:589–598.
50. Gorman JH, Gorman RC, Jackson BM, Enomoto Y, Edmunds LH Jr. (2004) The effect of regional ischemia on mitral valve annular saddle shape. *Ann Thorac Surg* 77:544–548.
51. Salgo IS, Gorman JH, III, Gorman RC *et al.* (2002) Effect of annular shape on leaflet curvature in reducing mitral leaflet stress. *Circulation* 106:711–717.
52. Anderson RH. (2000) Clinical anatomy of the aortic root. *Heart* 84:670–673.
53. Sutton JP, Ho SY, Anderson RH. (1995) The forgotten interleaflet triangles: a review of the surgical anatomy of the aortic valve. *Ann Thorac Surg* 59:419–427.
54. Hasdemir C, Aktas S, Govsa F, Aktas EO *et al.* (2007) Demonstration of ventricular myocardial extensions into the pulmonary artery and aorta beyond the ventriculo-arterial junction. *Pacing Clin Electrophysiol* 30(4):534–539.
55. Vesely TM, Cahill DR. (1986) Cross-sectional anatomy of the pericardial sinuses, recesses, and adjacent structures. *Surg Radiol Anat* 8:221–227.
56. Levy-Ravetch M, Auh YH, Rubenstein WA *et al.* (1985) CT of the pericardial recesses. *AJR Am J Roentgenol* 144:707–714.
57. Kodama F, Fultz PJ, Wandtke JC. (2003) Comparing thin-section and thick-section CT of pericardial sinuses and recesses. *AJR Am J Roentgenol* 181:1101–1108
58. Choi YW, McAdams HP, Jeon SC *et al.* (2000) The "high-riding" superior pericardial recess: CT findings. *AJR Am J Roentgenol* 175:1025–1028.
59. Winer-Muram HT, Gold RE. (1990) Effusion in the superior pericardial recess simulating a mediastinal mass. *AJR Am J Roentgenol* 154:69–71.
60. Protopapas Z, Westcott JL. (1995) Left pulmonic recess of the pericardium: findings at CT and MR imaging. *Radiology* 196:85–88.
61. Nesbitt T, Lemley A, Davis J, Yost MJ, Goodwin RL, Potts JD. (2006) Epicardial development in the rat: a new perspective. *Microsc Microanal* 12(5):390–398.
62. Ho E, Shimada Y. (1978) Formation of the epicardium studied with the scanning electron microscope. *Dev Biol* 66:579–585.
63. Shirani J, Berezowski K, Roberts WC. (1995) Quantitative measurement of normal and excessive (cor adiposum) subepicardial adipose tissue, its clinical significance, and its effect on electrocardiographic QRS voltage. *Am J Cardiol* 76:414–418.
64. Wheeler GL, Shi R, Beck SR *et al.* (2005) Pericardial and visceral adipose tissue measured volumetrically with computed tomography are highly associated in type 2 diabetic families. *Invest Radiol* 40:97–101.

2 Anatomical and Pathophysiological Classification of Congenital Heart Disease

Carla Frescura,[1] Emanuela Valsangiacomo Büchel,[2] Siew Yen Ho[3] & Gaetano Thiene[1]

[1]*University of Padua Medical School, Padua, Italy*
[2]*University Children's Hospital Zurich, Zurich, Switzerland*
[3]*Imperial College London, London, United Kingdom*

Introduction

Congenital heart diseases (CHD) basically consist of defects of the cardiac architecture that interfere with the venous drainage, septation of the cardiac chambers, and their sequences and regular function of the valve apparatuses without obstacles in blood flow [1–9]. Noninvasive imaging that is now available can perfectly detect in vivo cardiac abnormalities, thus providing precise diagnosis and rendering it feasible to plan optimal surgical/interventional repair. When approaching the diagnosis of any CHD, you have to keep in mind that the normal heart is like a three-storey building (atria, ventricles, and great arteries) (Figure 2.1): the atria are the platform, the ventricles the first floor, and the great arteries a second floor, each level connected to each other through valve orifices and each half is totally separated by septa, disposed in such a way to allow deoxygenated venous blood to go to the lungs through the pulmonary artery and the oxygenated venous blood to go to the systemic organs through the aorta. Small and great circulations are in sequence, with no connection to each other than the lung capillary network.

The aim of any surgical/interventional repair is to reconstruct a separate sequence of cardiac segments and to restore the regular physiology of blood circulation. CHD may be very complex in the combination of the cardiac segments: the key to sort out the puzzle is the segmental approach, essential to establish the sequential localization of the cardiac chambers.

Revisiting Cardiac Anatomy: A Computed-Tomography-Based Atlas and Reference, 1st edition. Edited by Farhood Saremi, Eloisa Arbustini, Stephen Achenbach and Jagat Narula.

Role of Magnetic Resonance Imaging for Imaging of Congenital Heart Disease

After echocardiography, which is still considered the first-line examination in congenital cardiology, cardiovascular magnetic resonance imaging (CV-MRI) is nowadays the most frequently used advanced imaging technique for delineation of the anatomy in CHD [10–12]. Because of its noninvasiveness, CV-MRI is replacing more and more cardiac catheterization for mere diagnostic purposes; moreover, the lack of radiation makes its use in young patients more advisable than computed tomography.

The most commonly utilized CV-MRI sequences for assessment of CHD are the Steady-State Free Precession sequence, so-called white-blood technique, which is usually performed without injection of contrast medium and the contrast-enhanced MR angiography. Particularly, MR angiography has dramatically revolutioned the noninvasive assessment of CHD: with one single peripheral injection of a gadolinium-based contrast medium, it allows multiplanar (views) visualization of all intrathoracic vessels and cardiac chambers. Three-dimensional reconstructions are most similar to patho-anatomic specimens and of great help for the surgeon, as they simulate exactly the picture that he is going to find intraoperatively.

The images presented in this chapter have been acquired in vivo by using both techniques described above in patients with CHD who had not yet been surgically corrected. The image orientation has been kept in the

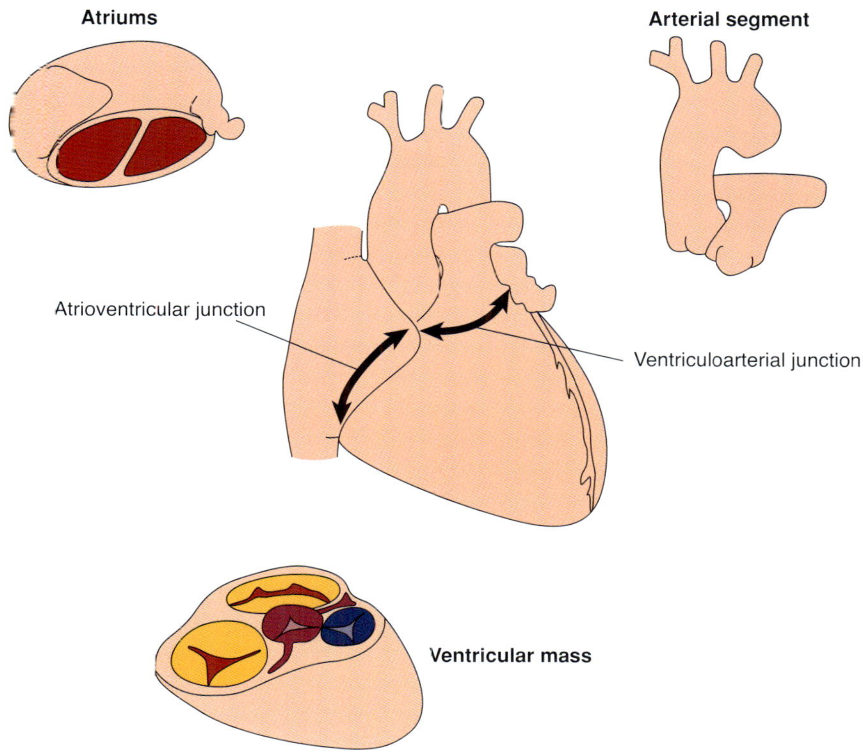

Figure 2.1 *The three-storey building concept of the heart.* The normal heart can be divided into three segments: atria, ventricles, and the great arteries joined together at two junctions atrioventricular and ventriculoarterial. In the normal anatomy, every junction posses two patent components (valves) and the septa are intact.

standard views that are clinically used for diagnostic purposes, and not always adapted to the anatomical views.

As most of CHD nowadays are being corrected within the first months of life, most of the images have been taken in newborns and young infants. The limited spatial resolution for imaging vascular structures, often smaller than few millimeters in these small patients, has caused blurring of the images in some cases. Nevertheless, demonstration of the anatomical findings is usually sufficient and the images are diagnostic for clinical decision making and for planning surgical therapy and many times can obviate the necessity of preoperative invasive procedures such as cardiac catheterization. In patients with CHD, CV-MRI is preferred to computed tomography in order to avoid radiation exposure, as these patients may require several follow-up examinations and interventions during their life.

Sequential Chamber Localization

The first step of any segmental approach to the diagnosis of CHD is to establish the platform of the heart, namely, the atrial situs and the venous drainage.

In *situs solitus* (Figure 2.2a and 2.3), the morphologically right atrium is located on the right side and the morphologically left atrium in the left side. The lungs and bronchi are concordant with such a position, with a trilobed lung and short bronchus on the right side and bilobed lung and long bronchus on the left side. In such a visceral asymmetry, the systemic venous blood (superior and inferior venae cavae) drains into the right atrium and the pulmonary veins into the left atrium. However, there are conditions in which partial or total pulmonary venous drainage may occur far away from the left atria into the systemic veins. Moreover, a left superior vena cava may persist and drain into the right atrium via the coronary sinus.

Situs inversus is the mirror image of the situs solitus, with the reversed position of the atria and lungs: morphologically right on the left side and morphologically left on the right side (Figure 2.2b).

There are conditions in which the situs is "ambiguus" (Figure 2.4–2.6) in so far as there is no laterality: both atria and lungs may exhibit right or left atriopulmonary isomerism. This visceral symmetry corresponds usually to asplenia and polysplenia syndromes, respectively, with heterotaxia of subdiaphragmatic organs. The agenesis of the spleen implies the lack development of left morphology, the genesis of multiple spleens (polysplenia) implies the lack of development of right morphology. In this setting, in *right isomerism* both atria show a right morphology and in *left isomerism* both atria show a left morphology. Thus, it is not casual that in right isomerism (asplenia syndrome) a totally anomalous pulmonary venous drainage, either supra or infra diaphragmatic, does occur

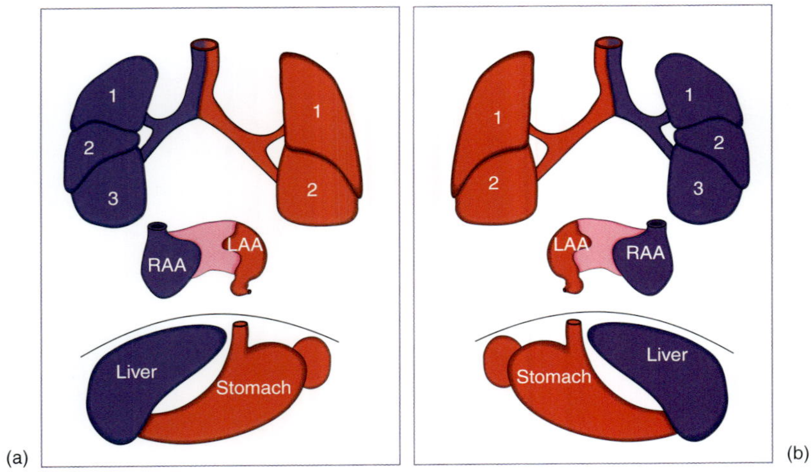

Figure 2.2 *Solitus (usual) and inversus (mirror image) atrial situs.* (a) In *situs solitus*, the morphologically right atrium is located on the right side and the morphologically left atrium in the left side, trilobed lung and short bronchus are on the right side and bilobed lung and long bronchus are on the left side. In such a visceral asymmetry, the superior and inferior venae cavae drain into the right atrium and the pulmonary veins in the left atrium. (b) The *situs inversus* is the mirror image of the situs solitus, with a reverse position of the atria and lungs: morphologically right atrium, trilobed lung and short bronchus on the left and morphologically left atrium, bilobed lung and long bronchus on the right. LAA, left atrial appendage; RAA, right atrial appendage.

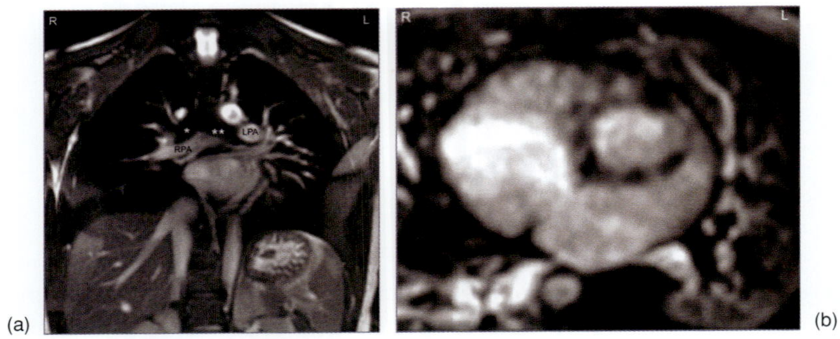

Figure 2.3 *Solitus (usual) atrial situs as visualized by magnetic resonance imaging.* (a) In situs solitus, the right short bronchus runs at the same level of the right pulmonary artery (epiarterial bronchus*); the left and long bronchus runs below the left pulmonary artery (hypoarterial bronchus**). (b) Axial view of both atria. The left atrial appendage appears in its typical long and narrow form; the right atrial appendage has a pyramidal shape and course trabeculations (pectinate muscles). L, left; LPA, left pulmonary artery; R, right; RPA, right pulmonary artery.

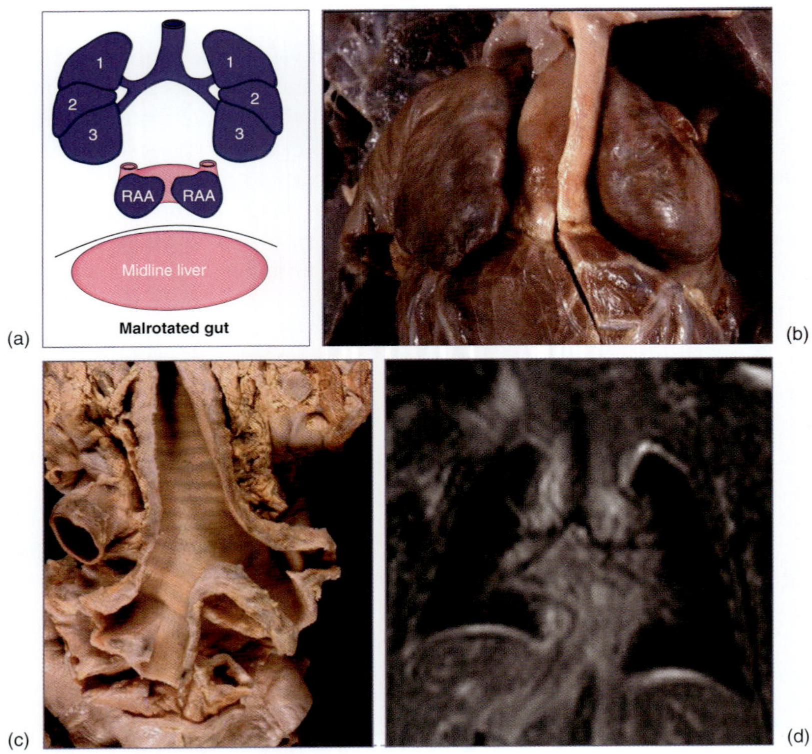

Figure 2.4 *Situs ambiguus: right atrial isomerism.* (a) Schematic representation. In right atrial isomerism, since there is no laterality, both atria are of right morphology, the lungs are bilaterally trilobed and the bronchi are short. Regularly anomalous pulmonary venous drainage is associated. Under the diaphragm usually there is heterotaxy of the abdominal organs, with midline liver and malrotated gut and the spleen tends to be absent (asplenia syndrome). (b) External view of the heart: both the appendages show right morphology. (c) Posterior view of the tracheal bifurcation: both the bronchi are short. (d) Coronal magnetic resonance imaging of right atrial isomerism with bilateral trilobed lungs showing short bronchi. RAA, morphologically right atrial appendage.

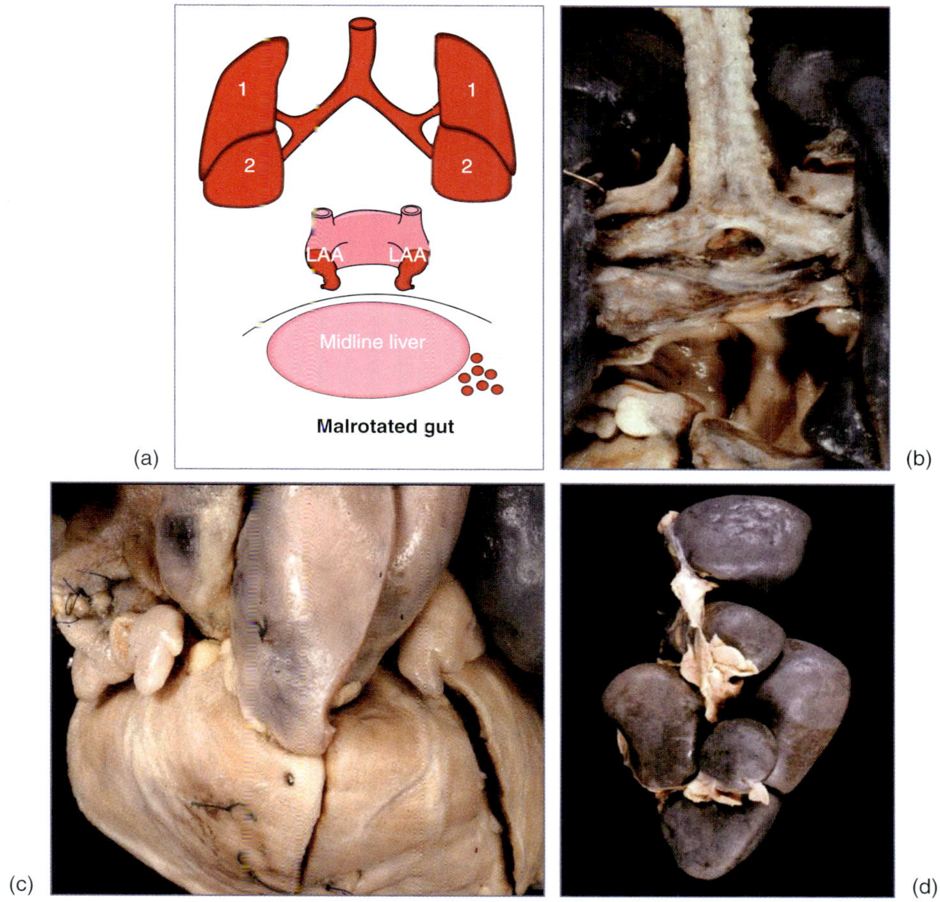

Figure 2.5 *Situs ambiguus: left atrial isomerism.* (a) Schematic representation. In left atrial isomerism, both atria present left morphology, the lungs are bilaterally bilobed with long bronchi. Frequently, a symmetric pulmonary venous drainage is present with two pulmonary veins draining in each atrium and interruption of the inferior vena cava with azygos continuation into the superior vena cava. Under the diaphragm there is heterotaxy of the abdominal organs, with midline liver and malrotated gut and multiple spleens (polysplenia syndrome). (b) Posterior view of the tracheal bifurcation: both the bronchi are long. (c) External view of the heart: both the appendages show left morphology. (d) Multiple spleens. LAA, left atrial appendage.

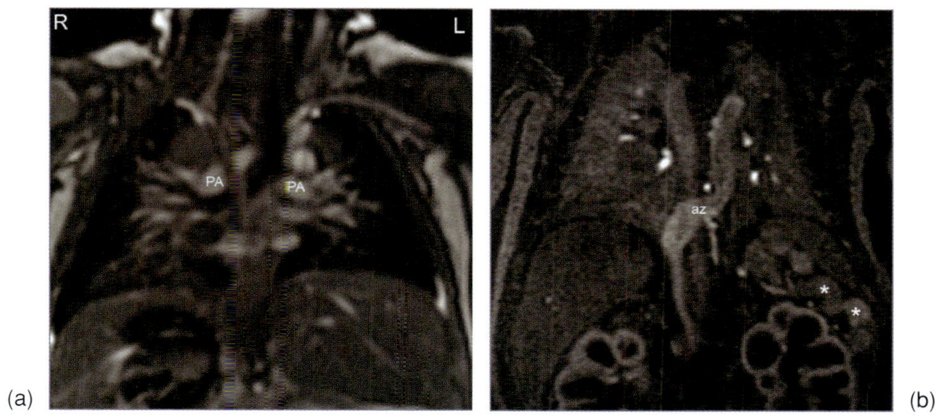

Figure 2.6 *Situs ambiguus: left atrial isomerism as visualized by magnetic resonance imaging.* Coronal images are presented. (a) In left atrial isomerism, the bronchi run below the pulmonary arteries bilaterally (hypoarterial bronchi). (b) Overview of the chest and the abdomen demonstrating the azygos vein (azygos continuation) and multiple spleens (*). az, azygos vein; L, left; PA, pulmonary artery; R, right.

because the absence of left atrial morphology implies an embryological "refusal" of the pulmonary veins to connect directly with the atria. On the opposite, in case of left isomerism (polysplenia syndrome), there is a direct continuation of the inferior vena cava with the azygos vein, thus draining into the superior vena cava system, since the absence of right atrial morphology means an embryological "refusal" of the inferior vena cava to connect directly with atria. In the other words, in the presence of situs ambiguus (right or left atrial isomerism) malformations do exist in the venous drainage and the clinician/surgeon should be aware of that, while reconstructing cardiac building.

Atrioventricular Connections

It is now necessary to establish the position of the ventricles and how they connect with the atria. The atrioventricular (AV) connection can be biventricular when the atria connect separately with the two ventricles or univentricular, when the atria mostly (>75%) connect with a sole ventricular cavity (single ventricle).

The *biventricular AV* connection may be *concordant* (Figure 2.7) when the right atrium connects with the right ventricle and the left atrium connects with the left ventricle, or *discordant* (Figure 2.8), when the right atrium connects with the left ventricle and the left atrium connects with the right ventricle (Figure 2.9), with the situs being either solitus or inversus. In case of situs ambiguus, in the setting of atrial isomerism, the connection is obviously indeterminate (biventricular connection in atrial isomerism) (Figure 2.9).

The *univentricular AV* connection may be absent right or left when the left or right AV orifice is atretic (*tricuspid and mitral valve atresia*, respectively) and *double inlet*, when both atria drain mostly (>75%) into a single ventricular chamber through two discrete (or a common) AV valves (Figure 2.10). Whatever the type of univentricular connection (absent right or left, double inlet), the main ventricular chamber may be of right or left morphology or, in exceptional cases, solitary/indeterminate (Figure 2.11–2.16).

In this regard, it should be underlined that a tiny, second ventricular chamber is most always existing and located anteriorly with right morphology ("outlet chamber"), when the main ventricular chamber is of left morphology ("single left ventricle") (Figure 2.15) and located posteriorly with left morphology ("inlet chamber"), when the main ventricular chamber is of right morphology ("single right ventricle") (Figure 2.12). Also in the setting of univentricular AV connection, the AV valve morphology may vary from two discrete AV valves, a common AV valve, straddling AV valves, one imperforated AV valve. As for the arterial pole, double inlet left ventricle is usually associated with transposition of the great arteries (discordant ventriculoarterial connections) and, more rarely, with concordant ventricular valve connection (so-called Holmes heart) (Figure 2.17).

Ventriculoarterial Connections

Having established the basement of the heart (atria and venous pole), and the first floor (ventricles), the sequence of the cardiac segments is completed by defining the ventriculoarterial (VA) connections, namely, the arterial outlet.

VA connection can be *concordant* when the right ventricle gives origin to the pulmonary artery and the left ventricle gives origin to the aorta (Figure 2.18) and can

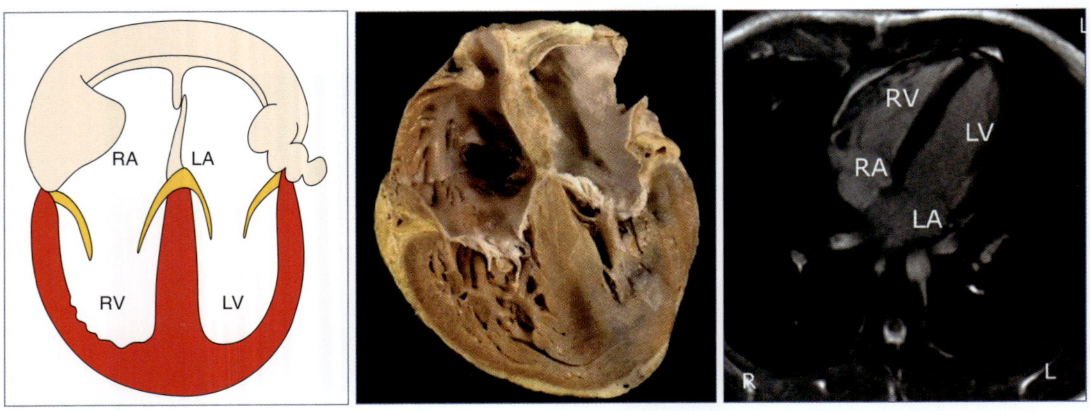

(a), (b) (c)

Figure 2.7 *Biventricular, concordant atrioventricular connection in situs solitus.* (a) Schematic representation. In the presence of two regular ventricular chambers, the atrioventricular connection is concordant when the right atrium connects with the right ventricle and the left atrium connects with the left ventricle, regardless the situs being solitus or inversus. (b) Corresponding anatomical specimen in four-chamber echocardiographic section. (c) Corresponding four-chamber view as visualized by magnetic resonance imaging white-blood sequence. L, left; LA, left atrium; LV, left ventricle; R, right; RA, right atrium; RV, right ventricle.

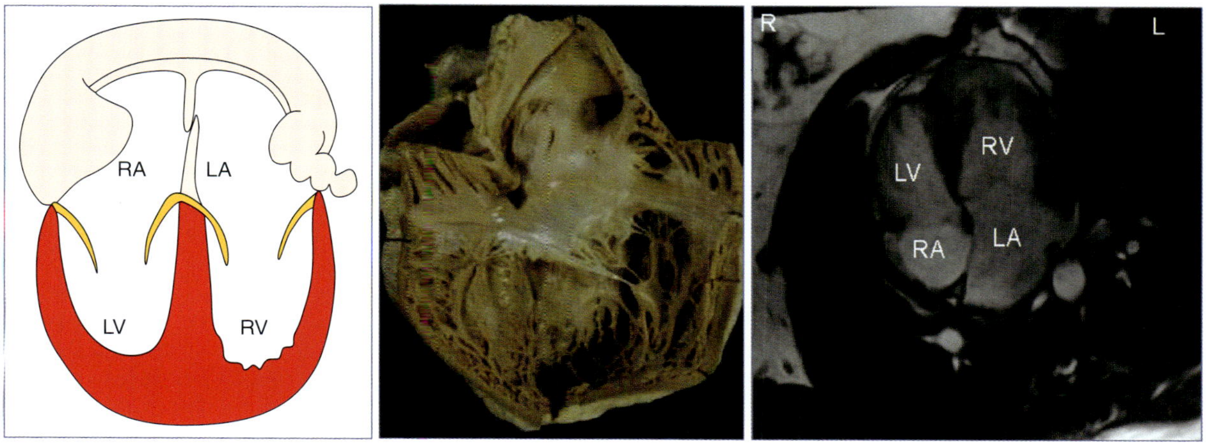

(a), (b) (c)

Figure 2.8 *Biventricular, discordant atrioventricular connection.* (a) Schematic representation. In the presence of two regular ventricular chambers, the atrioventricular connection is discordant when the right atrium connects with the left ventricle and the left atrium connects with the right ventricle, either the atrial situs being solitus or inversus. (b) Anatomical specimen: the morphologically right atrium is connected with a morphologically left ventricle through a mitral valve. (c) Corresponding four-chamber view showing atrioventricular discordance as visualized by magnetic resonance imaging white-blood sequence. L, left; LA, left atrium; LV, left ventricle; R, right; RA, right atrium; RV, right ventricle.

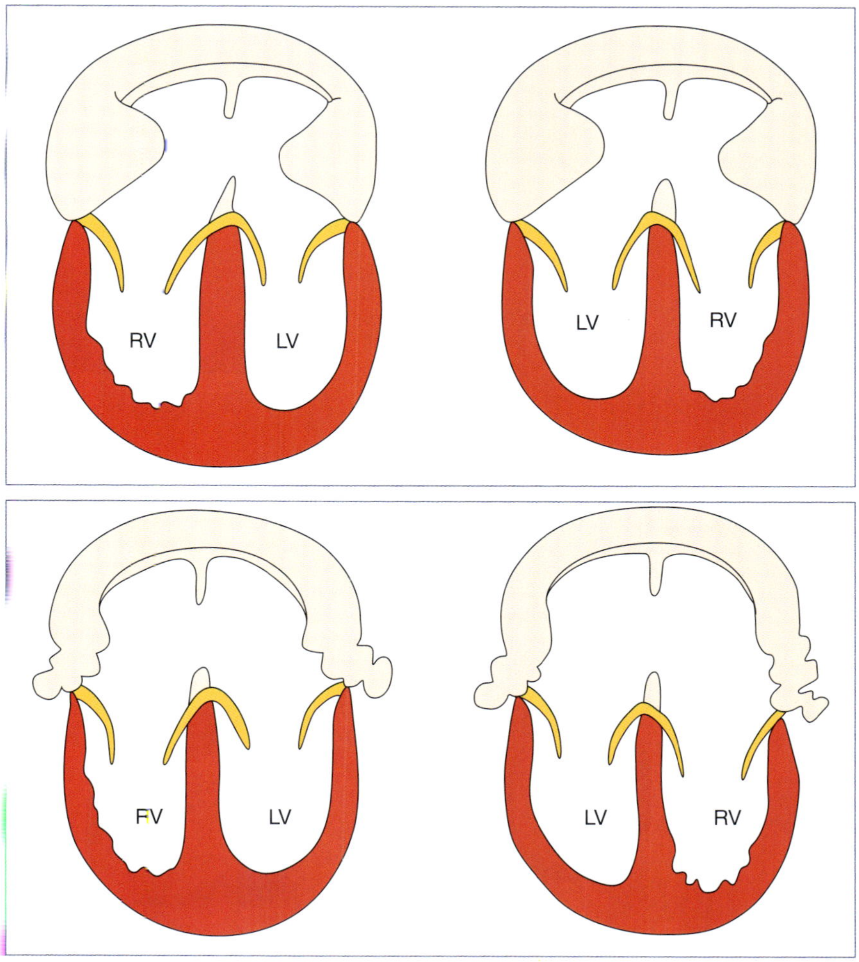

(a) (b)

Figure 2.9 *Biventricular atrioventricular connection in atrial isomerism.* In case of right or left isomerism and in the presence of two ventricles, it is not possible to use the terms concordant or discordant. The connection in these cases is only biventricular, and it is necessary to establish the spatial disposition of the ventricles. (a) Atrioventricular biventricular connection in right atrial isomerism. (b) Atrioventricular biventricular connections in left atrial isomerism. LV, left ventricle; RV, right ventricle.

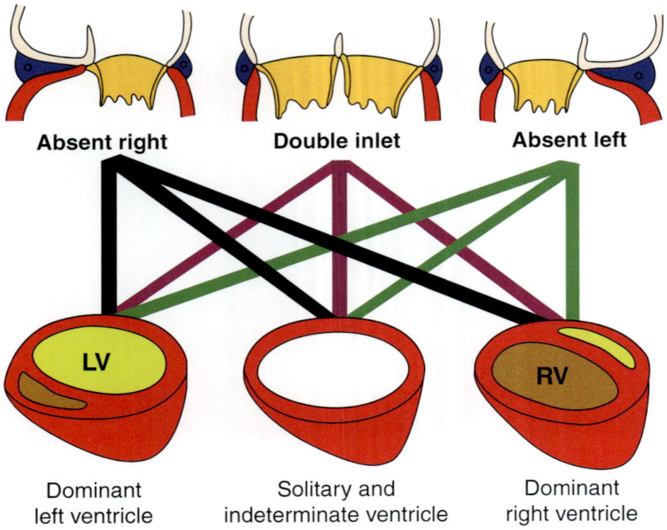

Figure 2.10 *Univentricular atrioventricular connection.* The blood flow from the atria can reach the dominant ventricle in the presence of two patent or a common atrioventricular valves (double inlet connection) or through a single patent valve in case of atretic mitral or tricuspid valve (absent right or left connection). In the former situation, the atrioventricular connection is univentricular when both atria drain mostly (>75%) into a single ventricular chamber. The dominant ventricle can show a left, right, or indeterminate morphology. LV, left ventricle; RV, right ventricle.

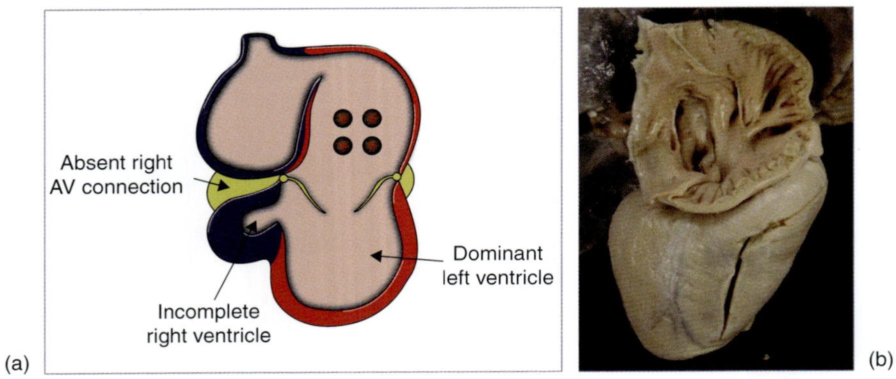

Figure 2.11 *Univentricular atrioventricular connection. Absent right atriventricular connection (tricuspid atresia).* (a) Schematic representation of absent right atrioventricular connection in solitus atrial situs. The blood from both the atria reaches the dominant left ventricle through the left atrioventricular valve. (b) Anatomical specimen: view from the right atrium with absent tricuspid valve orifice. AV, atrioventricular.

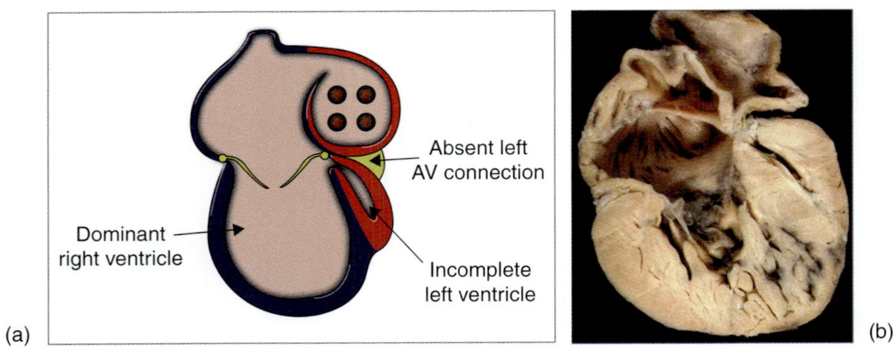

Figure 2.12 *Univentricular atrioventricular connection. Absent left atriventricular connection (mitral atresia).* (a) Schematic representation of absent left atrioventricular connection in solitus atrial situs. The blood from both the atria reaches the dominant right ventricle through the right atrioventricular valve. (b) Anatomical specimen in echocardiographic four chambers section: the mitral valve is absent and the left ventricle is severely hypoplastic. AV, atrioventricular.

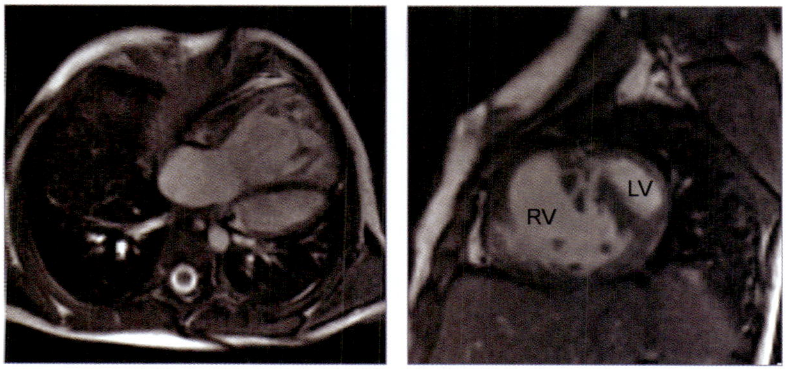

(a) (b)

Figure 2.13 *Univentricular atrioventricular connection and absent left atriventricular connection (mitral atresia).* (a) Four-chamber view of magnetic resonance imaging in mitral atresia and hypoplastic left ventricle. Note the enlarged and hypertrophic right ventricle. (b) Short-axis view showing the anteriorly located large right ventricle and the posterior hypoplastic left ventricle. LV, left ventricle; RV, right ventricle.

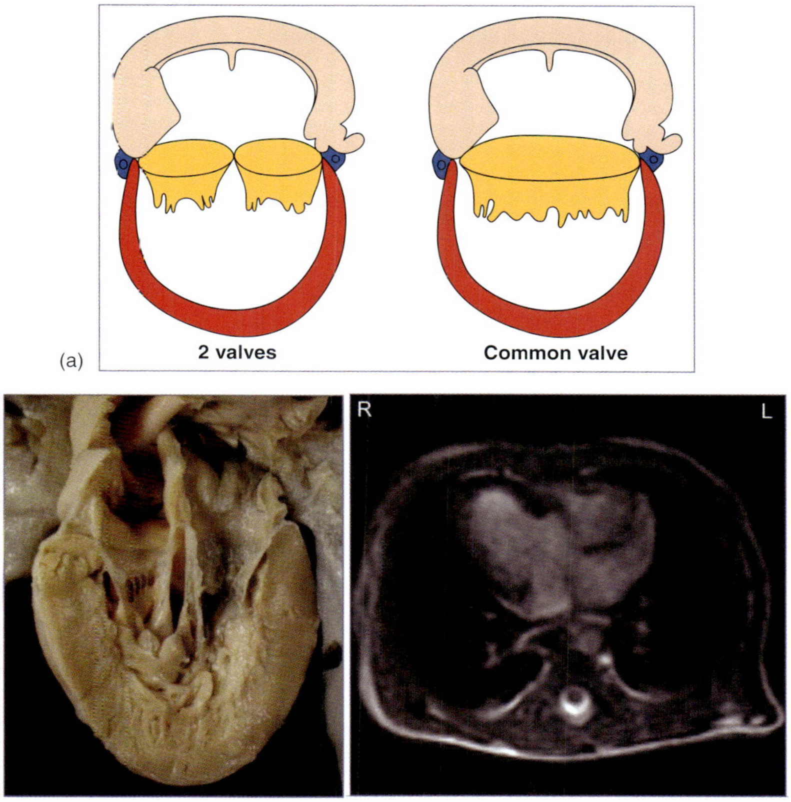

(a) (b) (c)

Figure 2.14 *Univentricular atrioventricular connection. Double inlet atrioventricular connection (double inlet left ventricle).* (a) The blood from both the atria reaches the dominant ventricle through two discrete atrioventricular valves or a common atrioventricular valve. (b) Anatomical specimen in echocardiographic four-chamber section: the blood from the atria drains into a dominant ventricle of left morphology, through two separate atrioventricular valves. (c) Axial image of magnetic resonance imaging in a patient with dextrocardia. Both atria connect to a single morphological left ventricle. L, left; R, right.

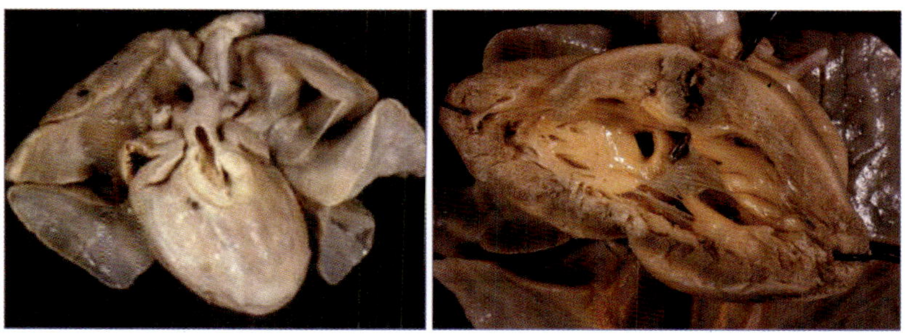

(a) (b)

Figure 2.15 *Univentricular atrioventricular connection. Double inlet atrioventricular connection: double inlet left ventricle with discordant ventriculoarterial connection.* (a) External view of the heart. A rudimentary anterior right ventricular chamber is present from which the aorta takes origin. (b) Both the atrioventricular valves drain into a morphologically left ventricle from which the pulmonary artery takes origin. Note the muscular ventricular septal defect (bulbo ventricular foramen) and the cleft in the mitral valve.

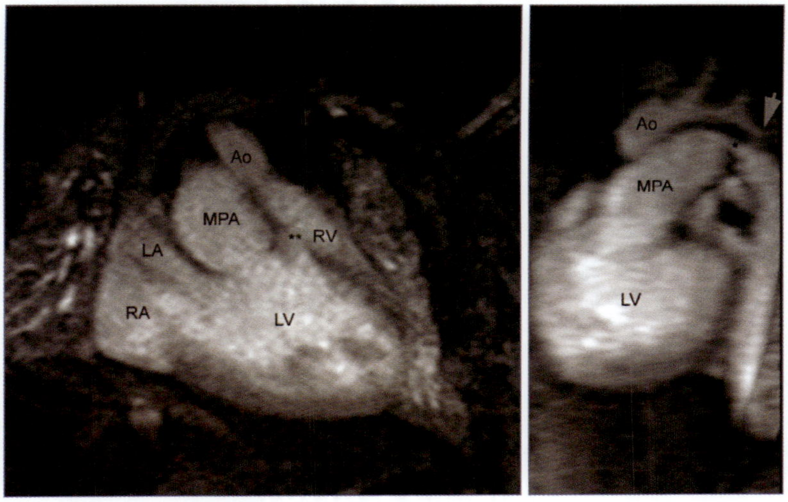

(a) (b)

Figure 2.16 *Univentricular atrioventricular connection as visualized by magnetic resonance imaging. Double inlet atrioventricular connection: double inlet left ventricle with discordant ventriculoarterial connection.* (a) Oblique view: both atria are emptying into a single left ventricle (double inlet); the pulmonary artery takes origin from the left ventricle and the aorta takes origin from an anteriorly located rudimentary right ventricle. Both ventricles are connected through a ventricular septal defect (bulbo ventricular foramen**). (b) The same patient presented with an aortic coarctation. The aortic arch is hypoplastic with a severe isthmal coarctation (arrow). The continuity to the descending aorta is warranted by a patent ductus arteriosus (*). Ao, aorta; LA, left atrium; LV, left ventricle; MPA, main pulmonary artery; RA right atrium; RV, right ventricle.

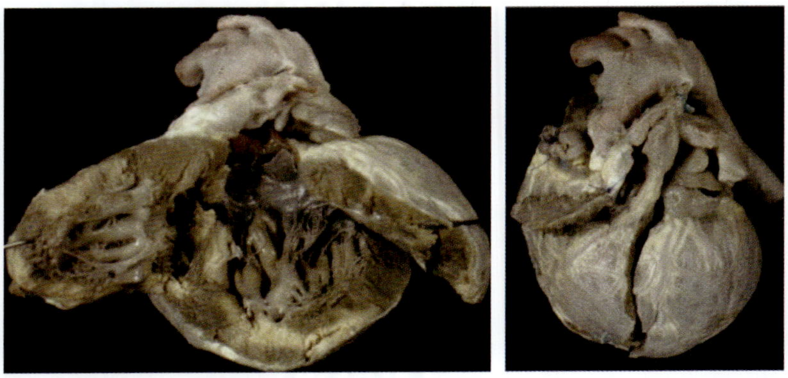

(a) (b)

Figure 2.17 *Univentricular atrioventricular connection. Double inlet atrioventricular connection: double inlet left ventricle with concordant ventriculoarterial connection (Holmes heart).* (a) View from the left ventricle from which the aorta takes origin. Both the atrioventricular valves drain into the left ventricle. (b) External view of the heart with normally related great arteries.

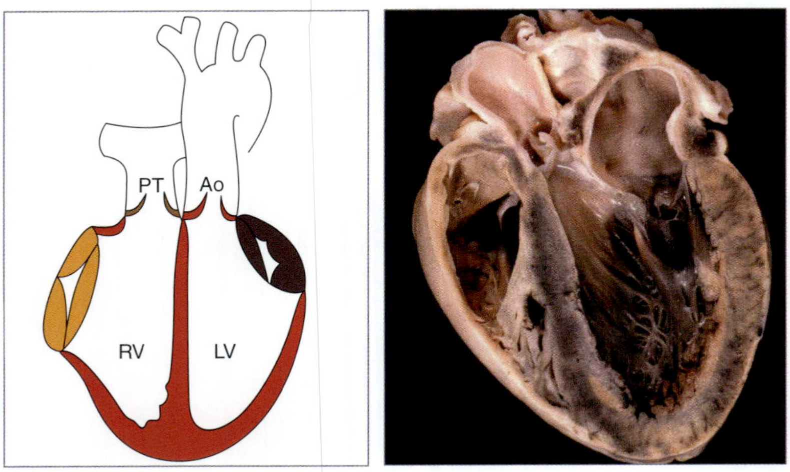

(a) (b)

Figure 2.18 *Concordant ventriculoarterial connections.* (a) Schematic representation: the ventriculoarterial connection is concordant, when the right ventricle gives origin to the pulmonary artery and the left ventricle to the aorta. (b) Corresponding anatomical specimen view in long axis. AO, aorta; LV, left ventricle; PT, pulmonary trunk; RV, right ventricle.

be *discordant* when the aorta takes origin from the right ventricle and the pulmonary artery from the left ventricle (Figure 2.19). A discordant VA connection (Figure 2.20) accounts for complete transposition of the great arteries in the presence of AV concordance (Figure 2.19) and to congenitally corrected transposition of the great arteries in the presence of AV discordance (Figure 2.21).

Double outlet VA connection is observed when both great arteries arise from only one ventricular cavity, either of right, left, or indeterminate morphology (double outlet ventricles) (Figure 2.22).

Single outlet VA connection occurs when only a patent great artery arises from the heart. It may be an aorta, in the setting of *pulmonary atresia* (Figure 2.23), a pulmonary artery, in the setting of *aortic atresia* (Figure 2.24), or a *common arterial trunk*, in the setting of persistent truncus arteriosus (Figure 2.25). The single arterial outlet may have a biventricular origin, astride the ventricular septum, or may arise mainly from the right, left, or indeterminate ventricle.

Establishing the sequence of cardiac segments is the prerequisite for planning a repair aimed to reconstruct the blood circulation with the pulmonary and systemic one in sequence each other, and completely separated this avoiding blood mixture.

The *spatial position* of the heart (ectopia cordis) (Figure 2.26) and cardiac apex (dextrocardia, mesocardia, levocardia) (Figure 2.27) is irrelevant to this purpose, although it may be indicative of some morbid entities. For instance, dextrocardia may suggest situs inversus or otherwise situs solitus with AV discordance (congenitally corrected transposition).

Pathophysiological Classification of Congenital Heart Disease

There are several ways to classify CHD: alphabetical order, cyanotic and noncyanotic, site of the defect (at the level of veins, atria, ventricles, septa, great arteries), etc. A pathophysiological classification seems more reasonable, namely, a classification based on the clinical consequences of structural defects impairing the physiology of blood circulation (Figure 2.28).

1 *CHD with increased pulmonary blood flow*. They correspond to septal defects without pulmonary obstruction and left-to-right shunt;
2 *CHD with decreased pulmonary flow*. They correspond to septal defects with pulmonary obstruction and right-to-left shunt;
3 CHD with obstruction to blood progression without septal defects and no shunt;
4 CHD so severe as to be incompatible with postnatal blood circulation; and
5 CHD silent until adult age.

CHD with Increased Pulmonary Blood Flow

The communication between left and right heart accounts for left-to-right shunt in postnatal circulation because of the progressive gradient of resistance in between the great and small circulations. The shunt may occur at:

1 *Venous pole*: This is the case of *anomalous pulmonary venous drainage*, like the "scimitar syndrome," with the

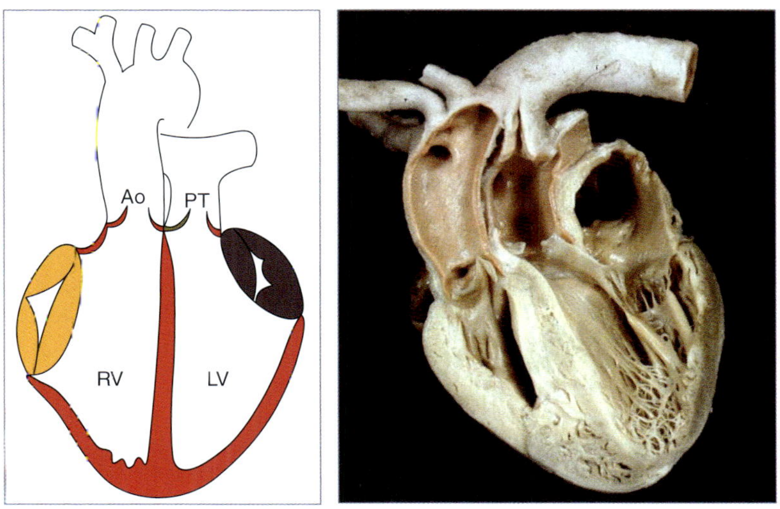

Figure 2.19 *Discordant ventriculoarterial connection: complete transposition of the great arteries.* (a) Schematic representation. The ventriculoarterial connection is discordant when the aorta takes origin from the right ventricle and the pulmonary artery from the left ventricle. In association with atrioventricular concordance, a discordant ventriculoarterial connection accounts of complete transposition for the great arteries. (b) Anatomic specimen in echocardiographic section: note the origin of the pulmonary artery from the left ventricle and the origin of the aorta from the right ventricle. The interventricular septum is intact. AO, aorta; LV, left ventricle; PT, pulmonary truck; RV, right ventricle.

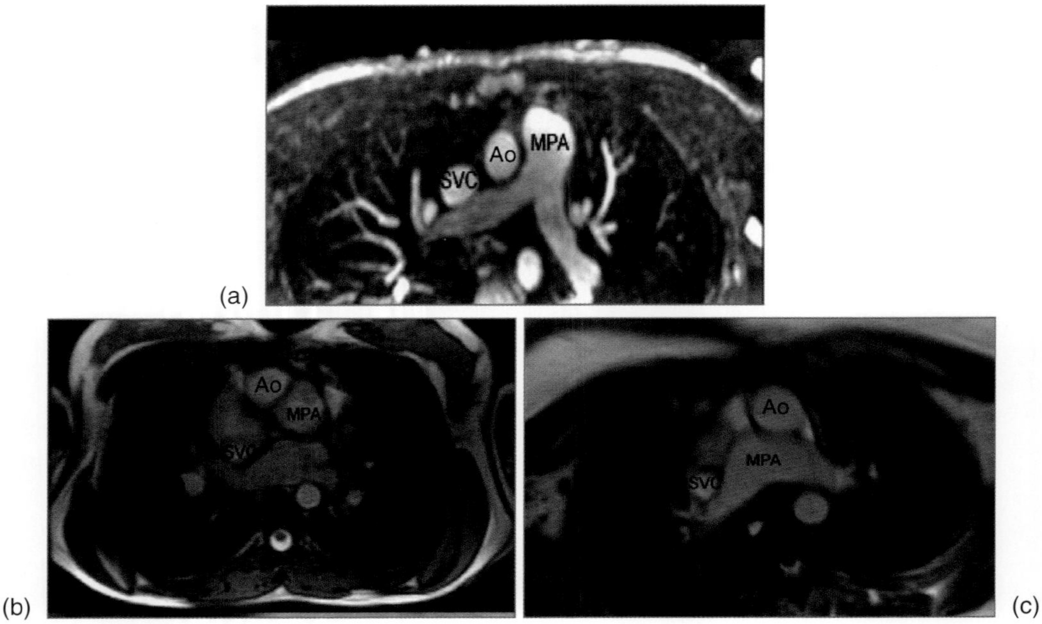

Figure 2.20 *Discordant ventriculoarterial connection as visualized by cardiac magnetic resonance.* Panel demonstrating the position of the great vessels to each other in an upper axial view (three-vessel view). (a) Normal position of the great arteries with right-sided posterior position of ascending aorta relative to the main pulmonary artery. (b) Discordant ventriculoarterial connection with right anterior position of the aorta (complete transposition of the great arteries, so-called d-transposition). (c) Discordant ventriculoarterial connection with left anterior position of the aorta (complete transposition of the great arteries, so-called l-transposition). Ao, aorta; MPA, main pulmonary artery; SVC, superior vena cava.

right pulmonary vein draining into the inferior vena cava (Figure 2.29) or partial anomalous pulmonary venous drainage into the superior vena cava district or coronary sinus.

2 *Atrial septum*: A communication between the two atria in the atrial septum is usually located at the level of the fossa ovalis [*"ostium secundum" or fossa ovalis type atrial septal defect* (ASD)] (Figure 2.30) or just over the AV orifices *("ostium primum" ASD)* in the setting of AV canal malformations (partial AV canal) (Figure 2.31).

More rarely the interatrial communication may be observed at the root of superior vena cava, associated with partial anomalous pulmonary venous drainage of the superior right pulmonary vein (*superior vena cava ASD*) (Figure 2.32) or with unroofed coronary sinus (*inferior vena cava ASD*).

3 *AV junction (AV septum)*: This is the case of *complete AV septal defect (complete AV canal)* where a common AV valve and orifice does exist. An interatrial and interventricular communication are just above and under the common AV valve (Figure 2.33). This is the largest septal defect inside the heart, accounting for a huge left-to-right shunt.

4 *Ventricular septum*: *Ventricular septal defects* (VSDs) (Figure 2.34) create an interventricular communication at the level or well around the membranous septum (*perimembranous VSD*) (Figure 2.35) or in the inlet, apical or outlet muscular part of the ventricular septum musculature (VSDs) (Figure 2.36). A peculiar VSD is that located in the distal infundibulum, just underneath the semilunar valves (*subarterial VSD*), and may or may not be extended to the membranous septum (Figure 2.37).

5 *Aortopulmonary septation: Persistent truncus arteriosus* is that condition in which the roots of great arteries are "in common" (common arterial trunk or truncus arteriosus communis). There is a common semilunar valve ("truncal valve") with a large communication under (ventricular septal defect) and over the common valve. From the common arterial trunk both systemic (including coronary) and the pulmonary arterial circulations take origin, the latter with or without the interposition of a pulmonary trunk (Figure 2.38 and 2.39).

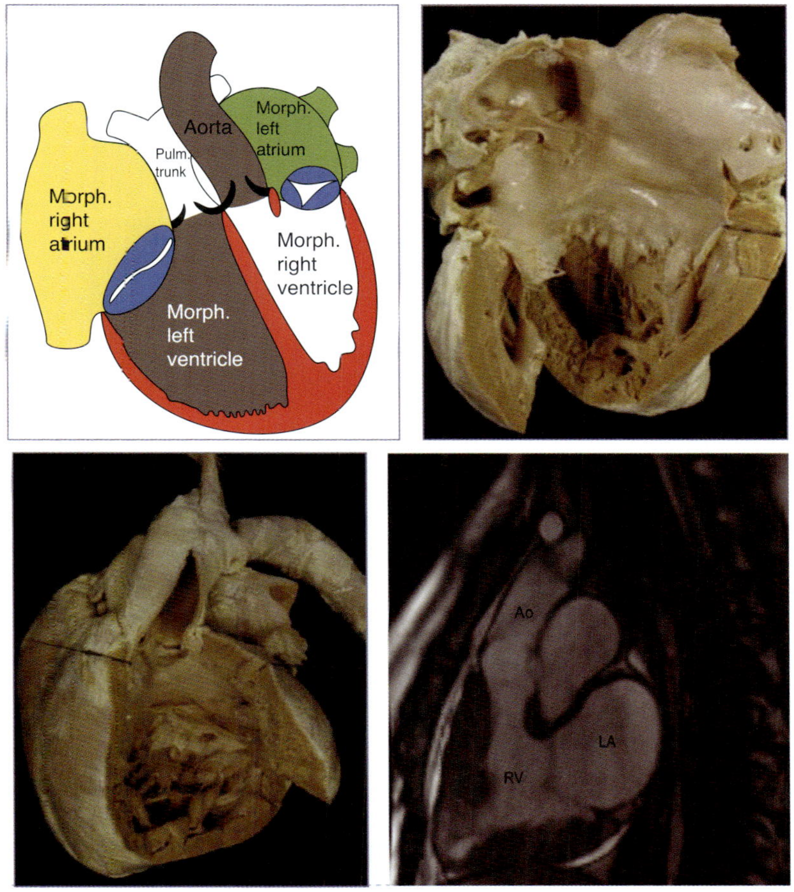

Figure 2.21 *Discordant ventriculoarterial connection: congenitally corrected transposition of the great arteries.* The association of atrioventricular and ventriculoarterial discordance accounts for congenitally corrected transposition of the great arteries. (a) Schematic representation: the right atrium is connected with the left ventricle from which a posterior right-sided pulmonary artery takes origin, and the left atrium is connected with the right ventricle from which an anterior left-sided aorta originates. This sequence of cardiac segments accounts for a normal physiology of blood circulation ("corrected" transposition). (b) Anatomic specimen in which the morphologically left atrium is connected to the left-sided right ventricle through a tricuspid valve. (c) In the same specimen, the aorta takes origin from the left-sided morphologically right ventricle. (d) Atrioventricular and ventriculoarterial discordance as visualized by magnetic resonance imaging: the left atrium is connected with the right ventricle and the ascending aorta arises from the right ventricle. Ao, aorta; LA, left atrium; RV, right ventricle.

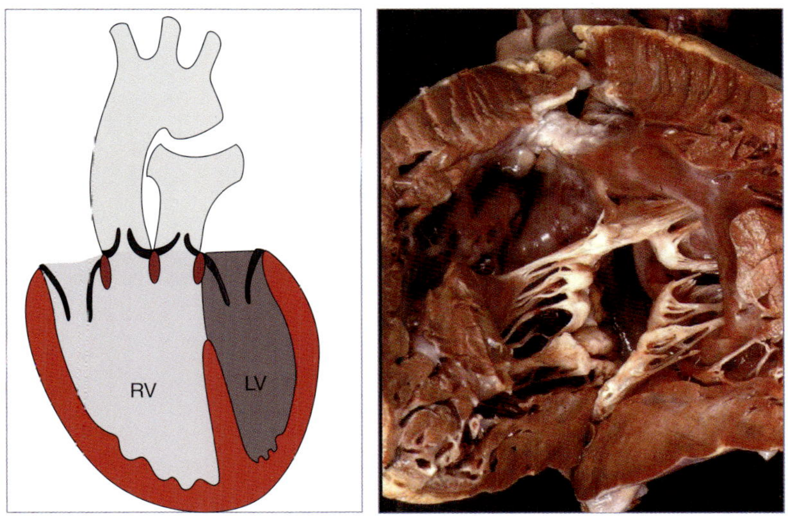

Figure 2.22 *Double outlet ventriculoarterial connection: double outlet right ventricle.* (a) Schematic representation: double outlet right ventriculoarterial connection is observed when both great arteries, or more than one and half, arise from the right ventricle. (b) View from the apex of the right ventricle: both the pulmonary artery and the aorta take origin from the same ventricle of right ventricular morphology (double outlet right ventricle). Note the presence of a common atrioventricular valve connecting both the atria with the right ventricle (double inlet right ventricle). LV, left ventricle; RV, right ventricle.

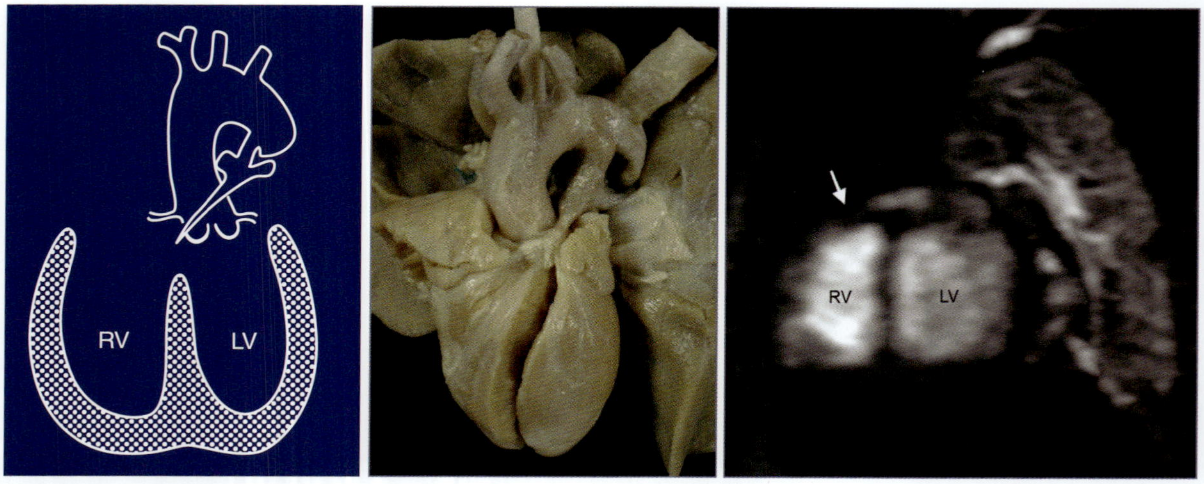

(a), (b) (c)

Figure 2.23 *Single outlet ventriculoarterial connection: pulmonary atresia.* (a) Schematic representation of a case of pulmonary atresia in which the atretic pulmonary artery is potentially connected with the right ventricle and the patent aorta with the left ventricle. (b) External view of heart and lungs: the pulmonary trunk and branches are hypoplastic. The blood can reach the pulmonary artery and the lungs through a ductus arteriosus. (c) Anterolateral view of cardiac magnetic resonance: the proximal segment of the pulmonary trunk (arrow) arising from the right ventricle can be barely visualized. The hypoplastic main pulmonary artery is retrogradely perfused from a patent ductus arteriosus (not on the figure). LV, left ventricle; RV, right ventricle.

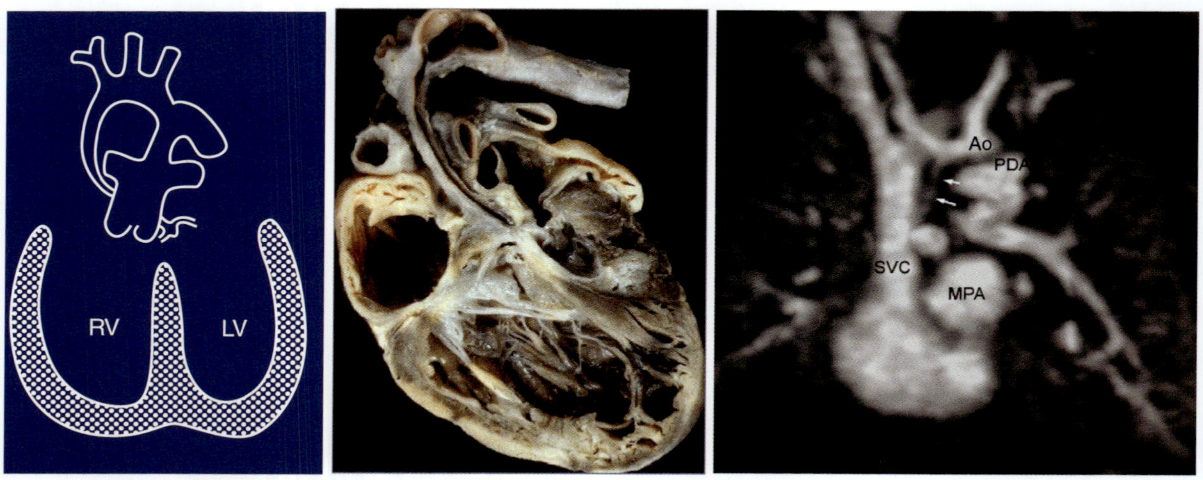

(a), (b) (c)

Figure 2.24 *Single outlet ventriculoarterial connection: aortic atresia.* (a) Schematic representation of a case of aortic atresia in which the atretic aorta potentially takes origin from the left ventricle and the patent pulmonary artery from the right ventricle. (b) Anatomic specimen of hypoplastic left heart: note the hypoplasia of the left cardiac chambers (atrium and ventricle), the absence of the aortic valve and the tinny ascending aorta. (c) Hypoplastic left heart syndrome with aortic atresia as visualized by cardiac magnetic resonance. The severely diminutive ascending aorta is indicated by the arrows. The hypoplastic aortic arch is retrogradly perfused by a patent ductus arteriosus. Ao, aorta; LV, left ventricle; MPA, main pulmonary artery; PDA, patent ductus arteriosus; RV, right ventricle; SVC, superior vena cava.

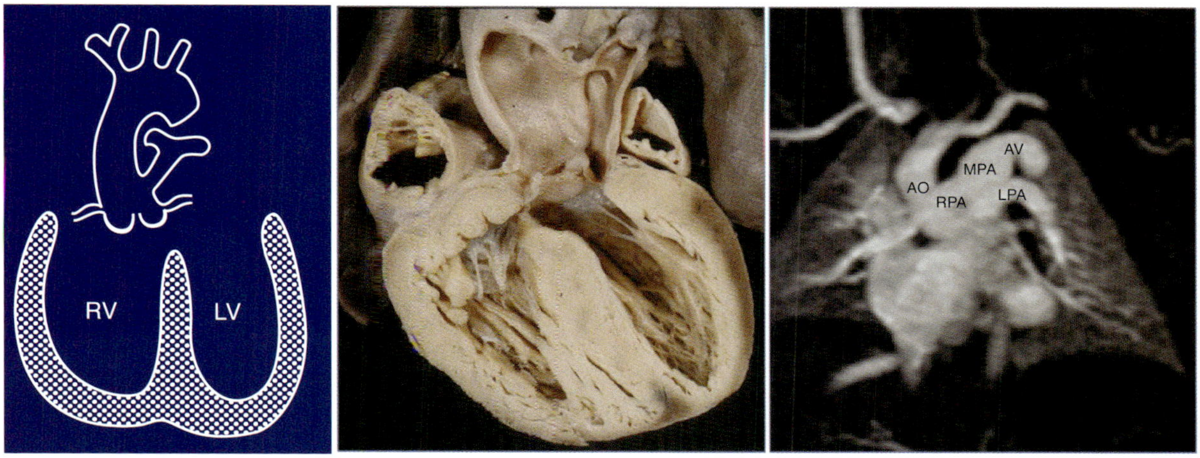

(a), (b) (c)

Figure 2.25 *Single outlet ventriculoarterial connection: common arterial trunk (persistent truncus arteriosus).* (a) A single arterial vessel arises from the heart and gives origin to systemic, pulmonary, and coronary circulations. An interventricular septal defect is usually associated. (b) Anatomical specimen: truncus arteriosus with a bicuspid truncal valve. (c) Cardiac magnetic resonance imaging of a newborn with truncus arteriosus and interrupted aortic arch. A common trunk arises from the heart; after a short common segment it divides into the ascending aorta and the main pulmonary artery and its side branches. The aortic arch is interrupted and a patent ductus arteriosus (**) provides continuity to the descending aorta. Ao, aorta; LPA, left pulmonary artery; LV, left ventricle; MPA, main pulmonary artery; RPA, right pulmonary artery; RV, right ventricle.

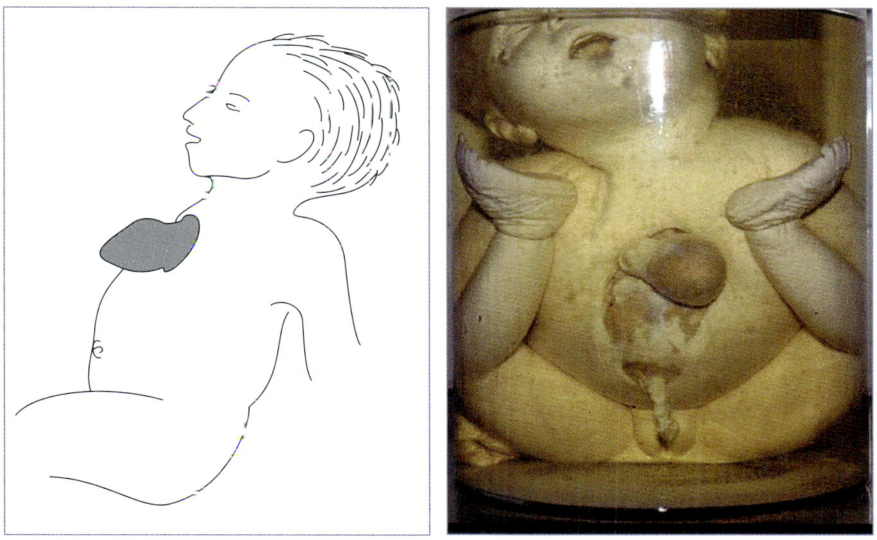

(a) (b)

Figure 2.26 *Ectopia cordis.* (a) Schematic representation. (b)Anatomical specimen of the Museum of the University of Padova. The heart is outside the chest.

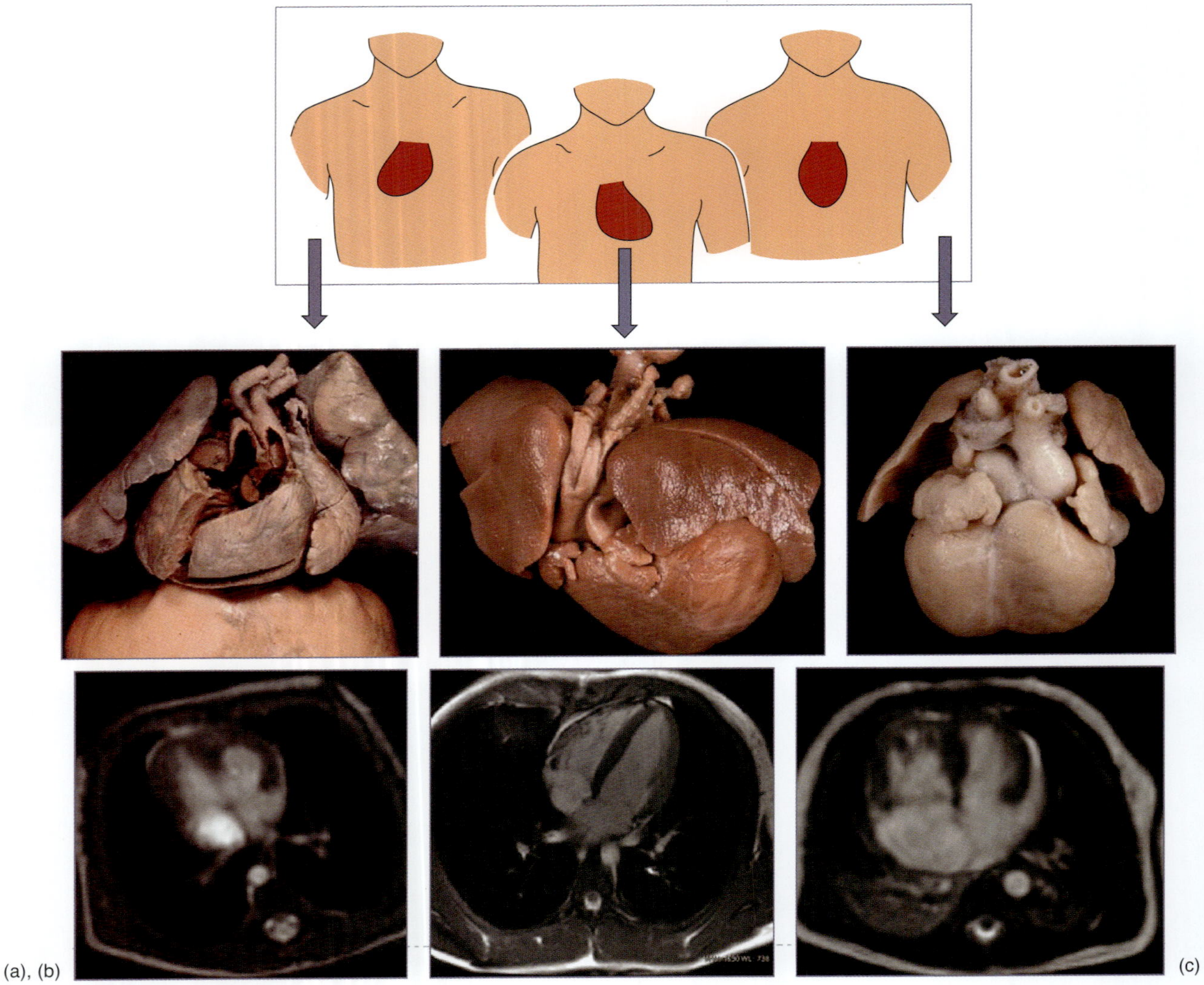

Figure 2.27 *Position of the heart. Dextrocardia* is the situation in which the heart is predominantly in the right part of the chest with a right-sided apex (a). *Levocardia* means that the heart is predominantly in the left part of the chest with a left-sided apex (b). *Mesocardia* is present when the heart is located in the middle of the chest with a midline apex (c). Upper panel: anatomical view of the heart and the lungs. Lower panel: axial views of cardiac magnetic resonance imaging.

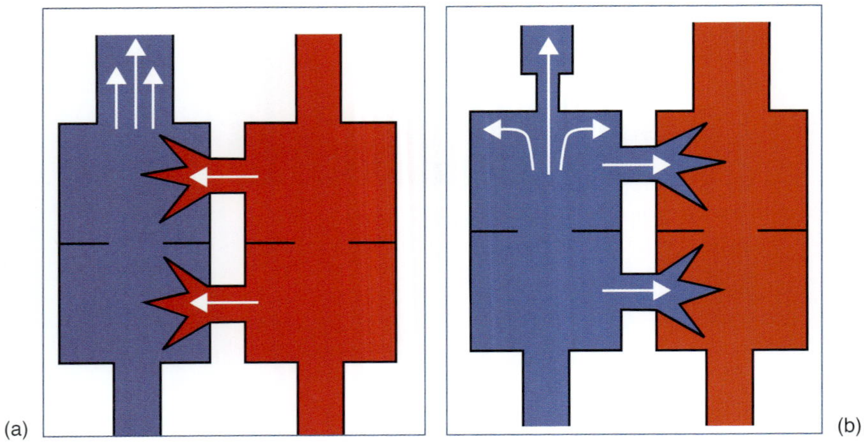

Figure 2.28 *Pathophysiological classification of congenital heart disease: septal defects.* (a) Congenital heart diseases with increased pulmonary blood flow. They correspond to septal defects without pulmonary obstruction and left to right shunts. (b) Congenital heart diseases with decreased pulmonary blood flow. They correspond to septal defects with pulmonary obstruction and right to left shunts.

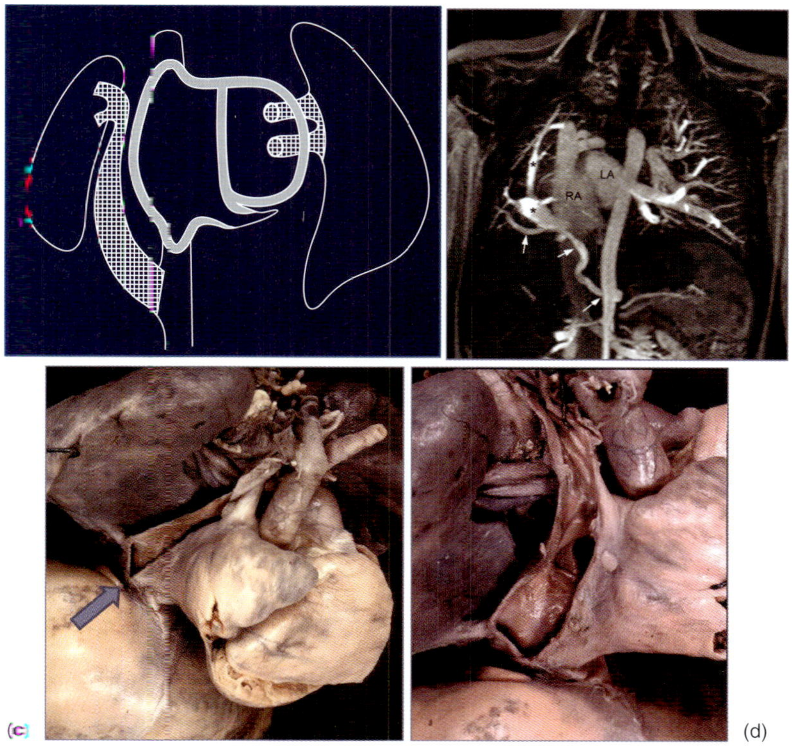

(a) (b) (c) (d)

Figure 2.29 *Congenial heart disease with increased pulmonary blood flow. Anomalous pulmonary venous drainage to inferior vena cava* ("Scimitar syndrome"). (a) Schematic representation: the right inferior pulmonary vein drains into inferior vena cava showing a radiologic aspect of "scimitar." (b) Cardiac magnetic resonance angiography provides an overview of all intra thoracic and intra abdominal vessels. The scimitar vein (*) drains all right pulmonary veins into the inferior vena cava merging into the right atrium. In scimitar syndrome, an anomalous systemic artery from the abdominal aorta to the right lung (arrow) can be found; this is often associated with a lung sequestration. (c) Anatomic specimen with a drainage of the right inferior pulmonary vein into the inferior vena cava (arrow). (d) The same specimen with opened sinus part of the right atrium. LA, left atrium; RA, right atrium.

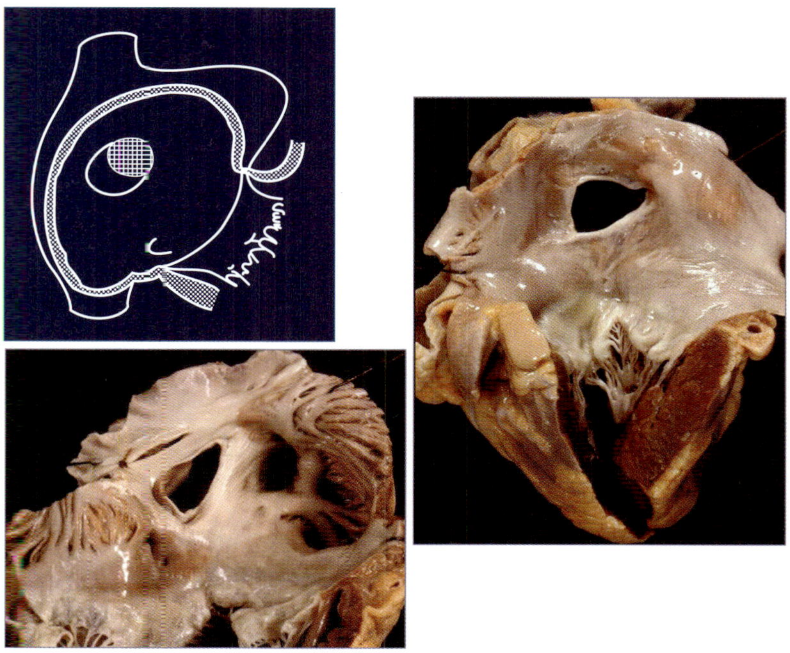

(a) (b) (c)

Figure 2.30 *Congenial heart disease with increased pulmonary blood flow. Atrial septal defect ostium secundum or fossa ovalis type.* (a) A communication between the two atria may does exist in the atrial septum at the level of the fossa ovalis: "ostium secundum" or fossa ovalis atrial septal defect. (b) View from the right atrium: a large interatrial communication is present at the level of the fossa ovalis. (c) Same defect viewed from the left atrium.

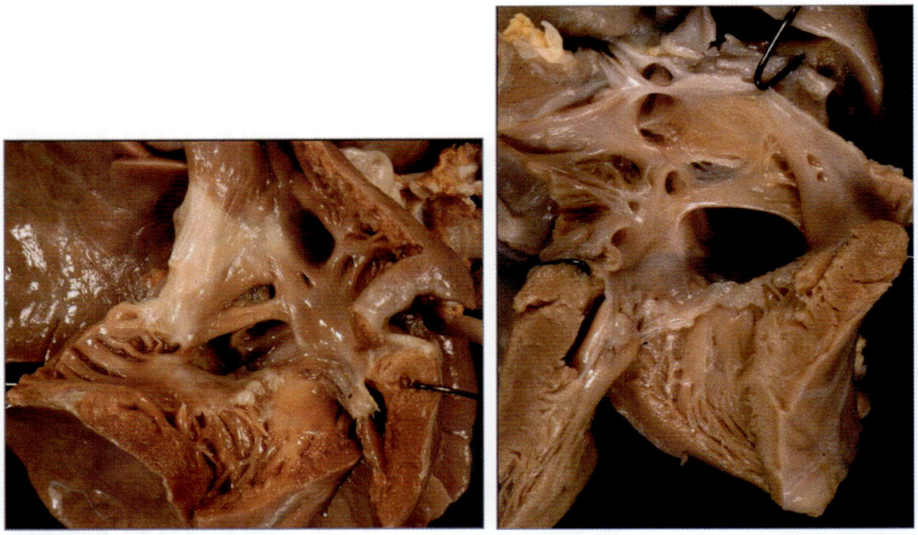

(a) (b)

Figure 2.31 *Congenial heart disease with increased pulmonary blood flow. Atrial septal defect ostium primum type (partial atrioventricular defect).* A communication between the two atria does exist in the atrial septum just over the atrioventricular orifices, "ostium primum" atrial septal defect, in the setting of partial atrioventricular defect. (a) View from the right cardiac chambers: the defect is far from the fossa ovalis and located at the atrioventricular junction. (b) View from the left cardiac chambers: note the large atrial septal defect and the association with a cleft in the anterior leaflet of the mitral valve.

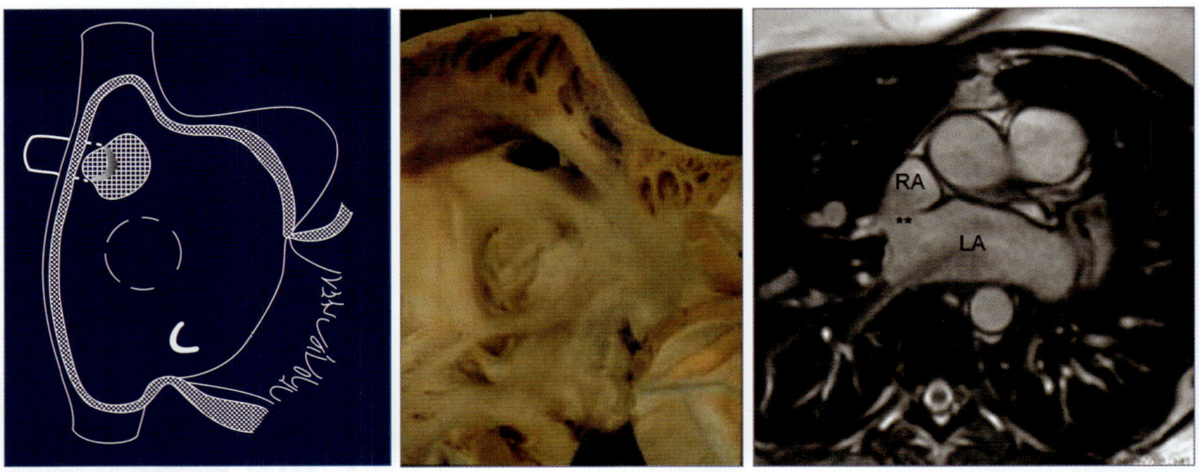

(a), (b) (c)

Figure 2.32 *Congenial heart disease with increased pulmonary blood flow. Atrial septal defect superior vena cava type.* Rarely the interatrial communication may be observed at the root of superior vena cava, associated with partial anomalous pulmonary venous drainage of the superior right pulmonary vein. (a) Schematic representation seen from the right atrium. (b) Corresponding anatomical specimen. (c) Corresponding axial cardiac magnetic resonance image. The interatrial communication is indicated by **. LA, left atrium; RA, right atrium.

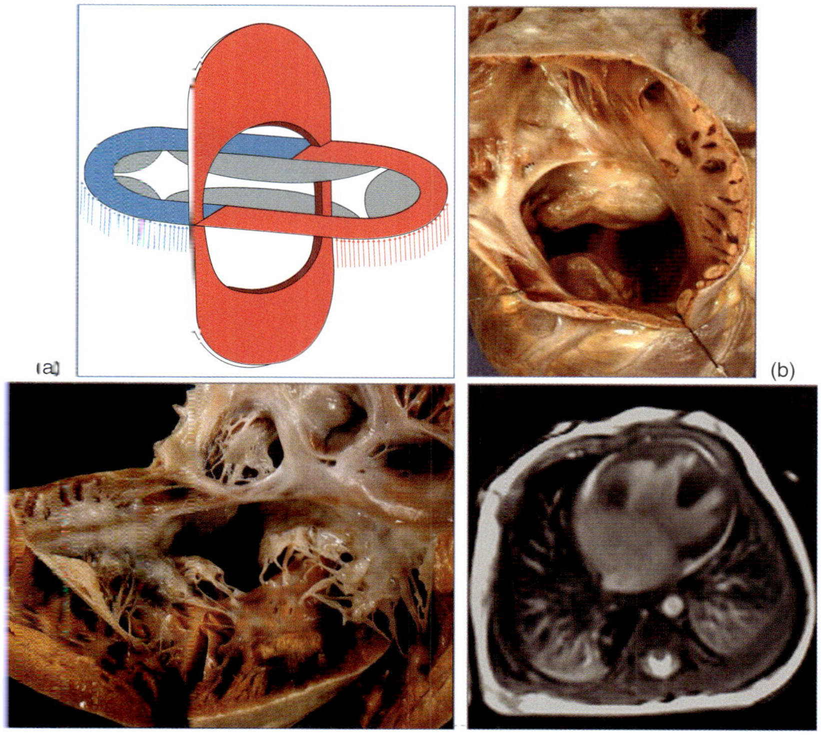

Figure 2.33 *Congenial heart disease with increased pulmonary blood flow. Complete atrioventricular septal defect.* (a) Schematic representation: a common atrioventricular valve is present and associated with a large atrioventricular septal defect with interatrial and interventricular communication. (b) View from the above: the common atrioventricular valve shows anterior (superior) and posterior (inferior) leaflets straddling the interventricular septum. (c) View from the right cardiac chambers: a complete form of atrioventricular septal defect is present with a common atrioventricular valve and a large communication at atrial and ventricular level. The anterior leaflet of the common valve shows cordae tendineae attached to the interventricular septum. (d) Four-chamber view as visualized by cardiac magnetic resonance imaging: this heart presents with a large interatrial communication, a common atrioventricular valve, and a large interventricular septal defect.

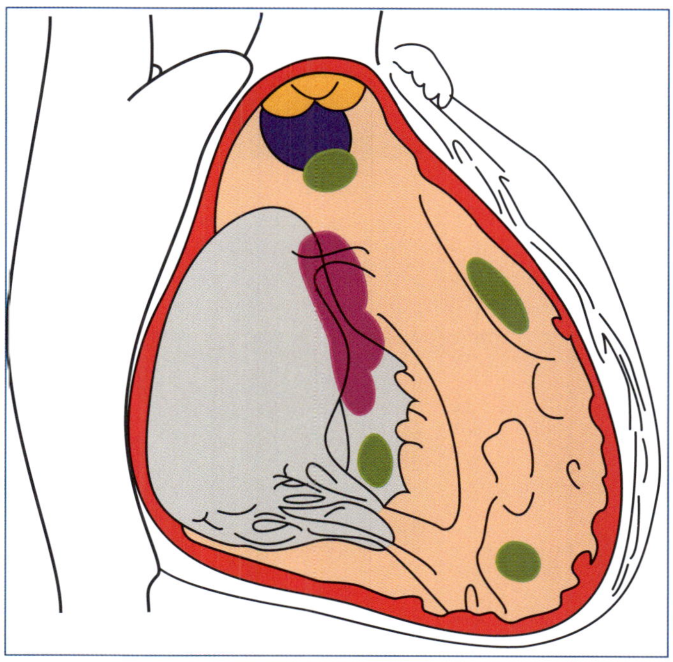

Figure 2.34 *Congenial heart disease with increased pulmonary blood flow. Ventricular septal defect.* Ventricular septal defects can be *perimembranous* (violet color) when located at the level of or well around the membranous septum or *muscular* (green color) if located in the muscular part of the setpum, whether in its inlet, apical, or outlet components. A peculiar type of ventricular septal defect is the *subarterial* (blue color) located in the distal infundibulum, just underneath the semilunar valves.

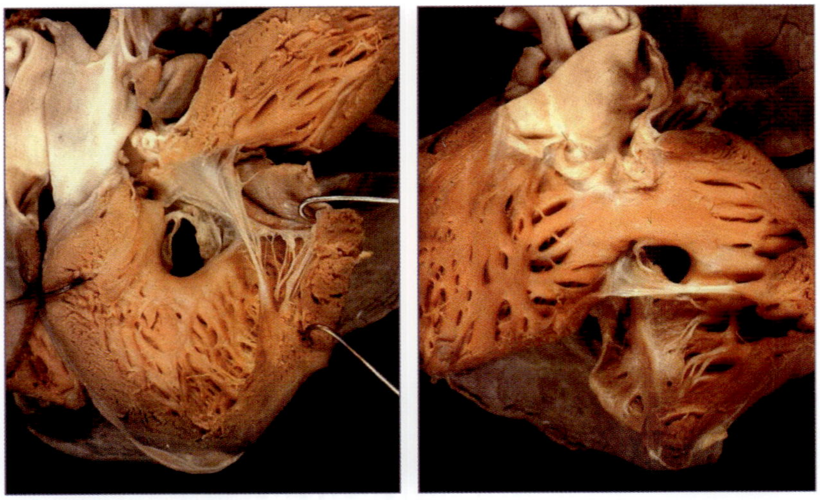

(a) (b)

Figure 2.35 *Congenial heart disease with increased pulmonary blood flow. Perimembranous ventricular septal defect.* (a) View from the left ventricle: the rim of the perimembranous defect is partially muscular and partially fibrous at the level of mitroaortic-tricuspid continuity. In this site (the posteroinferior rim of the defect), the atrioventricular conduction system is located and at risk of lesion during surgical closure. (b) View from the right ventricle: the defect is located under the septal leaflet of the tricuspid valve. The muscle of Lancisi, located on the superior rim of the defect, indicates a posterior extension of the defect.

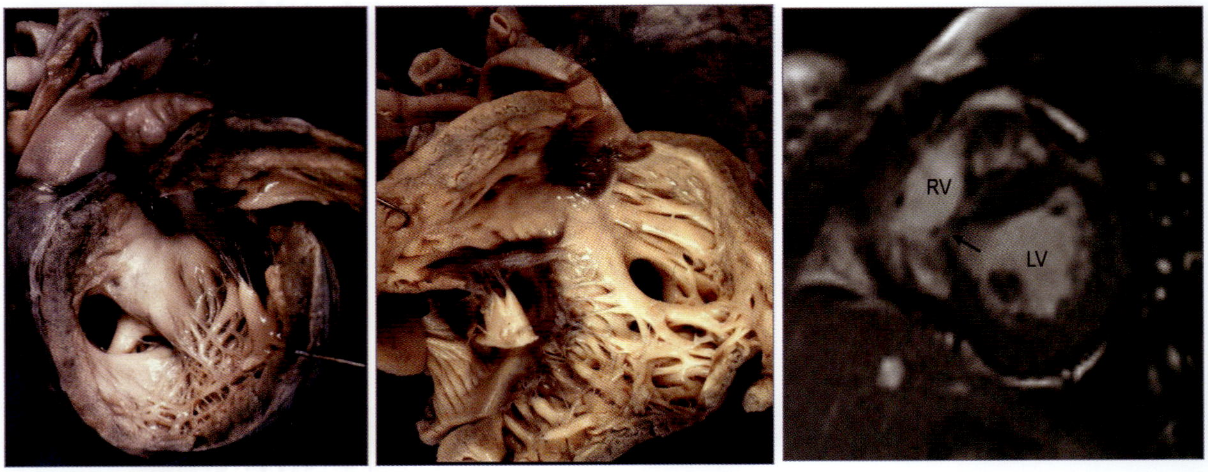

(a), (b) (c)

Figure 2.36 *Congenital heart disease with increased pulmonary blood flow. Muscular ventricular septal defect*: (a) View from the left ventricle. A large ventricular septal defect is present in the muscular trabecular portion of the interventricular septum. The defect is crossed by the trabecula septo-marginalis of the right ventricle. (b) View from the right ventricle of the same defect. (c) Short-axis view of cardiac magnetic resonance imaging showing a muscular septal defect (arrow) between the left ventricle and the right ventricle. LV, left ventricle; RV, right ventricle.

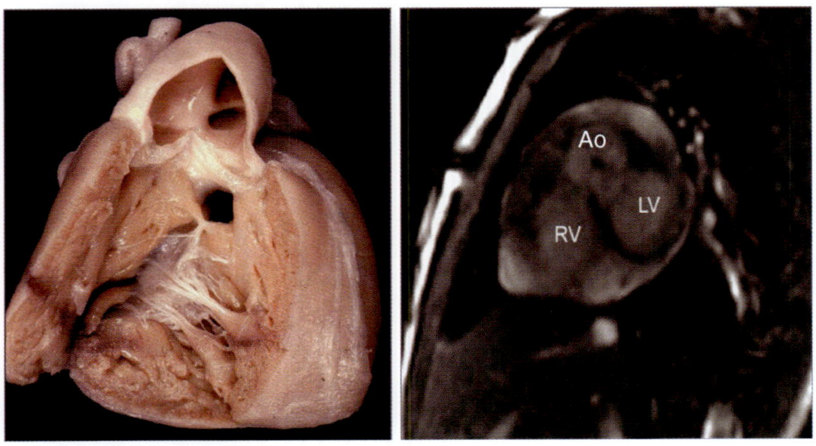

(a) (b)

Figure 2.37 *Congenial heart disease with increased pulmonary blood flow. Subarterial ventricular septal defect.* (a) View from the right ventricle with a ventricular communication, located in the infundibular septum, just underneath the semilunar valves. (b) Subarterial ventricular septal defect as visualized by magnetic resonance imaging: the aorta overrides the defect and arises from both the left and the right ventricles. Ao, aorta; LV, left ventricle; RV, right ventricle.

(a), (b)

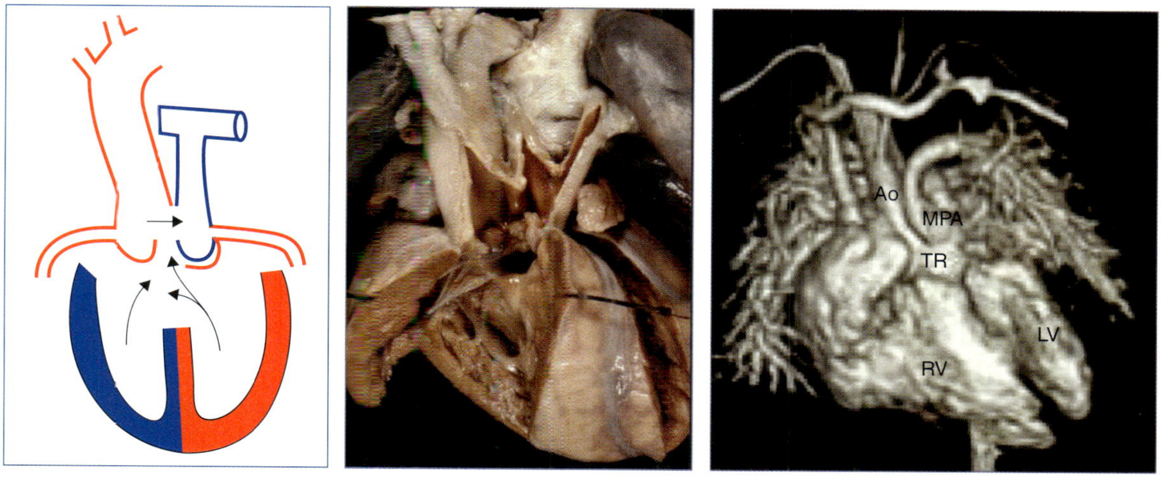

(c)

Figure 2.38 *Congenial heart disease with increased pulmonary blood flow. Persistent truncus arteriosus.* (a) Schematic representation: a single vessel arises from the heart and gives origin to systemic, pulmonary, and coronary circulations. A common truncal valve is present with a large communication over and under (ventricular septal defect). (b) View from the right ventricle: a single great vessel takes origin from the heart, overriding the interventricular communication. A dysplastic truncal valve is present. The pulmonary branches originate from a short common pulmonary trunk. (c) Anatomy of a persistent truncus arteriosus shown in a three-dimensional reconstruction of magnetic resonance angiography. Ao, aorta; LV, left ventricle; MPA, main pulmonary artery; RV, right ventricle; TR, truncus arteriosus

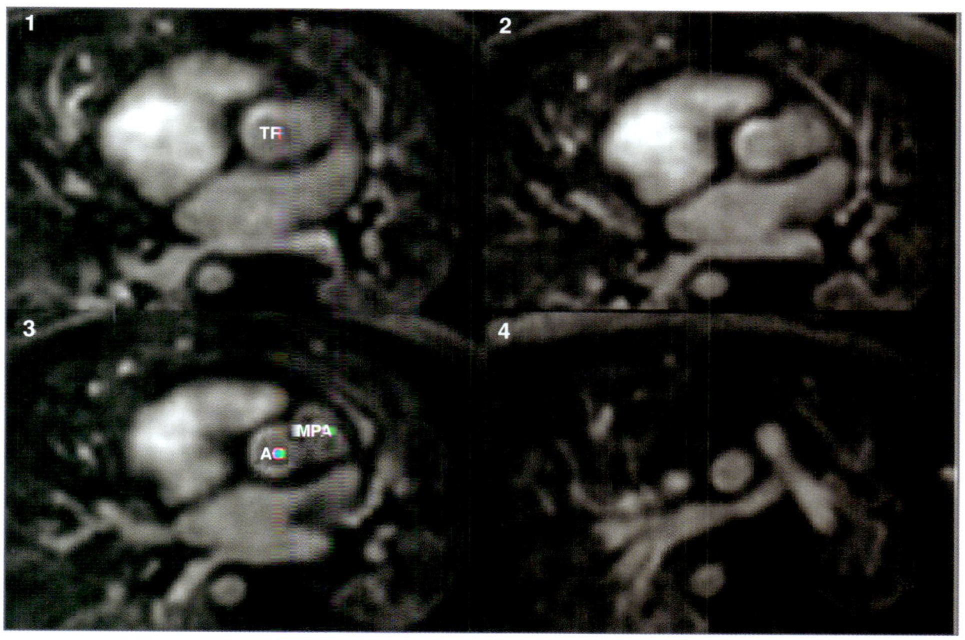

Figure 2.39 *Congenial heart disease with increased pulmonary blood flow. Persistent truncus arteriosus.* Stack of cardiac magnetic resonance axial views acquired from caudal (1) to cranial (4). At the base of the heart, a single vessel arises from both ventricles (1); after a common segment, both great arteries separate into the aorta and the main pulmonary artery. Ao, aorta; MPA, main pulmonary artery; TR, truncus arteriosus.

A peculiar isolated communication in between the aorta and the pulmonary trunk may be observed just above the two discrete semilunar valve apparatuses (so-called *aortopulmonary window*) (Figure 2.40). It may be associated with a subarterial VSD and obstructive lesions of the aortic arch.

The former communications at the level of arterial pole are inside the pericardiac cavity. *Patent ductus arteriosus* is instead a communication in the distal part of the arterial pole, between the pulmonary trunk bifurcation and the aortic arch isthmus, after the origin of the left subclavian artery (Figure 2.41). It corresponds to a patent fetal ductus arteriosus.

The increased pulmonary blood blow, due to left-to-right shunt, accounts with time for damage of the small pulmonary arteries and arterioles with obstructive intimal proliferations, arteritis and necrosis of the arterial wall, aneurismal dilatation, and glomoid-like plexiform lesions. These obstructive lesions (pulmonary vascular diseases) increase the pulmonary resistance to such an extent, as to decrease or even reverse the previous left-to-right into right-to-left shunt, converting the congenital cardiac defect into a cyanotic disease (Eisenmenger syndrome). Such a reaction of the pulmonary vasculature may occur very early, even in infancy (Figure 2.42). This is the reason why these defects should be closed within 1–2 years of age in order to prevent the onset of irreversible lesions that may jeopardize the surgical repair.

CHD with Decreased Pulmonary Blood Flow

When septal defects coexist with a significant obstruction to the pulmonary blood flow, a physiopathologic condition develops with right-to-left shunt, accounting for

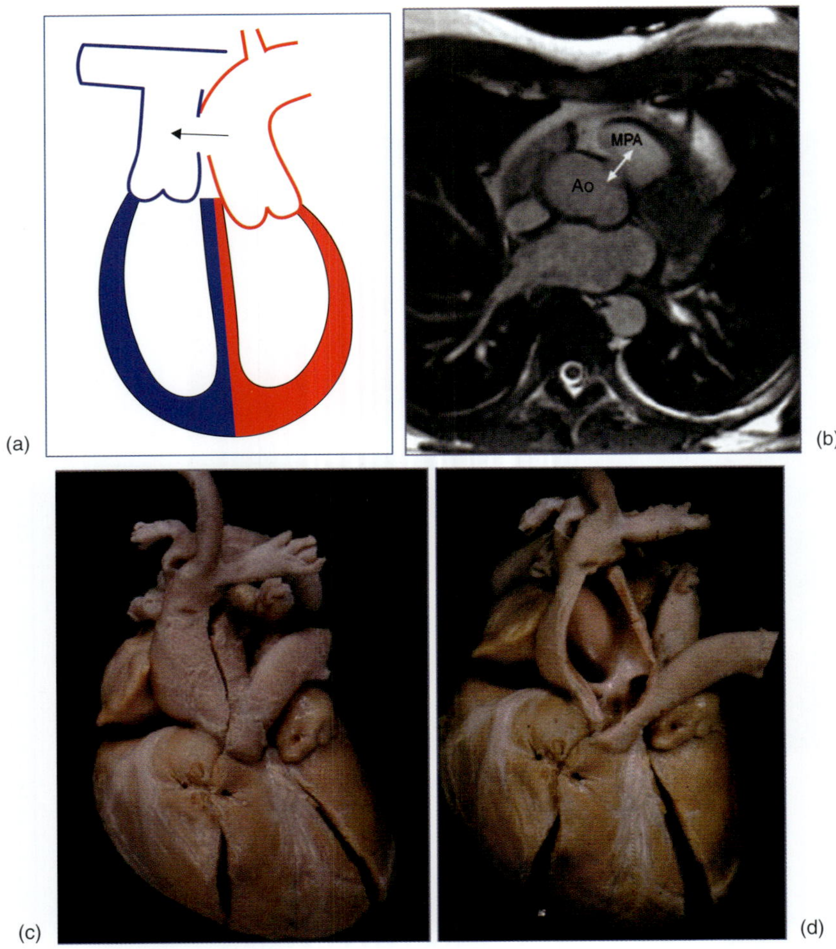

Figure 2.40 *Congenial heart disease with increased pulmonary blood flow. Aortopulmonary window*. (a) Schematic representation: a communication exists between the ascending aorta and the pulmonary trunk in the presence of two discrete semilunar valves. (b) Aortopulmonary window as visualized by magnetic resonance imaging: the communication between both great arteries is indicated by an arrow. (c) External view of the heart: the aspect of the great arteries is similar to truncus arteriosus. (d) At the opening of the great arteries, a communication is present between ascending aorta and common pulmonary trunk, with two separate semilunar valve apparatus. Ao, aorta; MPA, main pulmonary artery.

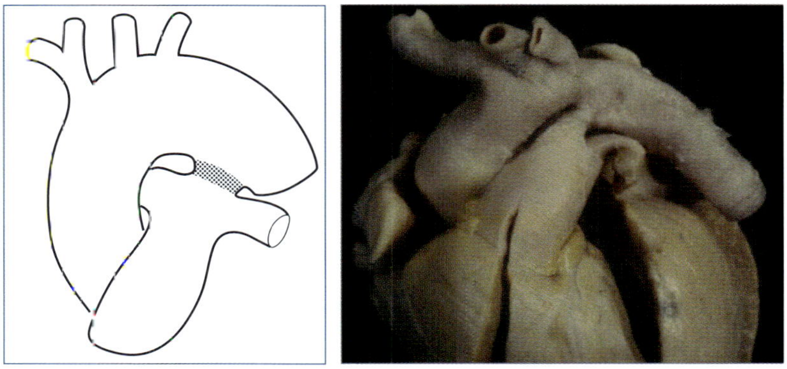

Figure 2.41 *Congenial heart disease with increased pulmonary blood flow. Patent ductus arteriosus.* (a) The ductus arteriosus represents a communication between the pulmonary trunk and the aortic arch in the isthmal level after the origin of the left subclavian artery. It corresponds to a patent fetal ductus arteriosus, which does not close after the birth. (b) Corresponding anatomical specimen.

congenital cyanosis, since part of the deoxygenated blood of the right heart is forwarded into the systemic circulation:

1 *Pulmonary valve stenosis with ASD*: The obstruction is located at the level of the pulmonary valve because of cusps dysplasia or dome-like acommissural cusp. The high pressure in the right atrium maintains open and progressively enlarges the foramen ovale as to create an interatrial communication with right-to-left shunt (Figure 2.43). This complex is also known with the eponym of trilogy of Fallot.
2 *Pulmonary stenosis with VSD (tetralogy of Fallot)*: An embryonic maldevelopment of the trunco-conal region determines a malseptation of the ventricular outflows at the expenses of the pulmonary infundibulum. The infundibulum septum appears deviated anteriorly, dislocated outside the septomarginal band, as to create an infundibular stenosis and a VSD (Figure 2.44). Also, the pulmonary valve may appear stenotic and it is frequently bicuspid due to malseptation at the truncal level. The right-to-left shunt through the VSD, with blood flow partially forwarded from the right ventricle into the aorta, accounts with dextroposition of the aorta, its overriding across the ventricular septum and biventricular origin as well as systemic right ventricle with right ventricular hypertrophy.

The complex (tetralogy of Fallot) may present frequently with associated lesions: right aortic arch, AV canal, anomalous coronary arteries. These defects, however, do not alter the basic physiopathology.

The obstruction to the pulmonary blood flow may be so severe as to create pulmonary atresia (*tetralogy of Fallot with pulmonary atresia*). The source of the pulmonary blood flow, in this setting, may be a patent ductus arteriosus (see CHD incompatible with postnatal blood circulation due to the postnatal closure of the ductus) or otherwise systemic collateral arteries arising from the descending thoracic aortic due to persistence of embryonic systemic-pulmonary arterial circulation (Figure 2.45). These arteries are functional (not nutritive like bronchial arteries) and may create paradoxically an increased pulmonary blood flow due to left-to-right shunt, at risk of obstructive pulmonary vascular disease.

3 *Tricuspid atresia*: The right AV orifice is atretic and the systemic venous blood return, through the venae cavae and coronary sinus, is shunted through the patent foramen ovale into the left atrium and left ventricle, from where it is ejected by large part into the aorta and in a small portion into the pulmonary infundibulum and artery through a restrictive VSD (in the setting of VA concordance) (Figure 2.46). The right-to-left shunt at the atrial level together with the pulmonary stenosis creates a condition for cyanotic CHD. The decreased

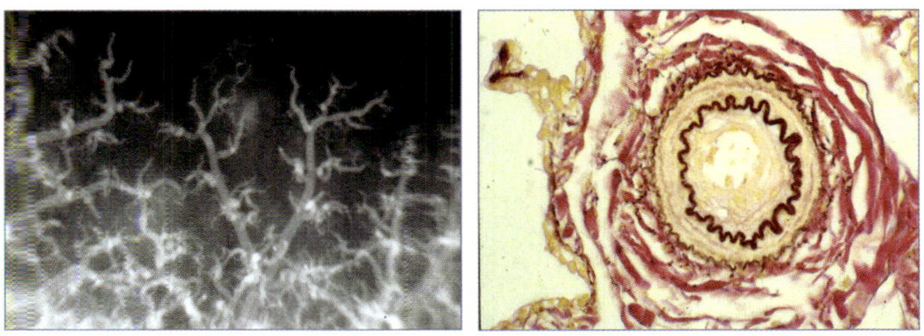

Figure 2.42 *Congenial heart disease with increased pulmonary blood flow. Pulmonary vascular disease.* Pulmonary vascular disease in an 8-month-old infant affected by complete atrioventricular septal defect and Down's syndrome. (a) Postmortem injection of contrast material in the lungs: note the typical "winter tree" aspect of the distal arterial circulation. (b) Histology of the lungs of the same patient showing subocclusion of the lumen of a small artery due to concentric fibrosis (pulmonary vascular disease grade III of Heath-Edwards classification).

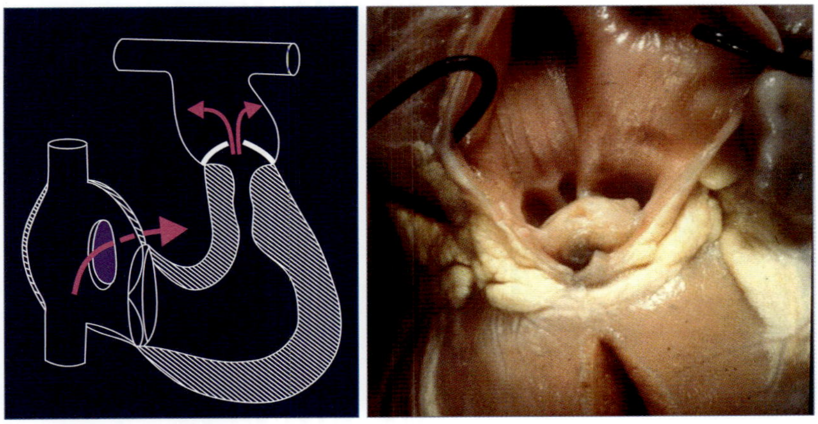

(a) (b)

Figure 2.43 *Congenital heart disease with decreased pulmonary blood flow. Pulmonary valvular stenosis with atrial septal defect.* (a) The obstruction is located at the level of the pulmonary valve. The high pressure in the right atrium maintains open and progressively enlarges the foramen ovale as to create an interatrial communication with right-to-left shunt. (b) Anatomical specimen: at the opening of the pulmonary trunk, the pulmonary valve shows a dome-like aspect with tiny central orifice.

blood flow to the lung is the prerequisite of a low pulmonary vascular resistance, ideal for atriopulmonary or cavopulmonary anastomosis for a Fontan operation.

In tricuspid atresia, when the VA connection is discordant, there is, on the opposite, an increased blood flow to the lungs and the pulmonary artery should be banded, in view of a Fontan operation, in order to protect the pulmonary arterial vasculature and to prevent the onset of high pulmonary vascular resistance.

4 *Ebstein's anomaly of the tricuspid valve*: When the tricuspid valve is maldeveloped with downward displacement of the septal and posterior dysplastic leaflets, the valve is usually stenotic, hindering the transfer of the systemic venous blood toward the pulmonary artery. In

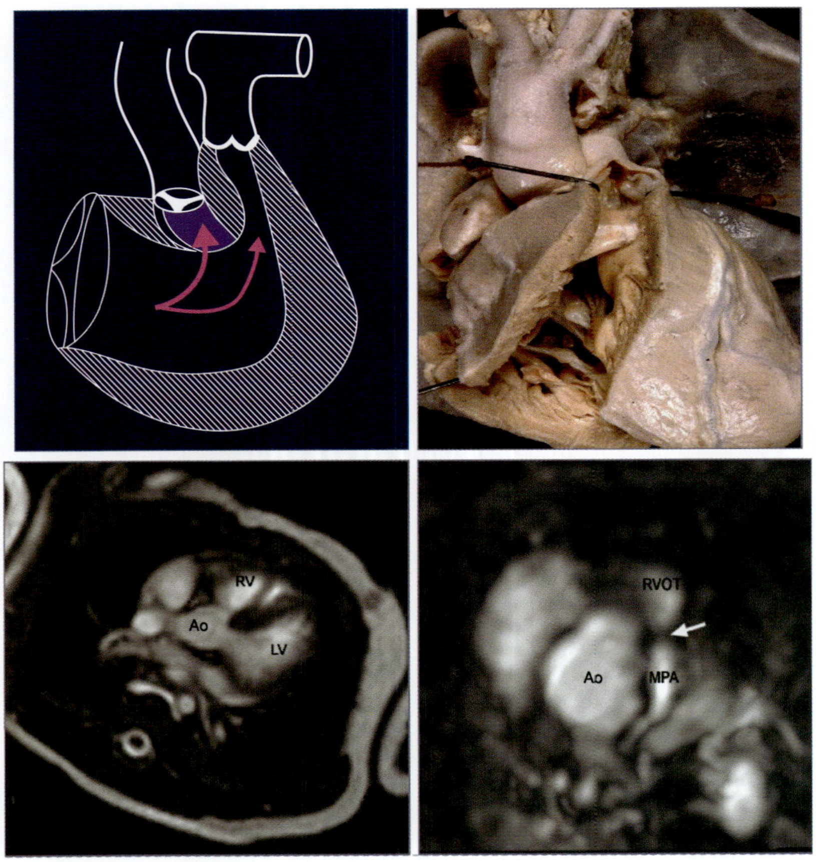

(a) (b) (c) (d)

Figure 2.44 *Congenital heart disease with decreased pulmonary blood flow. Pulmonary stenosis with ventricular septal defect (tetralogy of Fallot).* (a) The tetralogy of Fallot is characterized by association of four different cardiac anomalies: infundibular pulmonary stenosis, ventricular septal defect, dextroposition and overriding of the aorta, and right ventricular hypertrophy. (b) Anatomical specimen showing the stenotic right ventricular outflow tract due to anterior deviation of the infundibular septum. (c) Magnetic resonance imaging: axial view showing the ventricular septal defect with overriding aorta and the right ventricular hypertrophy. (d) Severe case of tetralogy of Fallot as visualized by magnetic resonance imaging with an extreme stenosis of the pulmonary valve (functional pulmonary atresia) (arrow) and severe hypoplasia of the main pulmonary artery and its side branches. Ao, aorta; LV, left ventricle; MPA, main pulmonary artery; RV, right ventricle; RVOT, right ventricular outflow tract.

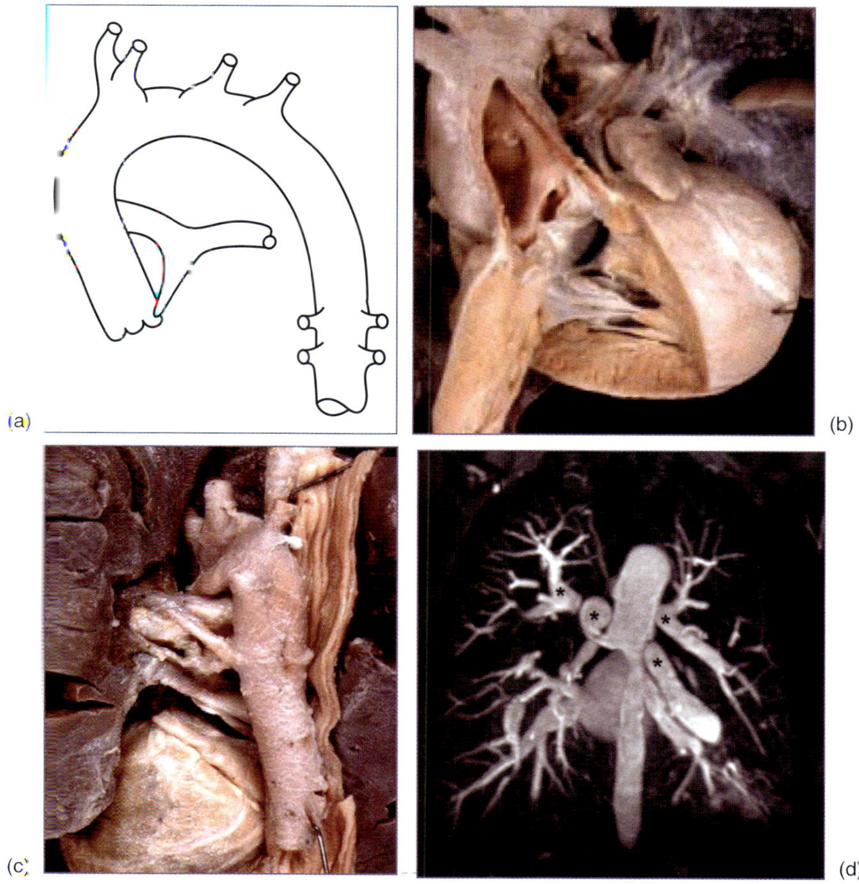

Figure 2.45 *Congenital heart disease with decreased pulmonary blood flow: Pulmonary atresia with ventricular septal defect.* (a) The obstruction of the pulmonary blood flow may be so severe as to create a pulmonary atresia (tetralogy of Fallot with pulmonary atresia). The source of the pulmonary blood flow, in this setting, may be systemic collateral arteries arising from the descending aorta. These arteries, when large, may create paradoxically an increased pulmonary blood flow due to left-to-right shunt at risk of obstructive pulmonary vascular disease. (b) View from the right ventricle: a blind end infundibulum is present. The aorta overrides the ventricular septum with a biventricular origin. (c) Posterior view of the specimen: multiple collateral arteries arise from the descending aorta and reach the left pulmonary hilum. (d) Magnetic resonance angiography can visualize all aortopulmonary collaterals. In this patient with pulmonary atresia and multifocal lung arterial connections, several large aortopulmonary collaterals (*) arise from the descending aorta and perfuse both lungs.

this condition, the foramen ovale may remain patent, thus creating an interatrial communication and a right-to-left shunt and cyanosis (Figure 2.47).

5 *Single (double inlet) ventricles with pulmonary stenosis*: The AV connection with both atria draining in the same ventricular cavity (double inlet ventricle) is such that by definition a mixture of oxygenated or deoxygenated blood occurs in the single ventricular cavity. Moreover, if a pulmonary stenosis is associated in the setting of transposition of the great arteries, as it usually occurs, an additional right-to-left shunt does exist as to explain the moderate-to-severe cyanosis frequently observed in these patients (Figure 2.48). The combination of defects (double inlet ventricle with pulmonary stenosis) is an ideal prerequisite for Fontan operation, considering that the pulmonary arterial circulation is protected by the pulmonary stenosis. On the contrary, there are cases of double inlet ventricle, without pulmonary stenosis and increased pulmonary blood flow, which necessitates early pulmonary banding in view of Fontan operation, to prevent increased pulmonary vascular resistance.

CHD with Obstruction to Blood Progression and No Septal Defect (No Shunt)

The obstacle to the systemic or pulmonary blood progression is not associated with upstream septal defects, thus there are no shunts, either right to left or left to right. A major problem is the ventricular overload with concentric myocardial hypertrophy of the left or right ventricle.

1 *Aortic stenosis*: It may be *subvalvular*, usually with a discrete cardiac diaphragm (Figure 2.49) or tunnel-like shape, valvular (unicuspid, bicuspid, tricuspid valve with dysplastic cusps) (Figure 2.50), or *supravalvular* (discrete diaphragm, hourglass, hypoplastic ascending aorta) (Figure 2.51). The latter condition is usually a genetic disorder due to deletion in elastin gene, with or without William's syndrome.

2 *Coarctation of the aorta*: This is the so-called *"adult" type of coarctation*, which may become symptomatic in the adolescence or even in the adult age. There is a plication of the aortic wall, soon after the insertion

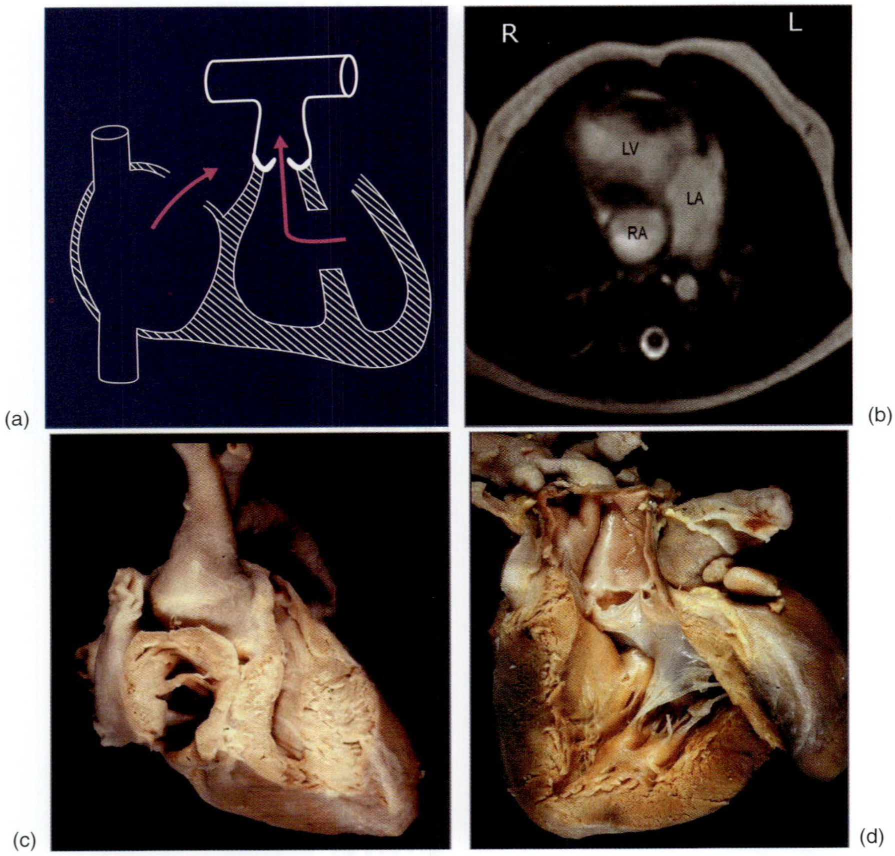

Figure 2.46 *Congenital heart disease with decreased pulmonary blood flow. Tricuspid atresia.* (a) When the tricuspid valve is atretic, the systemic venous blood return is shunted through the patent foramen ovale into the left atrium and left ventricle and can reach the pulmonary circulation crossing a usually restrictive ventricular septal defect. (b) Axial view cardiac magnetic resonance in a case of dextrocardia with tricuspid atresia and hypoplastic right ventricle. The right atrium has no connection to any ventricle. (c) Anatomical view of the right cardiac chambers: there is no connection between the right atrium and the right ventricle. Note the diminutive size of the right ventricle. (d) A mitral valve exists in the left ventricle, normal in size, from which the aorta takes origin. L, left; LA, left atrium; LV, left ventricle; R, right; RA, right atrium.

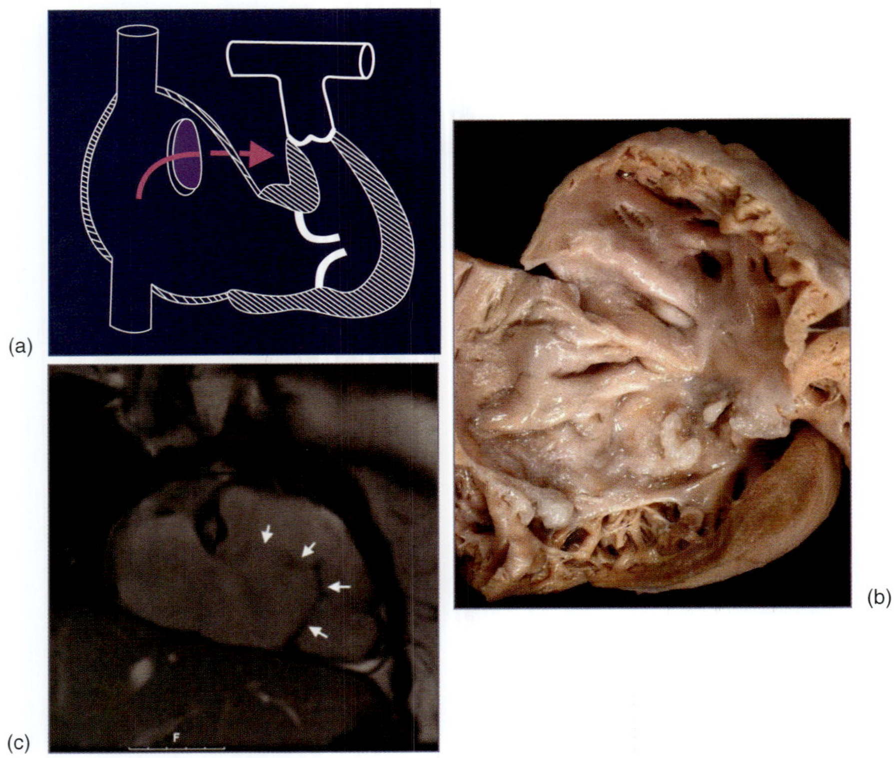

Figure 2.47 *Congenial heart disease with decreased pulmonary blood flow. Ebstein's anomaly of the tricuspid valve.* (a) In Ebstein's anomaly, the septal and posterior tricuspid leaflets are displaced downward into the right ventricular cavity. The displaced tricuspid valve divides the ventricle in two pars: one integrated with the right atrium and one functioning as right ventricle. High right atrial pressure maintains open the foramen ovale and accounts for right-to-left shunt. (b) Anatomical view of the right cardiac chambers: the dysplastic tricuspid leaflets are displaced inside the right ventricle. Note the dilatation of the right atrium and the small residual part of the right ventricle. (c) Cardiac magnetic resonance imaging: the arrows indicate the downward displacement of the tricuspid valve into the right ventricular cavity.

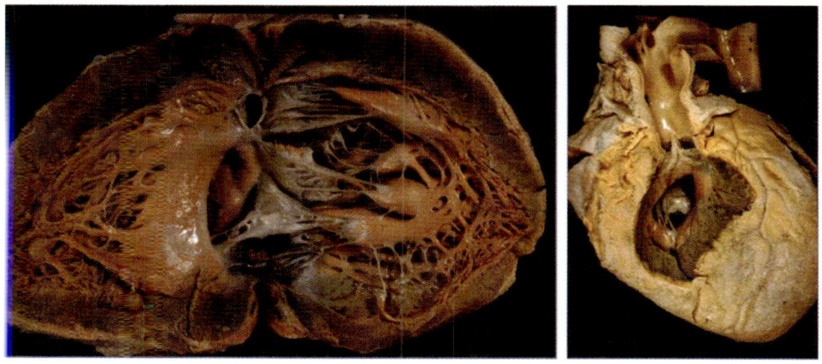

Figure 2.48 *Congenial heart disease with decreased pulmonary blood flow. Double inlet left ventricle with pulmonary stenosis.* (a) View from the apex of the left ventricle in which both the atrioventricular valves drain. The pulmonary artery takes origin from the left ventricle (discordant ventriculoarterial connection). Note the presence of a discrete subpulmonary stenosis. A cleft is present in the anterior mitral valve leaflet. (b) Anterior view of the heart. A rudimentary right ventricular chamber gives origin to the aorta. Note the large interventricular septal defect (bulbo ventricular foramen).

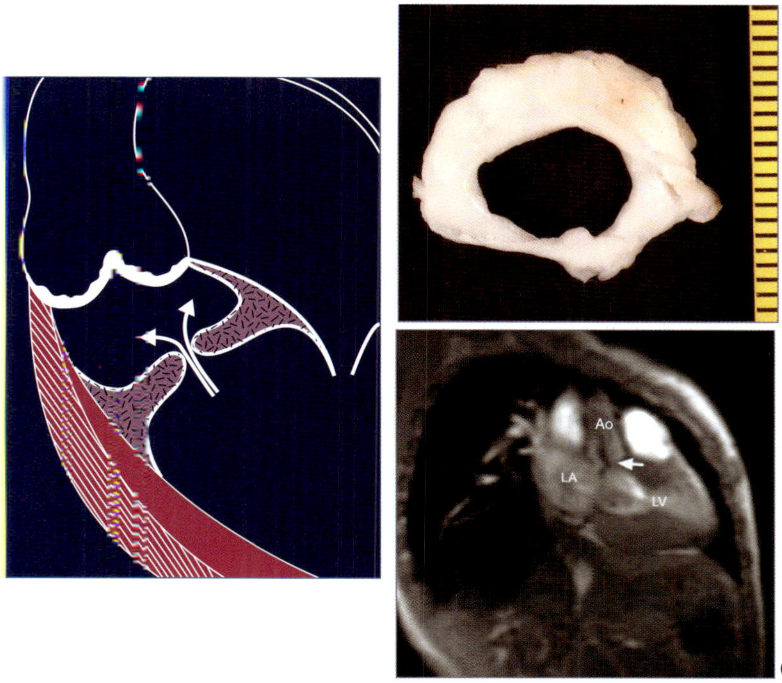

Figure 2.49 *Congenital heart disease with obstruction to blood progression and no septal defect (no shunt). Subvalvular discrete subaortic stenosis.* (a) A fibrous membrane (discrete diaphragm) is present under the aortic valve obstructing the left ventricular outflow tract. Frequently, the aortic valve is damaged as the consequence of jet lesions. (b) Fibrous diaphragm surgically relieved in a case of discrete subaortic stenosis. (c) Anterolateral view of cardiac magnetic resonance showing a discrete subaortic narrowing (arrow) caused by a fibrous membrane located immediately below the aortic valve. Note the significant hypertrophy of the left ventricle. Ao, aorta; LA, left atrium; LV, left ventricle.

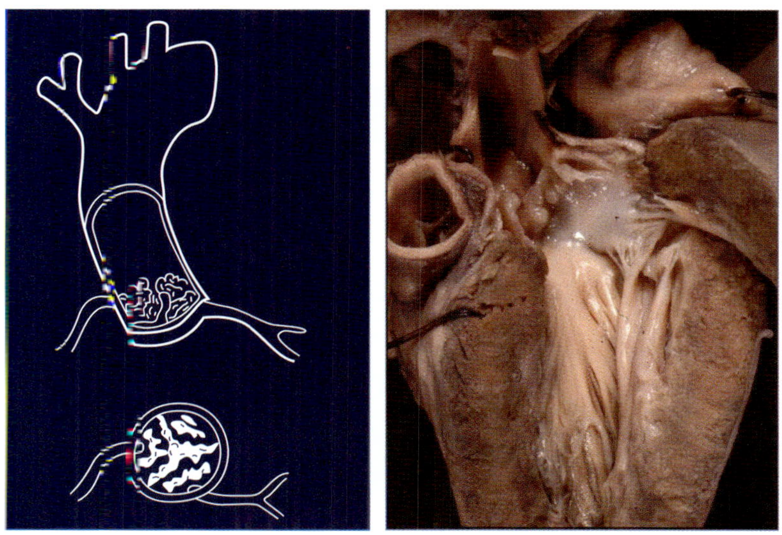

Figure 2.50 *Congenital heart disease with obstruction to blood progression and no septal defect (no shunt). Aortic valvular stenosis.* (a) Diagram illustrating aortic stenosis due to dysplastic cusps. (b) Outflow tract of the left ventricle with severely stenotic and dysplastic aortic valve.

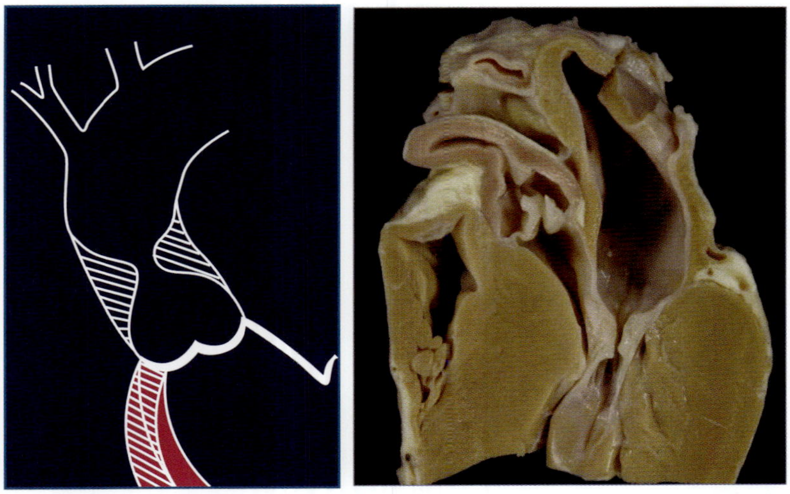

Figure 2.51 *Congenital heart disease with obstruction to blood progression and no septal defect (no shunt). Supravalvular aortic stenosis.* (a) The supravalvular stenosis can present as an hourglass shape of the ascending aorta. (b) Anatomic specimen presenting severe supravalvular stenosis with hourglass ascending aorta. A subaortic muscular stenosis is also present due to left ventricular septal hypertrophy.

of the ligamentum arteriosus (residual of the ductus arteriosus), most probably due to extension of ductal tissue, which creates a progressively severe stenosis at isthmal level (Figure 2.52). Collateral circulation of the aorta, before and after the coarctation, is provided mostly by internal mammary and intercostal arteries. The risk of coarctation, left unrepaired, is the underdevelopment of legs, systemic hypertension with left ventricular hypertrophy, accelerated coronary atherosclerosis, aortic dissection and stroke. About 40–50% of cases show an association with bicuspid aortic valve (BAV).

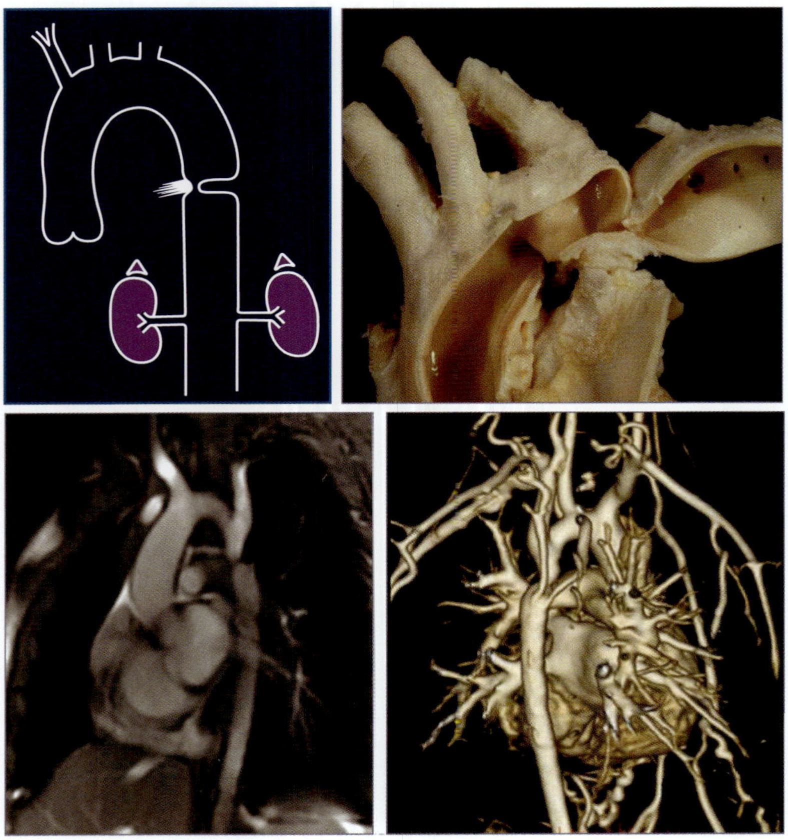

Figure 2.52 *Congenital heart disease with obstruction to blood progression and no septal defect (no shunt). Adult-type aortic arch coarctation.* (a) Schematic representation. (b) Anatomical specimen: a severe aortic coarctation is present in the isthmal region after the insertion of the ligamentum arteriosus. (c) Magnetic resonance angiography image. (d) Right posterior view of a 3D reconstruction. In presence of a significant coarctation, which has not been corrected in early age (adult type), a collateral circulation develop through both mammary arteries, the intercostal arteries as well as between the aortic arch and the descending aorta

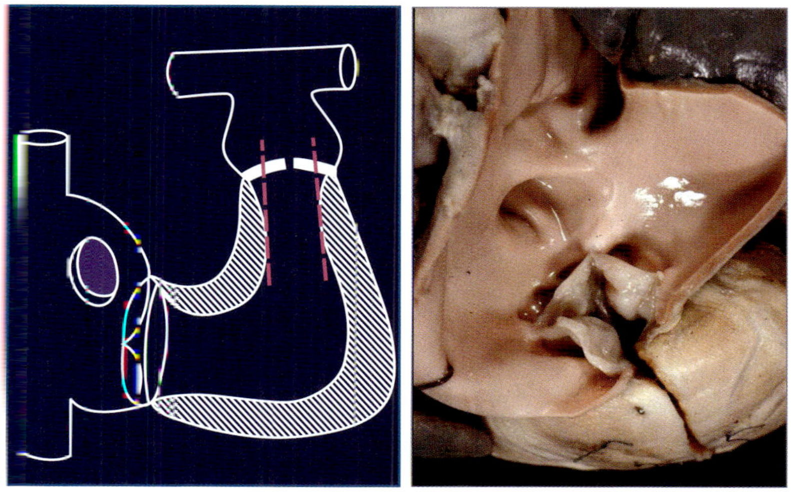

(a) (b)

Figure 2.53 *Congenital heart disease with obstruction to blood progression and no septal defect (no shunt). Pulmonary valvular stenosis.* (a) Schematic representation: the obstruction is located at valvular level with a stenotic and dysplastic valve. Poststenotic dilatation of the pulmonary trunk and hypertrophy of the right ventricle are secondary associated lesions. (b) View from the pulmonary artery of a stenotic and dysplastic tricuspid pulmonary valve. Note the severe dilatation of the pulmonary trunk.

3 *Pulmonary stenosis*: It may be subvalvular, usually due to prominent septo-parietal muscular bands; valvular with dome-shaped valve or thickened dysplastic cusps (Figure 2.53); *supravalvular* in the setting of William's syndrome or similar genetic disorders.

CHD Incompatible with Postnatal Blood Circulation

One of the most amazing features of CHD is that even very severe forms, such as complete transposition of the great arteries, total anomalous pulmonary venous drainage, aortic or pulmonary atresia, and interruption or atresia of the aortic arch, are perfectly compatible with fetal circulation, full-term pregnancy, and a baby with normal weight at birth. The paradox finds an explanation on the peculiarity of the blood circulation in the fetus, where the lungs do not work and the placenta acts for respiratory, renal, and intestinal functions (Figure 2.54).

The lung circulation is almost entirely bypassed, thanks to the interatrial shunt through foramen ovale and the pulmonary-aortic shunt through the ductus arteriosus. As said by the same Harvey in the De Motu Cordis, in the fetus the two great arteries behave like two aortae to transfer the blood from both ventricles to the descending aorta. Whether the aorta arises from the left or right ventricle or, vice versa, whether the pulmonary artery from the right or left ventricle, does not matter and does not affect fetal growth. By the way, the blood crossing the umbilical vein, full of oxygen and nourishment, bypasses the hepatic circulation via the ductus venosus of Arantius, which joins directly the umbilical vein to the suprahepatic inferior vena cava.

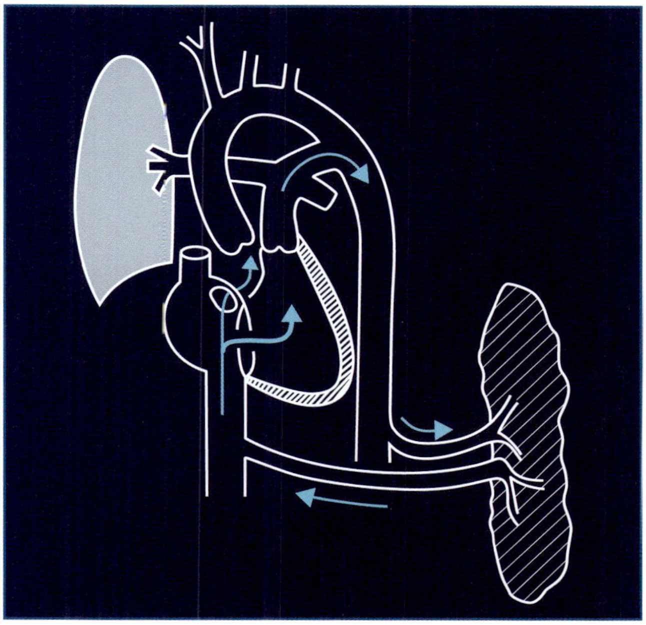

Figure 2.54 *Congenital heart disease incompatible with postnatal blood circulation. Fetal circulation.* In the fetus, the lungs are not active and the placenta acts for respiratory, renal, and intestinal functions. The lung arterial circulation is almost entirely bypassed, thanks to the interatrial shunt through foramen ovale and the pulmonary-aortic shunt through the ductus arteriosus. Both aorta and pulmonary arteries in the fetus transfer the blood from both ventricles to the descending aorta, irrespective of their origin. By the way, the blood crossing the umbilical vein, full of oxygen and nourishment, bypasses the hepatic circulation through the ductus venosus of Arantius, which joins directly the supraepatic inferior vena cava. At birth, the activation of lung ventilatory function as well as the pulmonary arterial circulation, the increase of pulmonary venous blood return, the closure of ductus arteriosus and ductus venosus, as well as the restriction of the foramen ovalis, can precipitate unstable conditions in case of peculiar congenital heart disease.

At birth, with the activation of lung ventilatory function with breathing as well as of the pulmonary arterial circulation, there is an increase of pulmonary venous blood return with the restriction of the foramen ovale, as well as the closure of ductus arteriosus and ductus venosus. The blood circulation changes suddenly, thus precipitating unstable conditions in case of peculiar CHD.

1 *Ductus-dependent CHD* (pulmonary atresia, aortic and mitral atresia, interrupted or atretic aortic arch): *In pulmonary atresia (with or without VSD)*, the source of the pulmonary arterial circulation may be the ductus arteriosus (Figure 2.55). Soon after birth, the spontaneous closure of the ductus interrupts the pulmonary arterial supply, jeopardizing the lung respiratory function.

In *aortic or mitral atresia/severe stenosis*, it is the systemic circulation that depends on the patency of the ductus arteriosus, which represents the only way for blood to reach the systemic arterial circulation (Figure 2.56). Its closure at birth interrupts the only source of blood for brain and all other vital systemic organs, thus creating a sort of heart without outlet. By the way, the massive return of venous blood from the lungs finds an obstacle both in the hypoplastic left heart and in the valve of the foramen ovale which, pushed from left to right, entraps the blood in the left atrium and the lungs.

In *aortic arch obstructions*, severe coarctation (Figure 2.57), interruption/atresia (Figure 2.58), which are usually associated with VSD and obstructive lesions in the inflow/outflow of the left ventricle, the descending aorta is perfused during fetal life by the ductus arteriosus. Its closure at birth is catastrophic for subdiaphragmatic organs with acute renal failure.

Clearly, in all these conditions the extrauterine life is ductus dependent and prostaglandin therapy is mandatory to maintain ductal patency, until surgical or interventional palliative procedures (aortopulmonary shunt, Norwood intervention, balloon atrial septostomy) are carried out.

2 *Parallel systemic and pulmonary circulation* (complete transposition of the great arteries): In *complete transposition of the great arteries*, the aorta takes origin from the right ventricle and the pulmonary artery from the left ventricle (VA discordance in AV concordance). The circulations become clearly in parallel at birth, with the deoxygenated systemic venous blood being forwarded to the aorta and the oxygenated pulmonary venous blood forwarded again to the lungs via the pulmonary artery (Figure 2.59). If no other defect like VSD and/or pulmonary stenosis is associated to facilitate blood mixing, the condition is clearly incompatible with the postnatal

(a) (b) (c) (d)

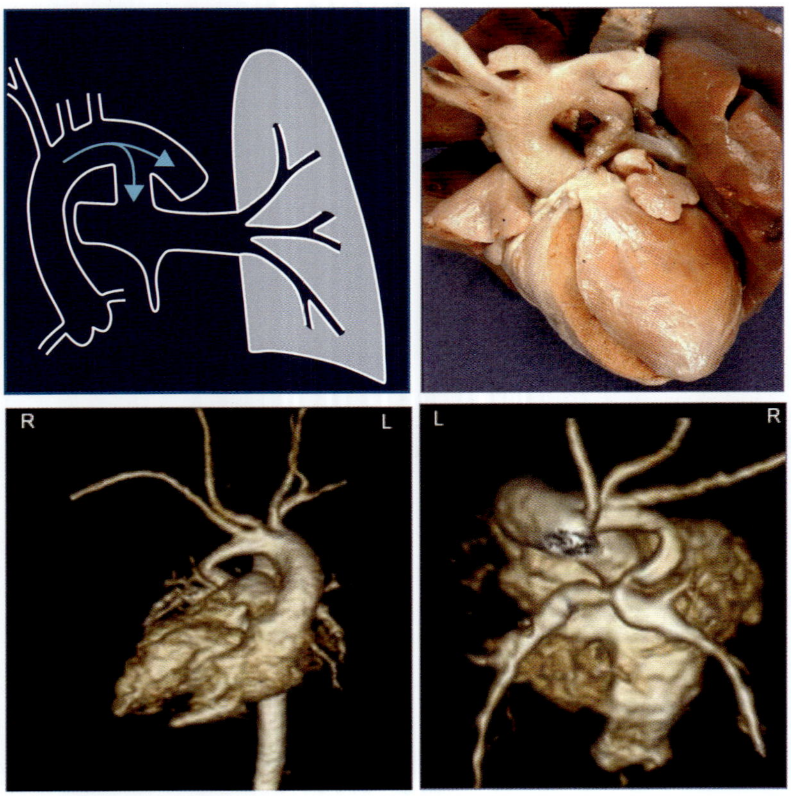

Figure 2.55 *Congenital heart disease incompatible with postnatal blood circulation: ductus-dependent pulmonary circulation. Pulmonary atresia.* (a) In pulmonary atresia (with or without ventricular septal defect), the pulmonary circulation may depend on the patency of the ductus arteriosus, which represents the only way for blood to reach the pulmonary arterial circulation. (b) External view of the heart in a case of pulmonary atresia with intact septum: note the hypoplasia of the pulmonary trunk and branches and the patent ductus arteriosus. (c) Cardiac magnetic resonance angiography in a three-dimensional reconstruction view. Anterior view showing a single vessel (aorta) arising from the left ventricle. The pulmonary artery is missing. (d) The image corresponds to a posterior view in which the ductus arteriosus supplying the right and the left pulmonary artery can be recognized. L, left; R, right.

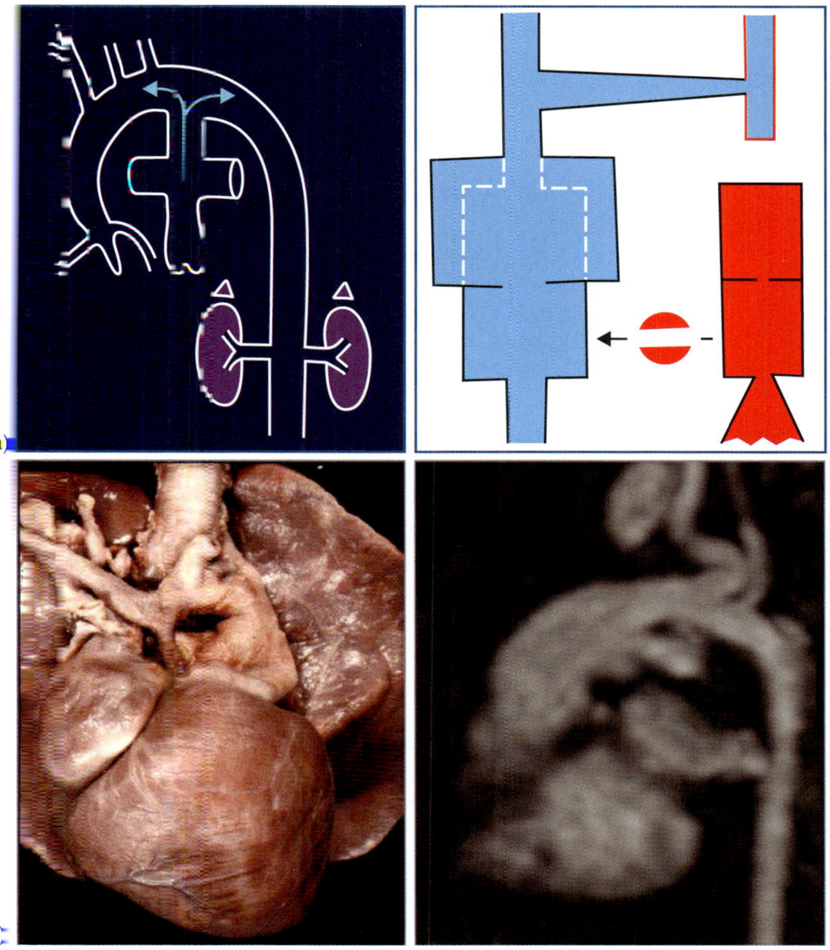

Figure 2.56 *Congenital heart disease incompatible with postnatal blood circulation: ductus-dependent systemic circulation. Aortic atresia.* (a) In aortic or mitral atresia/severe stenosis, the systemic circulation depends on the patency of the ductus arteriosus, which represents the only way for blood to reach the systemic arterial circulation. (b) Schematic representation. In aortic atresia, the venous blood from the lungs finds an obstacle in the hypoplastic left heart and in the valve of foramen ovalis. The pulmonary venous blood is entrapped in the left atrium and in the lungs. (c) External view of the heart in a case of mitroaortic atresia: note the extreme hypoplasia of the ascending aorta and aortic arch and the ductus arteriosus connecting the pulmonary trunk with the aortic arch. (d) As visualized by cardiac magnetic resonance imaging, the ductus arteriosus connects the main pulmonary artery to the descending aorta and therefore warrants the systemic circulation.

physiology. A prompt procedure is to create some mixing with atrial balloon Rashkind septostomy or maintaining patent the ductus with prostaglandins. If severe aortic arch obstruction lesions, like interrupted aortic arch, are associated, a ductus-dependent circulatory condition will aggravate the parallel circulation.

3 *Anomalous connection/obstruction of the pulmonary veins*: The lungs are not working in the uterus, with the fetus immersed in the amniotic fluid and his life and growth are totally dependent on the placenta. Pulmonary arterial supply is limited (nearly 8–10% of all cardiac output), and the destiny of the pulmonary venous return is irrelevant to the fetal physiology.

When at birth the small circulation starts with left and right heart completely separated, the amount of blood forwarded to the aorta normally is the one drained from the lungs. The presence of total anomalous pulmonary venous drainage or a severe obstruction of the pulmonary veins may overturn the physiology of the blood circulation.

In *total anomalous pulmonary venous drainage*, all the pulmonary venous blood, instead of entering the left atrium, is forwarded to the caval veins system (Figure 2.60) and then to the right atrium, thus mixing with the systemic venous blood. To reach the left atrium and the left ventricle, the blood has to cross the foramen ovale, which after birth may become restrictive. The great amount of the mixed venous blood drains into the right ventricle and the pulmonary artery and may reach the descending aorta through the ductus arteriosus (ductus-dependent circulation). A peculiar condition does exist when the total anomalous pulmonary venous damage occurs subdiaphragmatically into the portal system, usually the gastric veins (Figures 2.56 and 2.61). With the postnatal spontaneous closure of the ductus venosus of Arantius, there is no possibility for the anomalous pulmonary venous drainage to bypass the liver and thus it is forced to cross the "rete mirabilis" of the hepatic sinusoids, which act like a barrier.

By the way, the anomalous venous conduit presents frequently an obstruction, which concurs to aggravate the situation, creating blood entrapment into the lungs.

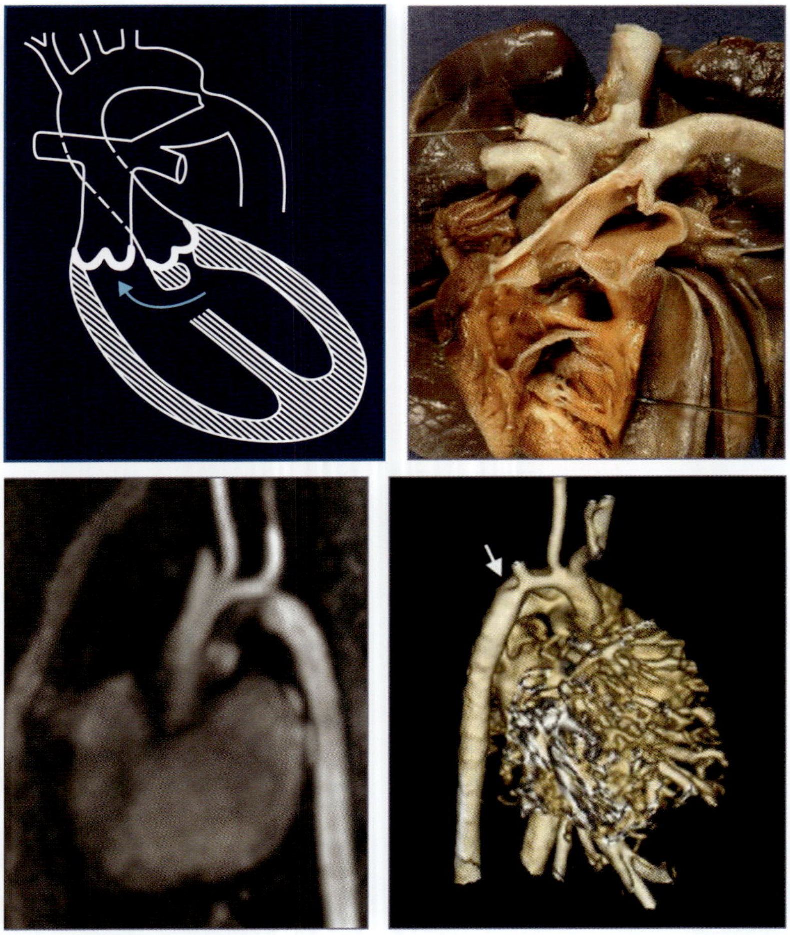

(a) (b) (c) (d)

Figure 2.57 *Congenital heart disease incompatible with postnatal blood circulation: ductus-dependent systemic circulation. Infantile-type aortic coarctation.* (a) The infantile type of aortic coarctation is characterized by the association of the aortic obstruction with intracardiac anomalies such as interventricular septal defect and/or stenosis in the inflow or outflow tract of the left ventricle. (b) Anatomical view: a severe obstruction of the aortic arch is present in isthmal region associated with a large ventricular septal defect. A ductus arteriosus connects the pulmonary artery to the descending aorta. Its closure jeopardizes the perfusion of the subdiaphragmatic organs with renal failure. (c) Hypoplasia of the distal aortic arch and severe obstruction in the isthmal region as visualized by cardiac magnetic resonance imaging. (d) Right posterior view: the patent ductus arteriosus (arrow) connects the pulmonary artery to the descending aorta.

Cor triatriatum sinister is a congenital morbid entity consisting of a diaphragm in the left atrium, in between the sinusal portion and the body of the left atrium. The diaphragm is above the foramen ovale and does not interfere with the blood fetal circulation (Figure 2.62).

This morbid entity becomes dramatic at birth, with the activation of the lung function and the pulmonary arterial circulation, with the pulmonary venous blood flood suddenly draining into the obstructed left atrium, thus precipitating pulmonary edema. A similar pathophysiological condition may occur in hypoplastic left heart and in congenital stenosis/atresia of the pulmonary veins.

CHD Silent Until Adult Age

There are some CHDs that are not symptomatic until adult age or may be observed incidentally either with in vivo imaging or at autopsy in patients who die for extracardiac causes.

1 *BAV*: Although BAV may be associated with other CHD (see for instance coarctation of the aorta with or without VSD), it may be an isolated defect. The malformation consists of two semilunar aortic cusps, with either side-by-side (latero-lateral) or anteroposterior (ventrodorsal) position, which are most probably the result of an embryonic defect of truncal cushions fusion. Two cusps fail to differentiate, resulting in a single semilunar cusp with a raphe ("aborted commissure"). BAV is frequently associated with dilatation of ascending aorta and cystic medial necrosis of the tunica media at risk of aortic dissection and sudden, unexpected death (Figure 2.63). Young subjects with BAV show a mean diameter of the aortic root significantly larger than age matched people with three cuspal aortic valves, as well as less elasticity, in keeping with loss of elastic lamellae of the tunica media, as occurring in Marfan patients. Different from the latter, BAV patients do not exhibit a mutation of fibrillin gene, although the disease may be occasionally familial. Like other CHD, BAV is at risk of infective endocarditis, thus

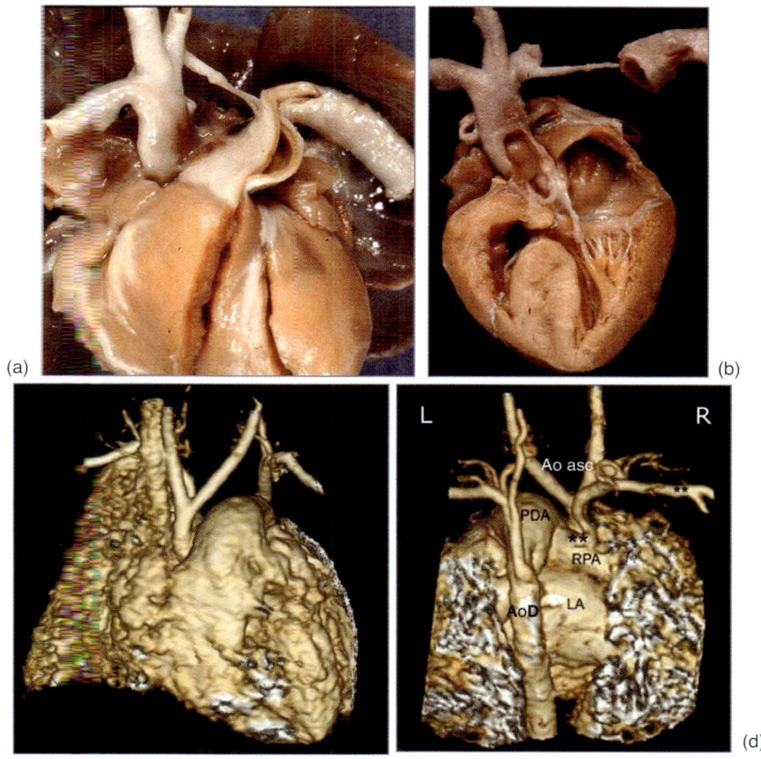

Figure 2.58 *Congenital heart disease incompatible with postnatal blood circulation: ductus-dependent systemic circulation. Atretic aortic arch.* (a) External view of the heart with atresia of the aortic arch in the isthmic region between the subclavian artery and the ductus arteriosus. The perfusion of descending aorta is ductus arteriosus dependent. (b) Same anatomical specimen in echocardiographic section: note the atretic aortic arch in association with a ventricular septal defect and subaortic obstruction. (c) Interrupted aortic arch as visualized by magnetic resonance imaging. Anterior view showing the hypoplastic ascending aorta and the enlarged pulmonary trunk. The aortic arch is interrupted after the origin of the left carotid artery. (d) Posterior view of a case of interrupted aortic arch. The perfusion of the descending aorta and of the lower body depends on the patency of the ductus arteriosus. In this particular case, the left subclavian artery arises from the right pulmonary artery (**). Ao asc, ascending aorta; AoD, descending aorta; L, left; LA, left atrium; PDA, patent ductus arteriosus; R, right; RPA, right pulmonary artery.

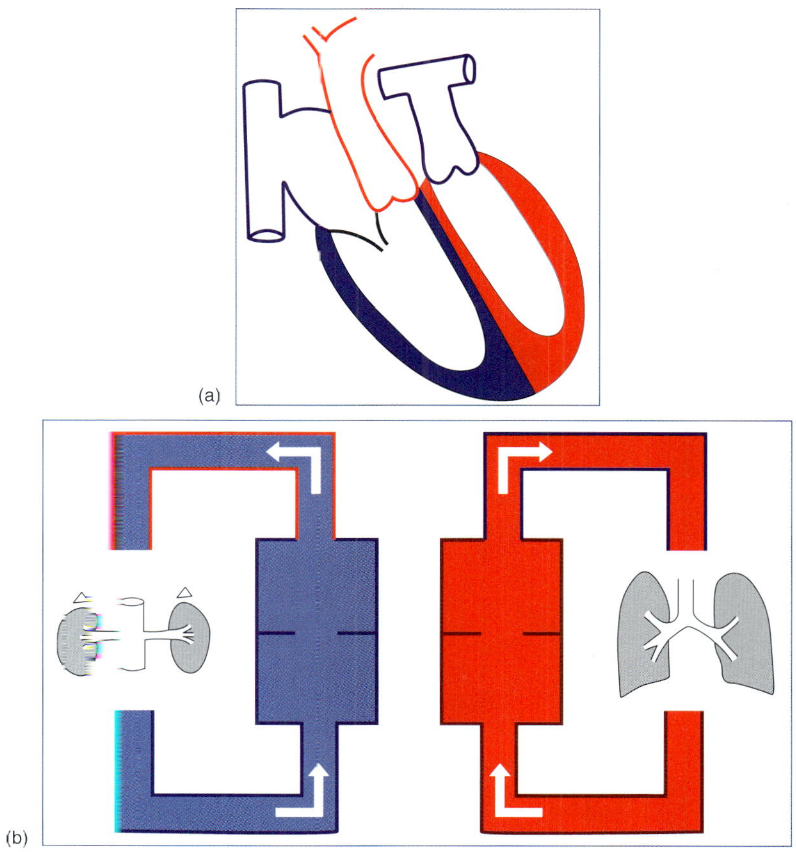

Figure 2.59 *Congenital heart disease incompatible with postnatal blood circulation: parallel systemic and pulmonary circulation.* (a) In complete transposition of the great arteries, the aorta takes origin from the right ventricle and the pulmonary artery from the left ventricles (ventriculoarterial discordance in atrioventricular concordance). (b) This type of circulation, compatible with the fetal life, becomes clearly in parallel at birth, with the deoxygenated systemic venous blood being forwarded to the aorta and the oxygenated pulmonary venous blood forwarded again to the lungs via the pulmonary artery. If no other lesions like ventricular septal defect or pulmonary stenosis do exist, the condition is clearly incompatible with the postnatal physiology.

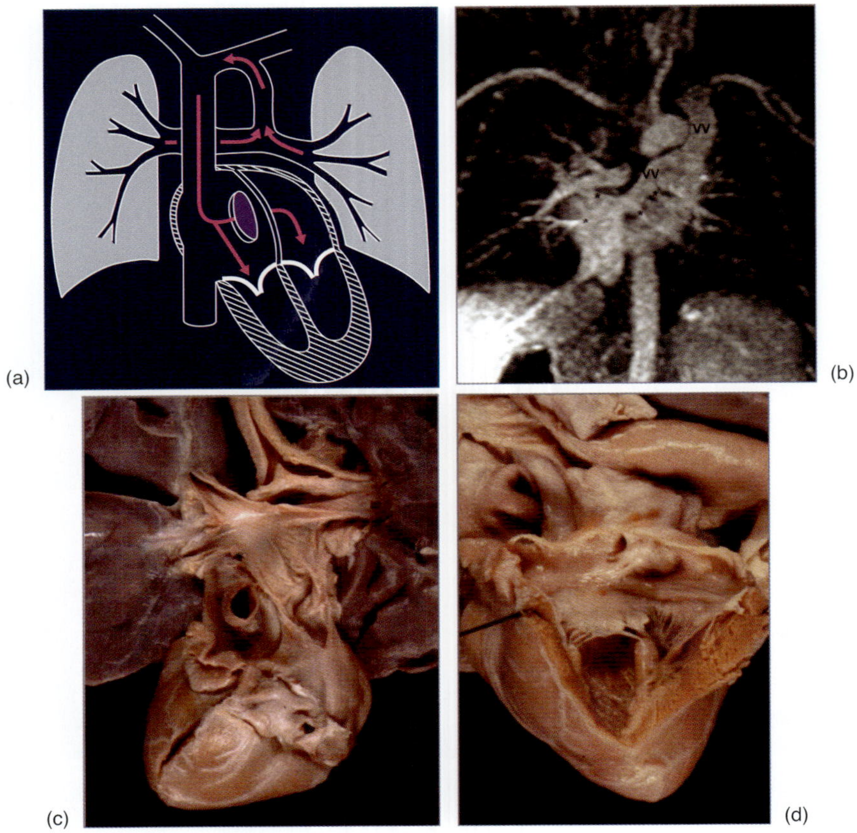

Figure 2.60 *Congenital heart disease incompatible with postnatal blood circulation: anomalous connection or obstruction of the pulmonary veins. Total anomalous pulmonary venous drainage into the superior vena cava.* (a) Schematic representation: all the pulmonary veins join the superior vena cava via a common duct and then the right atrium. A restrictive foramen ovale hinders the passage of the blood from right to left cavity. (b) As visualized by magnetic resonance imaging, all four pulmonary veins (*) merge into a vertical vein, which runs cranially and drains into the innominate vein. (c) Posterior view of the heart. All the pulmonary veins merge in a single trunk that drains into the superior vena cava. (d) View from the left cardiac chambers: note the restrictive foramen ovale that hinders the transfer of blood from the right atrium to the left atrium (foramen ovale dependent circulation). VV, vertical vein.

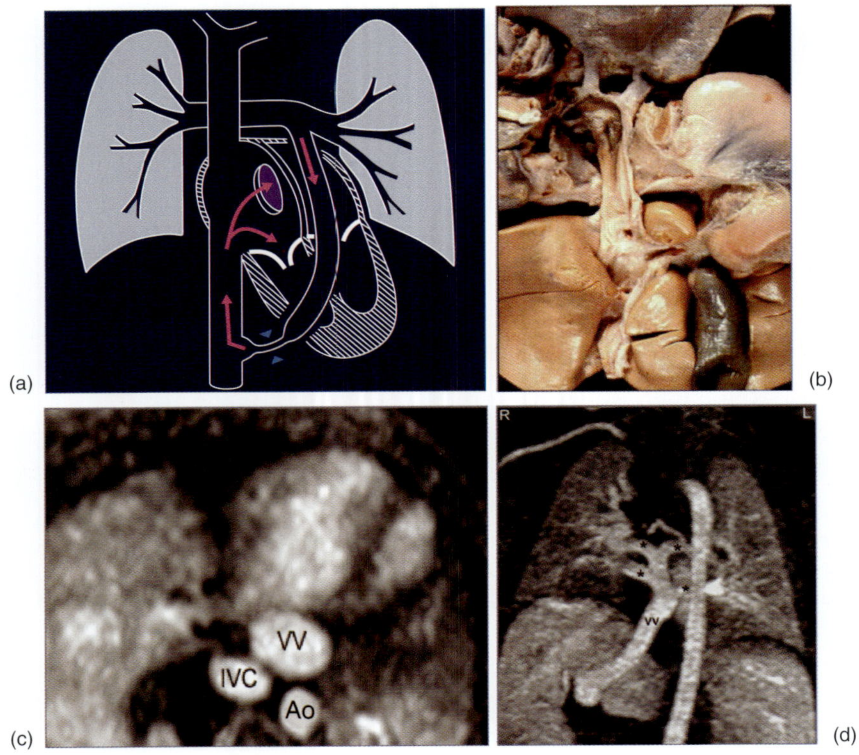

Figure 2.61 *Congenital heart disease incompatible with postnatal blood circulation: anomalous connection or obstruction of the pulmonary veins. Subdiaphragmatic total anomalous pulmonary venous drainage.* (a) Schematic representation: all the pulmonary veins join a vertical vein that crosses the diaphragm and reach the portal system. With the postnatal spontaneous closure of the ductus venosus of Arantius, there is no possibility for the anomalous pulmonary venous drainage to bypass the liver and thus it is forced to cross the "rete mirabilis" of the hepatic sinusoids, which act like a barrier. (b) Corresponding anatomical specimen: the vertical vein drains the pulmonary veins and reaches the hepatic hilum. (c) Cardiac magnetic resonance imaging: axial view at the level of the diaphragm. The vertical vein is typically situated beyond the heart and in front of the descending aorta. This additional vessel can be visualized in this way at echocardiography or cross-sectional imaging. (d) All four pulmonary veins (*) merge in a common vessel, which runs caudally, crosses the diaphragm, and drains into the portal system. AoD, descending aorta; IVC, inferior vena cava; L, left; R, right; VV, vertical vein.

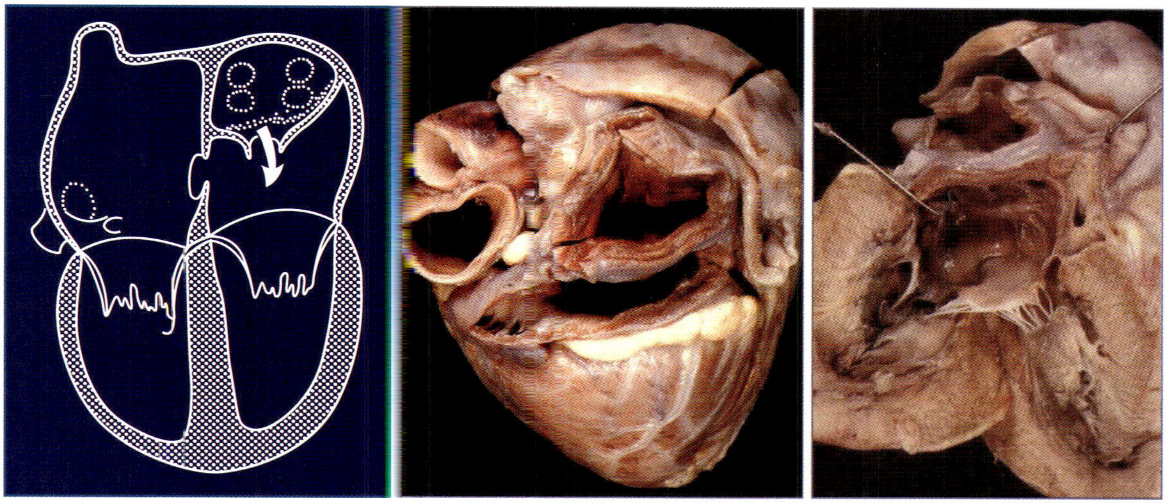

(a), (b) (c)

Figure 2.62 *Congenital heart disease incompatible with postnatal blood circulation: anomalous connection or obstruction of the pulmonary veins. Cor triatriatum.* (a) Cor triatriatum sinister is a congenital malformation characterized by a diaphragm in the left atrium in between the sinusal portion and the body of the left atrium. The diaphragm is over the foramen ovale and does not interfere with the blood fetal circulation. (b) Posterior view of the heart showing the subdivided left atrium. (c) View of the left cardiac chambers with a normal mitral valve, the subdivided left atrium, and the foramen ovale below the diaphragm.

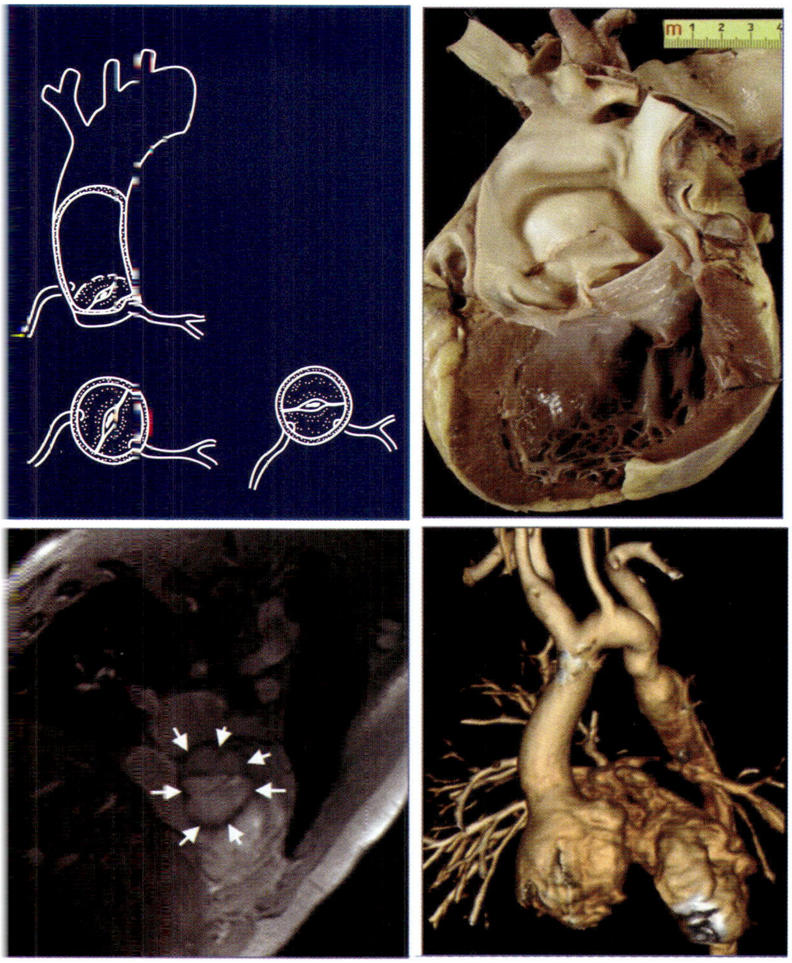

(a) (b) (c) (d)

Figure 2.63 *Congenital heart disease silent until adult age. Bicuspid aortic valve.* (a) Schematic representation: the malformation consists of two semilunar aortic cusp, either with side-by-side (latero-lateral) or anteroposterior (ventro-dorsal) position. (b) View from left ventricular outflow tract: a bicuspid aortic valve is present and associated with dilatation of ascending aorta, wall tear, and dissection. (c) Bicuspid aortic valve with one ventral and one dorsal cusp as visualized by cardiac magnetic resonance imaging. (d) Severe isolated dilatation of the aortic root in the same patient with bicuspid aortic valve. Coarctation of the aorta is a frequent concomitant finding, like in this case.

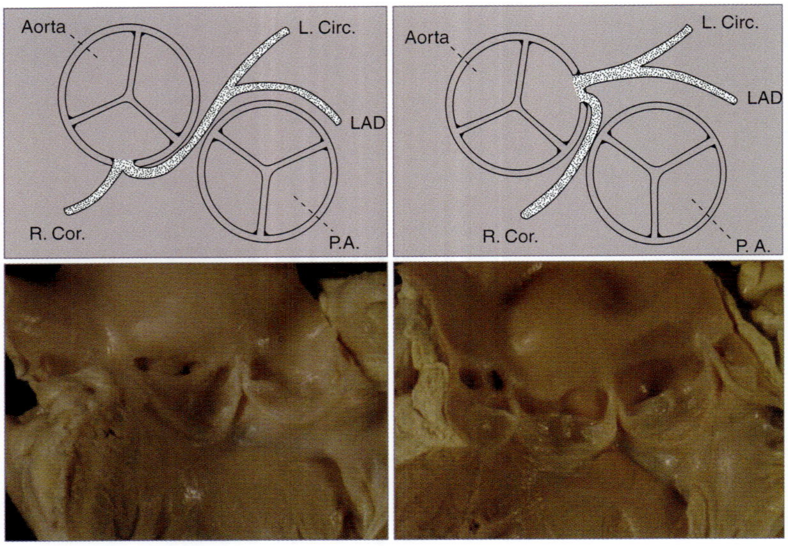

(a) (b)

Figure 2.64 *Congenital heart disease silent until adult age. Congenital anomalies of coronary arteries.* (a) Schematic representation and anatomical specimen of anomalous origin of left coronary artery from the right aortic sinus. (b) Schematic representation and anatomical specimen of anomalous origin of right coronary artery from the left aortic sinus. In both cases, the anomalous coronary artery runs in between the aorta and the pulmonary artery, with an intramural aortic course and a slit-like lumen, which acts as an obstruction precipitating coronary insufficiency during effort. LAD, left anterior descending; PA, pulmonary artery.

requiring prophylactic antibiotic treatment before dental, intestinal, or urethral procedures. Dystrophic calcification with aortic stenosis is another peculiar complication of BAV, with mineralization occurring much earlier then in senile aortic stenosis with tricuspid aortic valve.

2 *Congenital anomalies of coronary arteries*: A part from anomalous origin of the left (or right) coronary artery

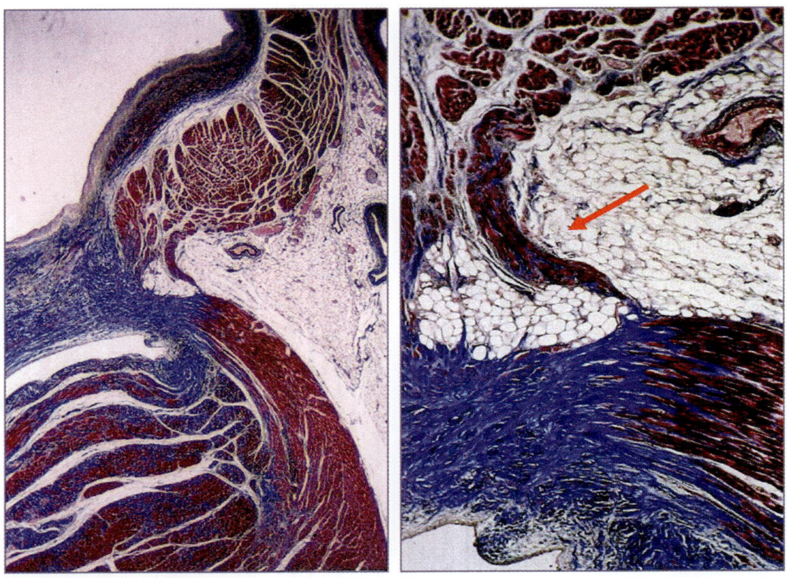

(a) (b)

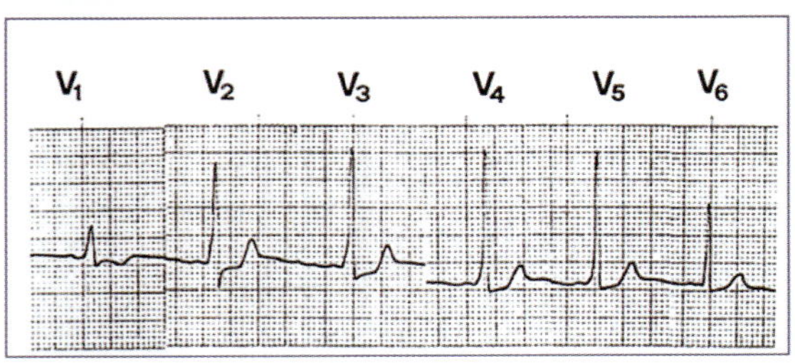

(c)

Figure 2.65 *Congenital heart disease silent until adult age. Wolf Parkinson White syndrome.* Ventricular pre-excitation occurs, because of an anomalous fascicle of working myocardium joining the atrial to the ventricular musculature, outside the regular specialized conduction system. (a–b) Histology in a case of WPW syndrome: note the presence of an abnormal small fascicle of working myocardium (arrow) joining the left atrial with the left ventricular musculature. Its location is close to the endocardium behind the fibrous annulus of the posterolateral mitral ring, and it renders ablation easily. (c) ECG recording with short PQ and delta wave.

from the pulmonary trunk, which usually becomes symptomatic early in infancy because of coronary blood steal from the aorta to the pulmonary artery, there are several congenital anomalies of the coronary arteries with origin from the aorta itself, which are apparently minor but may abruptly precipitate sudden death during effort.

This is the case, for instance, of *anomalous origin of right or left coronary arteries from the opposite (wrong) aortic sinus* (Figure 2.64). The anomalous coronary artery runs in between the aorta and the pulmonary artery, with an intramural aortic course and a slit like lumen, which act as an obstruction precipitating coronary insufficiency during effort, when there is an increased coronary blood flow demand. This CHD is one of the major causes of SD in athletes.

High take-off origin of a coronary artery (>1 cm above the sinotubular junction) accounts for a similar physiopathological condition, due to a vertical, intramural course of the first tract of the anomalous coronary artery.

Origin of the *left circumflex coronary artery from the right coronary artery* or directly from the right aortic sinus, with a retroaortic course, is usually considered a benign variant of the coronary arterial pattern. However sometimes, due to acute angle origin and aberrant course, this anomaly may precipitate acute myocardial ischemia during effort, triggering myocardial infarction and/or ventricular fibrillation with sudden death.

3 *Wolff-Parkinson-White syndrome*: It accounts for ventricular pre-excitation, due to an anomalous fascicle of working myocardium, joining the atria to the ventricle outside the regular specialized conduction system. It is recorded on ECG with short PQ and delta wave (Figure 2.65). Onset of supraventricular tachycardia may occur through a reentrant mechanism of the electrical impulse along with the anomalous fascicle. The accessory pathway (200–300 micron thick) can be regarded as the smallest CHD, defined as a structural defect present at birth. Its location close to the endocardium, usually behind the fibrous annulus of the posterolateral mitral ring, renders catheter ablation quite feasible.

4 *Congenitally corrected transposition of the great arteries*: Congenitally corrected transposition of the great arteries (AV and VA discordance), in the absence of associated lesions, may be completely asymptomatic for years.

The right atrium is connected through a mitral valve with the left ventricle from which a posterior right-sided pulmonary artery takes origin, and the left atrium is connected through tricuspid valve with the right ventricle from which an anterior left-sided aorta originates (Figure 2.21). This sequence of cardiac segments accounts for a normal physiology of blood circulation ("corrected" transposition). The systemic (left-sided) position renders the tricuspid valve vulnerable to regurgitation, progressively with time. The anteriorly displaced specialized AV junction (AV node and His bundle), with His bundle located in the subendocardium of the pulmonary outflow tract, accounts for progressive wearing and tearing and AV block, the onset of which may be abrupt as to account for cardiac arrest and sudden death. Congenitally corrected transposition is a rare cause of sudden death in adults, believed to have a normal heart, and represents an unexpected discovery at autopsy.

References

1. Anderson RH, Becker AE. (1986) *Cardiac Anatomy: An Integrated Text and Colour Atlas*. Gower Medical Publishing, Churchill Livingstone, Edinburgh.
2. Anderson RH, Becker AE. (1992) *The Heart—Structure in Health and Disease*. Gower Medical Publishing, London.
3. Anderson RH, Baker EJ, Macartney FJ, Rugby ML, Shinebourne EA, Tynan M. (2002) *Paediatric Cardiology* (2nd edition). Churchill Livingstone, London.
4. Becker AE, Anderson RH. (1981) *Pathology of Congenital Heart Disease*. Butterworths, London.
5. Frescura C, Ho SY, Thiene G. (1997) *La collezione anatomica delle cardiopatie congenite dell'Università di Padova*. Edizioni CLEUP, Padova.
6. Ho SY, Baker EJ, Rigby ML, Anderson RH. (1995) *Colour Atlas of Congenital Heart Disease*. Mosby-Wolfe, London.
7. Marino B, Thiene G. (1990) *Atlante di anatomia ecocardiografica delle cardiopatie congenite*. USES, Firenze.
8. Pistolesi GF, Thiene G, Casolo F. (1985) *L'imaging diagnostico del cucre*. Edizioni Libreria Cortina, Verona.
9. Thiene G, Frescura C. (1985) *Codificazione diagnostica ed atlante delle cardiopatie congenite*. Edizioni LINT, Trieste.
10. Kellenberger CK, Yoo SJ, Valsangiacomo Büchel ER. (2007) Cardiovascular MR imaging in neonates and infants with congenital heart disease. *Radiographics* 27:5–18.
11. Fratz S, Hess J, Shuchbaeck A *et al.* (2008) Routine clinical cardiovascular magnetic resonance in paediatric and adult congenital heart disease: patients, protocols, questions asked and contribution made. *J Cardiovasc Magn Reson* 10:46.
12. Valsangiacomo Büchel ER, DiBernardo S, Bauersfeld U, Berger F. (2005) Contrast-enhanced magnetic resonance angiography of the great arteries in patients with congenital heart disease: an accurate tool for planning catheter-guided interventions. *Int J Cardiovasc Imaging* 21:313–322.

3 CT in Pediatric Heart Disease

Hyun Woo Goo

University of Ulsan, Seoul, Korea

Introduction

Background knowledge on cardiac anatomy is the first important step in understanding congenital heart disease [1, 2]. The vast amount of the knowledge has been traditionally acquired through anatomical dissections and correlation with catheter angiocardiographic findings [3]. Recent developments in multidetector CT (MDCT) techniques enable us to see anatomic structures in the heart in more detail and under more physiologic conditions [4–6]. Highly flexible ECG synchronization with either retrospective gating or prospective triggering, high temporal resolution, and low radiation dose are key factors for these technical improvements of cardiac CT [7–9]. In this chapter, normal cardiac anatomy and typical examples of cardiac defects in congenital heart disease on MDCT images are described. Most cardiac CT examinations were performed with a dual-source 64-slice CT scanner. Various scan techniques including non-ECG-synchronized scan, retrospectively ECG-gated scan, and prospectively ECG-triggered scan are used depending on clinical questions and cooperative capability of a patient.

Cardiac Segments

The heart consists of three segments: atria, ventricles, and great arteries. It should be noted that each segment is defined by its specific morphologic features rather than its spatial orientation in the body. A solid understanding of these morphologic features is required for the accurate diagnosis of congenital heart disease, particularly in complicated cases.

Revisiting Cardiac Anatomy: A Computed-Tomography-Based Atlas and Reference, 1st edition. Edited by Farhood Saremi, Eloisa Arbustini, Stephen Achenbach and Jagat Narula.

Atria

The atrium is a thin-walled sac consisting of the atrium proper and the atrial appendage. Two atria are placed side by side on the base of the ventricles, the plane on which cardiac valves lie, and they are separated by the interatrial septum (Figure 3.1). The pectinate muscle is present in the atrial appendage and its extent is the most accurate anatomic determinant for atrial situs and thoracic situs: situs solitus, situs inversus, right isomerism, and left isomerism. The accurate determination of atrial situs has been thought to be feasible only by anatomic dissections because the pectinate muscle is not clearly seen on CT images using conventional scan techniques. However, the common knowledge has been changed because the pectinate muscle is typically delineated on MDCT images using current cardiac scan techniques. When atrial situs based on the extent of the pectinate muscle is unclear at CT, we may rely on the relationship between the upper lobar bronchus and the pulmonary artery: eparterial or hyparterial bronchus [1, 5]. Hemodynamically, venous blood enters the atrium and subsequently goes out to the corresponding ventricle.

The right atrium is morphologically characterized by a broad, triangular atrial appendage, the conspicuous crista terminalis (an inner vertical ridge between the right atrium proper and the right atrial appendage), and connections with the superior vena cava, the inferior vena cava, and the coronary sinus (Figure 3.1). The pectinate muscles in the right atrial appendage extend to the corresponding atrioventricular junction and then the atrium can be specified as the morphological right atrium (Figure 3.1). Valve-like ridges, the so-called Eustachian and Thebesian valves, are formed between the right atrium and the systemic veins, e.g., the inferior vena cava and the coronary sinus, respectively. Chiari network is a normal web-like structure in the right atrium in close proximity to the entrance of the inferior vena cava (Figure 3.2). These normal structures should be distinguished from lesions in the right atrium such

(a), (b)

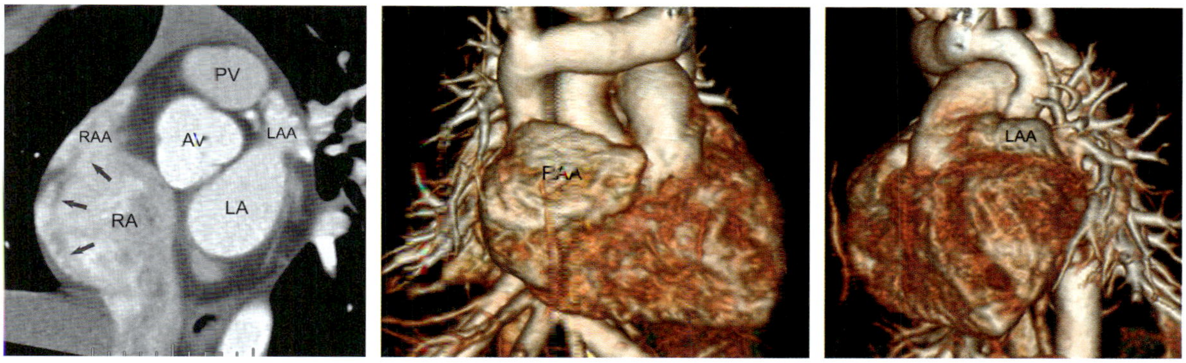

(c)

Figure 3.1 Morphologic features of the atria demonstrated on CT images. The shape is different between the right and left atria and the sidedness of the atrium is determined most accurately by the extent of the pectinate muscles (a–c). The right atrial appendage has a broader opening and a triangular configuration. In addition, the pectinate muscles in the right atrial appendage reach the tricuspid valve annulus. In the right atrial appendage, the comb-like pectinate muscles arise from the crista terminalis (arrows in (a)). The pulmonary valve is located anterior and left to the aortic valve in (a), which is the normal relationship of the great arteries. AV, aortic valve; LA, left atrium; LAA, left atrial appendage; PV, pulmonary valve; RA, right atrium; RAA, right atrial appendage.

as thrombus, vegetation, and tumor when they are prominent.

In contrast, the morphological left atrium is specified by a narrow, hooked, crenellated atrial appendage, the absence of the crista terminalis, connections with the pulmonary veins, and a limited extent of the pectinate muscles in the appendage that do not reach the corresponding atrioventricular junction (Figure 3.1).

Ventricles

The ventricle is a muscular pouch pumping blood to the great arteries. Like the atria, two ventricles are placed side by side under the base of the ventricles and they are separated by the atrioventricular septum and the interventricular septum (Figure 3.3). The apex of the heart is the most inferior external part of the heart that is normally formed by both ventricles and is normally on the left side of the thorax (levocardia). The shape of the cardiac apex can be abnormal: it may be elevated in right ventricular hypertrophy and it may show downward and leftward elongation in left ventricular enlargement. Clockwise rotation of the cardiac apex is commonly seen in cases with enlarged right cardiac chambers. Besides levocardia, the apex of the heart may be directed to the middle (mesocardia) or the right (dextrocardia) of the thorax. Hypoplastic ventricle may not contribute to form the cardiac apex. The crux cordis is defined as a crossing point between the atrioventricular and posterior interventricular sulci. A rudimentary ventricle touching the crux cordis is classically considered to be the morphological left ventricle. Each ventricle has supporting structures for the corresponding atrioventricular

(a), (b)

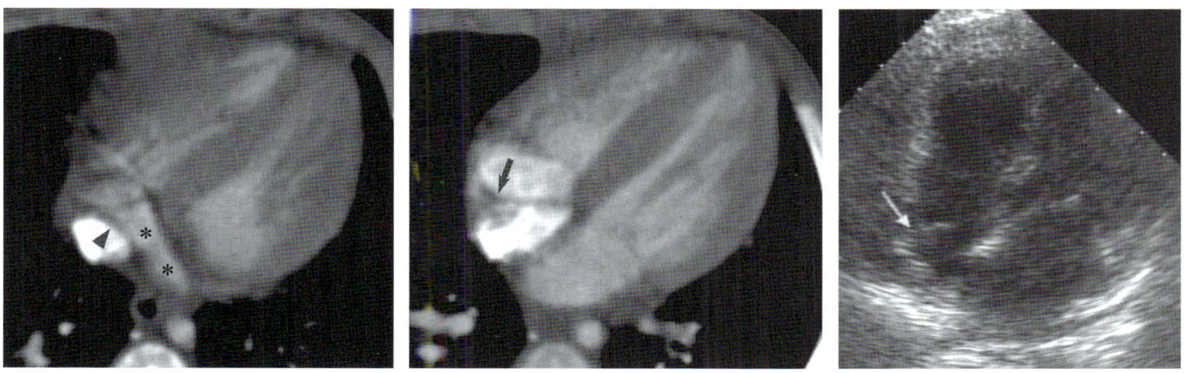

(c)

Figure 3.2 A prominent Chiari network may mimic a lesion in the right atrium. (a) The Eustachian valve (arrowhead) is shown anterior to the inferior vena cava. The coronary sinus (asterisks) draining into the right atrium is also seen. (b) CT image just above the level of (a) shows a hypodense structure adjacent to the junction of the inferior vena cava and the right atrium that is the normal Chiari network (arrow). (c) The corresponding structure is identified as an echogenic band (arrow) at the same location on echocardiographic image. Without sound knowledge on normal cardiac anatomy, the structure may be mistaken as a thrombus or vegetation in the right atrium.

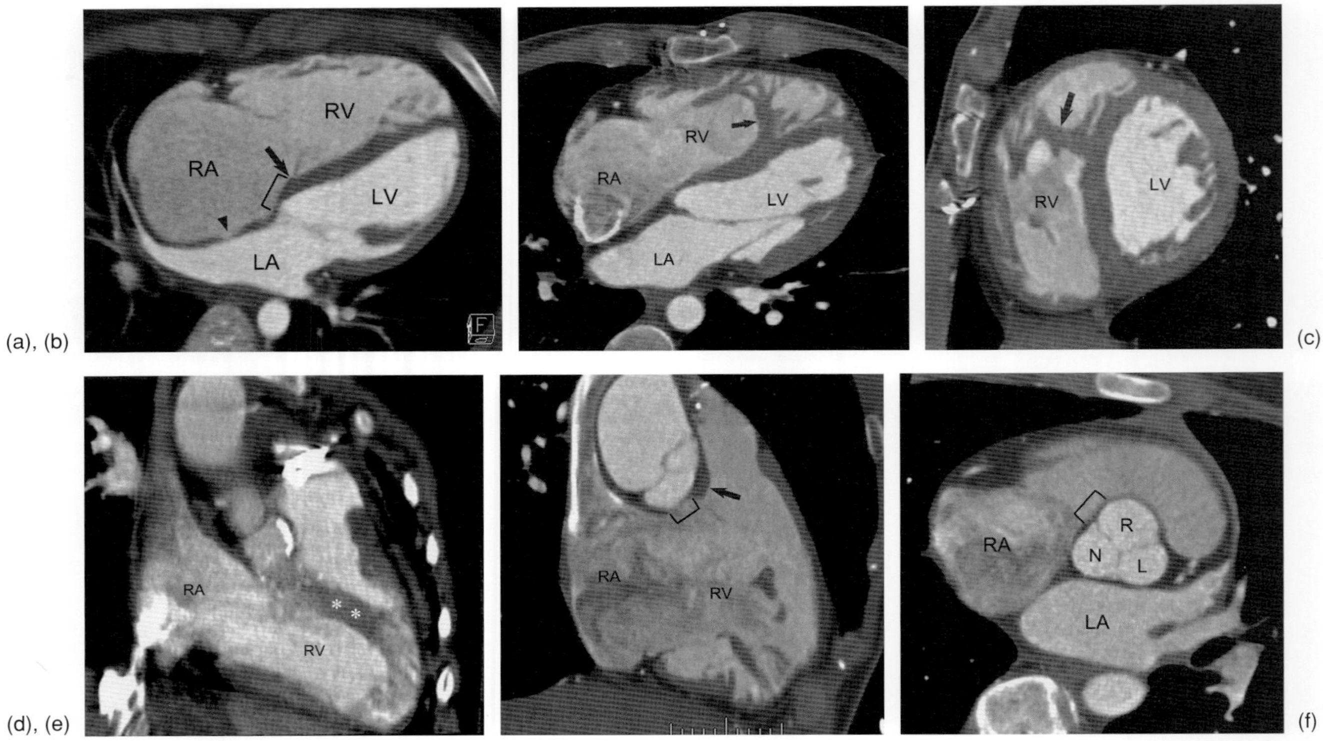

Figure 3.3 Morphologic features of the cardiac septum and right ventricle demonstrated on CT images. (a) Four-chamber view shows four cardiac chambers and their normal spatial relationships. Concordant atrioventricular connections are also shown: the right atrium is connected to the right ventricle and the left atrium is connected to the left ventricle. The CT image also shows the septum of the heart consisting of the interatrial, atrioventricular, and ventricular components. The septal attachment of the tricuspid valve (arrow) is slightly displaced to the cardiac apex, as compared to that of the mitral valve. This offset between the two atrioventricular valves results in the atrioventricular septum (bracket) between the right atrium and the left ventricle. The fossa ovalis (arrowhead) is also noted in the mid-portion of the interatrial septum. (b–f) Anatomic features of the right ventricle including moderator band (arrow in (b) and (c)), the trabecula septomarginalis (asterisks in (d)), and the crista supraventricularis (arrow in (e)) are shown. Thus, the pulmonary valve is separated from the tricuspid valve by the muscular outflow tract of the right ventricle. The membranous portions (bracket in (e) and (f)) of the atrioventricular and interventricular septa have a direct contact to the right and noncoronary aortic cusps. L, left aortic cusp; LA, left atrium; LV, left ventricle; N, noncoronary aortic cusp; R, right aortic cusp; RA, right atrium; RV, right ventricle.

valves: the papillary muscles and the tendinous cords. The right ventricle has three, e.g., the anterior, posterior, and medial, papillary muscles for the tricuspid valve, while the left ventricle has two, e.g., the anterolateral and posteromedial, papillary muscles for the mitral valve.

Morphological characteristics of the right ventricle include heavy trabeculations, coarse septal surface, moderator band, the infundibulum (the crista supraventricularis), and a tricuspid-pulmonary discontinuity (Figure 3.3). The trabecula septomarginalis is the stoutest septal trabeculation consisting of a body and anterior and posterior limbs (Figure 3.3). It contains the right branch of the bundle of His, a part of cardiac conduction system. The medial papillary muscle is attached to the septal surface of the right ventricle at the junction of the anterior and posterior limbs of the trabecula septomarginalis. Because of its small size, the medial papillary muscle is not frequently identified on MDCT images. Moderator band is a muscle bundle extending from the lower part of the trabecula septomarginalis to the right ventricular free wall around the base of the anterior papillary muscle (Figure 3.3). The crista supraventricularis is a saddle-shaped muscular crest separating the tricuspid valve from the pulmonary valve (Figure 3.3).

The right ventricular free wall is normally thinner than that of the left ventricle. The difference is not surprising because each ventricle is normally subject to a different pressure overload. The right ventricular wall becomes hypertrophic in cases with outflow obstruction, pulmonary arterial hypertension, and transposition of the great arteries (TGA). Of note, mild right ventricular hypertrophy is normally seen in neonates and young infants because it usually takes several months for dropping normally elevated pulmonary vascular resistance to the adult level.

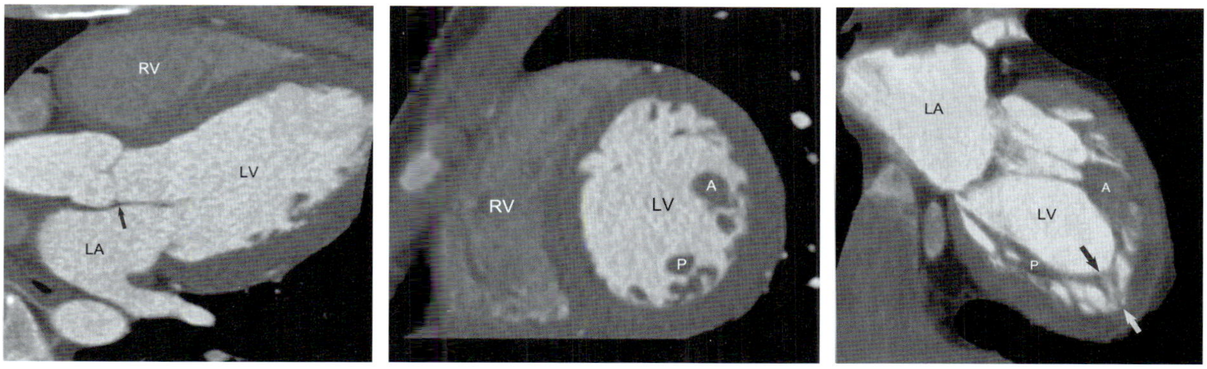

(a), (b) (c)

Figure 3.4 Morphologic features of the left ventricle demonstrated on CT images. (a) Vertical long-axis view of the left cardiac chambers shows smooth trabeculation of the left ventricle and a mitral-aortic fibrous continuity (arrow). (b) Short-axis view reveals smooth septal surface and two, e.g., anterolateral and posteromedial, papillary muscles of the left ventricle. (c) Another vertical long-axis view of the left cardiac chambers reveals trabeculations, papillary muscles, and tendinous cords attached to the mitral valve leaflets. Two-layered apical myocardium, inner noncompacted (arrows) and outer compacted layers, is clearly shown, which is within normal limits. A, anterolateral papillary muscle; LA, left atrium; LV, left ventricle; P, posteromedial papillary muscle; RV, right ventricle.

The left ventricle is morphologically specified by smooth trabeculations, smooth septal surface, and a mitral-aortic fibrous continuity (Figure 3.4). Myocardial noncompaction is regarded as a rare cardiomyopathy that is thought to represent an arrest in endomyocardial morphogenesis. The myocardial abnormality may occur with or without congenital heart diseases and involves the left ventricle more commonly than the right ventricle. The involved left ventricle shows an abnormally thickened layer of inner noncompacted myocardium with variable extent of the abnormality from the cardiac apex [10].

The atrioventricular valve is designated according to the ventricle morphology (e.g., the tricuspid valve for the morphological right ventricle, the mitral valve for the morphological left ventricle).

Great Arteries

Great arteries can be specified simply by their arterial branches. The great artery determines the semilunar valve (e.g., the pulmonary valve for the pulmonary artery, the aortic valve for the aorta). The semilunar valve is normally tricuspid but it may be unicuspid, bicuspid, quadricuspid, and so on in association with various congenital heart diseases. The truncal portion of a great artery consists of the annulus, sinus, sinotubular junction, and tubular portion.

Connections of Cardiac Segments

Two types of connections are present among three cardiac segments: atria, ventricles, and great arteries. They are atrioventricular and ventriculoarterial connections.

Atrioventricular Connection

Normally, the right atrium has a connection with the right ventricle and the left atrium has a connection with the left ventricle in a parallel manner, which is appreciated well on four-chamber view (Figure 3.3). This normal atrioventricular connection is defined to be concordant. In contrast, the connection is defined to be discordant when it is reversed as in congenitally corrected TGA. The atrioventricular connection is rarely twisted in which four cardiac chambers cannot be identified in single imaging plane, e.g., four-chamber view [3]. In the twisted atrioventricular connection, the typical relationship of two ventricles is superior–inferior and usually the superiorly located ventricle is the right ventricle. As in tricuspid atresia, one of the two atrioventricular connections may be absent (Figure 3.5). In association with a defect involving the atrioventricular connection, one atrium may override two ventricles. In addition, the tension apparatus of the atrioventricular valve may cross the ventricular septum through the defect and attach to the septal surface of the opposite ventricle. This condition is called as straddling and it is very important in congenital heart disease because of its great impact on surgical planning.

Ventriculoarterial Connection

Ventriculoarterial connection is defined to be normal or concordant when the pulmonary artery arises from the right ventricle and the aorta originates from the left ventricle (Figure 3.5). Discordant ventriculoarterial connection is shown in TGA (Figure 3.5). When both great arteries arise primarily from one ventricle, it is stated as double outlet ventricle (Figure 3.5). Double outlet right ventricle (DORV) is more commonly encountered than double

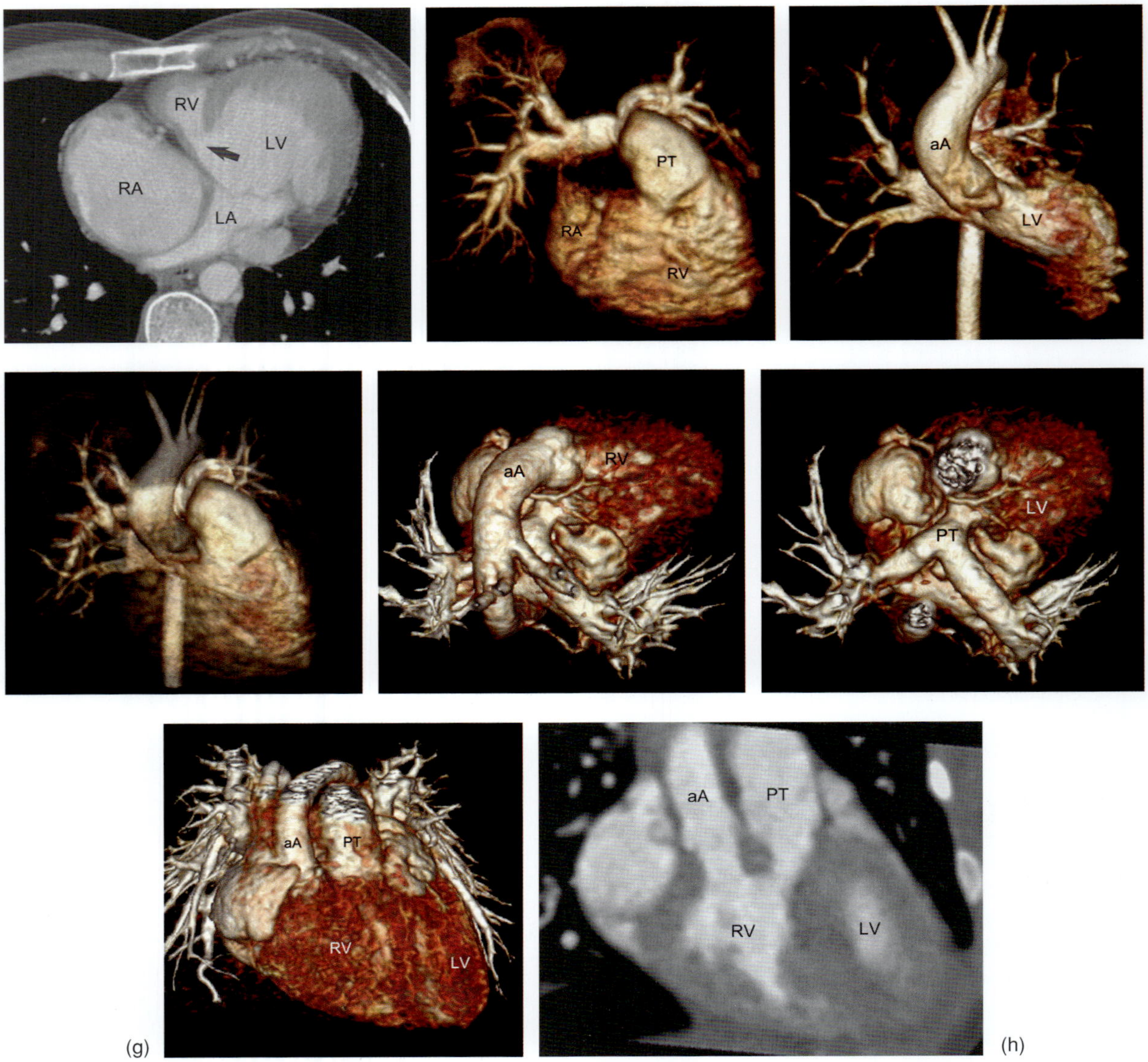

Figure 3.5 Connections of cardiac segments. (a) Axial CT image shows an absent right atrioventricular connection that is compatible with tricuspid atresia. Typically, the right atrioventricular sulcus is deep and is filled with the epicardial fat and the right coronary artery. The right atrium is dilated because of the restrictive atrial septal defect (not shown). A bulboventricular foramen (arrow) is noted between the dominant left and rudimentary right ventricles. (b–d) Volume-rendered images demonstrate normal right (b) and left (c) ventriculoarterial connections. They are related to each other in spiral fashion. Therefore, the great arteries or outflow tracts of the structurally normal heart cannot be shown in single imaging plane. (e, f) Volume-rendered images demonstrate discordant ventriculoarterial connections and d-malposition of the great arteries that are typical for transposition of the great arteries (TGA). (g, h) In double outlet right ventricle (DORV), both great arteries originate principally from the right ventricle and the semilunar valves commonly have bilateral conus. aA, ascending aorta; LA, left atrium; LV, left ventricle; PT, pulmonary trunk; RA, right atrium; RV, right ventricle.

outlet left ventricle. A 50% rule, in which more than a half of each great artery arises from the corresponding ventricle, should be fulfilled for this ventriculoarterial connection. Single outlet is found in truncus arteriosus, single pulmonary trunk with aortic atresia, and single aortic trunk with pulmonary atresia.

Relationships of the Great Arteries

The relationships of the great arteries are a spectrum. Nevertheless, they are typically divided into three categories: normal, d-malposition, and l-malposition. In normal relationship, the pulmonary trunk is anterior and left to the ascending aorta (Figures 3.1 and 3.3). In contrast, the ascending aorta is anterior to the pulmonary trunk in malposition of the great arteries, either on the right (d-malposition, typical of complete TGA) (Figure 3.5) or on the left (l-malposition, typical of congenitally corrected TGA).

Septum of the Heart

The septum of the heart consists of three components: the interatrial, the atrioventricular, and the interventricular septa (Figure 3.3). The atrioventricular septum is resulted from a trivial offset between the septal attachments of the tricuspid (more apical) and mitral valves. Hence, the atrioventricular septum is located between the left ventricle and the right atrium.

Atrial Septal Defect

The interatrial septum is formed by a sequential embryological evolution of the septum primum and the septum secundum. The fossa ovalis is a thinner part of the septum (the septum primum) bordered by the limbus of the septum secundum (Figure 3.3). Patent foramen ovale (PFO) that is resulted from a failure to close the foramen ovale may cause paradoxical embolism by means of a right-to-left shunt (Figure 3.6) [11]. Types of atrial septal defects (ASD) classified by their locations comprise secundum, ostium, and sinus venosus (superior and inferior subtypes) defects (Figure 3.6). The diagnosis of the secundum ASD should be carefully made at MDCT because the fossa ovalis may be so thin as to be mistaken as the ostium secundum defect or the interatrial septum may not be clearly delineated on non-ECG-synchronized CT images. Sinus venous defects are frequently associated with

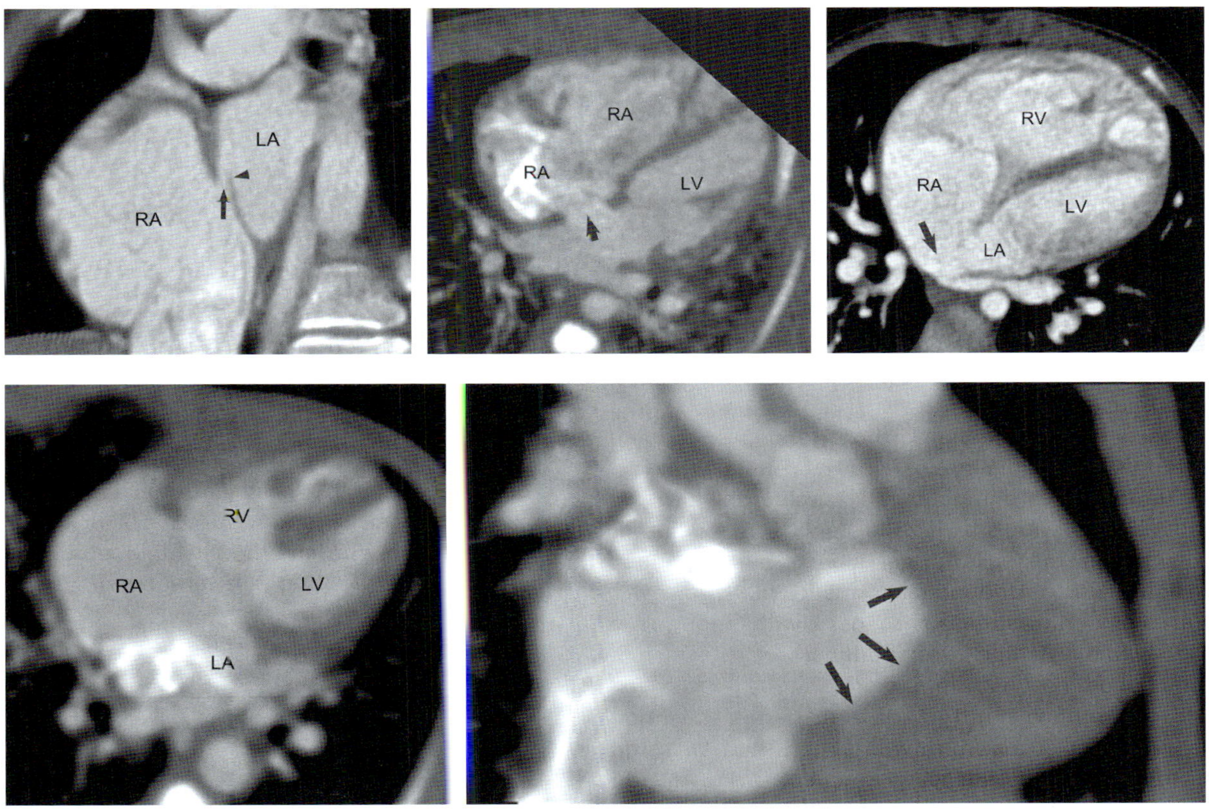

Figure 3.6 Various shunt lesions at the levels of the atrial and atrioventricular septa. (a) Patent foramen ovale (arrow) is identified between the superior septum secundum and the inferior septum primum. A short free flap valve (arrowhead) is noted, which predisposes to free bidirectional shunt. (b) Secundum atrial septal defect (arrow, ASD) is seen around the fossa ovalis with clear borders of the defect. (c) Sinus venosus defect (arrow) involves the posterior part of the interatrial septum. Thus, the posterior atrial surface is entirely smooth due to the absent posterior interatrial groove. The degree of enlargement of the right cardiac chambers is greater than that of a usual secundum ASD due to a greater shunt resulting from a combined partial anomalous venous return in addition to a large sinus venosus defect. (d, e) In this case, the atrioventricular septal defect (AVSD) is a compete type involving the septum primum, the atrioventricular septum, and the inlet part of the interventricular septum. In addition, the interatrial septum is almost absent. On an en-face view in (e), a typical "scooped" appearance of the defect (arrows) is nicely illustrated. LA, left atrium; LV, left ventricle; RA, right atrium; RV, right ventricle.

partial anomalous pulmonary venous connection. There is no discernible posterior interatrial groove in the sinus venosus defect (Figure 3.6). A left-to-right or right-to-left shunt through PFO or ASD can be shown as a contrast jet on MDCT images [11–13].

Atrioventricular Septal Defect

The atrioventricular septal defect (AVSD) presents with a wide range of abnormalities involving the atrioventricular septum. Typically, the defects are divided into partial and complete forms depending on the presence of interventricular communication in addition to primum ASD. Ventricular component of the defect involves the inlet portion accounting for its typical scooped appearance (Figure 3.6). Other cardiac anatomic features associated with AVSD include unwedged aorta at the base of the ventricles, shortened left ventricular inlet, elongated left ventricular outlet responsible for the so-called gooseneck deformity, and more closely opposed papillary muscles of the left ventricle [3]. Because of a greater shunt through the defect, patents with AVSD are more vulnerable to pulmonary vascular disease and a larger amount of contrast agent is needed to achieve sufficient cardiovascular enhancement at CT.

Ventricular Septal Defect

The ventricular septal defect (VSD) is a defect or defects in the ventricular septum between the right and left ventricles. The ventricular septum consists of the membranous and muscular parts. The membranous part is immediately below the right and noncoronary cusps of the aortic valve (Figure 3.3). The muscular part is divided into the inlet, trabecular, and outlet components. The size of the defect has the greatest clinical impact and thus it should be always described. There are various classification systems for VSD. In a commonly used classification system after modifying the originally proposed system [14], VSDs are classified into perimembranous, juxta-tricuspid and non-perimembranous, doubly committed juxta-arterial, and muscular defects [1, 4, 5]. The perimembranous defect is the most common type involving the membranous part of the interventricular septum and variable extents, e.g., inlet extension, trabecular extension, outlet extension, or combination of them, of the adjacent muscular septum (Figure 3.7). The size and location of a VSD is well delineated on an en-face view (Figures 3.6 and 3.7). Septal aneurysm formation is frequently responsible for the spontaneous closure of a perimembranous VSD or a gradual reduction of shunt flow via the defect (Figure 3.7). This aneurysm-like pouch is formed by the adhesion of the tricuspid valve leaflet to the rim of a perimembranous defect. Another mechanism limiting a perimembranous defect is a prolapse of the aortic sinus toward the defect that leads to the development of aortic regurgitation.

In addition, a VSD may be developed by the malaligned outlet septum, the so-called malalignment defect. Anterior malalignment defect, a more common type, is observed in patients with tetralogy of Fallot (TOF) (Figure 3.7), while the posterior type may occur in association with coarctation of the aorta or interrupted aortic arch.

Coronary Arteries

The normal coronary artery consists of the right and left coronary arteries arising from the corresponding facing sinus of Valsalva separately. The right coronary artery is dominant in approximately 70% of cases by giving rise to the posterior descending artery and the posterolateral branch. The left anterior descending artery and the posterior descending artery run along the anterior and posterior interventricular grooves, respectively, while the right coronary artery and the left circumflex artery run along the corresponding atrioventricular groove. Detailed descriptions about side branches are the beyond the scope of this chapter.

Anomalies and Clinically Important Anatomy

ECG-synchronized CT is the most accurate diagnostic imaging modality for coronary artery abnormalities. Various coronary artery anomalies that are more common in patients with congenital heart disease can be accurately characterized with MDCT (Figure 3.8) [9]. In addition to hemodynamically significant anomalies, it should be noted that hemodynamically insignificant anomalies and other variants may be clinically meaningful in patients with congenital heart disease (Figure 3.8) [9].

Typical Congenital Cardiac Defects

As in coronary arteries, cardiac anatomy can be accurately defined with ECG-synchronized CT. Consequently, MDCT is increasingly requested for characterizing common intracardiac defects including TOF, TGA, and DORV.

Tetralogy of Fallot

In TOF, the right ventricular outflow tract (RVOT) and the pulmonary arteries demonstrate variable degrees of obstruction and hypoplasia. Anterior malalignment VSD, the key pathology of TOF, results in infundibular narrowing, overriding of the aorta, and right ventricular hypertrophy (Figure 3.7) [1, 3–6, 15].

(a), (b) (c) (d), (e) (f)

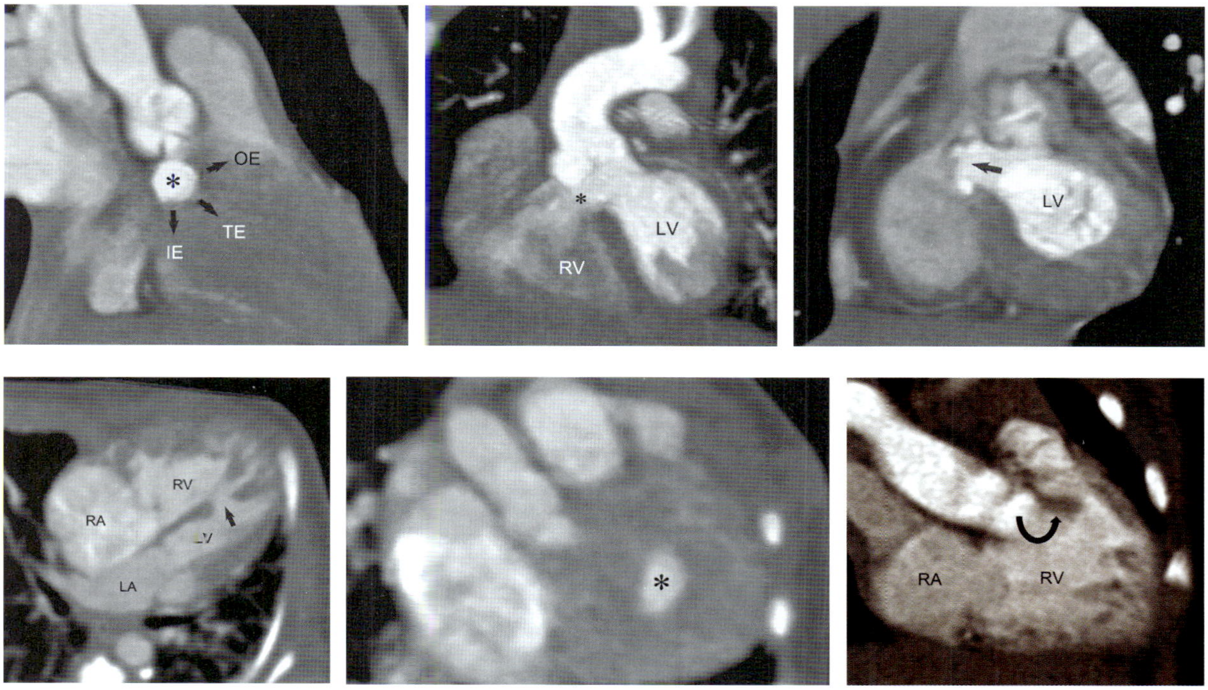

Figure 3.7 Various types of ventricular septal defect (VSD). (a–c) The location of a perimembranous VSD (asterisk in (a) and (b)) is demonstrated well on an en-face view. The defect always involves the membranous part of the interventricular septum and may show various extensions (arrows in (a)). A left-to-right shunt is seen as a contrast jet through the defect in (b). The tricuspid valve leaflet forms an aneurysm-like sac, the so-called septal aneurysm (arrow in (c)) for a perimembranous VSD. No shunt flow through the defect is observed at both CT and echocardiography. (d, e) Muscular VSD (arrow in (d) and asterisk in (e)) may be single or multiple and can be found in any parts of the muscular septum. The defect must be totally encircled by the myocardium ((e) reconstructed image through the muscular defect show the exact size of the defect). The morphologic evaluation of the defect with CT becomes important to assess the feasibility of VSD occlusion device. (f) In the anterior malalignment type of VSD, the outlet septum (arrow) is displaced in anterior and left directions, which results in right ventricular outflow tract (RVOT) obstruction. This type of VSD is typically encountered in patients with tetralogy of Fallot. Muscular hypertrophy of the anterior free wall of the RVOT also contributes to the infundibular narrowing. IE, inlet extension; LA, left atrium; LV, left ventricle; OE, outlet extension; RA, right atrium; RV, right ventricle; TE, trabecular extension.

(a), (b) (c)

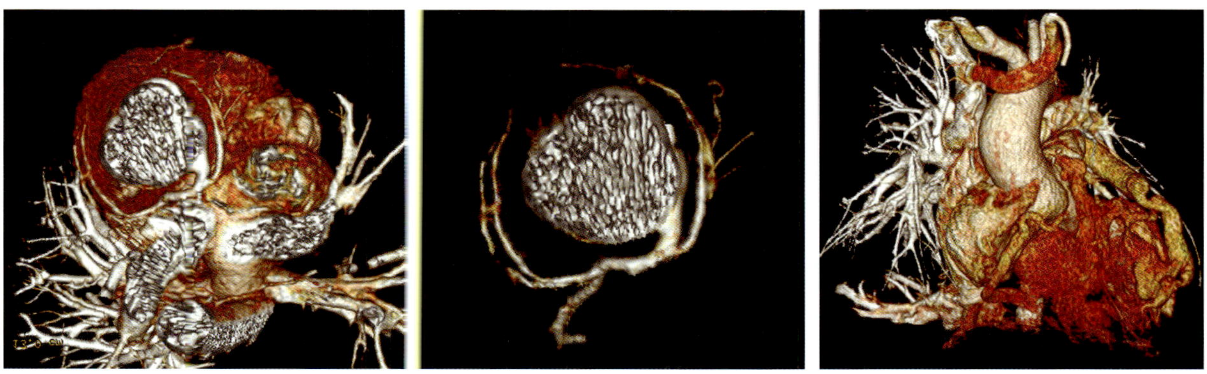

Figure 3.8 Coronary artery anomalies on CT images. (a, b) Single coronary artery is identified on MDCT images in a patient with functional single ventricle. (c) Volume-rendered CT image reveals extensive coronary artery fistulas, one of hemodynamically significant coronary artery anomalies, in a patient with pulmonary atresia and intact ventricular septum.

Transposition of the Great Arteries

TGA is ubiquitously characterized by ventriculoarterial discordance (Figure 3.5). Conotruncal and coronary artery anatomy should be accurately delineated prior to arterial switch operation, the most commonly performed operation for TGA repair. MDCT can be used to identify postoperative complications including coronary artery stenosis [16], dilatation of the switched great arteries, and outflow tract obstruction.

Double Outlet Right Ventricle

DORV is straightforwardly diagnosed by the definition in which both great arteries originate from the right ventricle (Figure 3.5). However, we should know that DORV is a collection of heterogeneous cardiac defects both anatomically and physiologically. DORV may have various anatomic relationships between the great arteries, and between VSD and the great arteries. These anatomic varieties result in various physiologic presentations ranging from VSD to TGA. MDCT may be helpful in planning surgical strategies by delineating these anatomic varieties [1,4–6,17].

References

1. Goo HW, Park IS, Ko JK *et al.* (2003) CT of congenital heart disease: normal anatomy and typical pathological conditions. *Radiographics* 23:S147–S165.
2. O'Brien JP, Srichai M, Hecht EM *et al.* (2007) Anatomy of the heart at multidetector CT: what the radiologists needs to know. *Radiographics* 27:1569–1582.
3. Freedom RM, Mawson JB, Yoo SJ *et al.* (1997) *Congenital Heart Disease: Textbook of Angiocardiography*. Futura, Armonk, NY.
4. Goo HW, Park IS, Ko JK *et al.* (2005) Computed tomography for the diagnosis of congenital heart disease in pediatric and adult patients. *Int J Cardiovasc Imaging* 21:347–365.
5. Leschka S, Oechslin E, Husmann L *et al.* (2007) Pre- and postoperative evaluation of congenital heart disease in children and adults with 64-section CT. *Radiographics* 27:829–846.
6. Sena L, Goo HW. (2008) Computed tomography in congenital heart disease. In Donoghue V. (ed.) *Radiological Imaging of the Neonatal Chest* (2nd revised edition), pp. 319–346. Springer, New York.
7. Weustink AC, Mollet NR, Pugliese F *et al.* (2008) Optimal electrocardiographic pulsing windows and heart rate: effect on image quality and radiation exposure at dual-source coronary CT angiography. *Radiology* 248:792–798.
8. Stolzmann P, Leschka S, Scheffel H *et al.* (2008) Dual-source CT in step-and-shoot mode: noninvasive coronary angiography with low radiation dose. *Radiology* 249:71–80.
9. Goo HW, Seo DM, Yun TJ *et al.* (2009) Coronary artery anomalies and clinically important anatomy in patients with congenital heart disease. *Pediatr Radiol* 39:265–273.
10. Goo HW, Park IS. (2007) Left ventricular noncompaction detected at non-ECG-gated heart CT in an infant. *Pediatr Radiol* 37:217–220.
11. Saremi F, Channual S, Raney A *et al.* (2008) Imaging of patent foramen ovale with 64-section multidetector CT. *Radiology* 249:483–492.
12. Kim YJ, Hur J, Choe KO *et al.* (2008) Interatrial shun detected in coronary computed tomography angiography: differential features of a patent foramen ovale and an atrial septal defect. *J Comput Assist Tomogr* 32:663–667.
13. Funabashi N, Asano M, Sekine T *et al.* (2006) Direction, location, and size of shunt flow in congenital heart disease evaluated by ECG-gated multislice computed tomography. *Int J Cardiol* 112:399–404.
14. Soto B, Becker AE, Moulaert AJ *et al.* (1980) Classification of ventricular septal defects. *Br Heart J* 43:332–343.
15. Wang XM, Wu LB, Sun C *et al.* (2007) Clinical application of 64-slice spiral CT in the diagnosis of the tetralogy of Fallot. *Eur J Radiol* 64:296–301.
16. Ou P, Celermajer DS, Marini D *et al.* (2008) Safety and accuracy of 64-slice computed tomography coronary angiography in children after the arterial switch operation for transposition of the great arteries. *JACC Cardiovasc Imaging* 1:331–339.
17. Chen SJ, Lin MT, Liu KL *et al.* (2008) Usefulness of 3D reconstructed computed tomography imaging for double outlet right ventricle. *J Formos med Assoc.* 107:371–380.

4 Mitral and Aortic Valves Anatomy for Surgeons and Interventionalists

Horia Muresian

San Donato Milan, Italy and University Hospital of Bucharest, Bucharest, Romania

The Position of the Valves

The atrioventricular and the ventriculoarterial junctions together with the corresponding valves lie in close contact, as readily apparent in short-axis views of the heart (Figure 4.1). However, only three of the four structures share a common fibrous sustain, and this latter structure is not an extensive fibrous skeleton as previously considered. In fact, the centrally located aortic root represents the anatomical element with which the other cardiac structures share more or less fibrous continuity. Thus, the left and the nonfacing leaflets of the aortic valve (and corresponding sinuses) share fibrous continuity with the anterior (hence, better called "aortic") leaflet of the mitral valve; the two thickened ends of this area are attached to ventricular musculature. The two thickened fibrous portions are the left and, respectively, the right fibrous trigones. The right trigone together with the adjacent membranous septum and with the tendon of Todaro—due to their collective conspicuous outline and location—constitutes the so-called *central fibrous body of the heart* (a clinical term, not homologated in the International Anatomical Nomenclature). This latter structure represents the only true fibrous portion of the tricuspid "*annulus*." The pulmonary valve leaflets are supported by musculature (the free-standing subpulmonary infundibulum). The attachments of the mitral valve leaflets follow the posterior extensions of the left and right fibrous trigones (*filia coronaria Henle*); however, incomplete structures in the posterior part in correspondence to the mural leaflet of the mitral valve. Roughly two thirds of the aortic root takes origin from the left ventricular musculature. Consequently, there is no fibrous skeleton of the heart comprising an aortic, mitral, or tricuspid "*annulus*," but only two major fibrous condensations (Figure 4.2).

Moreover, the four valvar orifices are not contained within the same plane, and their inflow–outflow axes are not parallel. In an *apical-to-basal* direction, the tricuspid valve is the most apical (*"the most inferior"*) of the four valves, followed by the mitral, the aortic, and the pulmonary valves, respectively. The mitral valve is also the most posterior, while the pulmonary valve the most anterior.

The Collective Description of the Mitral and Aortic Valves

There is a notable difference between the left ventricle and the right ventricle. In the left ventricle, the angle between the inflow and outflow compartments is acute, while in the right ventricle, this angle appears more open (i.e., between 45 and 60°). The right ventricle depicts a tubular shape and seems to wind around its left counterpart. Hence, the right ventricular inflow is widely separated from the outflow tract. The left ventricle appears more conical in shape, with the inflow and the outflow compartments adjacent, almost superimposed, and only transitory and functionally separated by the aortic leaflet of the mitral valve (Figure 4.3).

In the L-shaped right ventricle, the tricuspid and the pulmonary valves are separated. In the V-shaped left ventricle, the mitral and the aortic valves are adjoining structures: in fact, the base of the conical left ventricle has a double orifice bordered by an atrioventricular valve (mitral) and, respectively, by an arterial valve (aortic). The entire disposition of the left ventricle allows a more efficient active diastolic suction of blood and filling of the coronary arteries [1], and, respectively, a more efficient and forceful systolic ejection of blood. The tauter outline

Revisiting Cardiac Anatomy: A Computed-Tomography-Based Atlas and Reference, 1st edition. Edited by Farhood Saremi, Eloisa Arbustini, Stephen Achenbach and Jagat Narula.

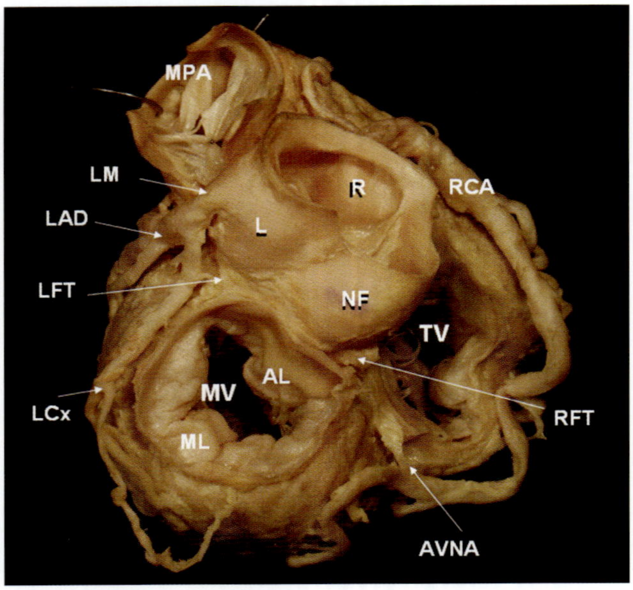

Figure 4.1 Basal view of a heart (from the top) specimen (analogous to the short-axis view). Note the central location of the aortic root with the three sinuses: R, right; L, left and NF, nonfacing ("noncoronary") and the two fibrous trigones (LFT and RFT). The left main (LM) coronary artery and its circumflex branch (LCx) wind around the mitral valve (MV) orifice; in an analogous manner, the right coronary artery (RCA) winds around the tricuspid valve (TV) orifice. The four heart valves are obviously not contained within the same plane and their inflow-outflow axes are not parallel. AL, aortic leaflet of mitral valve; AVNA, atrioventricular node artery; LAD, left anterior descending (the anterior interventricular branch); LFT, left fibrous trigone; ML, mural leaflet; MPA, main pulmonary artery; RFT, right fibrous trigone.

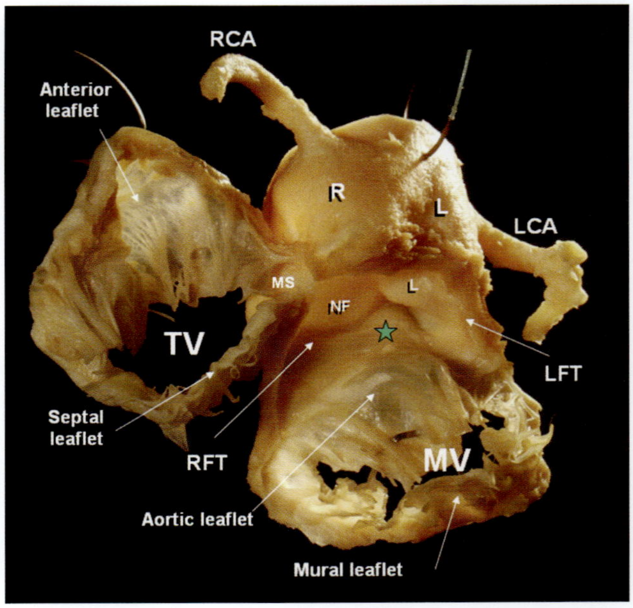

Figure 4.2 Apical and endoventricular ("*inferior*") view of the aortic root and associated structures. The aortic sinuses and corresponding leaflets are visible from below. The muscular portion of the aortic root skirts anteriorly from the membranous septum (MS) toward the left fibrous trigone (LFT). The remainder part is fibrous corresponding to the mitral-aortic curtain (green star) and to the aortic leaflet of the mitral valve (MV). The tricuspid "*annulus*" is of purely muscular nature except the area of the membranous septum (MS) between the anterior and the septal leaflets. L, left and NF, nonfacing ("noncoronary") aortic sinuses or leaflets; LCA, left coronary artery; R, right; RCA, right coronary artery; RFT, right fibrous trigone; TV, tricuspid valve.

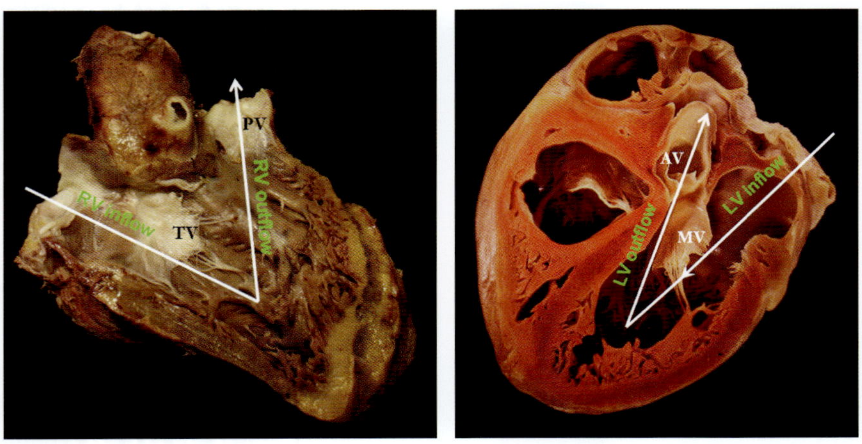

(a) (b)

Figure 4.3 A comparison between the disposition of the right and left ventricular inflow-outflow axes. Part (a) depicts the right ventricular side of the septum. The position of the tricuspid valve (TV) is suggested by the remnant septal leaflet of the tricuspid valve. The angle between the inflow and outflow portions is about 45–60°; the right ventricle (RV) has a more tubular shape and seems to wind around its left counterpart. Part (b) illustrates the disposition in the case of the left ventricle (LV). The angle between the two afore-mentioned compartments is acute with the aortic leaflet of the mitral valve (MV) interposed and actually belonging to both chambers that can be neatly separated only functionally during the phases of the cardiac cycle by the swinging aortic leaflet. AV, aortic valve; PV, pulmonary valve. (Reproduced with permission from Muresian H. (2009) The Clinical Anatomy of the Coronary Arteries. An Anatomical Study on 100 Human Heart Specimens. Ed. Enciclopedica).

of the left ventricular valves is readily apparent both at macroscopic as well as at microscopic level.

Because of its particular disposition and building, the mitral valve is not solely an atrioventricular valve, as it also takes part in the make-up and function of the left ventricular outflow tract and of the aortic root [2]. Consequently, the aortic leaflet of the mitral valve is not directly attached to the ventricular septum (although some false cords crossing the left ventricular outflow tract, indirectly attach the valve to the septum) [3].

The aortic leaflet of the mitral valve and the mitral-aortic curtain change their shape during the phases of the cardiac cycle, allowing on one hand, the passage of blood into the left ventricle, and on the other hand, the ejection of blood from the left ventricle [2]. Pathologic modifications of these particular structures impede either or both of the aforementioned processes, for example, the systolic anterior motion of the mitral valve, perforation of the aortic leaflet of the mitral valve, and of the mitral-aortic curtain in endocarditis or the development of pseudoaneurysm at this very level [4]. The anterior (i.e., aortic) portion of the mitral "*annulus*" is not immobile, as it folds away during left ventricular ejection. The adjacent intertrigonal portion of the mitral and aortic "annulus" represents a dynamic structure varying in size in response to changes in hemodynamic loading and ventricular contractility [5,6].

The mitral-aortic curtain continues with the interleaflet triangle between the left and nonfacing sinuses of the aorta; the anterior wall of the left atrium comes into contact with these structures from which it can be easily separated during the surgical act. The interleaflet triangle represents a portion of the left ventricular outflow tract in potential communication with the pericardial cavity [7,8]. Dissecting aneurysms of the aortic root can thus open either in the left or right atria, or in the pericardial cavity. The area of fibrous continuity allows the surgical enlargements of the aortic root; this area also carries the most hazards during percutaneous aortic valve plasty and replacement, as fracturing and tearing of this area may generate the same complications as above.

The Mitral Valvar Complex

The atrioventricular valves (mitral and tricuspid) are different from the arterial valves (aortic and pulmonary) in their constitution and physiology. The former are highly asymmetric structures having a septal and a mural leaflet and a well-developed subvalvar apparatus. The latter have a more symmetrical tripartite outline (though not perfectly symmetrical) with the three leaflets suspended in a particular milieu consisting of the corresponding sinuses, interleaflet triangles, commissures, and the

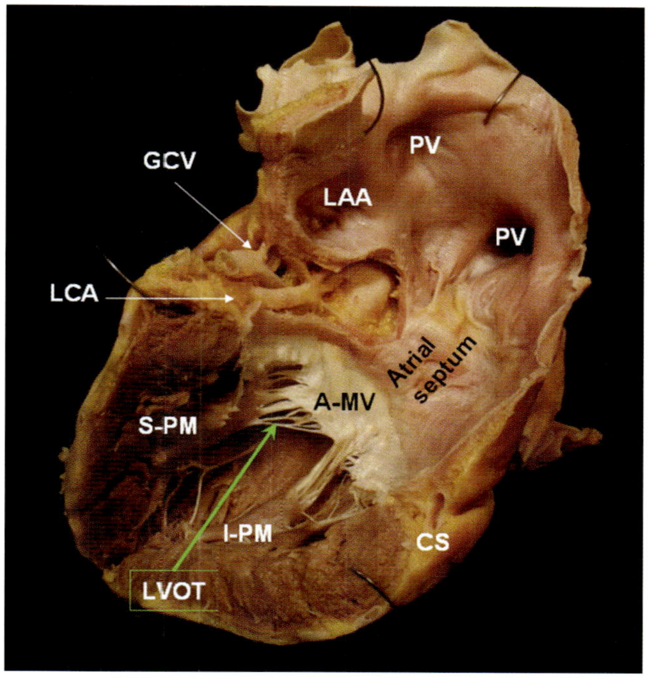

Figure 4.4 Left view of a heart specimen opened along its left aspect. All the components of the mitral va var complex are visible. Note the actual position of the papillary muscles (PM): superior (S) ("*anterolateral*") and inferior (I) ("*posteromedial*"). The relationship with the great cardiac vein (GCV), the left coronary artery (LCA), the left circumflex artery, and the coronary sinus (CS) are of clinical and surgical relevance (see text for details). LAA, left atrial appendage. LVOT, left ventricular outflow tract; PV, pulmonary veins. (Reproduced with permission from Muresian H. (2009) The Clinical Anatomy of the Coronary Arteries. An Anatomical Study on 100 Human Heart Specimens. Ed. Enciclopedica).

coronet-shaped insertion of the leaflets themselves—together forming the arterial root. The function of the arterial valves depends mostly on hemodynamic factors.

It is more appropriate to consider the atrioventricular valves (mitral and tricuspid) together with their adjacent interdependent elements that form the so-called valvar complex [9]. *The mitral valvar complex* (Figure 4.4) includes the valve leaflets, "*the annulus*," the subvalvar apparatus (cords and papillary muscles), the endocardium of the left atrium and left ventricle, the left atrial myocardium, the left ventricular myocardium, and the mitral-aortic curtain (Table 4.1). All these elements must function in a coordinated manner. Moreover, the concept of an active valve has recently emerged [10].

The Mitral Valve Leaflets

The valve leaflets form a continuous structure, however, divided from didactic and practical reasons into an anterior and posterior portion. The anterior leaflet skirts

Table 4.1 The mitral valvar complex

Valve leaflets	Aortic leaflet Mural leaflet
Subvalvar apparatus	Papillary muscles Tendinous cords
Mitral-aortic curtain Endocardium* Left atrial myocardium Left ventricular myocardium	

*The endocardium represents a continuous structure sheathing the interior of the left atrium, of the left ventricle, being continued over the valve leaflets and over the elements of the subvalvar apparatus.

between the two fibrous trigones, occupying roughly one third of the circumference. Because of its location and physiologic roles, it is more correct to be designated as *the aortic leaflet of the mitral valve*. The remainder two thirds of the mitral circumference gives origin to the posterior leaflet, a scalloped structure, generally consisting of three uneven portions. Going around the circumference of the mitral valve and following the disposition of the posterior leaflet, this is found to skirt actually from the lateral to the posterior and partially septal portions of the "*annulus*"; thus, the more correct denomination is *the mural leaflet of the mitral valve*. The two leaflets coapt along a solitary zone of apposition, which however does not extend to reach the "*annulus*," in a similar way to the clefts between the scallops of the mural leaflet. The valvar commissures are no more than the ends of this zone of apposition. The clefts and commissures act as pleats, allowing the sphincteric mechanism characteristic to the mural leaflet, which closes the mitral orifice by abutting against the elevated aortic leaflet in ventricular systole [11]. The mural leaflet bears higher systolic stress is narrower than the aortic leaflet and gets additional cordal support. In spite of their different shape and length of circumferential insertion, the mitral aortic and mural leaflets share similar areas [9,12].

Each leaflet has a thinner clear zone and a tauter rough zone, a peripheral insertion, and a free margin. The valve leaflets coapt at the level of their rough zones with the free margins located underneath the annular plane. The resultant *coaptation triangle* [2] can be accurately measured; its surgical restoration is *sine qua non* of the mitral plasty procedures. The mural leaflet has an additional basal zone, reinforced by the basal cords and left atrial myocardium. The mitral leaflets overlap between 6 and 8 mm toward the central portion of the valve; *the coaptation surface* can be precisely quantified during ultrasound interrogation and should also be included in the routine measurements performed after mitral valve repair.

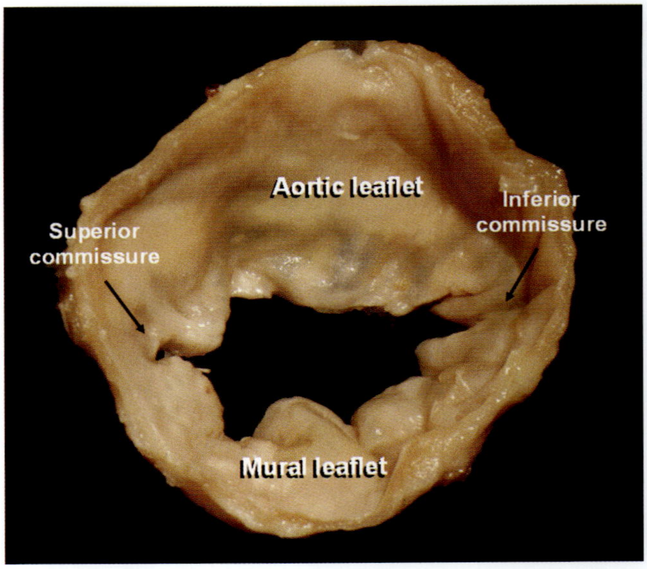

Figure 4.5 The mitral leaflets form a continuous structure; the commissural and cleft areas depicting a concave free margin and narrower leaflet material—functioning as pleats and allowing the sphincteric mechanism of the valve. The valve is funnel-shaped and the aperture between the leaflets has an ovoid shape.

The valve normally appears as funnel-shaped and this disposition becomes even more evident in case of mitral stenosis (Figure 4.5). The precise measurement of the anatomic mitral aperture is mandatory during ultrasound interrogation, as the cutting level may not be positioned at the level of the minimal mitral aperture if not aided by the Doppler examination by which the area of maximal turbulence can be located. The passage of blood takes place not only through the aperture between the mitral leaflets but also through the so-called *secondary spaces*, i.e., between the cords and the papillary muscles. The anatomical area indicates the mitral orifice; the functional area (as determined by the pressure half time parameter) measures the passage of blood through the main and through the secondary orifices; the two parameters are thus not identical but must be, however, similar in the given patient (Figure 4.6).

In the most accepted and currently used classification of the valve leaflets [13], each scallop of the mural leaflet is designated as P1, P2, and P3 starting from the left trigone and proceeding in a counter clockwise direction toward the right fibrous trigone—for reasons of terminological consistency, the denomination followed here is M1, M2, and M3. Although the aortic leaflet is an undivided structure, three corresponding portions can be analogously assigned to it, A1, A2 and A3—in relation with each of the three scallops of the mural leaflet. This classification makes sense not only because it follows the ultrasound planes of section but also because the papillary and cordal sustain

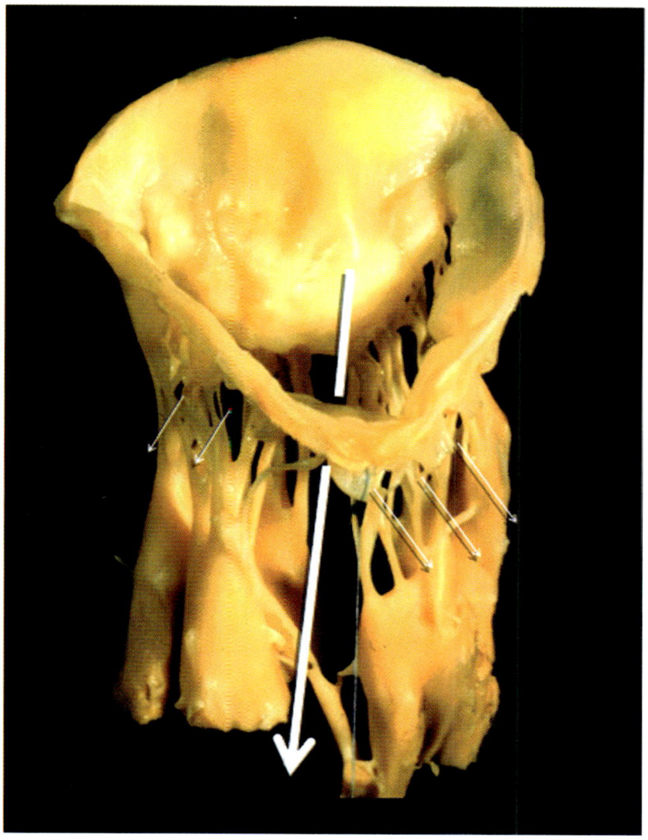

Figure 4.6 The funnel-shaped disposition of the mitral valve is again apparent. The figure depicts the main orifice (i.e., between the valve leaflets) and the secondary spaces (i.e., between the cords and the papillary muscles) that are normally traversed by the blood. Cordal and papillary muscle agglutination (as in mitral stenosis) or papillary muscle hypertrophy (as in hypertrophic cardiomyopathy), significantly reduce these spaces.

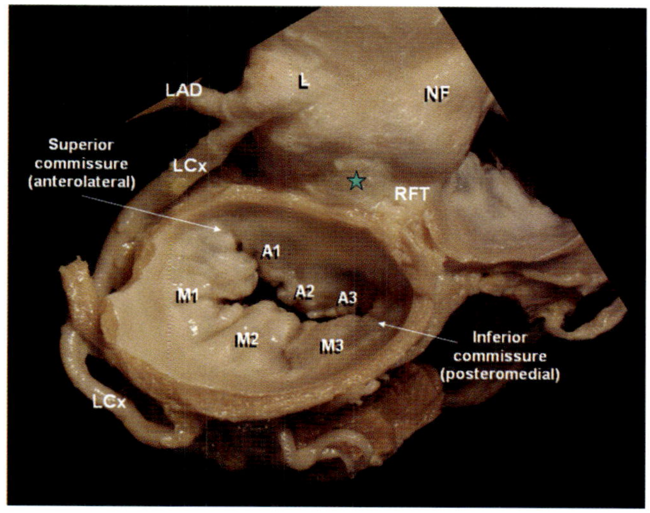

Figure 4.7 Left atrial ("superior") view of the mitral valve in closed position depicting the scallops of the mural leaflet (M1–M3). A1–A3 are the corresponding portions of the aortic leaflet, in spite of the fact that it is an undivided structure. Note also the not straightforward classification of the scallops of the mural leaflet: between the M1 and M2 scallops, there is an accessory scallop. If this latter one should be named as M1, then, the larger remaining scallop must be labeled as "*commissural cusp*." Or else, the mural leaflet must be defined as having four scallops. The confusing terminology and subsequent contradictory classifications can be, however, settled in the surgical setting, following the corresponding cords and their insertions, as well as the disposition of the papillary muscles. Blue star, Mitral-aortic curtain; L, left coronary sinus; LAD, left anterior descending artery; LCx, left circumflex artery, NF, nonfacing coronary sinus; RFT, right fibrous trigone.

is distributed to complementary portions of the two mitral leaflets, i.e., those portions that will directly coapt in ventricular systole. Consequently, three pairs of scallops result allowing a more precise quantification of the severity of mitral prolapse and insufficiency on a scale ranging from 1 out of 6 to 6 out of 6 scallops (1/6–6/6) [14] (Figure 4.7). Commissural prolapse when present must be mentioned, as this is of surgical relevance too. The doubtful existence of the so-called *commisural cusps* is of no practical value, only adding more ambiguities and confusion [15].

The Left Atrioventricular Orifice: The Mitral "Annulus"

There is no definite structure as a "*ring*" or "*annulus*" at the level of the atrioventricular junction. The fibrous tissue extending posteriorly from the left and right trigones is largely replaced by myocardium [16], while the anterior intertrigonal area is completed by the mitral-aortic curtain. Ultrasound interrogation identifies the annulus at the valvar hinge and precise measurements revealed the existence of a nonplanar structure, in fact a hyperbolic paraboloid having the "lowest" points at the level of the commissures [17]. During surgery, a transition between the whitish endocardium and the brownish myocardium is usually visible indirectly defining the position of the "*annulus*." However, disease processes may alter all these landmarks hindering or making more difficult the precise localization of the "*annulus*." Discordant findings regarding annular dimensions, form and dynamics, appear to be the result of the different methods of measurement [18]. Moreover, in mitral regurgitation the "*annulus*" dilates and flattens.

Neither "*ring*" nor "*annulus*" correctly define the atrioventricular orifice, as this latter structure appears ovoid or D-shaped (but not circular): the longer of the diameters joins the two commissures, while the shorter connects the aortic midpoint with the mural midpoint of the mitral orifice. The former is currently referred to as the *intercommissural diameter* (C-C), while the latter is called

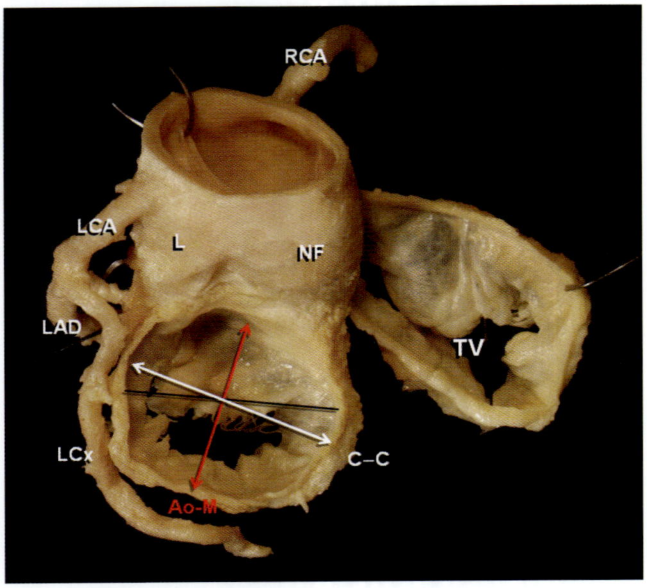

Figure 4.8 The axes of the mitral orifice. Note the ovoid shape of the mitral orifice ("*annulus*") and the position of the commissural areas with the specimen in anatomically correct orientation. Thus, the septal-to-lateral diameter black line) skirts closer to the intercommissural diameter (C-C; white double headed arrow). Consequently, it is more correct referring to the aortomural diameter (Ao-M; red double headed arrow), i.e., the line joining the midpoints of the aortic and mural leaflets. The normal values are given in text. L, left coronary sinus; LAD, left anterior descending artery; LCA, left coronary artery; LCx, left circumflex artery; NF, nonfacing coronary sinus; RCA, right coronary artery; TV, tricuspid valve.

septal-to-lateral diameter (S-L); in fact the septal-to-lateral diameter skirts closer to the intercommissural one, as depicted in Figure 4.8. It is thus more correct referring to the *aortomural diameter* (Ao-M). Body-weight corrected data pertaining to these dimensions are 0.39–0.59 mm/kg (C-C) and, respectively, 0.32–0.48 mm/kg (Ao-M) [19]. The proportion between the two diameters must be restored in mitral valve repair procedures, as orifice circumference reduction alone will not prevent mitral insufficiency [20]. The intercommissural diameter roughly corresponds to the diameter as determined in two-chamber view, while the aortomural diameter roughly corresponds to the diameter in three-chamber view [21].

The area of the mitral orifice depicts complex changes in shape during the phases of the cardiac cycle. *The sphincteric mechanism* designates the 23–40% systolic-to-diastolic variation in annular circumference [22]. *The excursion* or *annular descent* is the movement in apical-to-basal direction. The annular excursion volume strongly correlates with the left ventricular stroke volume [23]. *The rotation* indicates the torque movement of the left atrioventricular junction, while the complex three-dimensional modifications in shape are called *folding of the annulus*. All these changes in shape are diminished or abolished in disease or after surgery especially with the use of rigid annuloplasty rings, with extensive reduction of the mural leaflet, or with conspicuous postoperative fibrosis. The aortic (anterior) intertrigonal portion corresponding to the mitral-aortic curtain also changes in response to modifications in hemodynamic loading and left ventricular contractility [5].

The mitral orifice ("*annulus*") establishes significant anatomical relationships with important elements. Proceeding from the left fibrous trigone toward the atrial septum, the circumflex branch of the left coronary artery and the greater cardiac vein mark the external position of the annulus. After passing underneath the left atrial appendage (left auricle) and after receiving the oblique vein of the left atrium (Marshall), the great cardiac vein becomes the coronary sinus. On its way toward the right atrium, the coronary sinus receives important venous tributaries among which veins of the left aspect of the heart, the middle cardiac vein (posterior interventricular vein), and in some cases, the lesser cardiac vein. At the point of junction with these veins and at the level of its entrance into the right atrium, the coronary sinus has valves that sometimes can impede the retrograde passage of catheters. The retrograde coronary sinus route is used in electrophysiology for left ventricular stimulation and during surgery for the retrograde delivery of cardioplegia. The presence of a Chiari network can impede such maneuvers or entangle catheters [24]. Both the coronary sinus and the circumflex branch can be distorted or injured during surgery after substantial excision of the mural leaflet and extensive reduction of the annulus or with the too deep insertion of stitches. Lesions of the coronary sinus are as severe as those of the circumflex branch. Removal of conspicuous calcifications of the posterior annulus can be also hazardous, as the thinner portion of the posterior left ventricle can be easily torn and as such lesions are very difficult to repair. In such cases, the insertion of a supra-annular mitral prosthesis is indicated. The coronary sinus is usually located in a more atrial position ("*superior*") with respect to the circumflex branch as the great cardiac vein crosses either the left anterior descending or the circumflex branch (or both), either superficial or deep—in order to get its definitive position in the coronary sulcus where it will become the coronary sinus [25–27]. The crossing point(s) is (are) relevant for percutaneous mitral ring annuloplasty, as the ring may distort the circumflex branch [21]. Again, the concept of a "*mitral annulus*" might be more misleading than of any real clinical or surgical value.

A physiologic balance exists among the area of the mitral orifice ("*annulus*"), the total area of the leaflets, and the aperture between the leaflets. Annular area values superior to 2.3 cm^2/m^2 BSA are accepted as normal. Reflecting the funnel-shaped outline of the valve, the total area of the leaflets is 1.5–2 times the annular area. The difference between the two parameters appears in the coaptation surface (the systolic amount of leaflet overlapping)—an important element in mitral repair procedures that must be surgically restored and that can be adequately measured by intraoperative transesophageal echocardiography or during the postoperative follow-up of the patient. The aperture between the valve leaflets is normally ovoid in shape and measures roughly two thirds of the annular area [27]. The aperture becomes crescent-shaped in mitral stenosis or after rigid ring annuloplasty and fixation of the mural leaflet. In the case of particular mitral repair procedures, such as *the edge-to-edge technique*, the aperture becomes a double orifice, usually consisting of two asymmetric orifices. Ultrasound interrogation must allow the distinction between the two new apparently stenotic mitral orifices and an actual obstruction of blood flow—in a valve rendered competent by this technique.

The proportion between total leaflet area on one hand and the area of the annulus on the other is of surgical relevance: excessive, redundant leaflet material would inevitably lead to systolic anterior motion of the aortic leaflet and obstruction of the left ventricular outflow tract; the reverse will manifest as poor coaptation.

The Mitral Subvalvar Apparatus: Cords and Papillary Muscles

The mitral subvalvar apparatus represents the reciprocal connection between the valve leaflets and the ventricular wall; it depicts great individual variability in shape, disposition, and dimensions. As a consequence, numerous classifications have been elaborated during the time, aiming toward a more straightforward and practical categorization.

The papillary muscles belong to the trabecular system of the left ventricle. Their origin and vascularization is difficult to be neatly differentiated from those of the adjoining left ventricular wall and parietal trabeculae. Indeed, as evident in ischemic cardiac disease or in cardiomyopathies, a dysfunction of the papillary muscles actually represents a dysfunction of the neighboring left ventricular wall.

The papillary muscles continue unperceivable with the tendinous cords; the degree of cordal development displays also numerous variations even in the same individual. Muscular cords in the adult heart are considered as remnants of the embryological process during which the muscular tissue is being replaced by fibro-elastic elements toward the valve leaflets. Such muscular cords may lodge aberrant conduction pathways—a purported cause for dysrhythmias and sudden cardiac death [28–31]. The tendinous cords contain a central (inner) portion composed of tightly-bound collagen enclosed by an outer portion consisting of looser connective and elastic tissue and blood vessels: the latter have an alleged additional nutritional role for the leaflets [32]. The complex three-dimensional disposition of the collagen and elastic fibers offers both resistance and elasticity to the cords, with either of the two qualities prevailing with the type of cord considered (the strut cords bear the greatest tensional stress) and with the phase of the cardiac cycle (maximal tension is reached just prior to the ventricular systole) [33]. Nevertheless, an amount of tension is always present in the cords.

The cords proceed within the very substance of the valve leaflets, giving support to the fibrous framework of the latter. Some of the cordal extensions may reach the fibrous trigones and the peripheral portion of the leaflets ("*the annulus*"). Numerous fascicles intermingle in an arch-like manner and form the valvar rough zone. The more peripherally situated clear zone of the leaflets is traversed by some radially oriented cordal extensions. The contribution of each individual cord to leaflet support and to the fibrous framework of the leaflet is particularly variable, and hence, the significance of a cordal lesion is also highly different from individual to individual (Figure 4.9). Moreover, before reaching the leaflets, most cords give off ramifications toward the valvar-free edge, the rough zone, or between these. A more practical classification of the tendinous cords is offered in Table 4.2.

The complex disposition of the tendinous cords contribute not only to the internal fibrous framework of the valve leaflets but they also outline some hemodynamically significant *external* arrangements such as the gutter formed between the cords and their arch-like insertions on the ventricular aspect of the aortic leaflet—a structure that constitutes an important portion of the left ventricular outflow tract [35] (Figure 4.10).

In a similar way to the strings of a parachute, the mitral subvalvar apparatus must ensure on one hand, a circumferentially constant support of the leaflets and on the other; it must allow the passage of blood from the left atrium and inflow compartment of the left ventricle toward the outflow tract of the latter. The tendinous cords are arranged in groups traceable to the underlying papillary muscle heads or fascicles; some papillary muscle structures stand as clearly individualized and prominent elements within the cavity of the left ventricle. Others depict a bas-relief shape and sustain most of the basal cords of the mural leaflet. There are numerous individual variations of the papillary muscle heads which no classification so far can entirely encompass. Some constant features can be however revealed. Thus, each of the main papillary structures lies in relation to a valve commissure; additional secondary heads or fascicles correspond to the clefts of the mural leaflet. Tendinous cords originating from the very tip of the papillary muscles proceed

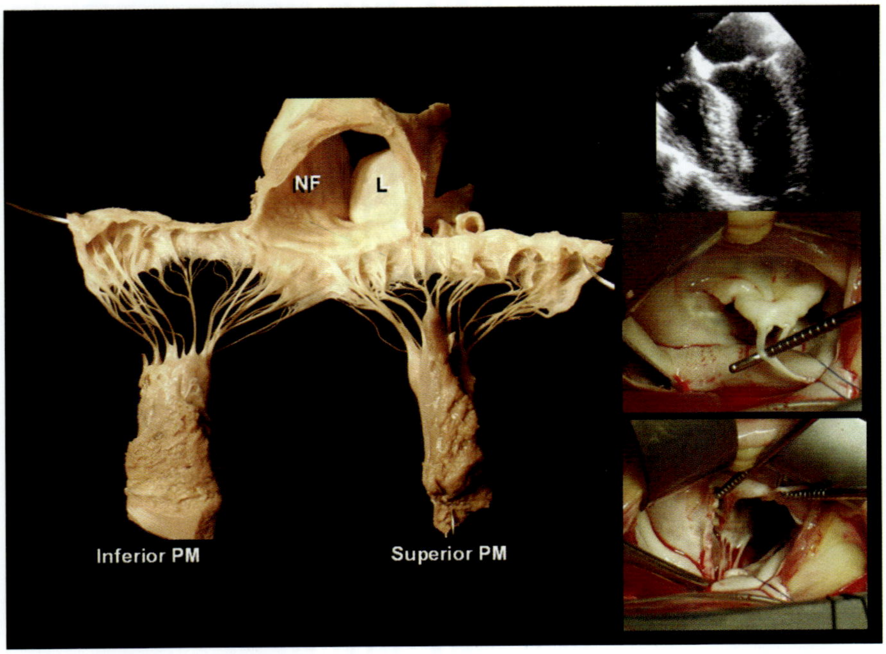

Figure 4.9 The individual variations of the cordal disposition and the contribution of each cord to the fibrous framework of the leaflets can explain the protean manifestations in disease. This example (right panels) illustrates the prolapse of the A2 scallop because of rupture of corresponding cords having origin only at the level of the inferior (*"posteromedial"*) papillary muscle (PM). The entire A2 was sustained by cords originating in the inferior muscle, thus envisaging the significance of the natural asymmetry of the mitral valve and the need for a precise diagnostic workup in the individual patient. L, left coronary sinus; NF, nonfacing coronary sinus.

toward the commissure or cleft and divide in a fan-like manner to sustain also the adjacent area possessing a concave free margin. Each of the remainder portions of the mitral valve leaflets depicting a convex free margin (i.e., the portions that will coapt with their rough zones) are sustained by tendinous cords originating from two different papillary muscle heads/fascicles (Figure 4.11). All the afore-mentioned papillary muscle heads are not isolated but grouped in a very individualized manner, giving the impression of the existence of two, three, or even more papillary muscles. However, a clear distinction is difficult to accomplish in most cases. The two papillary muscles represent both the ends of the more or less continuous column of papillary structures sustaining the mitral leaflets and that through a gap between them and underneath the aortic leaflet, allow the passage of blood toward the left ventricular outflow tract.

The classical denomination of *anterolateral* and, respectively, *posteromedial* papillary muscle bears more a clinical than an anatomical significance. Indeed, the anterolateral wall of the left ventricle is quite differently shaped and vascularized, as compared with the posteromedial (posteroseptal) wall. From a strictly anatomical point of view, the *anterolateral* papillary muscle group is actually located *superior*, posterior, parietal, and to the left with respect to the *posteromedial* muscle that is situated *inferior*, anterior, septal, and to the right (Figure 4.12). Consequently, the more useful terms *superior* and *inferior* indicating the true anatomical position of the papillary muscles in man, should be adopted by the surgeon and interventionalist should be implemented. The corresponding commissures take analogous names [2].

Particular Elements of the Mitral Valve: Commissures and Mitral-aortic Curtain

The commisural and the cleft areas of the mitral valve represent the narrower portions of the valve with a concave free margin, thinner leaflet material, and reduced

Table 4.2 Practical classification of the mitral tendinous cords

Type of cord	Major role	Equivalent term
Marginal cord	Essential for leaflet coaptation	First-order cord
Rough zone cord	Essential for maintaining leaflet geometry	Second-order cord
Strut (sustain) cord	Essential for maintaining the ventricular geometry [34]	Third-order cord
Basal cord	Reinforcement of the mural leaflet and posterior *"annulus"*	

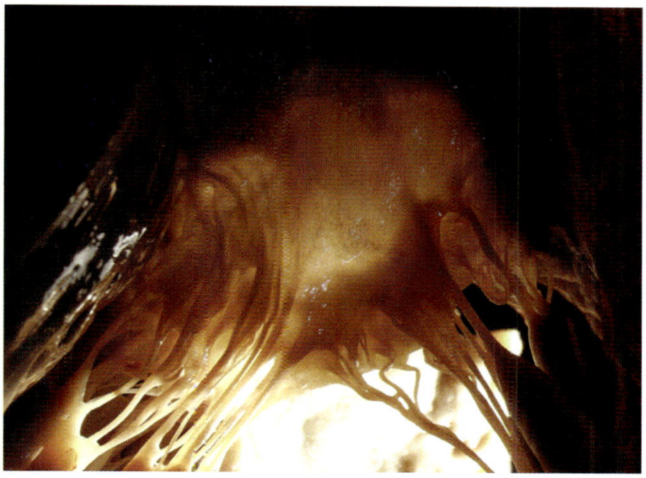

Figure 4.10 Endoventricular view of the aortic leaflet of the mitral valve. The arches and steps delineated by the cords inserting on the leaflet, collectively shape a hemodynamically important gutter that constitutes a portion of the left ventricular outflow tract.

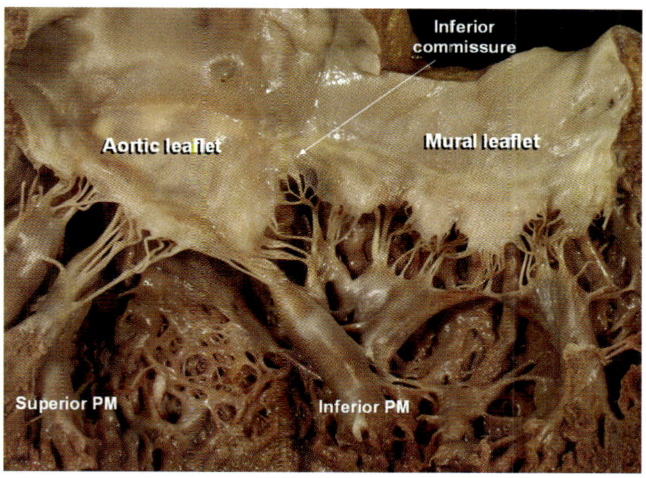

Figure 4.11 An overall view of the mitral valve opened at the level of the superior commissure. Both the superior and the inferior papillary muscles (PM) are constituted by more fascicles (heads). Note that the commissural and cleft cords originate in a muscular fascicle (head) located just underneath; the cords diverge as they approach these areas having a concave free margin. On the contrary, the portions of the mitral valve that will coapt in systole by apposition of their rough zones depict a convex outline and are sustained by cords originating in different papillary muscles fascicles (heads). Every scallop of the mural leaflet can be imagined from this point of view as a mini-aortic leaflet. Note the presence of four scallops of the mural leaflet in this specimen. The approximate location of the "*annulus*" is suggested by the transition between the whitish endocardium sheathing the leaflets and the brownish endocardium covering the left atrium. The intimate relationship among the papillary muscles, the left ventricular trabecular system, and the left ventricular wall proper is of clinical and surgical relevance. PM, papillary muscle.

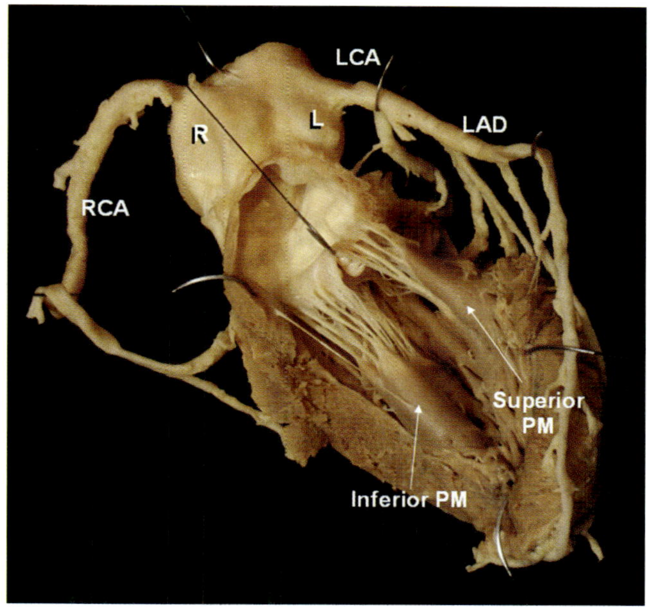

Figure 4.12 Advanced dissection of the left ventricle. The right heart chambers were removed; only the right coronary artery (RCA) being kept in its original position. The exact spatial disposition of the papillary muscles (PM) is depicted as "in situ." The anterolateral PM is in fact located superior, posterior, parietal, and to the left. The posteromedial PM is located inferior, anterior, septal, and to the right. Note also the details of the vascularization of the superior PM from branches originating in the left anterior descending (LAD) artery: diagonal and septal branches. Compare with figure 4.15. L, left coronary sinus; LCA, left coronary artery; R, right coronary sinus.

cordal sustain. The corresponding underlying cord divides dichotomously or in a fan-like manner before reaching the commissure (cleft). The submacroscopic arrangement of the commissures suggest their normal action during the phases of the cardiac cycle with alternating opening–closing movements, analogous to a fan, allowing these particular areas of the mitral valve to function as pleats and to adapt the valvar circumference to the systolic and, respectively, to the diastolic configuration of the valve. The disease processes changing either the mobility of the leaflets or their thickness alter the physiologic movements at commissural level favoring the scissoring stresses. Such stresses have a major impact on the commissures leading to earlier commissural involvement in disease. In mitral stenosis, the leaflets still maintain a degree of mobility during the earlier phases of the disease, while the modifications at commissural level are pregnant depicting fusion, calcification, and ulceration. The classical mitral commissurotomy is addressing this very stage of the disease. Only in the later stages of the disease, the valve becomes fibrosed or calcified as a whole (Figure 4.13). Higher than normal leaflet mobility—as encountered in fibro-elastic deficiency—especially at the level of

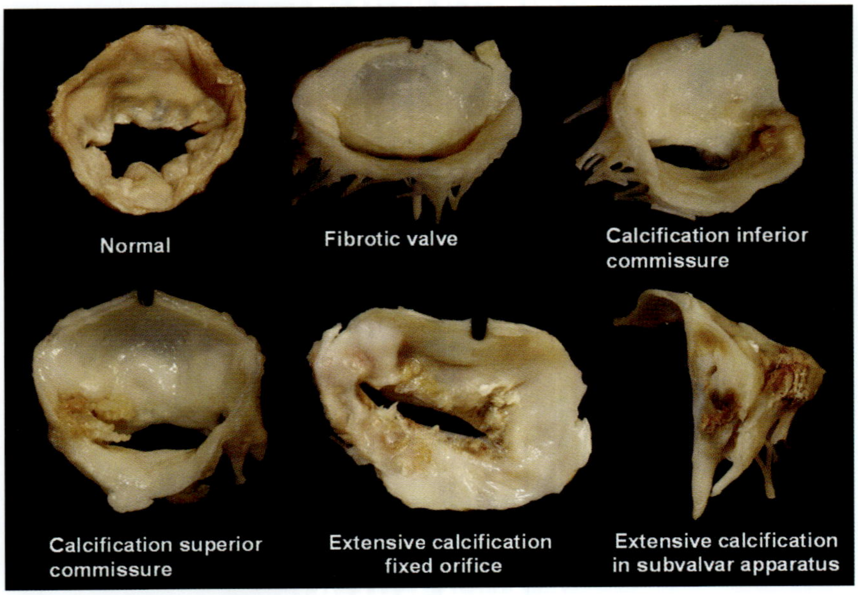

Figure 4.13 Pathologic changes in mitral stenosis. Excised valvar specimens depicting the natural evolution of the disease as compared with the normal disposition. The valve becomes fibrotic in the early stages of the disease (valve repair, plasty, are still possible). Scissoring stresses at the level of the commissures may be responsible for the earlier involvement of these areas. The natural asymmetry of the mitral valve may explain the predominant involvement of one of the commissures (more frequent the inferior commissure). At a later stage, both commissures will become involved; the valve eventually becomes rigid with a fixed orifice. The pathologic process and especially calcification will usually extend to the subvalvar apparatus, asking for more complex surgical repair techniques or directly indicating the mitral replacement.

the para-commissural scallops (A1 and M1 or A3 and M3) are accompanied by commissural prolapse or tearing.

In an analogous manner, scissoring stresses over the commissures may develop after mitral valve plasty, when only the aortic leaflet preserves its mobility, closing against a fixed mural leaflet. This particular might explain the premature failure of such techniques.

The mitral and the aortic valves share a common fibrous area called the mitral-aortic curtain. The curtain continues the aortic leaflet of the mitral valve and imperceptibly merges with the interleaflet triangle between the left and nonfacing sinuses of the aortic root. From this point of view, the curtain can be included among the elements of the fibrous framework of the heart. Being located at the border among the left atrium, the left ventricular outflow tract, and the aortic root, the curtain bears significant clinical relevance. The curtain may be involved in morbid conditions affecting the mitral valve, the aortic root, and valve: stenosis, calcification, endocarditis, perforation, and development of pseudoaneurysm. Endocarditis lesions with dehiscence of the aortic and mitral *"rings"* occur at this very level and surgical reconstruction represents a challenging procedure. Incisions through the curtain performed for aortic root enlargement must not proceed too deep into the aortic leaflet of the mitral valve, as this will alter the normal function of the latter.

The Normal Asymmetry of the Mitral Valve

The mitral valve depicts an asymmetric outline. The scallops of the mural leaflet are unequal and the central M2 scallop cannot be imaginary divided in two symmetrical portions. Both the aortic and the mural leaflets cannot be divided in two even segments. The two commissures also depict significant differences: the inferior (*"posteromedial"*) commissure has a longer circumferential length, and it is narrower as compared with the superior (*"anterolateral"*) commissure. The papillary muscle and the cordal support are also not symmetrically distributed over two imaginary halves of the valve. Such obvious dissimilarities can be frequently encountered in clinical practice and during surgery (Figure 4.14). Consequently, the superior (*"anterolateral"*) section of the valve is not the mirror imagine of the inferior one (*"posteromedial"*).

The complex actions of a normally asymmetric mitral valvar complex obviously ask for further clarifications and investigations [36, 37]. Indeed, beyond the macroscopic anatomical details relevant for the afore-mentioned asymmetry, there is also a physiologic regional nonuniformity of the left ventricle with a higher contribution to the endocardial ejection fraction of the inferior (*"posteroseptal"*) wall as compared with the lateral one [38].

The Vascularization of the Mitral Valve

The valve leaflets and the tendinous cords are considered avascular structures as blood vessels are not normally contained in their structure. Only the basal zone of the mural leaflet incorporates left atrial myocardium and associated small vessels. Valve leaflets get their nutrition and oxygenation by imbibition from neighboring structures possessing vascularization. Blood vessels in the tendinous cords may have additional nutritional role especially for

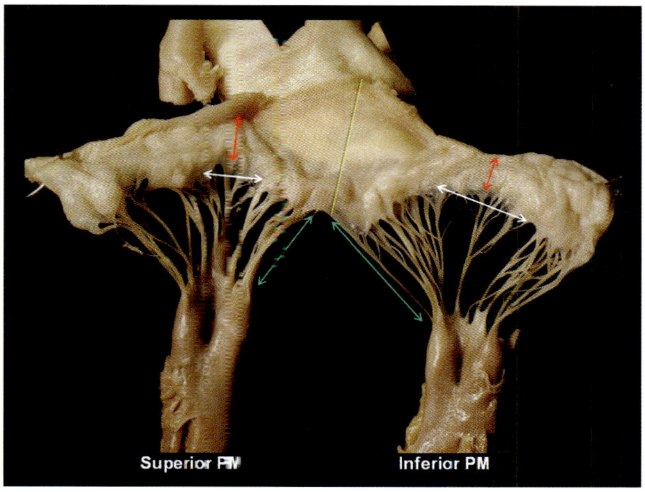

Figure 4.14 The natural asymmetry of the mitral valve. The valve cannot be divided in two even portions (imaginary yellow line at the level of the aortic leaflet). The inferior commissure (as compared with the superior one) has a longer circumferential length (white double-headed arrow) and narrower leaflet material (red double-headed arrow). Cords from the inferior papillary muscle (PM) are longer and more slender as compared with the cords from the superior papillary muscle (green double-headed arrows). See also text for details.

the aortic leaflet. The particular metabolism of the leaflets and tendinous cords permits numerous surgical procedures such as partial leaflet resection and suturing, cordal transfer, cordal reinsertion, etc.

The vascularization of the papillary muscles is closely related to that of the corresponding left ventricular walls depends on the coronary arterial typology and dominance and depicts numerous individual variations (Figure 4.15). Posteroinferior branches with origin in either or both coronary arteries vascularize the posteroinferior wall of the left ventricle, the inferior aspect of the septum, and the inferior papillary muscle group. Several arterial branches contribute to the vascularization of this particular area of the heart; moreover, the so-called *posteromedial* papillary muscle (i.e., inferior) is usually represented by numerous fascicles and their blood supply is not dependent on only one arterial source as previously thought (H. Muresian, 2006, personal communication). Ischemic injury of the inferior papillary muscle reflects the alterations and damages at the level of the posteroinferior left ventricular wall.

The superior papillary muscle group and the adjoining area of the left ventricular wall are usually vascularized by several arteries having their origin in the left anterior descending, diagonal, intermediate, or obtuse marginal branches. In some cases, however, a single conspicuous artery can represent the sole blood supply of this area of the left ventricle and the superior ("*anterolateral*") papillary muscle can become infracted even after the occlusion of a single diagonal branch [39].

Ischemic mitral regurgitation recognizes several conditions:

- Papillary muscle rupture, occurring with small myocardial infarctions, requiring mitral valve replacement and bearing a high risk and mortality;
- Acute myocardial infarction with normal global left ventricular function but with regional abnormalities

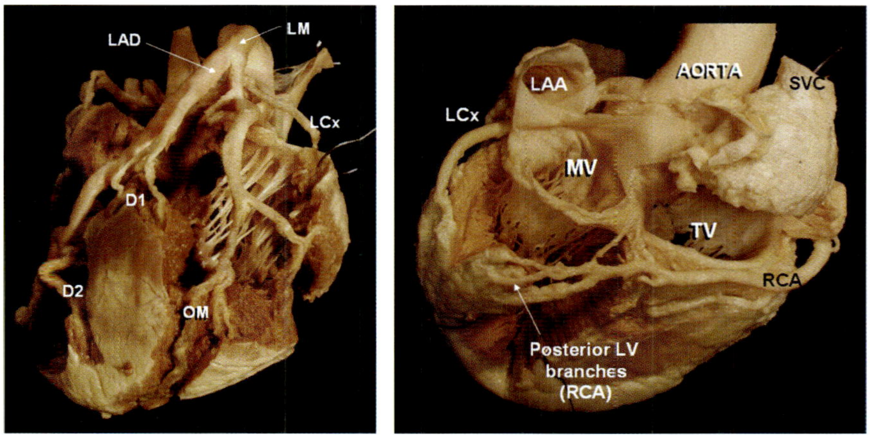

Figure 4.15 The vascularization of the papillary muscles. (a) Vascularization of the superior ("*anterolateral*") papillary muscle and adjacent left ventricular wall is accomplished by branches originating in the left anterior descending (LAD) artery (the first diagonal in this specimen) and the obtuse marginal (OM) branch. (b) Vascularization of the inferior ("*posteromedial*") papillary muscle and adjacent wall of the left ventricle. Note that these structures are located at the border zone between the territories of the left and right coronary arteries—being in fact the most distal coronary territory (i.e., the most distal from the aortic origin and the most distal as order of bifurcations). This area is more prone to ischemic dysfunction, and its vascularization depends more on coronary typology and anastomoses. D, diagonal branch; LAA, left atrial appendage; LCx, left circumflex; LM, left main; MV, mitral valve; RCA, right coronary artery; SVC, superior vena cava; TV, tricuspid valve.

(hypo- or akinesia), causing impaired mitral valve closure and regurgitation;

- Chronic ischemic disease, with normal resting left ventricular function and ischemia with exercise, producing mitral regurgitation or even flash pulmonary edema;
- End-stage ischemic disease, with remodeled ventricle, alterations of the ventricular geometry and distortion of the valvar apparatus. The increased tethering of the valve leaflets due to papillary muscle displacement generates mitral regurgitation even after mitral ring annuloplasty, consequently requiring more elaborate surgical procedures such as ventricular restoration or papillary muscle sling or repositioning.

Papillary muscle ischemia and ischemic dysfunction actually designate ischemia and dysfunction of the left ventricular wall—the two structures being interdependent from the anatomical and functional points of view.

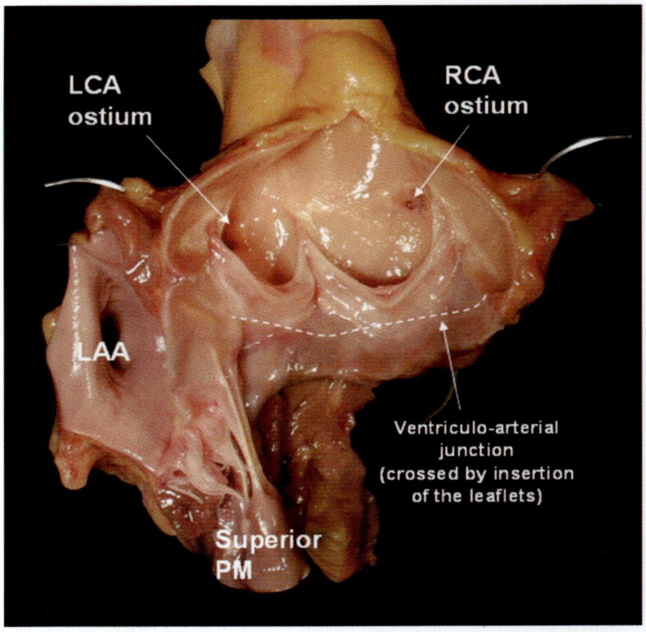

Figure 4.16 The muscular portion of the aortic root, as it appears on a fresh heart specimen, in correspondence with the right and the left sinuses. The anatomical ventriculoarterial junction is apparent only at the level of the muscular portion; this landmark is crossed by the insertion of the aortic valve leaflets. Two of the three interleaflet triangles are evident in this specimen. LAA, left atrial appendage; LCA, left coronary artery; PM, papillary muscle; RCA, right coronary artery.

The Aortic Root

The junction between the left ventricle and the tubular aorta is represented by the aortic root—a complex and particular structure that must receive the blood volume ejected by the left ventricle and assure its progression through the aortic system, preventing in the mean time its backflow into the ventricle. A complex valvar system and associated sinuses have developed at this level. The left ventricle ejects the blood into an already filled aorta, where the blood column is kept at a high pressure. The aortic root with its sinuses must therefore distend in order to accommodate the extra volume of blood and must assure its progression by elastic recoil and by transmission of the pulse wave in distal direction. Moreover, the aortic root must allow the systolic-diastolic rotating movements of the heart with respect to the relatively fixed aorta. On the other hand, the high energy of the ejected blood and the to-and-fro and torque movements of the cardiac base require the aortic root to be well attached to the ventricular mass. The aortic root appears thus as an elaborate system of interdependent elements, asking for a detailed presentation.

A prominent landmark is to be found at the distal limit of the aortic root and its "junction" with the ascending aorta proper: *the sinotubular junction* (supravalvar crest in the International Anatomical Nomenclature). The distal insertion of the aortic valve leaflets is located at this very level. The connection between the left ventricular myocardium and the aortic fibro-elastic tissue is represented by *the anatomical ventriculoarterial junction*. This landmark is apparent only in correspondence with the muscular portion of the aortic root (Figure 4.16).

The semilunar attachment of the three aortic valve leaflets skirts between the sinotubular junction and an area under the anatomical ventriculoarterial junction; the circle joining these lowest points is traditionally known as "the basal ring" although this notion designates an inexistent structure [8] still used, however, in the absence of a distinct proximal limit of the aortic root. The attachments of the aortic leaflets represent the hemodynamic ventriculoarterial junction, the pressure profile distal to it being characteristically aortic, while proximal to it, typically ventricular. The remnants of the leaflets are then used by the surgeon so as to anchor prostheses used to replace the diseased valve. It is these semilunar remnants that the surgeon then describes as "*the annulus*" [8].

The valve leaflets are enclosed by three corresponding sinuses, possessing distensibility in radial and longitudinal directions. The walls of the sinuses are primarily composed of elastic tissue and are thinner than the walls of the ascending aorta [40]. The aortic valve leaflets and sinuses are usually named according to the origin of the coronary arteries although the most pertinent and useful nomenclature is offered by the so-called Leiden convention [41] and will be followed here (Figure 4.17) Table 4.3.

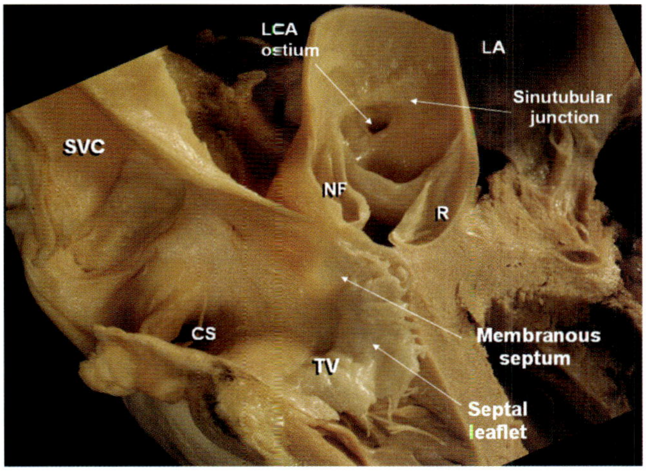

Figure 4.17 Anatomical relationships of the aortic root and of its main components. In this oblique section through the heart, the central location of the aortic root is readily apparent. The interleaflet triangle between the nonfacing (NF) and the right (R) aortic sinuses is in direct relationship with the membranous septum. The triangle of Koch corresponds to the area below the ostium of the coronary sinus (CS) and above the insertion of the septal leaflet of the tricuspid valve (TV). The bundle of His travels below the membranous septum. This latter structure is partly covered by the septal leaflet of the tricuspid valve. Only the atrioventricular portion of the membranous septum is evident in this picture. The interleaflet triangle between the right and the left aortic sinuses corresponds to the muscular portion of the aortic root and it represents a relatively safe area that can be used for root enlargement procedures. The third interleaflet triangle (between the left and nonfacing sinuses of the aorta) corresponds to the mitral-aortic curtain and is not evident in this picture (compare with Figure 4.2 and 4.8). LA, left atrium; LCA, left coronary artery; SVC, superior vena cava.

The valve leaflets depict a concave outline possess a fibrous layer (the fibrosa) toward the aortic aspect and an underlying layer of loose connective tissue (the spongiosa) toward the ventricular aspect. Both surfaces are covered by endocardium. Similar to the mitral valve, the leaflets of the aortic valve do not coapt with their free margins;

Table 4.3 Systematic classification of the sinuses of the aortic root*

Numeric nomenclature (Leiden)	Nomina Anatomica	Actual disposition in the adult heart
1	Right	Anterior
2	Left	Left posterior
Nonfacing	Posterior/noncoronary	Right posterior

*Adapted from Muresian [42].

instead, the free margins are located above the line of closure, are thinner (the so-called *lunulas*), may be fenestrated, and usually contain a collagenous aggregation (the node of Arantius). The systolic dilation of the aortic root with the consequent straightening of the valve leaflets and the inertia of the free margins provided by the presence of the nodes of Arantius, and the vortices created in the sinuses minimize the fluttering of the valve leaflets during ventricular ejection and prevent the valve leaflets from contacting the wall of the aortic root.

Because of its central location, the aortic root establishes important anatomical relationships with almost all the cardiac elements (Figures 4.1–4.3). The least covered part is the left aortic sinus (sinus 2).

The three *interleaflet triangles* are the remainder portions of the aortic root and represent extensions of the ventricular cavity in potential communication with the pericardial cavity. The triangles are composed mostly of fibrous tissue and represent the less distensible and less extensible portion of the aortic root anchoring the root to the tauter part of the left ventricular base. However, dilation of the triangles occurs in disease (annuloectatic disease or aortic aneurysm) and the basal portion of the aortic root including the triangles needs to be stabilized in aortic valve repair procedures (e.g., T. David procedure as compared with Yacoub technique).

Each of the three interleaflet triangles establishes particular anatomical relationships of clinical relevance (Figures 4.7 and 4.17). Thus, the interleaflet triangle between the nonfacing and the right aortic sinuses is continued in apical direction by the membranous septum. This area can be recognized in the living patient as corresponding to the normally occurring gap between the septal and the anterior leaflets of the tricuspid valve. The insertion of the valve leaflets divides the membranous septum into an atrioventricular and an interventricular portion. From the area of the triangle of Koch, the bundle of His courses below the membranous septum. The same pathway is followed by the atrioventricular node artery; distortion or interruption of this artery can occur in mitral valve surgery and especially when the artery originates in the left coronary artery [43,44]. The triangle between the left and the nonfacing aortic sinuses is in direct continuity with the mitral-aortic curtain and with the aortic leaflet of the mitral valve. The triangle between the left and the right aortic sinuses directly overlies the muscular portion of the aortic root. This is the safest area for performing incisions necessary for enlargements of the aortic root as in the Konno procedure or for the myotomy–myectomy operation (the Morrow procedure).

The origin of the *two coronary arteries* is located at the level of the right (sinus 1) and, respectively, of the left (sinus 2) aortic sinuses. Numerous anatomical variations and anomalies have been reported during the time, both in otherwise normal hearts as well as in congenitally malformed hearts [45]. Minor variations are, however, frequently encountered, regarding the origin of the coronary arteries with respect to the sinotubular junction (e.g., distal to this landmark) or with respect to one of the valve commissures. Although innocuous by themselves, such minor variations can render difficult, impede, or even contraindicate some surgical maneuvers. The precise identification of the coronary arterial origin and proximal tract is mandatory in redo operations on the aortic root and valve. The main trunk of the left coronary artery can depict various lengths up to its absence, rendering difficult the antegrade delivery of cardioplegia or the reimplantation of the left coronary button. The accessory right coronary artery (conspicuous conal/infundibular branch or the so-called *third coronary artery*) may originate either from the very proximal portion of the right coronary artery or from the right aortic sinus (sinus 1) and should be identified and preserved during surgery. At times, its mobilization prior to reimplantation of the right coronary trunk is mandatory as it may contribute to the kinking of the latter. The origin of either coronary artery from the nonfacing sinus of the aorta represents a rare event, usually associated with more complex cardiac malformations [46].

The aortic root represents the connecting structure interposed between the left ventricle and the aorta proper. At the proximal level, there is no neat demarcation between the ventricular structures and the aortic root. Moreover, the adjoining mitral valve and the presence of shared elements renders the picture even more complex—both from a strictly anatomical as well as from a functional point of view, with significant consequences in disease:

- Redundant mitral aortic leaflet with systolic anterior motion (SAM) and obstruction of the left ventricular outflow tract;
- Mitral stenosis with fibrosis and calcification encompassing the mitral-aortic curtain and adjacent aortic leaflets, and consequent aortic insufficiency;
- Aortic or mitral valve endocarditis extending to the adjacent valve and ring abscess or significant annular destruction;
- Aortic or mitral disease with heavy calcification involving the conduction tissue and heart block;
- Hypertrophic cardiomyopathy with jet lesions on the aortic leaflets plus SAM; and
- Aortic valve stenosis with calcifications extending into the mitroaortic curtain and aortic leaflet of the mitral valve (Figure 4.18).

The distal limit is represented by the sinotubular junction. Effacement of the sinotubular junction induces aortic valve insufficiency and its surgical restoration represents one of the main steps in aortic valve repair procedures.

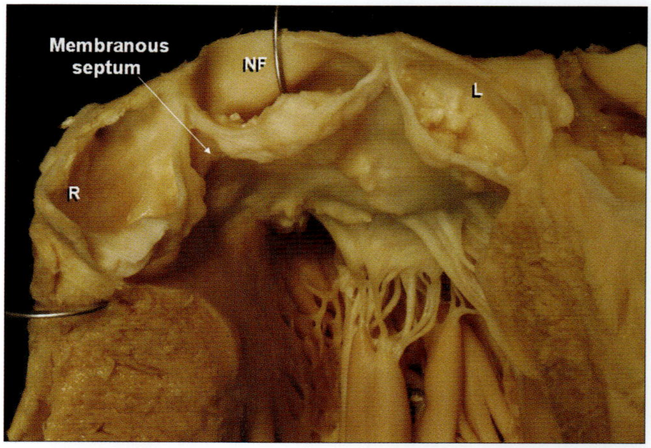

Figure 4.18 Disease processes affecting the adjacent mitral and aortic valves. This picture shows the extension of aortic valve calcifications into the aortic leaflet of the mitral valve, and not least, into the area of the membranous septum—explaining the development of heart block in these disease states. Similarly, infective endocarditis can lead to devastating lesions involving both left-sided heart valves, requiring challenging surgical techniques. L, left; NF, nonfacing aortic sinuses are shown; and R, right.

On the other hand, the proximal dilation of the aortic root as in annuloectatic disease will also produce aortic insufficiency. A proper ratio must be maintained between the diameters of the sinotubular junction and the "*basal ring*," as evident in aortic valve repair procedures or root replacement using the homograft or the pulmonary autograft (Ross procedure) [47].

The aortic root depicts a natural asymmetry with static differences between the three sinuses R>NF>L [48] and with different distensibilities: R>L>NF [49]. The ensuing "aortic tilt angle" was measured in humans (5.47°; anatomic study) and experimentally in sheep ($16.3 \pm 1.5°$ in diastole and $6.6 \pm 0.5°$ in ventricular ejection). The tilt angle diminishes during the ejection period, probably facilitating the ejection of blood; during diastole, the tilt angle increases, probably reducing the leaflet stress. The new artificial substitutes for the aortic root are currently under experimentation as the preserved aortic leaflets must be suspended and work in the most suited physiological milieu as possible. The naturally occurring asymmetry of the pulmonary root also dictates the proper mode of its insertion when used in aortic position [50,51].

The arterial roots (aortic and pulmonary) are adjacent structures, sharing only a limited portion of the septum (the outlet septum). Incisions performed at this level as for example in the Konno procedure [47] may easily lead to the outside of the heart if the strict anatomic landmarks are not followed.

The Vascularization of the Aortic Root

The aortic root represents a heterogeneous structure possessing a larger anterior muscular portion (roughly two thirds of the circumference), while being of a fibrous nature in the remainder posterior part in relation with the mitral valve (roughly one third of the circumference). The muscular segment of the aortic root actually represents the most distal part of the left ventricular outflow tract and is vascularized by the anterior and posterior septal branches with origin in the left, right, or both coronary arteries. Small collateral branches of the arteries vascularizing the left atrium travel across the mitral aortic curtain following the insertion of the left atrial myocardium. The aortic sinuses are vascularized by recurrent branches originating in the main coronary trunks or from their atrial [52] or infundibular branches [53] (Figure 4.19) (Table 4.4). The arterial branches originating in the right coronary artery vascularize both the aortic and pulmonary roots. The arteries to the aortic root can easily bleed with extensive dissection and such bleeding may resemble an anastomotic leak [47] after aortic root replacement or reimplantation of the coronary buttons. Incisions for enlargement of the aortic root performed at the level of the fibrous portion as in the Nicks [54] or Manouguian procedures [55] interfere very little with the vascularization of the aortic root. Aortoventriculoplasty—the Ross-Konno procedure [56]—requires ampler incisions in the muscular portion of the aortic root and septum with interruption of one or more septal arteries; the clinical consequences are still difficult to predict especially in the case of pediatric patients depending also on the number and caliber of the arteries interrupted.

The Normal Functioning of the Mitral and Aortic Valves

The mitral and the aortic valves constitute a dual structure located at the base of the left ventricle allowing both the inflow and, respectively, the proper outflow from the left ventricle; the valves share a common fibrous portion. Their measurable dimensions are related and correspond to the body shape and surface area [57]. The valves are richly innervated and contain contractile elements [58,59] providing for an active role, beside the well-known and well-documented passive flap role. Adjacent elements and tissues assist in the normal physiology of the mitral valve: almost 90% of annular reduction occurs before the ventricular systole on behalf of the left atrial myocardium [60] *"annular"* myocardial ablation does not lead to annular dilation but to delayed valve closure occurring at higher left ventricular pressures [61].

The mitral valve leaflets coapt by the apposition of their rough zones. Coaptation occurs "below" the level of the mitral *"annulus"*; the resultant coaptation triangle can be accurately measured and must be surgically restored in the mitral repair procedures. *The tenting volume* correlates better with the severity of functional mitral regurgitation as occurring in ischemic or dilated cardiomyopathy [62].

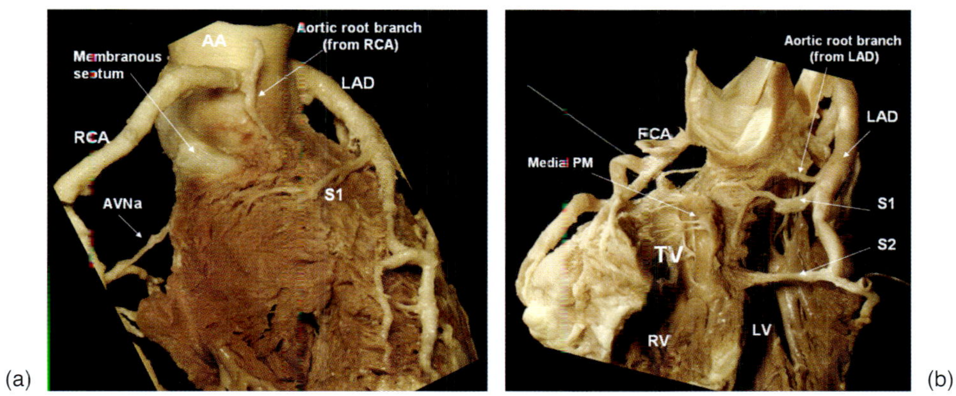

Figure 4.19 The vascularization of the aortic root. While the fibrous portion of the aortic root is relatively less vascularized by the contribution of small and inconstant arterial vessels (see text for details), the muscular portion of the aortic root is vascularized by important and more constant branches. Part (a) illustrates the contribution of the first septal artery (S1), the atrioventricular node artery (AVNa), and a branch from the right coronary artery (RCA)—together with their corresponding territories of vascularization below the right and the left aortic sinuses. The branches from the RCA frequently have a common origin with the right infundibular branches. Part (b) illustrates contributions of the first two septal arteries (S1 and S2) and an accessory branch arising directly from the left anterior descending (LAD) just below the interleaflet triangle between the right and left aortic sinuses (in this specimen, the three sinuses were scalloped and only the interleaflet triangles are visible. The coronary buttons are detached as in aortic root replacement procedures). Note also the contribution of the first septal arteries to the vascularization of the medial papillary muscle (PM) of the tricuspid valve (TV). AA, ascending aorta; LV, left ventricle; RV, right ventricle.

Table 4.4 Arterial vascularization of the aortic root*

Origin of the arterial branches to the aortic root	Characteristics	Territory vascularized R, L and NF†	Additional notes
Right coronary artery	Vessels of variable diameter	R	Constant
Accessory right coronary artery	May have a common origin with the right posterior infundibular artery	R	Constant
Right sinoatrial branch	May anastomose with the atrioventricular node artery and with the left sinoatrial branch (when present)	R, NF	Inconstant
Left coronary artery (main trunk or origin of the left anterior descending branch)	Minute branches; variable number and caliber	L	Inconstant
First and second anterior septal arteries	Conspicuous branches	R, L (partially) and the area of the outlet septum	Constant
Atrioventricular node artery	Minute branches	Area close to the membranous septum	Constant
Posterior septal arteries	Minute branches	Diaphragmatic aspect of the septum	Inconstant

*Adapted from Muresian [42].
†R, L, and NF indicate the right, left, and nonfacing aortic sinuses and the corresponding areas of the aortic root.

The mechanisms of normal valve closure are complex and still incompletely understood. The major processes are annular reduction (the sphincteric mechanism) followed by the apposition of the mural leaflet against the elevated aortic leaflet (that functions as a trap door), reduction of all left ventricular dimensions, and the subsequent creation of a pressure gradient between the ventricle and atrium that eventually brings the leaflets toward the annular plane. Many interesting details are emerging, including the contribution of the left ventricular architecture and contraction characteristics, the spatial disposition of the trabeculae and papillary muscles.

The mitral-aortic curtain represents a flexible element interposed between the left ventricular inflow and outflow compartments. The anterior intertrigonal distance also represents a dynamic structure. The normal function of the aortic valve depends more on hemodynamic factors but, however, in the context of adjacent anatomical components that together constitute the aortic root. The synchronous dynamic physiology of the aortic and mitral valves has recently been revealed with changes occurring in a reciprocal fashion [6]. *The aortomitral angle* changes during the cardiac cycle although such changes are not mediated through the anatomic fibrous continuity. Post-surgical excessive reduction of the aortomitral angle predisposes to systolic anterior motion of the mitral valve.

The left-sided heart valves depict characteristics related to the particular hemodynamic conditions in the systemic division of the circulation. Besides their tauter appearance and the higher pressure gradients these elements must experience, the mitral and the aortic valves are intimately coupled both from an anatomical as well as from a functional point of view—asking for a more elaborate clinical approach and requiring further investigation as well.

References

1. Davies JE, Whinett ZI, Francis DP *et al.* (2006) Evidence of a dominant backward-propagating "suction" wave responsible for diastolic coronary filling in humans attenuated in left ventricular hypertrophy. *Circulation* 113:1768–1778.
2. Muresian H. (2009) The clinical anatomy of the mitral valve. *Clin Anat* 22:85–98.
3. Loukas M, Louis RG Jr, Black B, Pham D, Fudalej M, Sharkees M. (2007) False tendons: An endoscopic and cadaveric approach. *Clin Anat* 20:163–169.
4. Espinosa-Caliani JS, Montijano A, Melero JM, Montiel A. (2000) Psuedoaneurysm in the mitral-aortic intervalvular fibrosa. A cause of mitral regurgitation. *Eur J Cardio Thorac Surg* 17:757–759.
5. Parish LM, Jackson BM, Enomoto Y, Gorman RC, Gorman JH 3rd. (2004) The dynamic anterior mitral annulus. *Ann Thorac Surg* 78(4):1248–1255.
6. Timek TA, Green GR, Tibayan FA *et al.* (2003) Aorto-mitral annular dynamics. *Ann Thorac Surg* 76(6):1944–1950.
7. Sutton JPI, Ho SY, Anderson RH. (1995) The forgotten interleaflet triangles: a review of the surgical anatomy of the aortic valve. *Ann Thorac Surg* 59:419–427.
8. Anderson RH. (2000) Anatomy: clinical anatomy of the aortic root. *Heart* 84:670–673.

9. Ho SY. (2002) Anatomy of the mitral valve. *Heart* 88(Suppl 4):iv5–iv10.
10. Williams TH, Jew JY. (2004) Is the mitral valve passive flap theory overstated? An active valve is hypothesized. *Med Hypotheses* 62:605–611.
11. Victor S, Nayak VM. (1994) Definitions and functions of commissures, slits and scallops of the mitral valve. Analysis of 100 hearts. *Asia Pacific J Thorac Cardiovasc Surg* 3:10–16.
12. Roberts WC, Perloff JK. (1972) Mitral valvular disease. A clinicopathologic survey of the conditions causing the mitral valve to function abnormally. *Ann Intern Med* 77:939–975.
13. Carpentier A, Branchini B, Cour JC *et al.* (1976) Congenital malformations of the mitral valve in children. Pathology and surgical treatment. *J Thorac Cardiovasc Surg* 72:854–866.
14. Muresian H, Diena M, Cerin G, Filipoiu F. (2006) The mitral valve: new insights into the clinical anatomy. *Maedica* 1:5–12.
15. Kumar N, Kumar M, Duran CM. (1995) A revised terminology for recording surgical findings of the mitral valve. *J Heart Valve Dis* 4:70–75.
16. Angelini A, Ho SY, Anderson RH, Davies MJ, Becker AE. (1988) A histological study of the atrioventricular junction in hearts with normal and prolapsed leaflets of the mitral valve. *Br Heart J* 59:712–716.
17. Levine RA, Handschumacher MD, Sanfilippo AJ *et al.* (1989) Three-dimensional echocardiographic reconstruction of the mitral valve, with implications for the diagnosis of mitral valve prolapse. *Circulation* 80:589–598.
18. Timek TA, Miller DC. (2001) Experimental and clinical assessment of mitral annular area and dynamics: what are we actually measuring? *Ann Thorac Surg* 72:966–974.
19. Fyrenius A, Engvall J, Janerot-Sjoberg B. (2001) Major and minor axes of the normal mitral annulus. *J Heart Valve Dis* 10:146–152.
20. Timek TA, Lai DT, Tibayan F *et al.* (2002) Septal-lateral annular cinching abolishes acute ischemic mitral regurgitation. *J Thorac Cardiovasc Surg* 123:881–888.
21. Choure AJ, Garcia MJ, Hesse B *et al.* (2006) In vivo analysis of the anatomical relationship of coronary sinus to mitral annulus and left circumflex coronary artery using cardiac multidetector computer tomography. *JACC* 48:1938–1945.
22. van Rijk-Zwikker GL, Delemarre BJ, Huysmans HA. (1994) Mitral valve anatomy and morphology: relevance to mitral valve replacement and reconstruction. *J Card Surg* 9(2 Suppl):255–261.
23. Carlhall C, Wigstrom L, Heiberg E, Karlsson M, Bolger AF, Nylander E. (2004) Contribution of mitral annular excursion and shape dynamics to total left ventricular volume change. *Am J Physiol Heart Circ Physiol* 287:H1836–H1841.
24. Bhatnagar KP, Nettleton GS, Campbell FR, Wagner CE, Kuwabara N, Muresian H. (2006) Chiari anomalies in the human right atrium. *Clin Anat* 19:510–516.
25. Bales GS. (2004) Great cardiac vein variations. *Clin Anat* 17:436–443.
26. Muresian H. (2005) Great cardiac vein variations. Letter to the editor. *Clin Anat* 18:313.
27. Tsakiris AG. (1976) The physiology of the mitral annulus. In Kalmanson D (ed.) *The Mitral Valve. A Pluridisciplinary Approach*. Edward Arnold, London, pp. 21–26.
28. Francia P, Pittalis MC, Ali H, Cappato R. (2008) Electrophysiological study and catheter ablation of a Mahaim fibre located at the mitral annulus-aorta junction. *J Interv Card Electrophysiol* 23(2):153–157.
29. Liew R, Ward D. (2008) Two cases of accessory pathways located at the aortomitral continuity: clues from the 12-lead ECG where the algorithms have failed. *Heart Rhythm* 5(8):1206–1209.
30. Dagres N, Wasmer K, Monnig G *et al.* (2009) Novel surface ECG criteria for differentiation between left- and right-sided manifest inferoseptal accessory pathways. *Int J Cardiol* 134(3):412–414.
31. Calo' L, Sciarra L, DeRuvo E, Franceschetti R, Pellegrini R, Liov E. (2007) Successful catheter ablation of a manifest left anterior accessory pathway. *J Cardiovasc Med (Hagerstown)* 8(12):1065–1068.
32. Ritchie J, Warnock JN, Yoganathan AP. (2005) Structural characterization of the chordae tendineae in native porcine mitral valves. *Ann Thorac Surg* 80:189–197.
33. Lomholt M, Nielsen SL, Hansen SB, Andersen NT, Hasenkam JM. (2002) Differential tension between secondary and primary mitral chordae in an acute in-vivo porcine model. *J Heart Valve Dis* 11:337–345.
34. Goetz WA, Lim HS, Lansac E *et al.* (2005) Anterior mitral basal "stay" chords are essential for left ventricular geometry and function. *J Heart Valve Dis* 14(2):195–202.
35. Nayak VM, Victor S. (2006) Steps, arches, and struts supporting the aortic leaflet of the mitral valve. *J Heart Valve Dis* 15:740–746.
36. Jimenez JH, Soerensen DD, He Z, Ritchie J, Yoganathan AP. (2005) Effects of papillary muscle position on chordal force distribution: an in-vitro study. *J Heart Valve Dis* 14:295–302.
37. Einstein DR, Kunzelman KS, Reinhall PG, Nicosia MA, Cochran RP. (2005) Non-linear fluid-coupled computational model of the mitral valve. *J Heart Valve Dis* 14:376–385.
38. Bogaert J, Rademakers FE. (2001) Regional non-uniformity of normal human adult left ventricle. *Am J Physiol Heart Circ Physiol* 280; H610–H620.
39. Kim TH, Seung KB, Kim PJ *et al.* (2005) Images in cardiovascular medicine. Anterolateral papillary muscle rupture complicated by the obstruction of a single diagonal branch. *Circulation* 112:e269–e270.
40. Hokken RB, Bartelings MM, Bogers AJ, Gittenberger-de Groot AC. (1997) Morphology of the pulmonary and aortic roots with regard to the pulmonary autograft procedure. *J Thorac Cardiovasc Surg* 113; 453–461.
41. Gittenberger-de Groot AC, Sauer U, Openheimer-Dekker A, Quagebeur J. (1983) Coronary arterial anatomy in transposition of the great arteries: a morphological study. *Pediatr Cardiol* (Suppl 1):15–24.
42. Muresian H. (2009) The Clinical Anatomy of the Coronary Arteries. An Anatomical Study on 100 Human Heart Specimens. Ed. Enciclopedica ISBN 978–973-45–0581-4, 43pp.
43. Berdajs D, Kunzli A, Schurr U, Zund G, Turina MI, Genoni M. (2006) Clinical anatomy of the atrioventricular node artery. *J Heart Valve Dis* 15(2):225–229.
44. Berdajs D, Schurr U, Wagner A, Seifert B, Turina MI, Genoni M. (2008) Incidence and pathophysiology of atrioventricular

block following mitral valve replacement and ring annuloplasty. *Eur J Cardiothorac Surg* 34(1):55–61.
45. Angelini P. (2002) Coronary artery anomalies: current clinical issues. *Tex Heart Instit J* 29:271–278.
46. Vlodaver Z, Neufeld HN, Edwards JE. (1975) *Coronary Arterial Variations in Normal Heart and in Congenital Heart Disease.* Academic Press Inc, New York; San Francisco, London, pp. 1–14.
47. Muresian H. (2006) The Ross procedure: new insights into the surgical anatomy. *Ann Thorac Surg* 81:495–501.
48. Berdajs D, Lajos P, Turina M. (2002) The anatomy of the aortic root. *Cardiovasc Surg* 10(4):320–327.
49. Lansac E, Lim HS, Shomura Y *et al.* (2005) Aortic root dynamics are asymmetric. *J Heart Valve Dis* 14:400–407.
50. Berdajs D, Lajos P, Zund G, Turina MI. (2005) Geometrical model of the pulmonary root. *J Heart Valve Dis* 14(2):257–260.
51. Berdajs D, Zund G, Schurr U, Camenisch C, Turina MI, Genoni M. (2007) Geometric models of the aortic and pulmonary roots: suggestions for the Ross procedure. *Eur J Cardiothorac Surg* 31(1):31–35.
52. Busquet J, Fontan F, Anderson RH, Ho SY, Davies MJ. (1984) The surgical significance of the atrial branches of the coronary arteries. *Int J Cardiol* 6:223–236.
53. Muresian H. (2001) The vascularization of the pulmonary infundibulum (Abstract). Verhandlungen der Anatomischen Gesellschaft—Münster 2001. *Ann Anat* 183:S125–S126.
54. Nicks R, Cartmill T, Bernstein L. (1970) Hypoplasia of the aortic root. The problem of aortic valve replacement. *Thorax* 25:339–346.
55. Monouguian S, Kirchhoff PG. (1996) Aortic and aortic-mitral annular enlargement. *J Thorac Cardiovasc Surg* 112: 207.
56. Erez E, Kanter KR, Tam VKH, Williams W. (2002) Konno aortoventriculoplasty in children and adolescents: from prosthetic valves to the Ross operation. *Ann Thorac Surg* 74:122–126.
57. Poutanen T, Tikanoja T, Sairanen H, Jokinen E. (2006) Normal mitral and aortic valve area assessed by three- and two-dimensional echocardiography in 168 children and young adults. *Pediatr Cardiol* 27(2):217–225.
58. Marron K, Yacoub MH, Pollak JM *et al.* (1996) Innervation of human atrioventricular and arterial valves. *Circulation* 94:368–375.
59. Filip DA, Radu A, Simionescu M. (1986) Interstitial cells of the heart valves possess characteristics similar to smooth muscle cells. *Circ Res* 59:310–320.
60. Glasson JR, Komeda M, Daughters GT *et al.* (1997) Most ovine mitral annulas 3-D size reduction occurs before ventricular systole and is abolished with ventricular pacing. *Circulation* 96:II115–II123.
61. Timek TA, Lai DT, Dagum P *et al.* (2003) Ablation or mitral annular and leaflet muscle: effects on annular and leaflet dynamics. *Am J Physiol Heart Circ Physiol* 285:H1668–H1674.
62. Tiabayan FA, Wilson A, Lai DT *et al.* (2007) Tenting volume: three-dimensional assessment of geometric perturbations in functional mitral regurgitation and implications for surgical repair. *J Heart Valve Dis* 16(1):1–7.

5 Clinical Applications of CT Imaging of the Aortic and Mitral Valves

Hatem Alkadhi, Lotus Desbiolles & Sebastian Leschka

University Hospital Zurich, Zurich, Switzerland

Introduction

The clinical mainstay in the diagnosis and quantification of cardiac valvular disease is echocardiography [1]. Although widely available and cost effective, echocardiography is limited by considerable dependency on the operator and on the patient constitution. Alternatively, transesophageal echocardiography (TEE) is an invasive procedure requiring sedation and has various contraindications, such as recent esophageal surgery, recent oral ingestion, unstable cervical spine injuries, and unevaluated gastrointestinal bleeding.

The primary indication for cardiac CT represents the noninvasive imaging of the coronary arteries with regard to the presence or absence of coronary artery disease [2, 3]. However, with each cardiac CT examination, cross-sectional imaging data are acquired containing high-quality information about the aortic and mitral valve apparatus [4–7]. Retrospective synchronization of the electrocardiogram (ECG-gating) allows for the reconstruction of data sets at various systolic or diastolic phases throughout the cardiac cycle. Images can thus be generated showing the open or closed valves in the respective part of the cycle [8].

Using this data, the normal and pathologic morphology of the aortic and mitral valve can be depicted with CT in an excellent quality [4–8]. This holds particularly true for valve thickening, calcifications [9, 10], or abnormalities associated with infective endocarditis [11]. Beyond the pure morphology, CT of the aortic valve can be also used for the quantitative assessment of the degree of stenosis and regurgitation through planimetric measurements of the valve opening or regurgitant orifice area [4–7, 12]. Thus, cardiac CT may serve as an alternative to the clinical reference standard modality echocardiography or to magnetic resonance imaging, particularly when these modalities fail, are not feasible, or provide inconclusive results [13, 14].

CT image quality during systole usually is lower than that in diastole, which is explained by the use of ECG-controlled tube current modulation (or ECG-pulsing) [15, 16]. This dose reduction technique delivers a normal tube current during diastole, but only 25% of the normal tube current during systole resulting in an increased image mottle.

CT Study of the Aortic Valve

CT provides information about the morphology of the aortic valve in different phases of cardiac cycle (Figure 5.1). CT allows a measurement of the "true" anatomic aortic valve orifice area (so-called planimetry) as well as assessment of the amount of calcification of the valve [4, 5, 12]. Detailed CT anatomy of normal valves is described in Chapter 1.

Aortic Orifice Area Assessment (Planimetry)

The area of the aortic valve will be measured in midsystole to evaluate aortic stenosis (AS). Using short-axis planes through the aortic valve, the plane that demonstrates the orifice with smallest opening during the phase of maximum valve opening is chosen (Figure 5.2). ECG dose modulation (dose reduction during systole) is not recommended by some authors, as in this specific setting increasing image noise may interfere with accurate measurements [12].

Revisiting Cardiac Anatomy: A Computed-Tomography-Based Atlas and Reference, 1st edition. Edited by Farhood Saremi, Eloisa Arbustini, Stephen Achenbach and Jagat Narula.

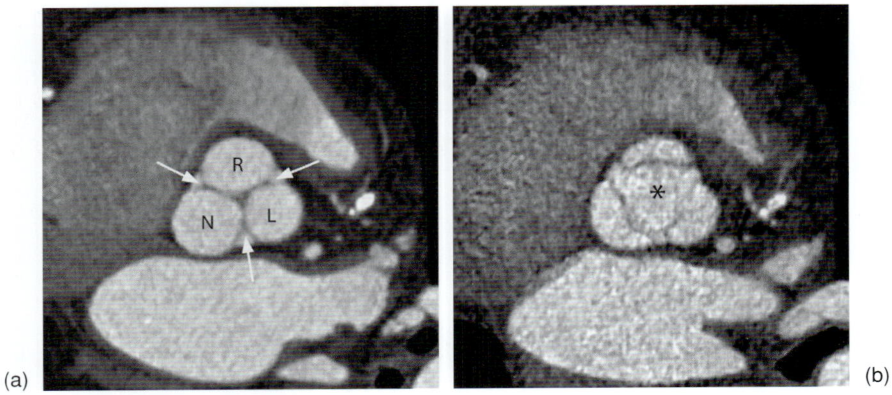

Figure 5.1 (a) Short-axis view parallel to the aortic valve during mid-diastole shows a tricuspid valve with smooth cusps. (b) Short-axis image during early systole shows normal opening (asterisk) of a tricuspid aortic valve. arrows, commissures; L, left coronary cusp; N, noncoronary cusp; R, right coronary cusp.

Planimetric measurements of the regurgitant orifice area of the aortic valve can be performed during diastole to assess severity of the aortic regurgitation [6].

Accurate valve area measurement in heavily calcified valves may be difficult is some patients. Compared to echocardiography, CT is suffering from relatively slow temporal resolution (75–165 ms) and lack of capability for hemodynamic valve study [13, 14, 17].

Aortic Root Morphology for Percutaneous Aortic Valve Replacement

Percutaneous aortic valve replacement is an emerging therapy for selected patients with severe AS who may not be candidates for conventional surgical valve replacement [18]. A bioprosthetic valve is placed within the native diseased stenotic aortic valve. Detailed knowledge of aortic valve and aortic root morphology, including the longitudinal distance from the aortic annulus to the coronary arteries and annular diameters, is important for preprocedural planning and device deployment. Owing to the large distribution of ostial locations and the dilatation of the aortic root, CT is recommended before the procedure in each patient [19, 20].

In a recent study, it was shown that the distance from the aortic valve annulus to the coronary artery ostia and sinotubular junction is reduced in patients with AS compared with controls [19]. In another study in patients with severe tricuspid AS, coronary ostial locations were similar to the controls, but a transverse remodeling of the aortic root was recognized [20] (Figure 5.3).

CT Anatomy of the Bicuspid Aortic Valve

A bicuspid aortic valve is composed of two cusps. Approximately 25% of the bicuspid aortic valves have no raphe, or fibrous ridge, representing the site of congenital fusion between the two conjoined cups [21] (Figure 5.4). With degeneration of aging valves, sclerosis and calcification commonly occur, and most bicuspid valves become stenotic or regurgitant.

A raphe can be found in about 75% of the bicuspid valves and is most commonly located between the right and left coronary cusps [21] (Figure 5.5).

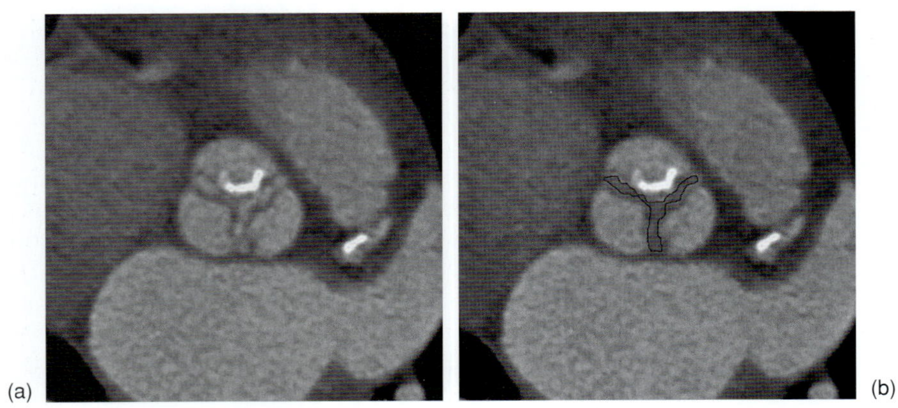

Figure 5.2 Plane selection for aortic valve CT planimetry in 56-year-old man with severe degenerative aortic stenosis. (a) Oblique axial CT reconstruction in early systole (at 10% of the RR interval) demonstrates the thickened and partially calcified aortic cusps with restricted opening. (b) Image shows inner contour of the opening of the aortic valve area manually outlined. The aortic valve area was 0.66 cm^2, which indicated severe aortic stenosis.

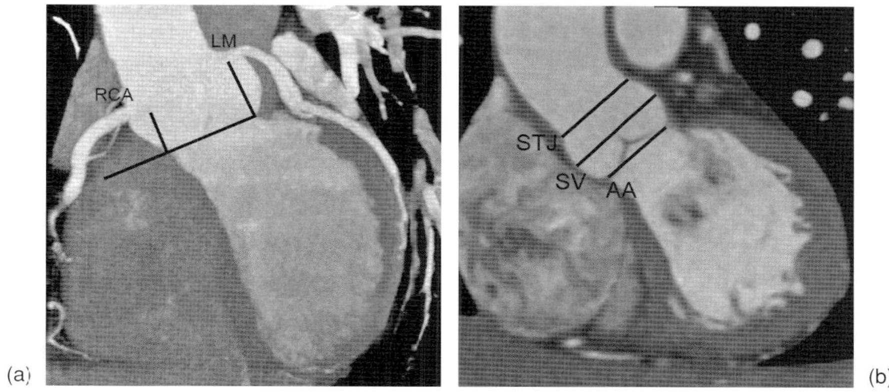

Figure 5.3 Measurements of coronary ostial locations and sinus heights with CT. Coronary ostial locations of the left main artery (LM) is localized on an oblique coronal reformation (a) orientated orthogonally to the plane of aortic annulus. LM measurements are made from the base of the aortic annulus (AA) perpendicularly up to the coronary ostium. The location of the right coronary artery (RCA) ostium is measured in a similar fashion. (b) The width of the AA, sinus of Valsalva (SV), and sinotubular junction (STJ) are measured on a parallel oblique coronal reformation.

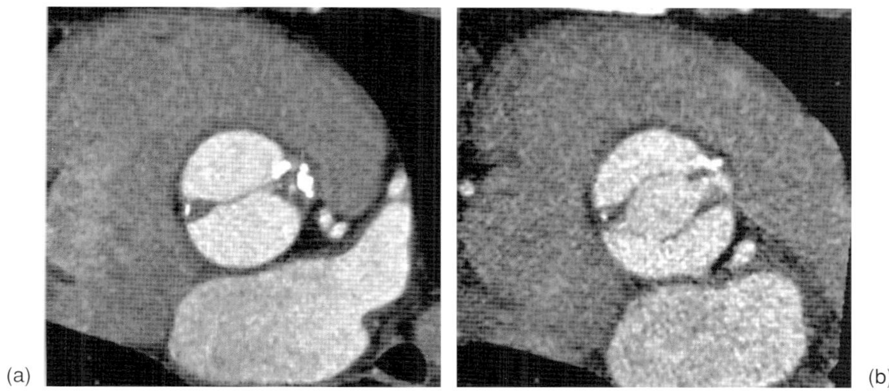

Figure 5.4 Bicuspid aortic valve without raphe. (a) Short-axis reconstruction at the level of the aortic valve during mid-diastole shows a closed aortic valve with two cusps. No raphe is present. (b) Short-axis reconstruction during systole shows the open bicuspid valve.

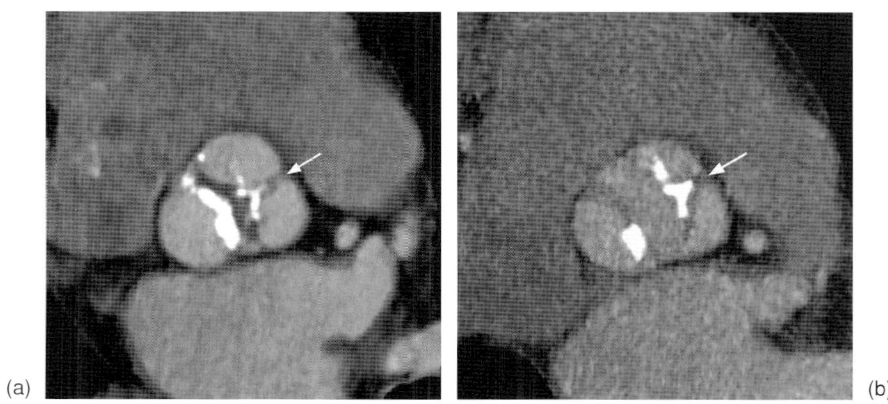

Figure 5.5 Bicuspid aortic valve with raphe. (a) Short-axis reconstruction during mid-diastole shows closed aortic valve with two cusps and a raphe (arrow). (b) Short-axis reconstruction during systole shows the open bicuspid valve. The bicuspid valve with raphe (arrow) can be most easily identified on images reconstructed in systole.

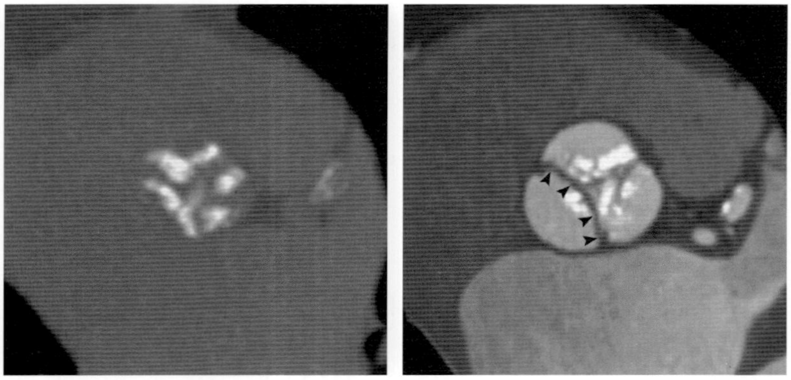

(a) (b) **Figure 5.6** (a) Precontrast short-axis reconstruction parallel to the aortic valve demonstrates the severe valve calcifications affecting all three cusps of the aortic valve. (b) Contrast-enhanced short-axis reconstruction shows both thickening (arrowheads) and calcification of the aortic valve apparatus.

CT Study of the Calcified Aortic Valve

Most of the aortic stenosis in elderly (>65) is the result of degenerative changes of the valve. Degenerative aortic valve disease is due to the thickening of the valve apparatus with deposition of calcium and is associated with stiffness and restricted movement of the cusps. The higher the degree of aortic valve calcifications, the more severe the degree of AS will be [9] (Figure 5.6). The amount of calcific deposits in the aortic valve correlates with the classical atherosclerotic risk factors and the severity of coronary artery sclerosis [10, 22].

If the normal aortic valve opening area of 3–4 cm^2 decreases to approximately one-fourth of that area, the stenosis becomes hemodynamically significant. Mild AS is present with a valve area of >1.5 cm^2 and severe AS with a valve area of 1.0 cm^2 or less [23].

Preoperative knowledge about aortic valve, morphologic characteristics, and extent of aortic valve calcification is desirable when one is planning surgical valve replacement [10]. For example, the presence or absence of a bicuspid aortic valve poses a risk factor for postoperative complications following aortic valve or root replacement [24]. Similarly, extensive valve calcification is associated with increased surgical difficulties for valve placement and fixation of the valve prosthesis into the annulus [25].

CT Anatomy of the Mitral Valve

Similar to the aortic valve, the data obtained from routine CT coronary angiography can be used to evaluate the morphology of the mitral valve in normal and pathological conditions (Figure 5.7).

Mitral Annulus Planimetry

The mitral annulus is a complex nonplanar structure [26]. In contrast to aortic valve, accurate imaging assessment of mitral annulus geometry and its dynamic motion can be a formidable challenge. The mitral annulus is a functional component of the mitral apparatus that contributes to normal valve closure [27]. Its size and sphincteric mechanism may have important effects on valve performance in health and in diseased states.

The dynamics of annular motion have been an area of active investigation for decades using different imaging modalities by animal experiments or in human subjects [26, 28–30]. Recently, CT has been used to define the annulus morphology in normal and pathological conditions [30].

Defining normal annular physiology and motion is important for designing more efficient annuloplasty ring

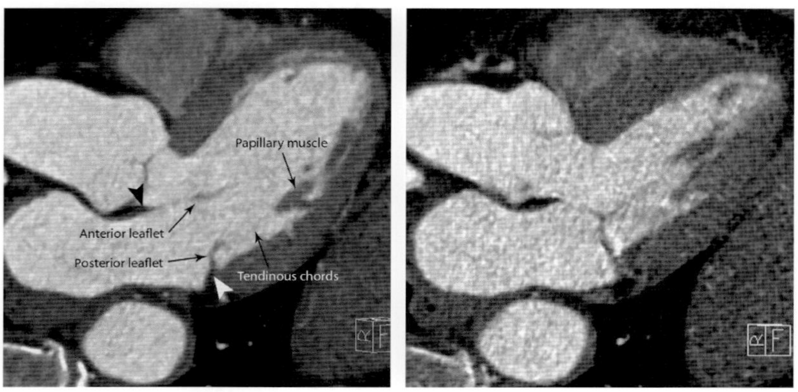

(a) (b) **Figure 5.7** (a) Long-axis reconstruction along the long axis of the left ventricle showing the opened mitral valve during mid-diastole. Arrowheads represent mitral annulus. (b) Long-axis reconstruction along the long axis of the left ventricle showing the closed mitral valve during systole. Again, image quality during systole is hampered by noise.

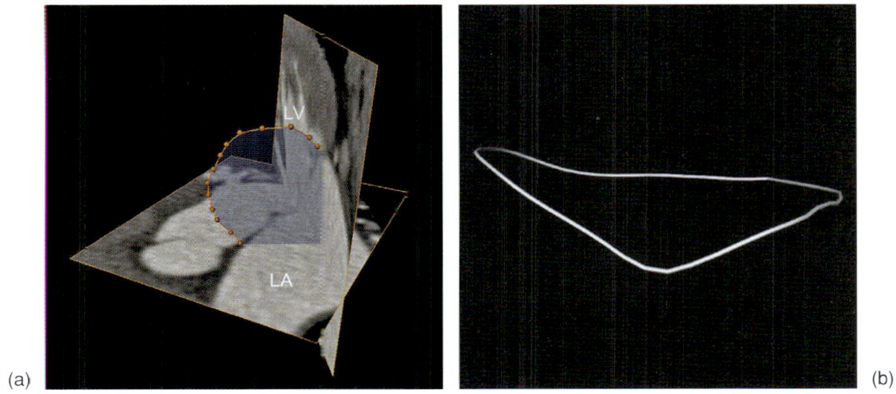

Figure 5.8 (a) Multiplanar reformation of the mitral annulus (dotted orange line). (b) The mitral annulus can be segmented from the volumetric CT data. Note the three-dimensional saddle-shape of the mitral annulus. LA, left atrium; LV, left ventricle.

prostheses. It may also have implications for transvenous mitral valve annuloplasty [31].

Annular area appears to be maximal in diastole and contracts to a minimum size in systole, with substantial presystolic (atrial contraction) area reduction observed in most human studies [27] (Figure 5.8). It is shown that annular dynamics are almost totally eliminated when annular size is decreased sufficiently with most ring annuloplasty techniques [32].

CT Demonstration of Mitral Annulus Calcification

Assessment of mitral annulus calcification with CT is accurate and straightforward. Extensive calcification of the mitral valve annulus is a pathologic entity frequently associated with degenerative valvular disease [33]. The calcification process usually is localized to the annulus (mainly posterior). However, it may extend to the underlying myocardium and interrupt normal conduction of the heart.

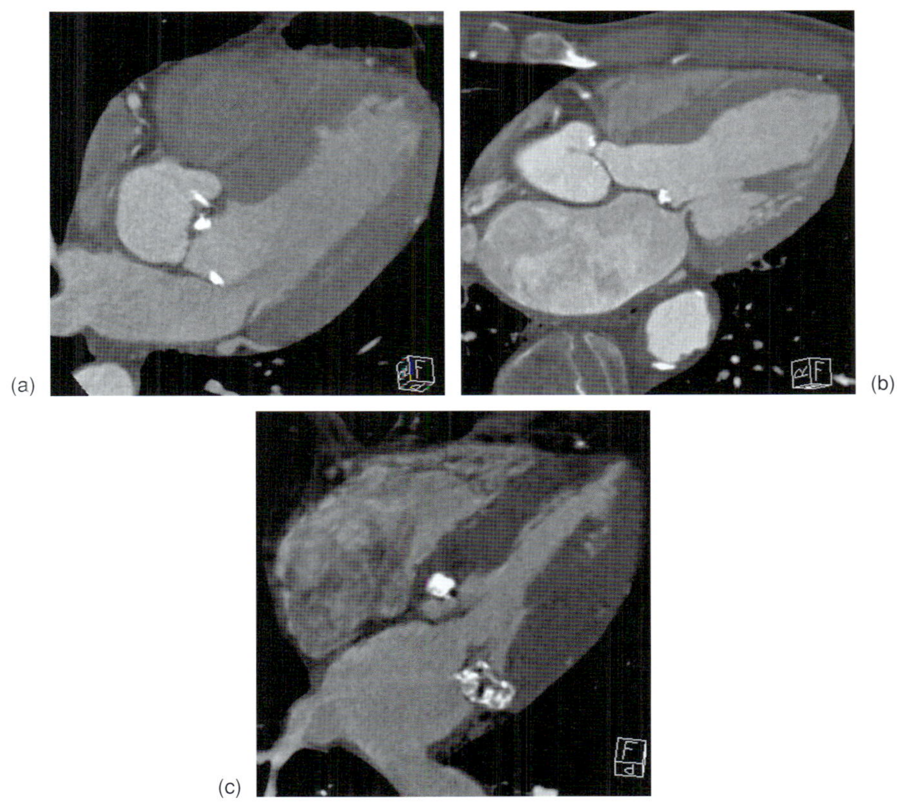

Figure 5.9 Oblique CT images through the long axis of the left ventricle and left atrium showing grade I (<2 mm) (a), grade II (>2 but ≤ 5 mm) (b), and grade III (>5 mm) (c) calcifications of the mitral valve.

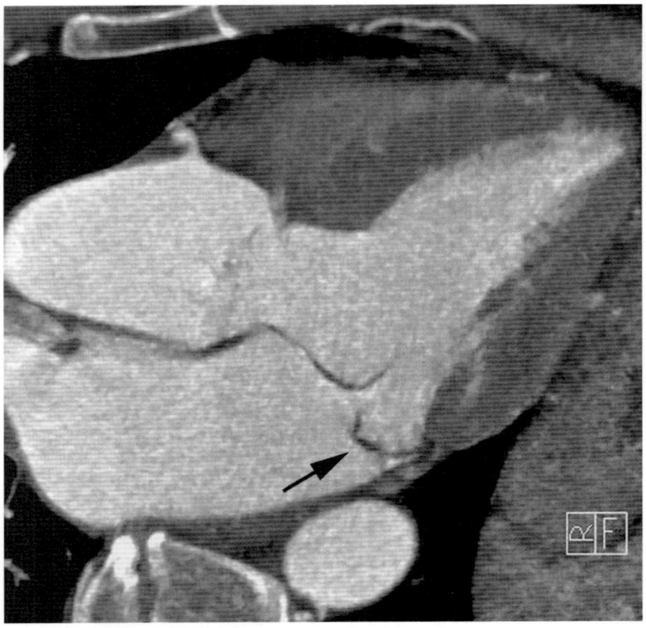

Figure 5.10 Three-chamber reconstruction during early systole shows prolapse of the posterior mitral valve leaflet (arrow). The anterior leaflet is in normal position.

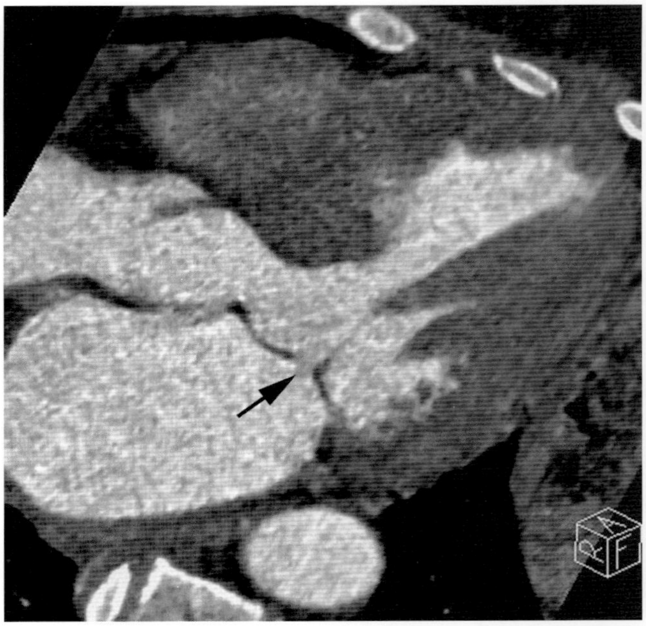

Figure 5.11 Oblique CT reconstruction through the long axis of the left ventricle and left atrium in a 61-year-old woman shows incompetent mitral valve closure during systole (at 15% of the RR interval); the leaflets create a regurgitant orifice (arrow). Echocardiography graded mitral regurgitation as moderate (grade 2).

Severe calcification can interfere with normal valve function. Dense calcification of the posterior leaflet, annulus, and chordae can cause great difficulty in the insertion of a prosthetic device, and is associated with a high frequency of technical complications [34] (Figure 5.9).

CT Anatomy of Mitral Valve Prolapse

Mitral valve prolapse (MVP) is defined as bowing of one or both mitral valve leaflets toward the left atrium during systole (Figure 5.10). The reported prevalence is about 2.3%, without gender or age predilection. MVP can be subdivided into *billowing*, defined as systolic displacement of the leaflet body below the mitral annulus plane $\geq$ 2 mm, and into *flail leaflet*, defined as systolic displacement of the free edge of the leaflet below the mitral annulus plane $\geq$ 2 mm.

CT study of Mitral Regurgitation

CT can accurately depict the common morphologic abnormalities of the valvular apparatus associated with mitral regurgitation except rupture of the tendinous cords. A correlation between regurgitant orifice size (Figure 5.11) at CT and the degree of mitral regurgitation was reported [7]. However, due to the severe and complex motion pattern of the mitral valve apparatus, CT often fails to depict the incompetent valve closure and hence is not able to accurately quantify the degree of mitral regurgitation.

References

1. Bonow RO, Carabello BA, Kanu C *et al.* (2006) ACC/AHA 2006 guidelines for the management of patients with valvular heart disease: a report of the American College of Cardiology/American Heart Association Task Force on Practice Guidelines (writing committee to revise the 1998 Guidelines for the Management of Patients with Valvular Heart Disease): developed in collaboration with the Society of Cardiovascular Anesthesiologists: endorsed by the Society for Cardiovascular Angiography and Interventions and the Society of Thoracic Surgeons. *Circulation* 114(5):e84–231.
2. Achenbach S, Giesler T, Ropers D *et al.* (2001) Detection of coronary artery stenoses by contrast-enhanced, retrospectively electrocardiographically-gated, multislice spiral computed tomography. *Circulation* 103:2535–2538.
3. Leschka S, Alkadhi H, Plass A *et al.* (2005) Accuracy of MSCT coronary angiography with 64-slice technology: first experience. *Eur Heart J* 26:1482–1487.
4. Alkadhi H, Wildermuth S, Plass A *et al.* (2006) Aortic stenosis: comparative evaluation of 16-detector row CT and echocardiography. *Radiology* 240:47–55.
5. Bouvier E, Logeart D, Sablayrolles JL *et al.* (2006) Diagnosis of aortic valvular stenosis by multislice cardiac computed tomography. *Eur Heart J* 27:3033–3038.
6. Alkadhi H, Desbiolles L, Husmann L *et al.* (2007) Aortic regurgitation: assessment with 64-section CT. *Radiology* 245:111–121.

7. Alkadhi H, Wildermuth S, Bettex DA *et al.* (2006) Mitral regurgitation: quantification with 16-detector row CT—initial experience. *Radiology* 238:454–463.
8. Baumert B, Plass A, Bettex D *et al.* (2005) Dynamic cine mode imaging of the normal aortic valve using 16-channel multidetector row computed tomography. *Invest Radiol* 40:637–647.
9. Koos R, Mahnken AH, Sinha AM, Wildberger JE, Hoffmann R, Kuhl HP. (2004) Aortic valve calcification as a marker for aortic stenosis severity: assessment on 16-MDCT. *AJR Am J Roentgenol* 183:1813–1818.
10. Messika-Zeitoun D, Aubry MC, Detaint D *et al.* (2004) Evaluation and clinical implications of aortic valve calcification measured by electron-beam computed tomography. *Circulation* 110:356–362.
11. Feuchtner GM, Stolzmann P, Dichtl W *et al.* (2009) Multislice computed tomography in infective endocarditis: comparison with transesophageal echocardiography and intraoperative findings. *J Am Coll Cardiol* 53:436–444.
12. Feuchtner GM, Müller S, Bonatti J *et al.* (2007) Sixty-four slice CT evaluation of aortic stenosis using planimetry of the aortic valve area. *AJR Am J Roentgenol* 189(1):197–203.
13. Pouleur AC, le Polain de Waroux JB, Pasquet A, Vanoverschelde JL, Gerber BL. (2007) Aortic valve area assessment: multidetector CT compared with cine MR imaging and transthoracic and transesophageal echocardiography. *Radiology* 244:745–754.
14. Habis M, Daoud B, Roger VL *et al.* (2007) Comparison of 64-slice computed tomography planimetry and Doppler echocardiography in the assessment of aortic valve stenosis. *J Heart Valve Dis* 16:216–224.
15. Jakobs TF, Becker CR, Ohnesorge B *et al.* (2002) Multislice helical CT of the heart with retrospective ECG gating: reduction of radiation exposure by ECG controlled tube current modulation. *Eur Radiol* 12:1081–1086.
16. Stolzmann P, Scheffel H, Schertler T *et al.* (2008) Radiation dose estimates in dual-source computed tomography coronary angiography. *Eur Radiol* 18:592–599
17. Pouleur AC, le Polain de Waroux JB, Pasquet A, Vancraeynest D, Vanoverschelde JL, Gerber BL. (2007) Planimetric and continuity equation assessment of aortic valve area: head to head comparison between cardiac magnetic resonance and echocardiography. *J Magn Reson Imaging* 26:1436–1443.
18. Lutter G, Ardehali R, Cremer J *et al.* (2004) Percutaneous valve replacement: current state and future prospects. *Ann Thorac Surg* 78:2199–2206.
19. Akhtar M, Tuzcu EM, Kapadia SR *et al.* (2009) Aortic root morphology in patients undergoing percutaneous aortic valve replacement: evidence of aortic root remodeling. *J Thorac Cardiovasc Surg* 137(4):950–956.
20. Stolzmann P, Knight J, Desbiolles L *et al.* (2009) Remodelling of the aortic root in severe tricuspid aortic stenosis: implications for transcatheter aortic valve implantation. *Eur Radiol* 19(6):1316–1323.
21. Sabet HY, Edwards WD, Tazelaar HD, Daly RC. (1999) Congenitally bicuspid aortic valves: a surgical pathology study of 542 cases (1991 through 1996) and a literature review of 2715 additional cases. *Mayo Clin Proc* 74:14–26.
22. Feuchtner GM, Muller S, Grander W *et al.* (2006) Aortic valve calcification as quantified with multislice computed tomography predicts short-term clinical outcome in patients with asymptomatic aortic stenosis. *J Heart Valve Dis* 15:494–498.
23. Wiegers SE, Herrmann HC, Plappert T, St John Sutton MG. (2004) Valvular heart disease. In St John Sutton MG, Rutherford JD (eds) *Clinical Cardiovascular Imaging: A Companion to Braunwald's Heart Disease*. Elsevier Saunders, Philadelphia, PA, pp. 280–338.
24. Russo CF, Mazzetti S, Garatti A *et al.* (2002) Aortic complications after bicuspid aortic valve replacement: long-term results. *Ann Thorac Surg* 74:S1773–S1776.
25. Mullany CJ. (2000) Aortic valve surgery in the elderly. *Cardiol Rev* 8:333–339.
26. Levine RA, Handschumacher MD, Sanfilippo AJ *et al.* (1989) Three-dimensional echocardiographic reconstruction of the mitral valve, with implications for the diagnosis of mitral valve prolapse. *Circulation* 1; 80:589–598.
27. Timek TA, Miller DC. (2001) Experimental and clinical assessment of mitral annular area and dynamics: what are we actually measuring? *Ann Thorac Surg* 72:966–974.
28. Tsakiris AG, von Bernuth G, Rastelli GS, Bourgeois MJ, Titus JL, Wood EG. (1971) Size and motion of the mitral valve annulus in anesthetized intact dogs. *J Appl Physiol* 30:611–618.
29. Glasson JR, Komeda M, Daughters GT *et al.* (1997) Most ovine mitral annular three dimensional size reduction occurs before ventricular systole and is abolished with ventricular pacing. *Circulation* 96(Suppl II):115–122.
30. Alkadhi H, Desbiolles L, Stolzmann P *et al.* (2009) Mitral annular shape, size, and motion in normals and in patients with cardiomyopathy: evaluation with computed tomography. *Invest Radiol* 44:218–225.
31. Webb JG, Harnek J, Munt BI *et al.* (2006) Percutaneous transvenous mitral annuloplasty: initial human experience with device implantation in the coronary sinus. *Circulation* 14;113(6):851–855.
32. Glasson JR, Green GR, Nistal JF *et al.* (1998) Mitral annular size and shape in sheep with annuloplasty rings. *J Thorac Cardiovasc Surg* 117:302–309.
33. Carpentier AF, Pellerin M, Fuzellier JF, Relland JY. (1996) Extensive calcification of the mitral valve annulus: pathology and surgical management. *J Thorac Cardiovasc Surg* 111(4):718–729.
34. Ng CK, Punzengruber C, Pachinger O *et al.* (2000) Valve repair in mitral regurgitation complicated by severe annulus calcification. *Ann Thorac Surg* 70(1):53–58.

6 Computed Tomography for Percutaneous Aortic Valve Replacement

Hursh Naik,[1] Niraj Doctor,[1] Gregory P. Fontana[1] & Raj R. Makkar[1,2]

[1]*Cedars-Sinai Medical Center, Los Angeles, CA, USA*
[2]*UCLA School of Medicine, Los Angeles CA, USA*

Introduction

Cardiothoracic surgeons have traditionally used CT to guide the treatment of aortic valve stenosis. With the recent advent of percutaneous aortic valve therapies for the treatment of aortic stenosis [1], CT imaging of the aortic valve and its surrounding structures have played an important role for interventional cardiologists as well. With this technology, imaging's role has grown tremendously, and is a necessary part of the workup of these patients.

Percutaneous aortic valve replacement first involves CT assessment at multiple levels:

1. The iliac and femoral vessels for caliber, tortuosity, and calcification.
2. The aorta for aneurysmal segments, tortuosity, and calcification, as well as arch configuration.
3. The sinotubular junction (STJ), aortic valve, and aortic annulus.
4. The mitral and aortic annular continuity.
5. Left ventricle wall thickness, particularly the septal wall.

Iliac and femoral Assessment

Iliac and femoral vessel anatomy is easily evaluated with CT [2–4]. The lumen size (diameter and area) is the first aspect that is important (Figure 6.1). At the time of this publication, the delivery sheaths for the transfemoral percutaneous approach range from 18 to 24°F [1,5,6]. The size depends on the style of and/or size of the valve. On the basis of the current experience, this translates to a minimum acceptable diameter of 6 mm. Figures 6.1 and 6.2 illustrate what surgeons and interventionalists look for when evaluating potential transfemoral percutaneous aortic valve patients.

Aortic Assessment

The second level of assessment involves the aorta. The amount of plaque and calcification is important (Figure 6.3). Studies have shown that atheroma and elevated aortic plaque burden are risk factors for stroke including the periprocedural time period [7–11]. The arch configuration is important. Especially in the elderly, the aorta becomes unfolded (type II and III arches). These aortas become troublesome when advancing the aortic valve around the arch (Figures 6.4–6.6).

Ventricular Wall Thickness, Sinotubular Junction, Aortic Valve, and Aortic Annulus

So far we have illustrated the imaging needed for safe delivery of the sheath and valve. Yet, if the position of the valve during deployment is to be accurate, understanding the STJ, aortic valve anatomy, mitral calcification, and ventricular septal thickness become critical [12–14]. With the advent of percutaneous valve replacement, CT has played a vital role not only in preparation for the procedure, but possibly for predicting events from aortic valve disease [15].

The STJ is quite important for positioning and deployment of the valve. First, large amount of calcifications in

Revisiting Cardiac Anatomy: A Computed-Tomography-Based Atlas and Reference, 1st edition. Edited by Farhood Saremi, Eloisa Arbustini, Stephen Achenbach and Jagat Narula.

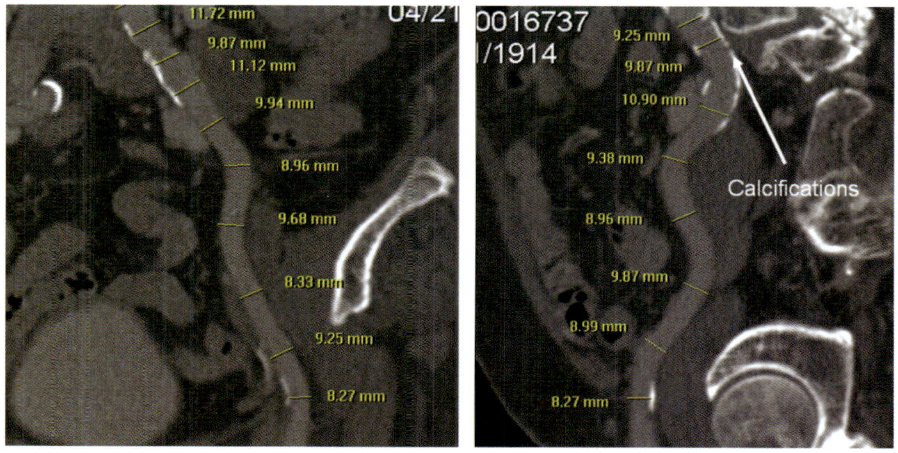

Figure 6.1 Left iliac and femoral system in orthogonal views. The caliber of vessels is appropriate for the current delivery sheaths that are available. Notice the lack of tortuosity and minimal calcification.

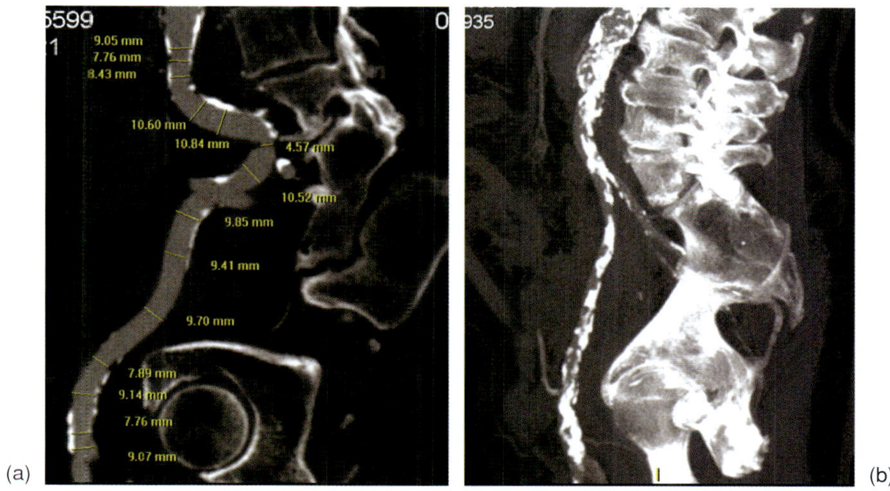

Figure 6.2 (a) Lateral orthogonal view demonstrates tortuosity and deep diving of the right external iliac artery. This tortuosity proves to be a risk factor for iliac complications during sheath placement and removal. (b) Example of heavy calcifications in the right iliac and femoral system. This amount makes the patient a nonideal candidate for transfemoral interventions.

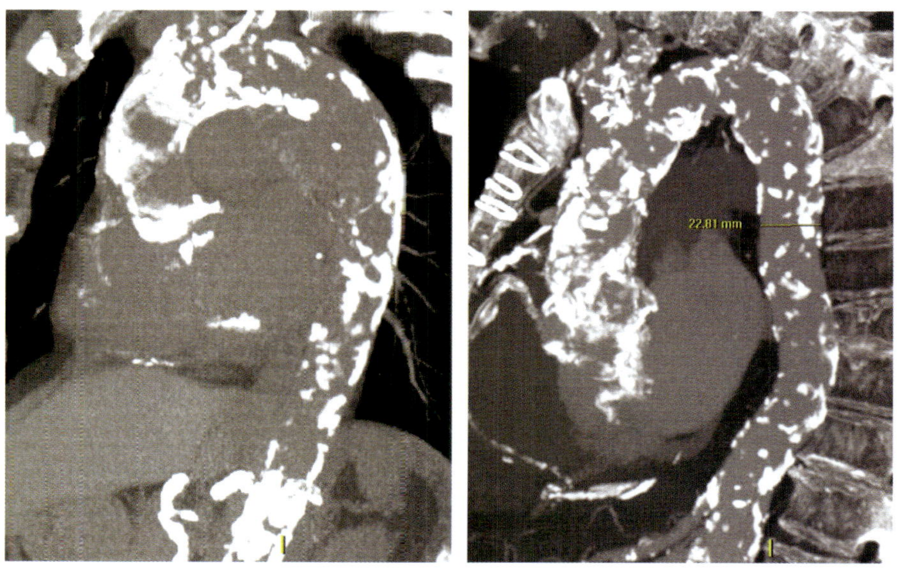

Figure 6.3 Examples of heavily calcified "porcelain" aortas. Eventually these cases will likely be referred for percutaneous valve replacement, as the calcification makes it difficult to cross-clamp the aorta during surgical valve replacement. The calcification burden in this aorta is a risk factor for embolic stroke with the transfemoral technique. Also, the delivery system has multiple segments in which it can be inhibited.

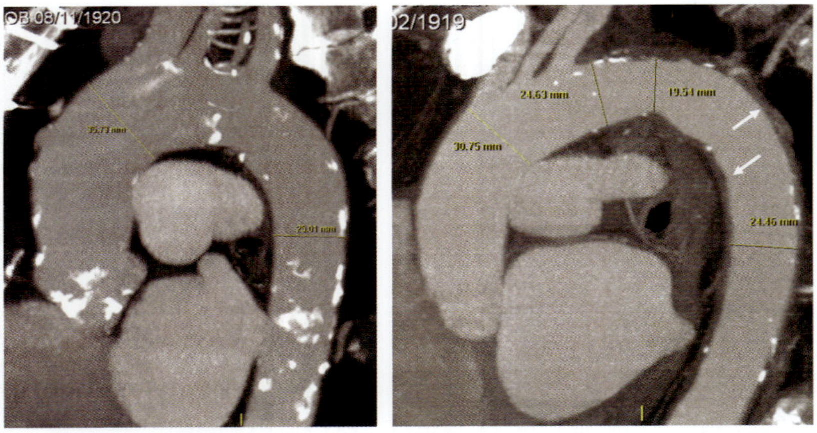

(a) (b)

Figure 6.4 (a) An example of a type I arch configuration. There is minimal plaque and calcification deposition in the descending aorta. Overall this is a favorable aortic configuration for advancement of the aortic. (b) An example of an unfolded aorta (type III arch). Negotiating this arch with current technology is more difficult. Also notice the amount of soft (minimal calcification) aortic plaques (arrows).

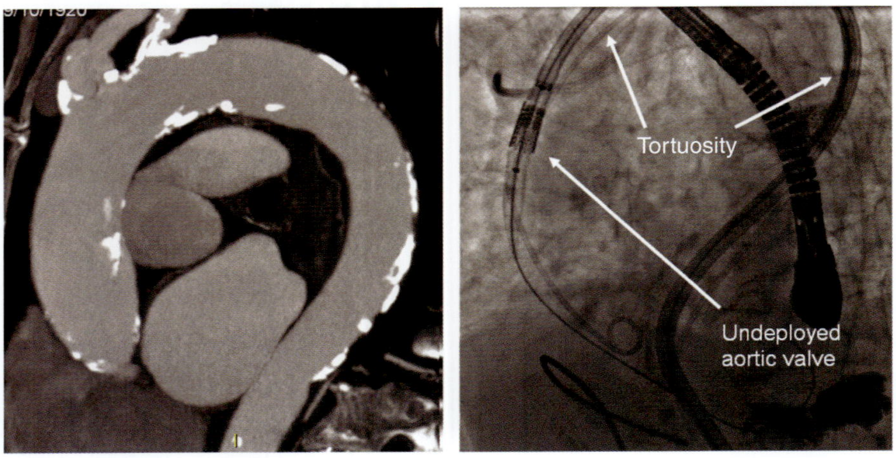

Figure 6.5 Extremely curved arch. The aorta also entered horizontally into the ventricle. This anatomy predicts the difficulty of advancing the catheter and the expected flexion one will need to enter the aortic annulus. A preprocedure CT would have been helpful in this case (not done) as the tortuosity almost proved prohibitive.

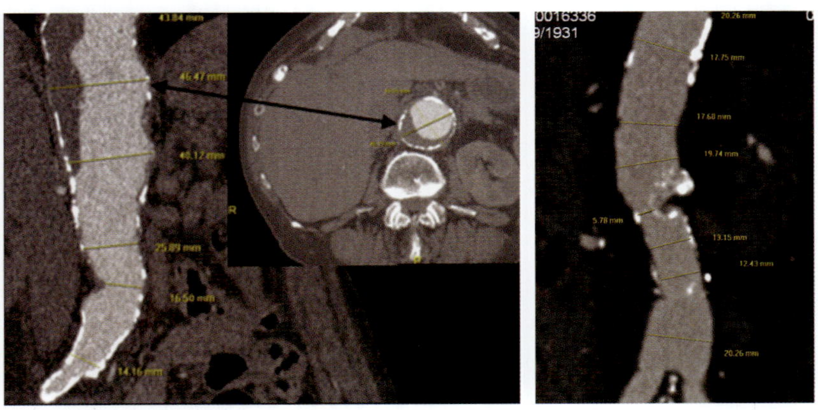

(a) (b)

Figure 6.6 (a) Aneurysmal aorta with clot formation. This has a risk of embolization during sheath advancement. (b) Tight stenosis of the aorta found on CT. Large diameter sheaths will not be able to traverse this stenosis. AP-CMPR, anteroposterior-multiplanar reconstruction.

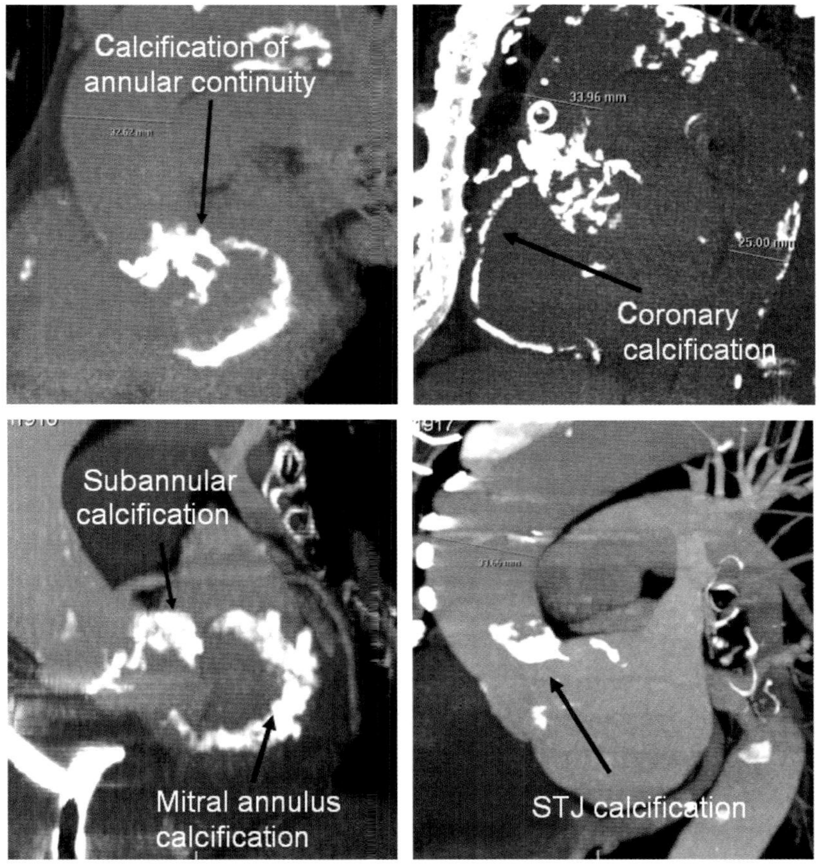

Figure 6.7 (a) An example of the continuity of calcifications of the mitral annulus and aortic annulus. This area can sometimes rupture with inflation of the valve within the annulus. (b) An example of continuity of calcifications with the sinotubular junction (STJ) and left main coronary artery. With aggressive expansion within the aortic annulus, there is a possibility of left main injury. (c) Subannular calcification that is very close to the mitral annulus calcification, but is not contiguous. There is one reported case of a ventricular septal defect creation after inflation of the valve in this area. (d) STJ calcifications limited to the medial side of the aorta. This type of calcification can lead to rupture with higher sized valves.

this area may lead to increased risk of rupture during deployment (Figure 6.7). It is also possible that large subannular calcifications can cause improper implantation of the prosthetic valve, which may result in aortic regurgitation (Figure 6.8). Second, the width of the STJ needs to be measured. A smaller diameter can lead to rupture and/or a large amount of movement during deployment, resulting in possible embolization (Figure 6.9). A wide STJ can lead to inappropriate apposition and embolization. Lastly, it is important to visualize the distance from the valve annulus to the coronary arteries, as in some percutaneous valve systems, covering the coronary artery can lead to an acute coronary occlusion (Figure 6.10).

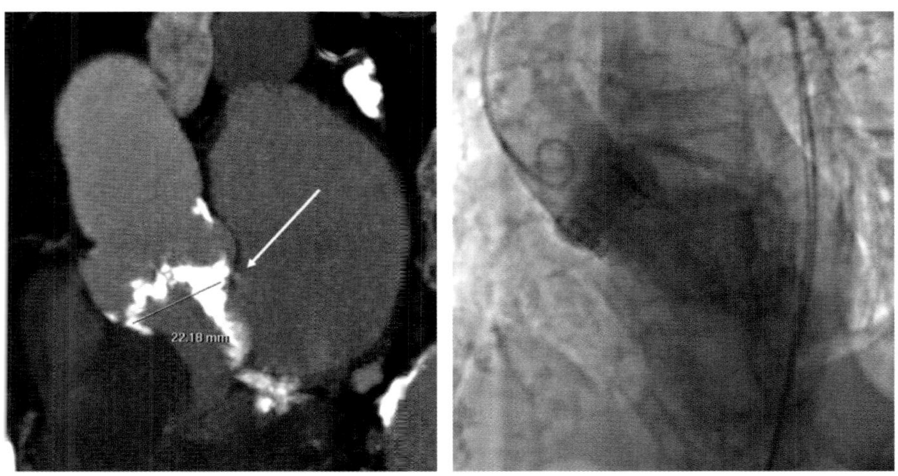

Figure 6.8 Large lower subannular calcifications (arrow) has caused eccentric implantation of the valve, and resulting aortic regurgitation as shown in the angiogram.

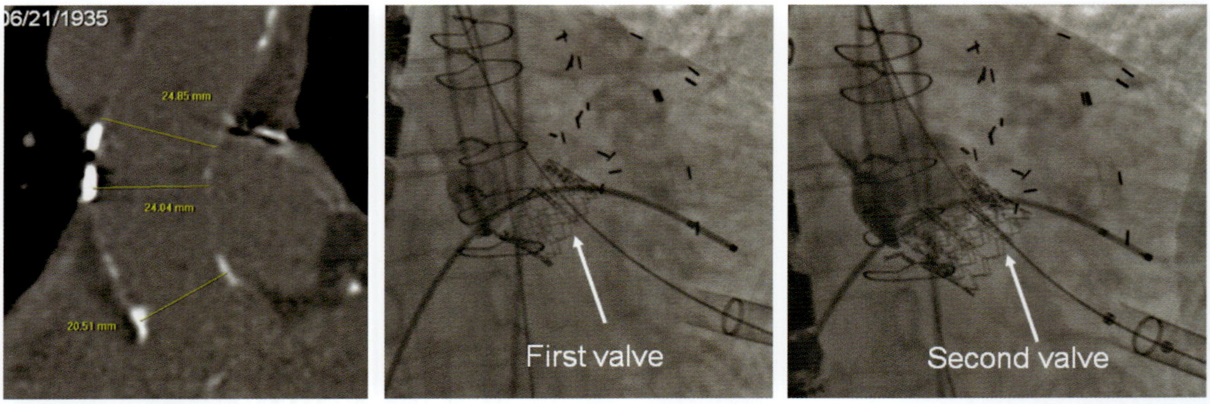

(a), (b) (c)

Figure 6.9 (a) An example of a narrow sinotubular junction. In balloon expandable systems, the balloon dilates to 23 mm or 26 mm. In a narrow sinotubular junction (STJ), the balloon can slip resulting in malposition. (b) The narrow STJ caused the valve to slip down during a transapical procedure (the iliacs were too narrow for a transfemoral approach). (c) A second attempt was made to stabilize the situation by placing another valve. However, this slipped as well. The patient then proceeded to emergent open heart surgery.

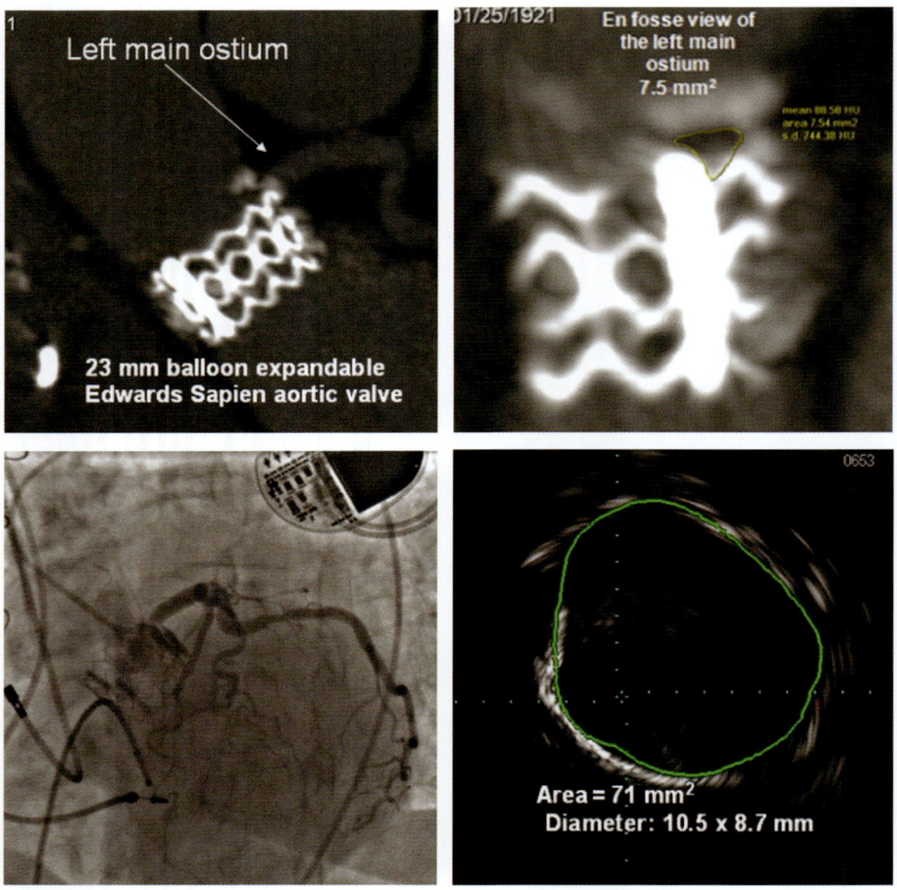

(a) (b) (c) (d)

Figure 6.10 The image illustrates the importance of measuring the annulus to coronary ostium measurements. (a) The valve impinges on the left main ostium. (b) Cross-sectional view of the left main ostium just above the valve. From this view, the area does not seem to be significantly compromised. (c) Angiographic image of the same patient. (d) Intravascular ultrasound of the ostial left main demonstrating no significant stenosis. Fractional flow reserve study (not shown) through the ostium of the left main demonstrated no evidence of hemodynamic disturbance.

(a), (b)

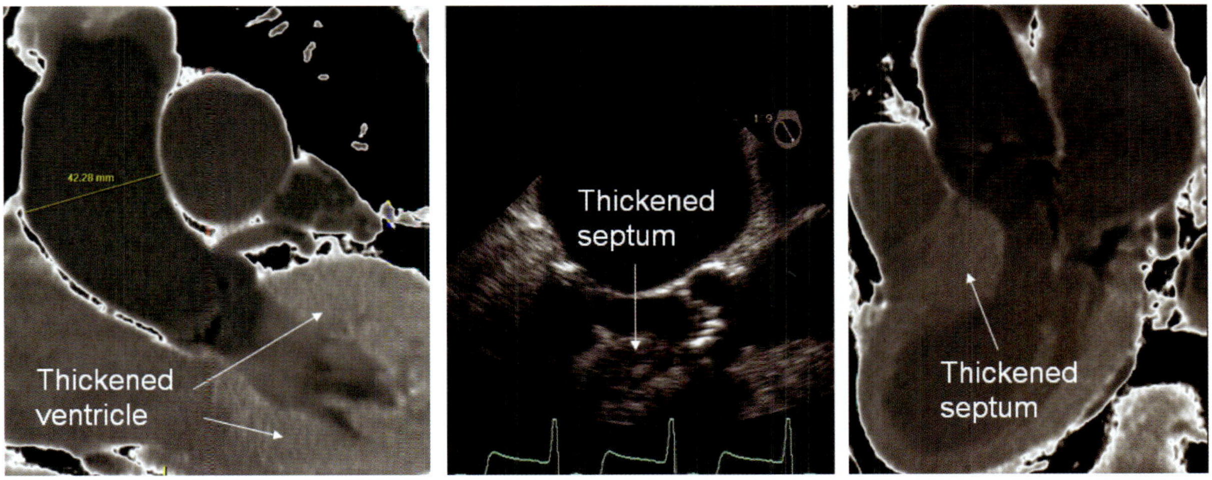

(c)

Figure 6.11 (a) An example of a thickened left ventricle wall resulting in narrowing of the area below the aortic annulus. Just as in the case of a narrowed STJ, the balloon can slip in this area causing malposition of the valve. (b) Intraprocedural transesophageal echocardiographic image of the same patient. CT allowed us to anticipate this issue during deployment. (c) A hypertrophied septum (different patient) that encroaches on the aortic annulus. This presents a challenge during deployment, and/or positioning of the valve.

Thickness of the left ventricle including interventricular septum can easily be assessed with CT at different phases of cardiac cycle (Figure 6.11)

Final anatomical assessment concerns the aortic valve itself (Figures 6.12–6.14). Analysis of the aortic valve involves assessment of calcification (leaflets and annulus), aortic valve area, cusp anatomy, and annulus dimension. It has been demonstrated that CT can assess calcification of the valve and corresponds well with echocardiography [14–16]. There is also promising data that indicate aortic valve area and correlate well with echocardiography [16].

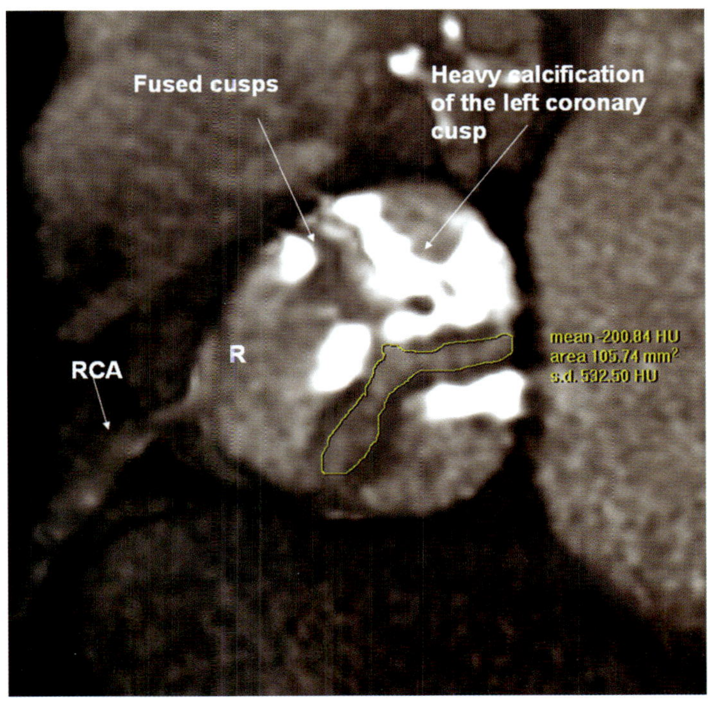

Figure 6.12 Short-axis view of the aortic valve. In our series, the aortic valve area (AVA) matches well with echocardiography. The AVA here is 1.05 cm^2. Three cusps are also seen with the right and left coronary cusps fused. R, right coronary cusp; RCA, right coronary artery.

(a), (b)
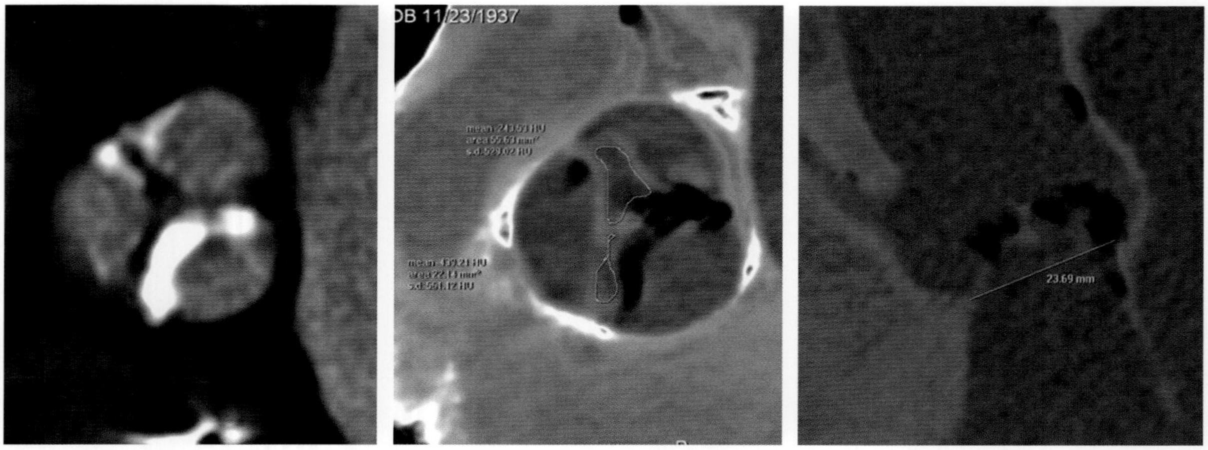

(c)

Figure 6.13 (a) Short axis of the valve during diastole. No contrast is visible through the valve. (b) Severe aortic stenosis. No calcification. This patient had low-gradient severe aortic stenosis (AS). After dobutamine infusion, the aortic valve area increased significantly. The lack of calcification is often a clue that pseudo AS exists. (c) Annulus measurements are critical in terms of sizing the valve during percutaneous procedures.

(a), (b)
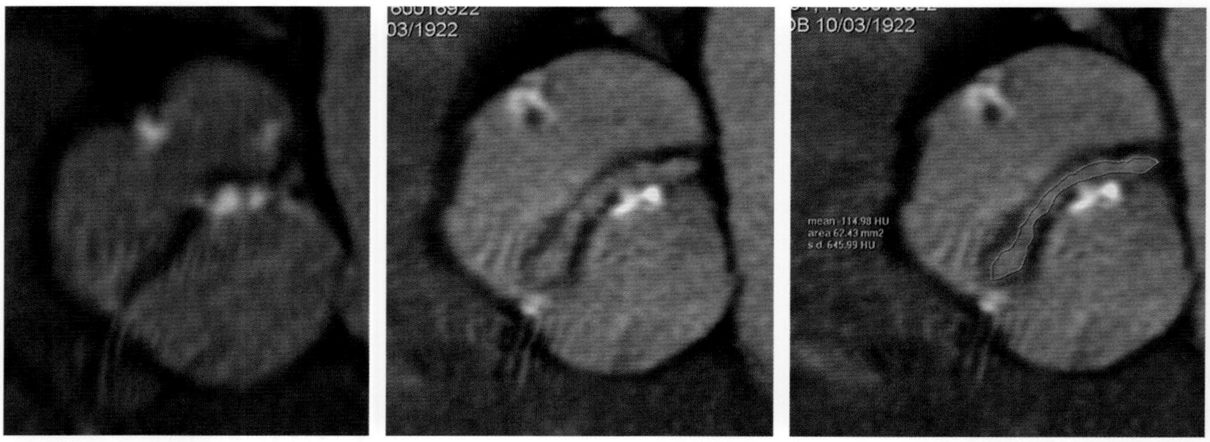
(c)

Figure 6.14 Cross-sectional views of a bicuspid aortic valve at diastole (a) and systole (b). (c) Aortic valve area of 0.62 cm^2. Notice minimal calcification. Bicuspid valves have been shown in cadaveric studies to prevent full expansion of balloon expandable valves. It is currently an exclusion criteria. Also these valves tend to have less calcification, which may prevent appropriate apposition.

With the advent of percutaneous technologies for valve repair/replacement, interventionalists and surgeons are working more closely together than ever before. Through the use of imaging, especially CT, we are learning from each other's strengths the planning and workup that is needed for the treatment of valvular patients.

References

1. Chiam PT, Ruiz CE. (2009) Percutaneous transcatheter aortic valve implantation: evolution of the technology. *Am Heart J* 157: 229–242.
2. Jilaihawi H, Spyt T, Chin D, Logtens E, Laborde JC, Kovac J. (2008) Percutaneous aortic valve replacement in patients with challenging aortoiliofemoral access. *Catheter Cardiovasc Interv* 72:885–890.
3. Kurra V, Schoenhagen P, Roselli EE *et al.* (2009) Prevalence of significant peripheral artery disease in patients evaluated for percutaneous aortic valve insertion: preprocedural assessment with multidetector computed tomography. *J Thorac Cardiovasc Surg* 137:1258–1264.
4. Lin PH, Bechara C, Kougias P, Huynh TT, LeMaire SA, Coselli JS. (2008) Assessment of aortic pathology and peripheral arterial disease using multidetector computed tomographic angiography. *Vasc Endovascular Surg* 42:583–598.
5. Del Valle-Fernandez R, Ruiz CE. (2008) Transcatheter heart valves for the treatment of aortic stenosis: state-of-the-art. *Minerva Cardioangiol* 56:543–556.

6. Eltchaninoff H, Zajarias A, Tron C *et al.* (2008) Transcatheter aortic valve implantation: technical aspects, results and indications. *Arch Cardiovasc Dis* 101:126–132.
7. Gottsegen JM, Coplan NL. (2008) The atherosclerotic aortic arch: considerations in diagnostic imaging. *Prev Cardiol* 11:162–167.
8. Harloff A, Strecker C, Frydrychowicz AP *et al.* (2007) Plaques in the descending aorta: a new risk factor for stroke? Visualization of potential embolization pathways by 4D MRI. *J Magn Reson Imaging* 26:1651–1655.
9. Kaya D, Yildiz E. (2009) Aortic atheromas in stroke subgroups detected by multidetector computed tomographic angiography. *Clin Neurol Neurosurg* 111:415–421.
10. Sen S. (2009) Aortic arch plaque in stroke. *Curr Cardiol Rep* 11:28–35.
11. Sen S, Hinderliter A, Sen PK *et al.* (2007) Aortic arch atheroma progression and recurrent vascular events in patients with stroke or transient ischemic attack. *Circulation* 2007; 116:928–935.
12. Berdajs D, Lajos P, Turina M. (2002) The anatomy of the aortic root. *Cardiovasc Surg* 10:320–327.
13. Akhtar M, Tuzcu EM, Kapadia SR *et al.* (2009) Aortic root morphology in patients undergoing percutaneous aortic valve replacement: evidence of aortic root remodeling. *J Thorac Cardiovasc Surg* 137:950–956.
14. Koos R, Mahnken AH, Kuhl HP *et al.* (2006) Quantification of aortic valve calcification using multislice spiral computed tomography: comparison with atomic absorption spectroscopy. *Invest Radiol* 41:485–489.
15. Feuchtner GM, Muller S, Grander W *et al.* (2006) Aortic valve calcification as quantified with multislice computed tomography predicts short-term clinical outcome in patients with asymptomatic aortic stenosis. *J Heart Valve Dis* 15:494–498.
16. Koos R, Kuhl HP, Muhlenbruch G, Wildberger JE, Gunther RW, Mahnken AH. (2006) Prevalence and clinical importance of aortic valve calcification detected incidentally on CT scans: comparison with echocardiography. *Radiology* 241:76–82.

7 Mitral Valve Disease Imaging

Javier G. Castillo, David H. Adams & Mario J. Garcia

The Mount Sinai School of Medicine, Los Angeles, CA, USA

Introduction

The human mitral valve is a very complex three-dimensional assembly of independent elements that constitute a dynamic functional structure [1]. The normal mitral valve function involves a coordinated interaction among the leaflets, the annulus, the subvalvular apparatus (chordae tendinae and papillary muscles), and the left ventricle [2,3]

Normal Anatomy

Mitral Annulus

The junction between the atrium and the valvular tissue creates a hinge where the motion of the valvular leaflet initiates [4]. The annulus, 2 mm external to the hinge, is a band of thin connective tissue located at the attachment of the posterior leaflet. This segment is not attached to any rigid structures and consequently it is prone to dilation [5]. Conversely, the attachment of the anterior leaflet is a continuation of the aortomitral curtain reinforced at the base by two fibrous structures: the right and left fibrous trigones. The annulus has a three-dimensional saddle-shaped configuration with two lowest (trigones) and highest (middle point of the anterior and posterior annulus) reference points [6,7]. The middle portion of the anterior annulus is higher than the mid-portion of the posterior annulus.

Revisiting Cardiac Anatomy: A Computed-Tomography-Based Atlas and Reference, 1st edition. Edited by Farhood Saremi, Eloisa Arbustini, Stephen Achenbach and Jagat Narula.

Mitral Leaflets and Commissures

The mitral valve has two leaflets with similar surface area, anterior and posterior, which are separated by two commissures [8]. An optimal closure and competency implies a precise fitting between the surface area of the leaflets and the orifice area of the mitral valve [9]. The anterior leaflet extends vertically (trapezoidal shape) is attached to one third of the annular circumference, and relates to the left ventricular outflow tract because of its continuity with the aortomitral curtain. The posterior leaflet extends transversally together with the commissures is attached to the remaining two thirds of the annular circumference, and is related to the parietal base (mural leaflet) of the left ventricle (peak concentration of systolic stress). Both leaflets present two zones from their base to the free margin: *the atrial zone* (smooth and translucent) and the *coaptation zone* (thicker and rough due to the attachment of numerous chordae). Both anterior and posterior coaptation zones come together in systole to create a curved "smiley" line known as the coaptation line [10] (Figure 7.1).

Additionally, the mitral valve is subdivided into eight anatomical segments. The anterolateral and posteromedial commissures are two segments by themselves. The posterior leaflet, as opposed to the anterior leaflet, presents two indentations in the free edge that allow full leaflet opening [11]. In turn, these indentations delimitate three scallops: the anterior (P1), middle (P2), and posterior (P3) leaflet segments (Figures 7.1 and 7.2) [12]. It is important to highlight the particular bulky shape of the posterior leaflet middle scallop due to the impact of systolic pressures, thus explaining the likeliness of this segment to prolapse [13]. By definition, the three corresponding segments of the anterior leaflet are A1 (anterior segment), A2 (middle segment), and A3 (posterior segment). This anatomical nomenclature, particularly after the introduction of real-time three-dimensional echocardiography and other advance imaging techniques, has led to a better valve analysis allowing precise location of the lesions [14,15].

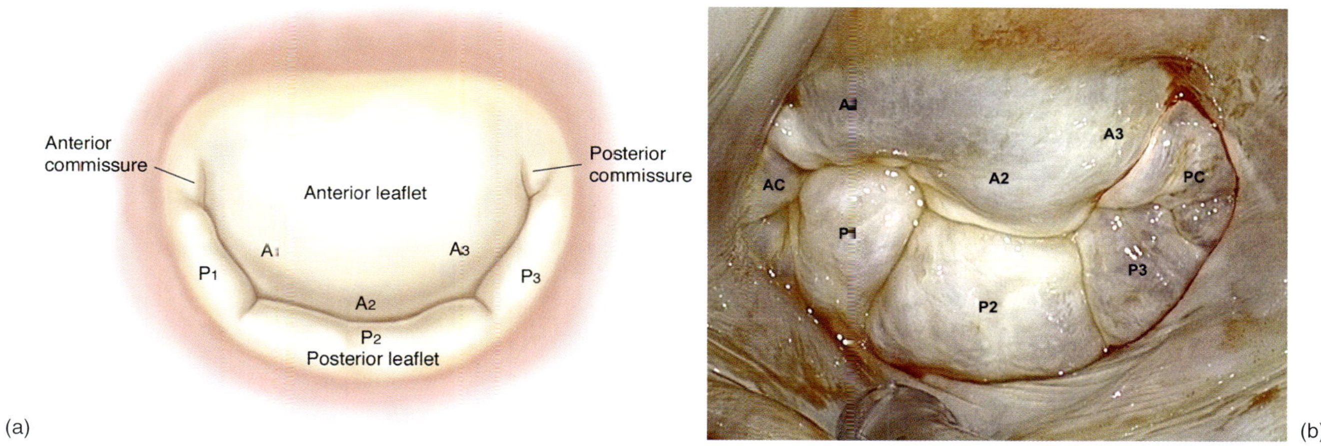

Figure 7.1 (a) Anatomical segmentation of the mitral valve leaflets. (b) Surgical view of a mitral valve with myxomatous degeneration and abnormal elongation of the posterior leaflet. A1–A3, anterior mitral leaflet segments 1 through 3; AC, anterior commissure; P1–P3, posterior mitral leaflet segments 1 through 3; PC, posterior commissure.

Subvalvular Apparatus

The subvalvular apparatus attaches the leaflets to the ventricular cavity creating a suspension system with two active roles: allowing full opening of the leaflets during diastole and preventing an excessive displacement of the leaflets above the annular plane during systole. Two anatomical structures compose the subvalvular apparatus: the papillary muscles (contractility) and the chordae tendinae (elasticity).

The chordae tendinae are classified according to their attachment between the free margin and the base of the leaflets as follows: (a) primary chordae, attached to the margin of the leaflets (marginal) (b) secondary chordae, attached to the ventricular side of the leaflet c) tertiary chordae, attached to the base (basal) of the leaflets (Figure 7.3) [16]. Each segment of the leaflets receives two or three chordae in proportional length to the length of the papillary muscles [17].

The papillary muscles arise from the ventricular wall at a junction located around one third from the apex and two thirds from the annulus; each group provides chordae to both leaflets, mainly to A2 and P2 segments. The anterolateral papillary muscle vasculature is supplied by the left anterior descending and the diagonal or marginal branch of the circumflex artery, whereas the posterior descending artery provides the blood supply to the posteromedial papillary muscle. The posteromedial papillary muscle is most commonly affected in the event of an ischemic insult because of its particular single blood vessel supply, playing an important role in ischemic mitral regurgitation [18,19].

The attachment of the papillary muscles to the ventricular wall grants the left ventricle with an important functional role in the mitral valve excursion, particularly in the setting of ischemic functional mitral regurgitation. Thus, progressive dilatation of the left ventricle in ischemic or nonischemic cardiomyopathies may result in functional regurgitation [20,21].

Mitral Valve Regurgitation

Acquired Mitral Valve Disease

Carpentier's classification has been consistently acquired and adapted by surgeons; however, a growing number of imaging specialists are familiar with the classification, mainly in terms of leaflet dysfunction (Table 7.1). Imaging techniques have traditionally played a very important role in the exact characterization of the resultant leaflet dysfunction [22]. In this line, Carpentier originally classified leaflet dysfunction into three types: type 1, normal leaflet motion; type II, excessive leaflet motion; and type III, restricted leaflet motion. After the recognition of ischemic ventricular remodeling in the pathogenesis of mitral regurgitation, type III was subdivided into type IIIA (restricted leaflet motion in diastole) and type IIIB (restricted leaflet motion in systole).

Carpentier's Type I Dysfunction

Type I dysfunction groups those patients with normal leaflet motion as the course of the leaflets between systole and diastole has a normal amplitude. The regurgitation is due to either a primary leaflet perforation or a lack of coaptation between leaflets due to annular dilation (Figures 7.4 and 7.5).

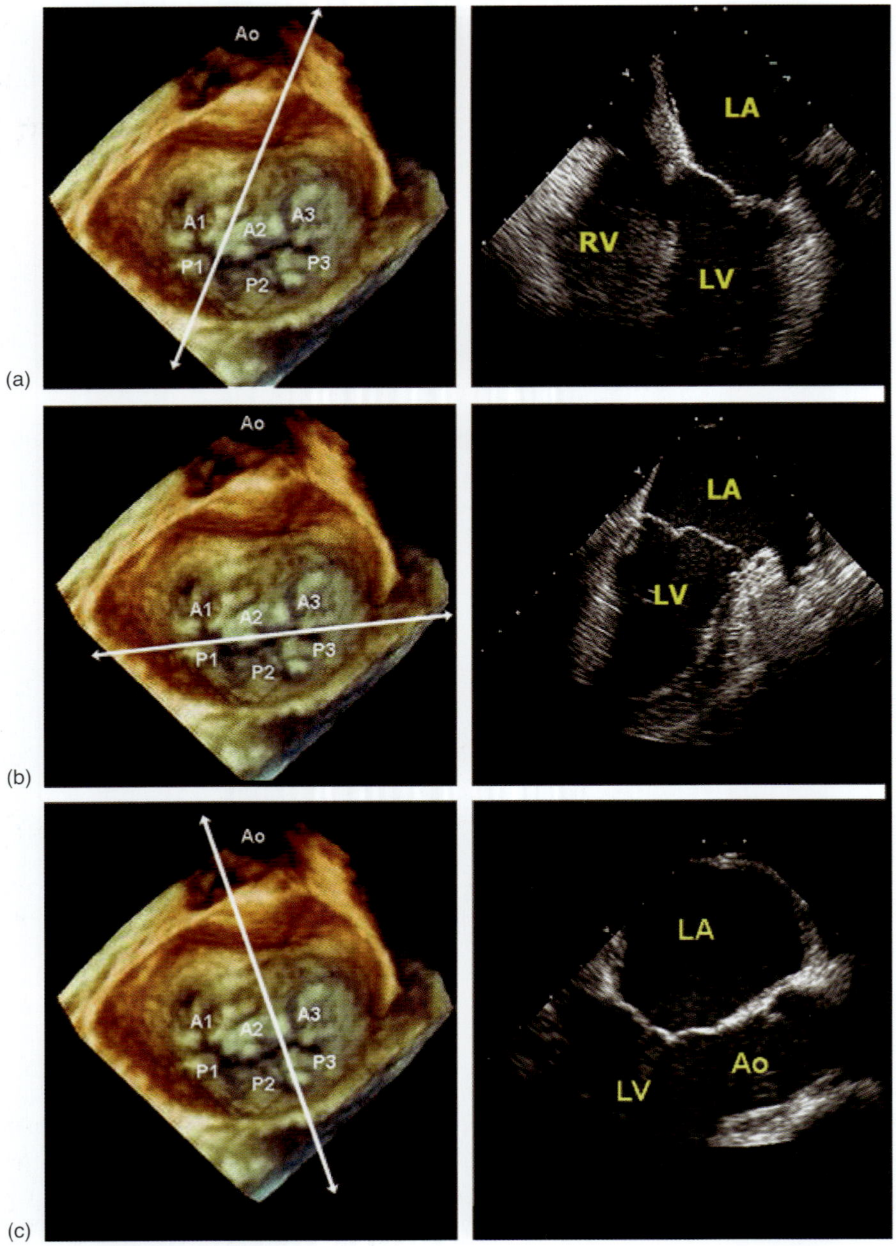

Figure 7.2 Transesophageal views of a normal mitral valve at three anatomic planes are shown: (a) four-chamber, (b) two-chamber, and (c) three-chamber planes. The orientations of these anatomic planes are shown on three-dimensional view of the mitral valve on the left panel. Ao, aorta; A1–A3, anterior mitral leaflet segments 1 through 3; LA, left atrium; LV, left ventricle; P1–P3, posterior mitral leaflet segments 1 through 3; RV, right ventricle.

Carpentier's Type II Dysfunction

Patients with type II dysfunction (Figure 7.6) present with an increased leaflet motion, which causes the free edge of the leaflet to override the plane of the annulus during systole (leaflet prolapse) [23, 24]. This condition is frequently associated with degenerative mitral valve disease, the most common cause of mitral regurgitation in western countries, which can be defined as a spectrum of conditions in which infiltrative tissue changes cause myxomatous degeneration (pathology) of the leaflets resulting in elongation or rupture of the mitral valve chordae and consequently leading to leaflet prolapse and annular dilatation (disease) [25].

The first entity of the spectrum of changes of degenerative mitral valve disease is fibroelastic deficiency (Figures 7.7–7.9) [26]. Clinically, fibroelastic deficiency features an older age patient (usually ≥50 years old) with a recent onset of a holosystolic murmur, and an absence of symptoms

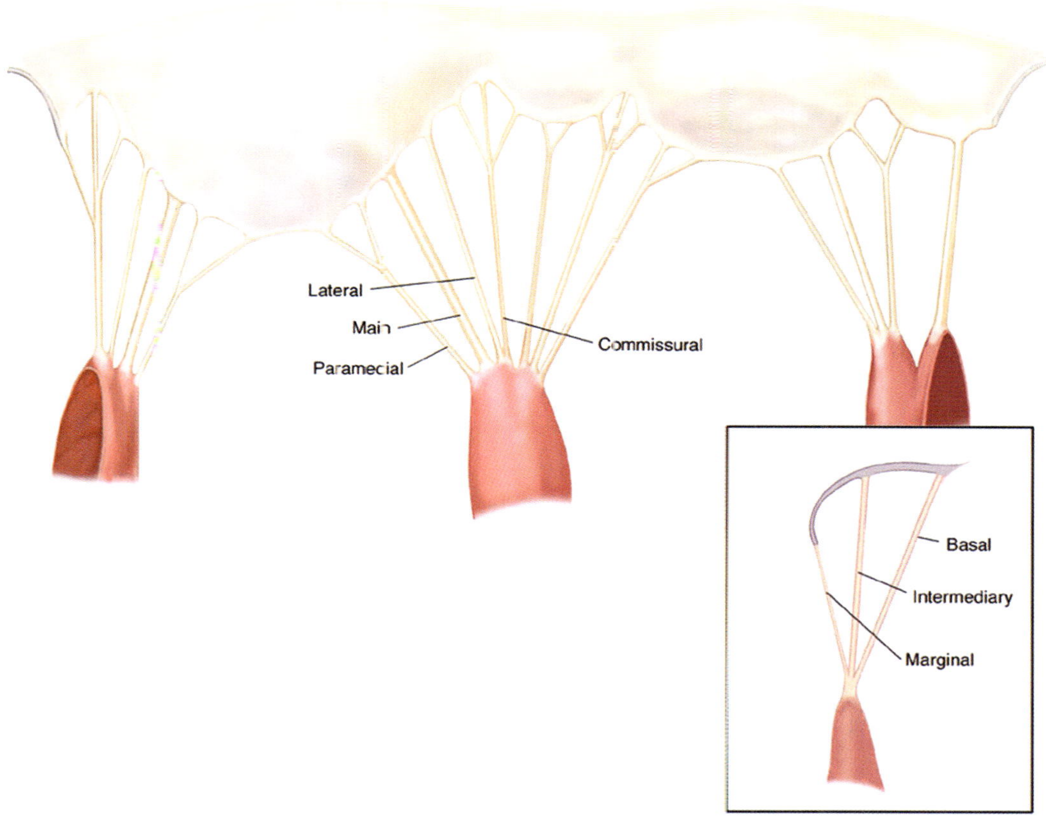

Figure 7.3 Illustration of the mitral valve subvalvular components: chordae tendinae.

until severe mitral regurgitation occurs (acute chordal rupture). Imaging studies usually show a single P2 prolapsed segment because of chordal rupture, no excess tissue, and mild to moderate symmetrical dilation of the annulus. Surgical inspection typically correlates with imaging findings and shows a single prolapsed segment and an otherwise normal valve with no excess tissue. Over time, secondary lesions may occur in the prolapsing segment resulting in an isolated myxomatous process leading to excess leaflet tissue and thickening [27].

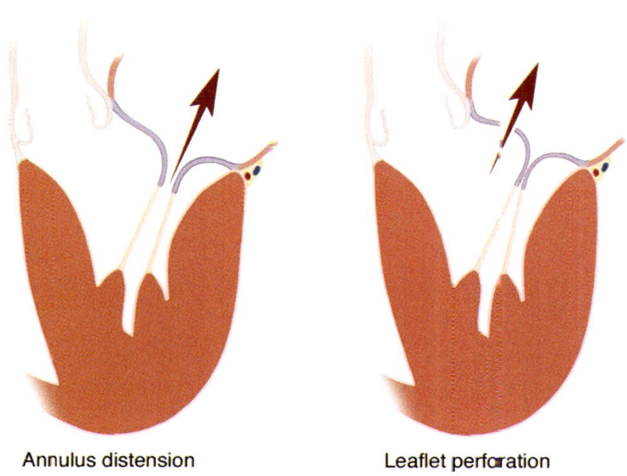

Figure 7.4 Carpentier's type I mechanisms of mitral valve dysfunction.

The opposite end of the degenerative mitral valve disease spectrum is Barlow's disease (Figures 7.10–7.12). The clinical diagnosis of Barlow's is generally established in a young patient with a mid-systolic click because of diffuse excess leaflet tissue frequently followed by a late systolic murmur [28,29]. Imaging studies are also the cornerstone in the diagnosis of Barlow's disease, displaying disease characteristic features such as diffuse severe leaflet thickening (leaflet prolapse into the left atrium during systole), severe annular dilation, and the presence of calcification along the posterior annulus although occasionally it may involve the entire annular surface and extend toward the subvalvular apparatus [30].

In the setting of Barlow's disease, surgical inspection may differ from imaging studies due to the complexity of the disease and lesions. As opposed to fibroelastic deficiency, leaflets present with diffuse excess tissue and multisegment irregular prolapse that gives the valve a cauliflower appearance with marked severe leaflet thickening in the coaptation area. Additionally, the

Table 7.1 Pathophysiologic triad used in Carpentier's classification of mitral regurgitation.

Dysfunction	Lesions	Etiology
Type I Normal leaflet motion	Annular dilatation Annular deformation Leaflet perforation	Ischemic cardiomyopathy Dilated cardiomyopathy Endocarditis
Type II Increased leaflet motion (leaflet prolapse)	Chordal elongation Chordal rupture Papillary muscle elongation Papillary muscle rupture	Degenerative mitral disease ■ Fibroelastic deficiency ■ Barlow's disease ■ Marfan's disease Endocarditis Rheumatic disease Trauma Ischemic cardiomyopathy
Type IIIA Restricted leaflet motion (restricted opening)	Leaflet thickening Leaflet retraction Chordal thickening Chordal retraction Chordal fusion Calcification Commissural fusion Ventricular fibrous plaque	Rheumatic disease Carcinoid disease
Type IIIB Restricted leaflet motion (restricted closure)	Leaflet tethering Papillary muscle displacement Ventricular dilatation Ventricular aneurysm Ventricular fibrous plaque	Ischemic cardiomyopathy Dilated cardiomyopathy

accumulated leaflet tension created by the severity and complexity of the lesions displaces the leaflet attachment toward the atrium subsequently creating a disjunction of the mitral annulus. Accordingly, the annulus is severely dilated, adapting a rounder shape in larger valves. The subvalvular apparatus analysis shows a thick, elongated, mesh-like chordae that may or may not be ruptured.

Carpentier's Type IIIA Dysfunction

Patients with type IIIA dysfunction have a restricted leaflet motion during both diastole and systole [19]. The most common lesions are leaflet thickening and retraction, chordal thickening and shortening or fusion, and commissural fusion; therefore, mitral regurgitation is most often associated with some degrees of mitral stenosis (Figures 7.13–7.15) [31]. Those mitral lesions that result in type IIIA dysfunction are mainly seen in two clinical settings: rheumatic disease and carcinoid heart disease.

Rheumatic heart disease leads to mitral regurgitation mainly secondary to ventricular dilation and restricted leaflet motion. Over time, an increased rigidity of the valve leaflets and the presence of shortening and fusion of the subvalvular apparatus results in leaflet scarring and consequently inadequate leaflet coaptation (Figure 7.14). In this setting, the misalignment of the papillary muscles further contributes to mitral regurgitation particularly in the setting of chronic rheumatic disease [32, 33]. When mitral stenosis coexists with mitral regurgitation, the classic leaflet opening with a doming "hockey stick" motion due to commissural fusion is frequently observed (Figure 7.15).

Carpentier's Type IIIB Dysfunction

Type IIIB mitral valve dysfunction is mostly represented by ischemic mitral valve disease and functional nonischemic mitral regurgitation secondary to ventricular dilatation (Figure 7.16) [34]. In the event of a myocardial infarction or chronic ischemia, left ventricular remodeling may occur, which, in turn, alters the geometrical conformation of the mitral subvalvular apparatus leading to mitral valve incompetence and miscoaptation [35,36].

Left ventricular changes after myocardial remodeling result in a spherical ballooned ventricle leading to an

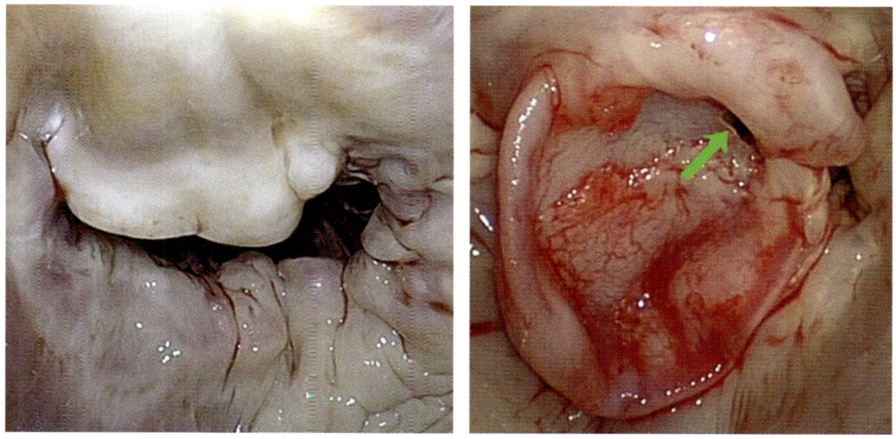

Figure 7.5 Surgical views of mitral valves with Carpentier's type I dysfunction. The mitral valve shown on the left panel has incomplete coaptation due to annular dilatation, whereas the valve shown on the right panel has a windsock deformity and a leaflet perforation caused by infective endocarditis.

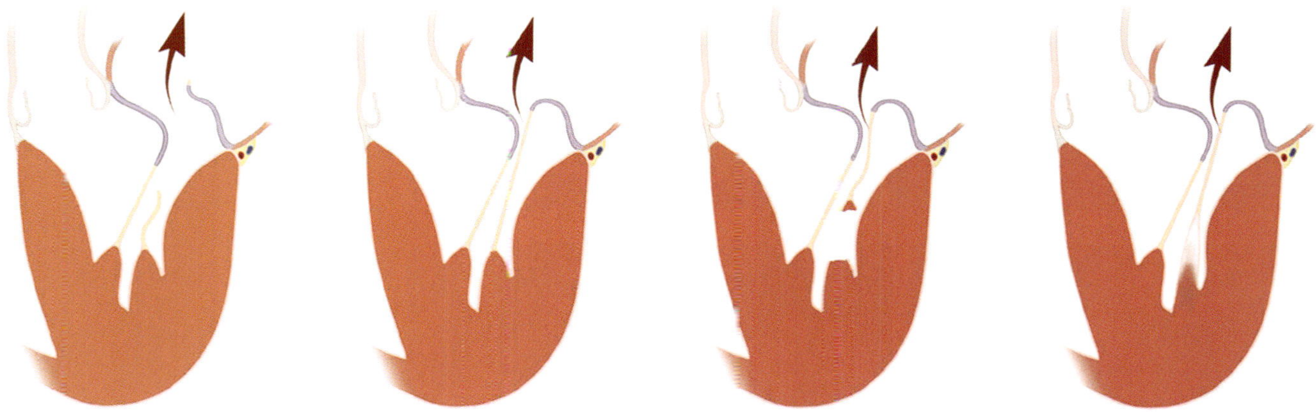

Figure 7.6 Carpentier's type II mechanisms of mitral valve dysfunction.

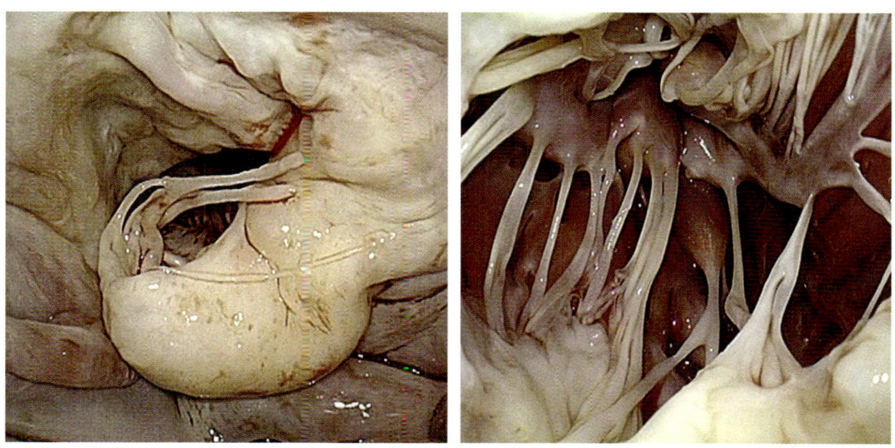

Figure 7.7 Surgical views of a mitral valve with Carpentier's type II dysfunction. The image shown on the left panel has thickened leaflets and a ruptured chord, whereas the image shown on the right panel shows chordal thickening and elongation.

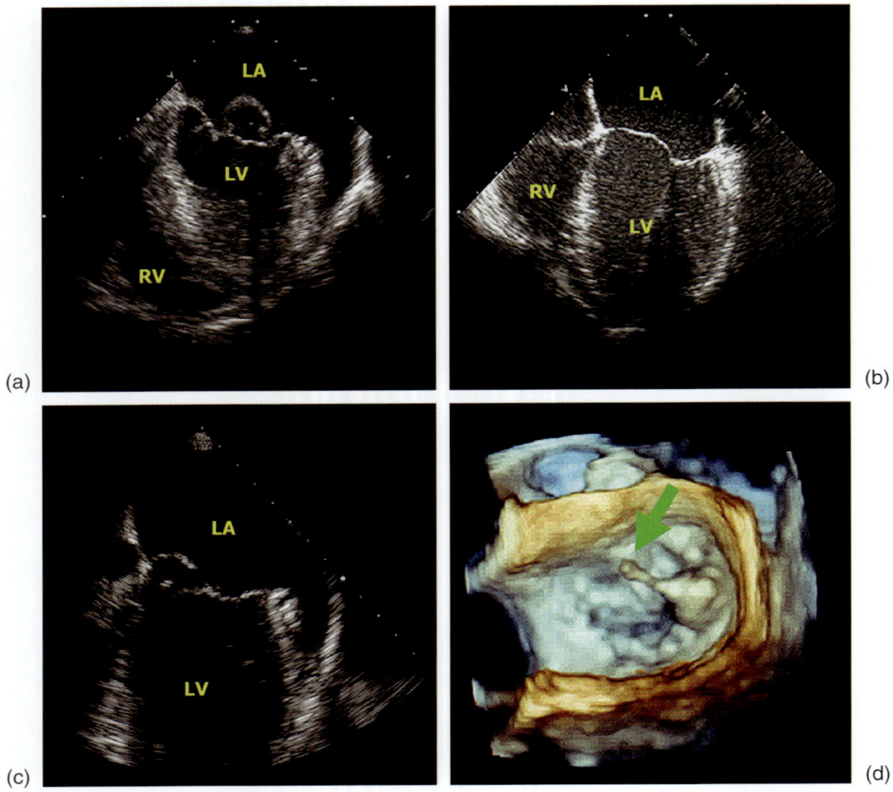

Figure 7.8 Transesophageal views of a mitral valve with Carpentier's type II dysfunction. (a) modified two-chamber view showing a prolapsing posterior leaflet middle scallop, (b) four-chamber view, (c) two-chamber view, and (d) three-dimensional view showing a ruptured chord (green arrow). LA, left atrium; LV, left ventricle; RV, right ventricle.

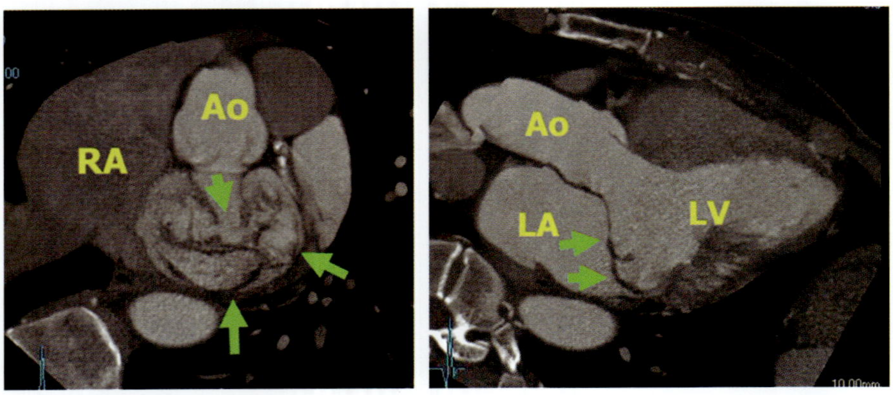

Figure 7.9 Cardiac computed tomography showing posterior leaflet prolapse (green arrows) from a short-axis (the left panel) and long-axis (the right panel) LV projections. Ao, aorta; LA, left atrium; LV, left ventricle; RA, right atrium.

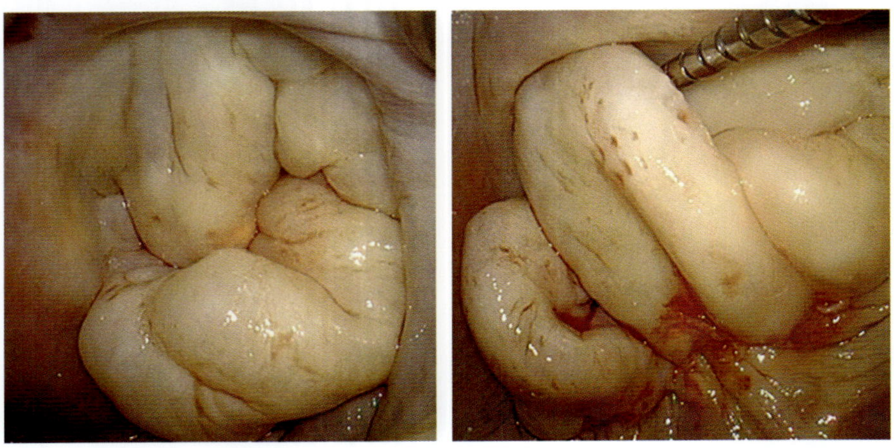

Figure 7.10 Surgical views of a mitral valve with Carpentier's type II dysfunction. The diffuse leaflet thickening and redundant tissue is characteristic of Barlow's disease.

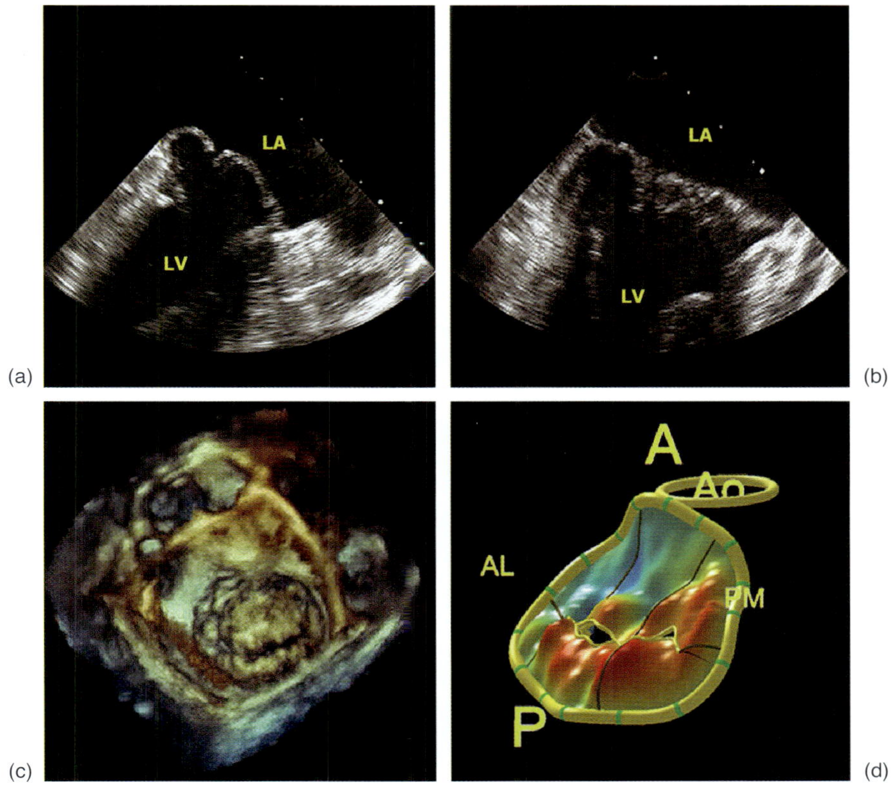

Figure 7.11 Transesophageal views of a mitral valve with Carpentier's type II dysfunction. (a) two-chamber view showing bileaflet prolapse, (b) modified two-chamber view, (c) three-dimensional view, (d) three-dimensional surface reconstruction demonstrating the location of the regurgitant orifices and the prolapsing surface highlighted in red. Ao, aorta; AL, anterolateral mitral commissure; LA, left atrium; LV, left ventricle; PM, posteromedial mitral commissure; A=anterior, P=posterior.

apical and lateral displacement of the papillary muscles further pulling the leaflets toward the ventricle (systolic tethering of mitral leaflets) [37]. Imaging studies will reveal restricted systolic leaflet motion and severe tenting of the mitral valve leaflets that is the area between the annulus and the leaflets and is considered the current reliable marker of severity.

Imaging has revealed two major patterns of leaflet tethering in the setting of ischemic mitral regurgitation: symmetric and asymmetric tethering. Asymmetric tethering is defined by the displacement of the posteromedial papillary muscle, causing posterior leaflet restriction and leading to an eccentric jet toward the posterior wall of the left atrium (Figure 7.17) [38].

As opposed to asymmetric tethering, symmetric tethering results from the displacement of both papillary muscles, and a central jet is typically observed. This symmetric pattern is the one observed in the setting of functional nonischemic mitral regurgitation secondary to dilated cardiomyopathy (Figures 7.18 and 7.19).

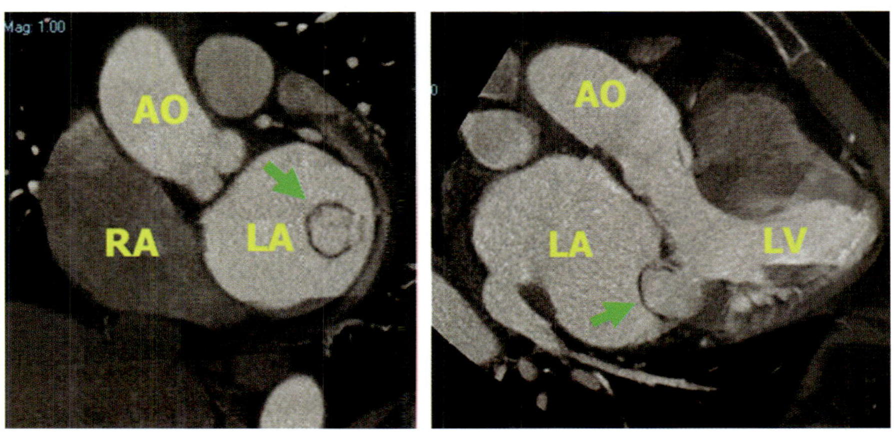

Figure 7.12 Cardiac computed tomography showing posterior bileaflet prolapse from a short-axis (the left panel) and long-axis (the right panel) LV projections. Ao, aorta; LA, left atrium; LV, left ventricle; RA, right atrium.

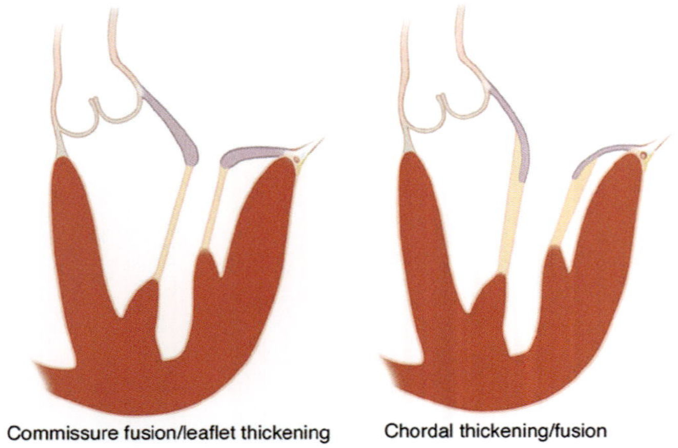

Figure 7.13 Carpentier's type IIIA mechanisms of mitral valve dysfunction.

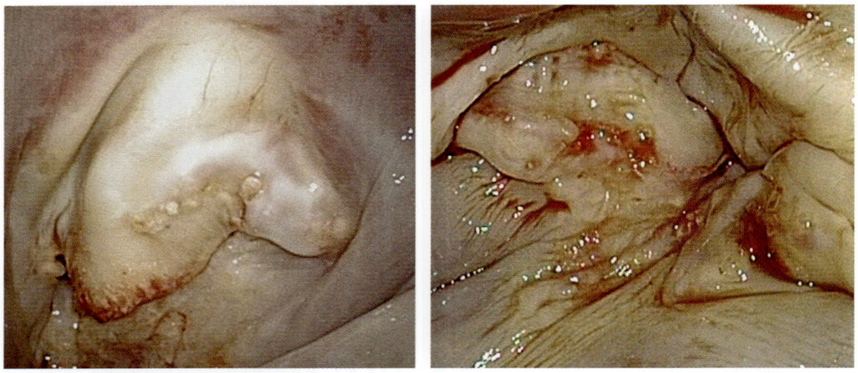

Figure 7.14 Surgical views of a mitral valve with Carpentier's type IIIA dysfunction. The leaflet deformation and retraction is characteristic of rheumatic disease.

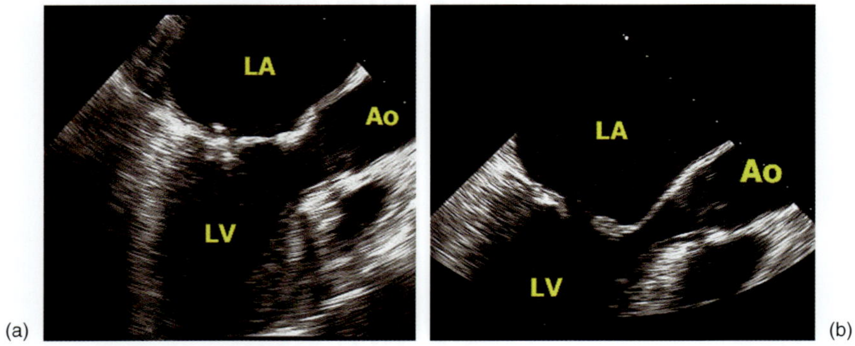

Figure 7.15 Transesophageal views of a mitral valve with Carpentier's type IIIA dysfunction caused by rheumatic disease. (a) Three-chamber view showing thickened leaflets at end-systole and (b) typical leaflet doming seen at end-diastole. Ao, aorta; LA, left atrium; LV, left ventricle.

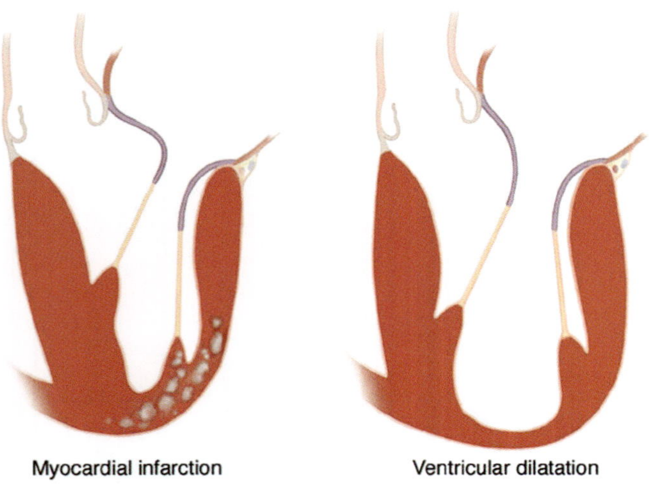

Figure 7.16 Carpentier's type IIIB mechanisms of mitral valve dysfunction

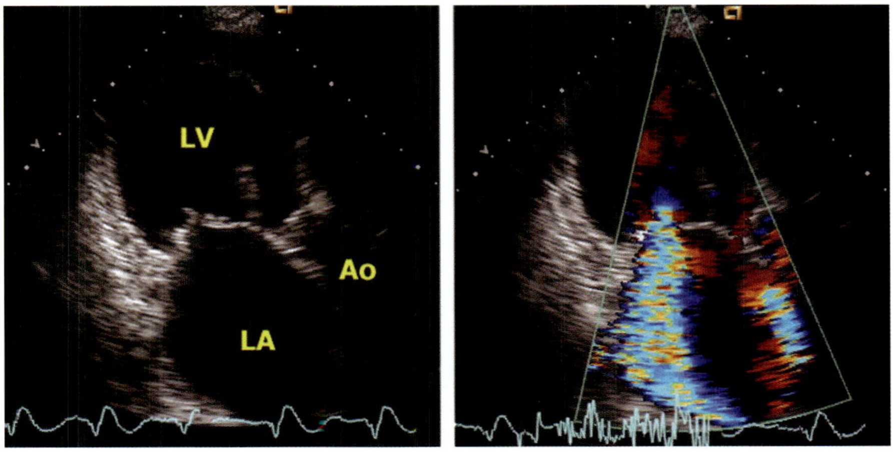

Figure 7.17 Transthoracic apical long-axis views obtained from a patient with Carpentier's type IIIB dysfunction. In the left panel, restricted motion of the posterior leaflet, caused by an inferolateral infarction, is apparent. In the right panel, a jet of severe mitral regurgitation is directed toward the restricted leaflet. Ao, aorta; LA, left atrium; LV, left ventricle.

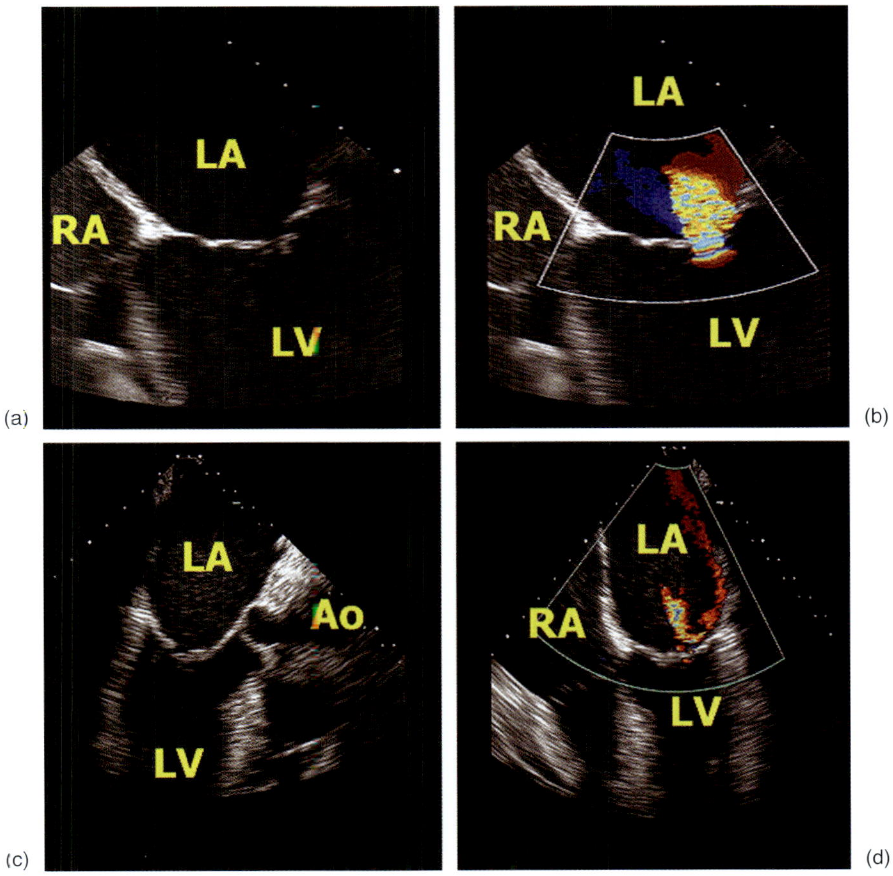

Figure 7.18 Transesophageal views of mitral valves with Carpentier's type IIIB dysfunction. (a) Four-chamber view obtained from a patient with dilated cardiomyopathy showing bileaflet tenting and incomplete leaflet coaptation, (b) four-chamber view showing moderate central regurgitation, (c) three-chamber view obtained from a different patient showing two chambers with a restricted posterior leaflet caused by an inferolateral infarct, and (d) four-dimensional view showing moderate eccentric regurgitation directed toward the restricted leaflet. Ao, aorta; LA, left atrium; LV, left ventricle; RA, right atrium.

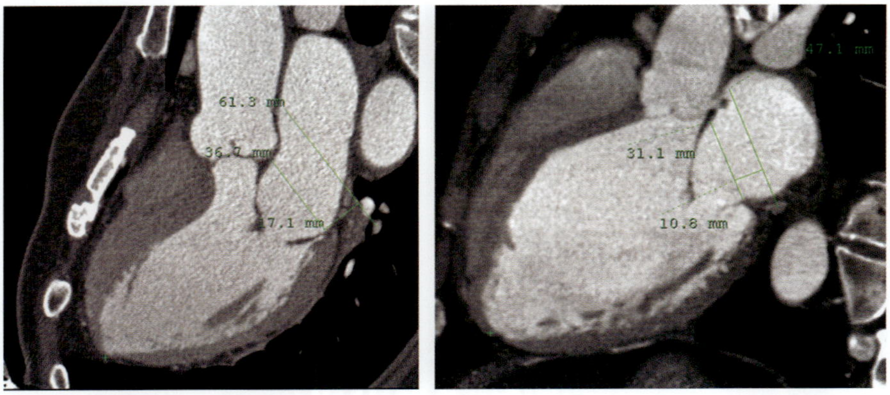

Figure 7.19 Cardiac computed tomography showing a normal (left) and a patient with dilated cardiomyopathy (right) showing posterior displacement of the plane of leaflet coaptation and tenting of the mitral valve leaflets.

Congenital Anomalies

Congenital malformations of the mitral valve are often associated with other cardiac or great vessel anomalies [39, 40]. Similar to acquired mitral valve disease, echocardiography and CT or magnetic resonance imaging allow classification of the malformations into functional groups (Figures 7.20 and 7.21) [41].

Mitral Valve Stenosis

Acquired Stenosis

The mitral valve orifice area is considered normal when it ranges from 4 to 6 cm^2. If mitral stenosis is present, it is considered mild when the area is <2 cm^2 and becomes critical when the valve area is <1 cm^2. A reduction in the mitral valve orifice area results in atrioventricular gradients and consequent elevation in left-sided pressures. The retrograde transmission of the elevated left atrial pressure leads to pulmonary arteriolar constriction, and pulmonary hypertension (chronic stages of the disease) often resulting in further tricuspid regurgitation. In this setting, rheumatic fever appears to be the leading cause of mitral stenosis as it is estimated that 25% of all patients with rheumatic heart disease have pure mitral stenosis.

Rheumatic Valve Disease

In the acute phase of the disease, exudative inflammatory reactions involve the connective tissue of the heart resulting in a slow progressing fibrous transformation of the leaflets and the subvalvular apparatus [42]. In this

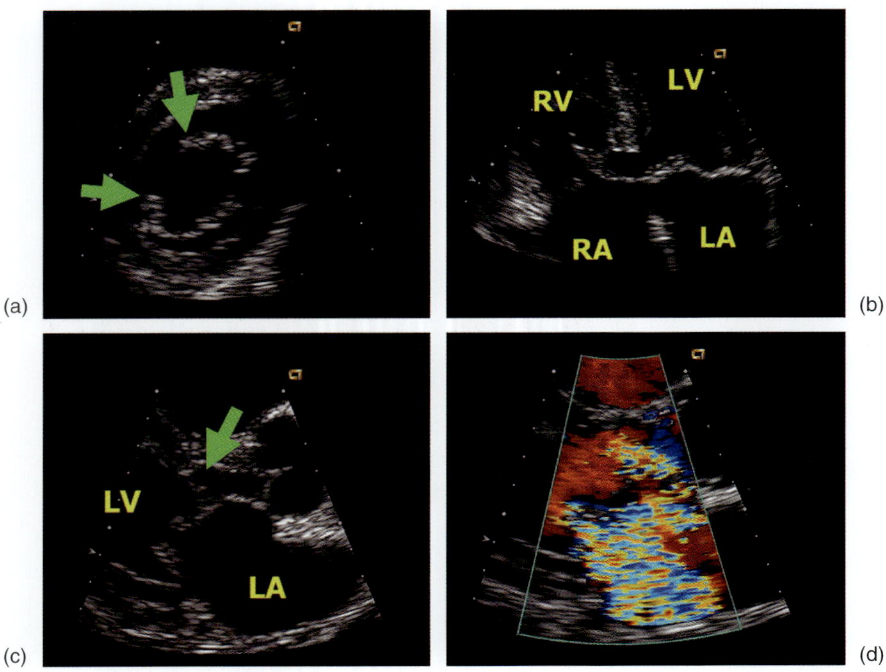

Figure 7.20 Cleft mitral valve seen by transthoracic echocardiography. (a) Short-axis view, (b) four-chamber view showing primum atrial septal defect and ventricular septal defect, (c) parasternal long-axis view showing abnormal septal chordal attachments, and (d) parasternal long-axis view showing severe regurgitation. LA, left atrium; LV, left ventricle; RA, right atrium; RV, right ventricle.

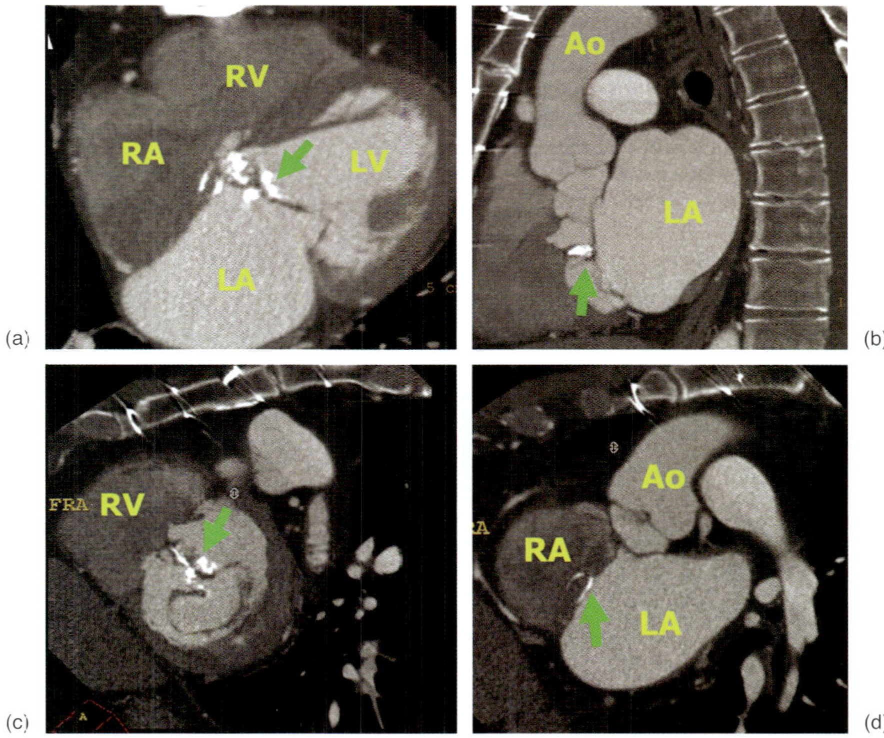

Figure 7.21 Cardiac computed tomography obtained in a patient with congenital mitral regurgitation caused by a cleft. (a) Axial view, (b) sagittal view showing calcified abnormal septal attachment, (c) short-axis view showing the anterior leaflet cleft, and (d) short-axis view showing a previously repaired primum atrial septal defect. Ao, aorta; LA, left atrium; LV, left ventricle; RA, right atrium; RV, right ventricle.

setting, the annulus of the mitral valve is severely dilated and deformed with an often asymmetrical dilation, predominant at the P3 segment and the posterior commissure. The leaflet tissue typically displays marked fibrotic changes leading to retraction and the leaflet indentations are no longer visible, particularly along the posterior leaflet (Figure 7.22). The anterior leaflet is less altered, and only the free edge is slightly prolapsed, thickened, and calcified. The chordae are shortened (reduced leaflet mobility) and often thickened and fused (reduced coaptation area). The commissural areas are always heavily fused. In the late stages of the disease, calcifications are particularly present, especially at the commissural edges producing a "fish mouth" like single central opening [32].

The diagnosis of mitral stenosis should be made with two-dimensional Doppler echocardiography (Figure 7.23) [43]. This examination evaluates the appearance and mobility of the mitral valve leaflets, commissures, and the subvalvular apparatus as well as the presence of calcifications. Echocardiography and cardiac magnetic resonance allow determination of the severity of mitral stenosis by measuring the mitral valve area, the trans-mitral gradient, and pulmonary artery pressures. However, cardiac computed tomography may also be very useful to assess the mitral valve orifice area by planimetry, measuring the degree of valvular calcification and leaflet thickening (Figure 7.24) [44].

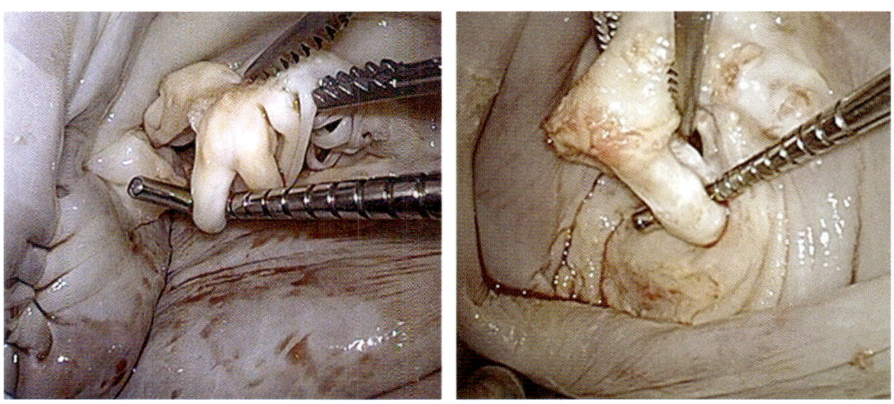

Figure 7.22 Surgical views of rheumatic valves showing thickened and fused chordae and fused commissures.

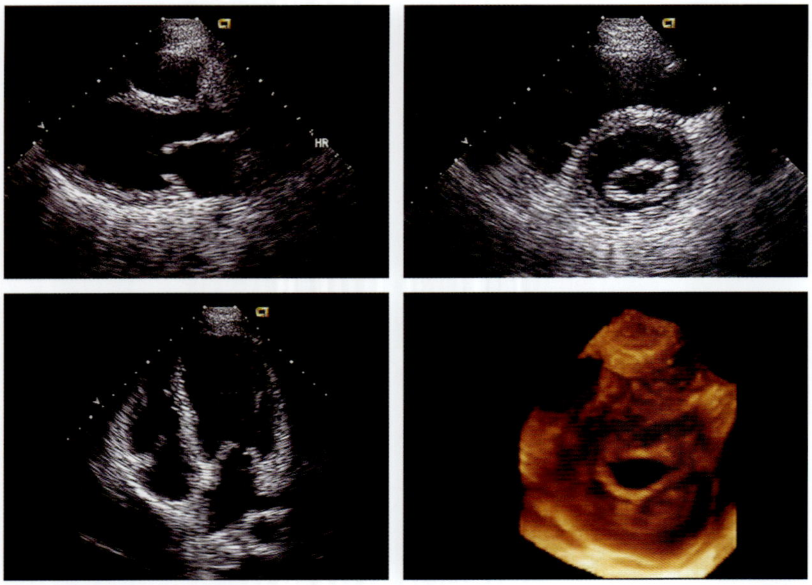

(a) (b) (c) (d)

Figure 7.23 Mitral stenosis seen by transthoracic echocardiography. (a) Parasternal long-view showing doming of the leaflets, (b) short-axis view showing fusion of the commissures and leaflet thickening, (c) apical four-chamber view showing restricted opening of the posterior leaflet, and (d) three-dimensional view showing the typical "fish-mouth" appearance.

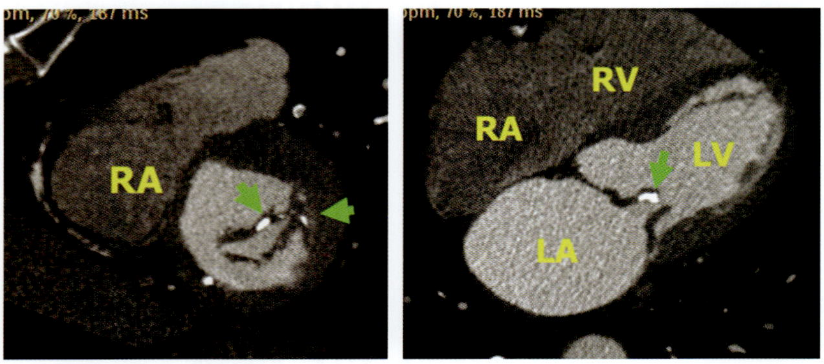

(a) (b)

Figure 7.24 Cardiac computed tomography obtained in a patient with mild rheumatic mitral valve stenosis. (a) Short-axis view and (b) four-chamber view. Arrows indicate location of calcification. LA, left atrium; LV, left ventricle; RA, right atrium; RV, right ventricle.

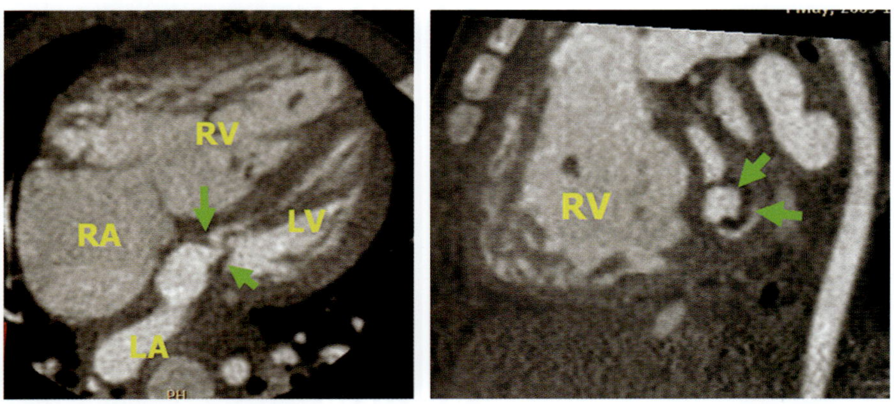

Figure 7.25 Cardiac computed tomography obtained in a 17-month patient with congenital mitral stenosis caused by a parachute valve. There is hypertrophy and dilatation of the RV. The thickened mitral valve leaflets lead to a common papillary muscle (the left panel). The restricted orifice measured 0.4 cm^2 by planimetry (the right panel). LA, left atrium; LV, left ventricle; RA, right atrium; RV, right ventricle.

Congenital Mitral Stenosis

Congenital mitral valve stenosis is uncommon and is usually diagnosed and treated early in infancy. Imaging is essential to establish the specific diagnosis and the presence of associated cardiovascular anomalies (Figure 7.25).

References

1. Chiechi MA, Lees WM, Thompson R. (1956) Functional anatomy of the normal mitral valve. *J Thorac Surg* 32:378–398.
2. Perloff JK, Roberts WC (1972) The mitral apparatus. Functional anatomy of mitral regurgitation. *Circulation* 46:227–239.
3. Quill JL, Hill AJ, Laske TG, Alfieri O, Iaizzo PA. (2009) Mitral leaflet anatomy revisited. *J Thorac Cardiovasc Surg* 137:1077–1081.
4. Glasson JR, Komeda MK, Daughters GT *et al.* (1996) Three-dimensional regional dynamics of the normal mitral annulus during left ventricular ejection. *J Thorac Cardiovasc Surg* 111:574–585.
5. Hueb AC, Jatene FB, Moreira LF, Pomerantzeff PM, Kallas E, de Oliveira SA. (2002) Ventricular remodeling and mitral valve modifications in dilated cardiomyopathy: new insights from anatomic study. *J Thorac Cardiovasc Surg* 124:1216–1224.
6. Jensen MO, Jensen H, Smerup M *et al.* (2008) Saddle-shaped mitral valve annuloplasty rings experience lower forces compared with flat rings. *Circulation* 118:S250–S255.
7. Nguyen TC, Itoh A, Carlhall CJ *et al.* (2008) The effect of pure mitral regurgitation on mitral annular geometry and three-dimensional saddle shape. *J Thorac Cardiovasc Surg* 136:557–565.
8. Ranganathan N, Lam JH, Wigle ED, Silver MD. (1970) Morphology of the human mitral valve. II. The value leaflets. *Circulation* 41:459–467.
9. He S, Fontaine AA, Schwammenthal E, Yoganathan AP, Levine RA. (1997) Integrated mechanism for functional mitral regurgitation: leaflet restriction versus coapting force: in vitro studies. *Circulation* 96:1826–1834.
10. Kumar N, Kumar M, Duran CM. (1995) A revised terminology for recording surgical findings of the mitral valve. *J Heart Valve Dis* 4:70–75; discussion 76–77.
11. Dent JM, Spotnitz WD, Nolan SP, Jayaweera AR, Glasheen WP, Kaul S. (1995) Mechanism of mitral leaflet excursion. *Am J Physiol* 269:H2100–H2108.
12. Carpentier AF, Lessana A, Relland JY *et al.* (1995) The "physio-ring": an advanced concept in mitral valve annuloplasty. *Ann Thorac Surg* 60:1177–1185; discussion 1185–6.
13. Pomerance A. (1969) Ballooning deformity (mucoid degeneration) of atrioventricular valves. *Br Heart J* 31:343–351.
14. Adams DH, Anyanwu AC, Sugeng L, Lang RM. (2008) Degenerative mitral valve regurgitation: surgical echocardiography. *Curr Cardiol Rep* 10:226–232.
15. Zegdi R, Khabbaz Z, Flecher E *et al.* (2006) Management of commissural lesions in native mitral valve endocarditis: long-term results of valve repair and partial homograft replacement. *J Heart Valve Dis* 15:356–359.
16. Lam JH, Ranganathan N, Wigle ED, Silver MD. (1970) Morphology of the human mitral valve. I. Chordae tendineae: a new classification. *Circulation* 41:449–458.
17. Nielsen SL, Nygaard H, Mandrup L *et al.* (2002) Mechanism of incomplete mitral leaflet coaptation—interaction of chordal restraint and changes in mitral leaflet coaptation geometry. Insight from in vitro validation of the premise of force equilibrium. *J Biomech Eng* 124:596–608.
18. Burch GE, De Pasquale NP, Phillips JH. (1963) Clinical manifestations of papillary muscle dysfunction. *Arch Intern Med* 112:112–117.
19. Godley RW, Wann LS, Rogers EW, Feigenbaum H, Weyman AE. (1981) Incomplete mitral leaflet closure in patients with papillary muscle dysfunction. *Circulation* 63:565–571.
20. Kono T, Sabbah HN, Rosman H, Alam M, Jafri S, Goldstein S. (1992) Left ventricular shape is the primary determinant of functional mitral regurgitation in heart failure. *J Am Coll Cardiol* 20:1594–1598.
21. Kono T, Sabbah HN, Stein PD, Brymer JF, Khaja F. (1991) Left ventricular shape as a determinant of functional mitral regurgitation in patients with severe heart failure secondary to either coronary artery disease or idiopathic dilated cardiomyopathy. *Am J Cardiol* 68:355–359.
22. O'Gara P, Sugeng L, Lang R *et al.* (2008) The role of imaging in chronic degenerative mitral regurgitation. *JACC Cardiovasc Imaging* 1:221–237.
23. Carpentier A, Deloche A, Dauptain J *et al.* (1971) A new reconstructive operation for correction of mitral and tricuspid insufficiency. *J Thorac Cardiovasc Surg* 61:1–13.
24. Lillehei CW, Gott VL, Dewall RA, Varco RL. (1958) The surgical treatment of stenotic or regurgitant lesions of the mitral and aortic valves by direct vision utilizing a pump-oxygenator. *J Thorac Surg* 35:154–191.
25. Fornes P, Heudes D, Fuzellier JF, Tixier D, Bruneval P, Carpentier A. (1999) Correlation between clinical and histologic patterns of degenerative mitral valve insufficiency: a histomorphometric study of 130 excised segments. *Cardiovasc Pathol* 8:81–92.
26. Nesta F, Leyne M, Yosefy C *et al.* (2005) New locus for autosomal dominant mitral valve prolapse on chromosome 13: clinical insights from genetic studies. *Circulation* 112:2022–2030.
27. Carpentier A, Chauvaud S, Fabiani JN *et al.* (1980) Reconstructive surgery of mitral valve incompetence: ten-year appraisal. *J Thorac Cardiovasc Surg* 79:338–348.
28. Gulotta SJ, Gulco L, Padmanabhan V, Miller S. (1974) The syndrome of systolic click, murmur, and mitral valve prolapse—a cardiomyopathy? *Circulation* 49:717–728.
29. Reduto LA, Gulotta SJ. (1976) Cardiology: prolapsed mitral valve syndrome. *Postgrad Med* 60:171–176.
30. Anyanwu AC, Adams DH. (2007) Etiologic classification of degenerative mitral valve disease: Barlow's disease and fibroelastic deficiency. *Semin Thorac Cardiovasc Surg* 19:90–96.
31. David TE (1997) The appropriateness of mitral valve repair for rheumatic mitral valve disease. *J Heart Valve Dis* 6:373–374.
32. Chauvaud S, Fuzellier JF, Berrebi A, Deloche A, Fabiani JN, Carpentier A. (2001) Long-term (29 years) results of reconstructive surgery in rheumatic mitral valve insufficiency. *Circulation* 104:I12–I15.

33. Zegdi R, Khabbaz Z, Chauvaud S, Latremouille C, Fabiani JN, Deloche A. (2007) Posterior leaflet extension with an autologous pericardial patch in rheumatic mitral insufficiency. *Ann Thorac Surg* 84:1043–1044.
34. Agricola E, Oppizzi M, Pisani M, Meris A, Maisano F, Margonato A. (2008) Ischemic mitral regurgitation: mechanisms and echocardiographic classification. *Eur J Echocardiogr* 9:207–221.
35. Hung J, Otsuji Y, Handschumacher MD, Schwammenthal E, Levine RA. (1999) Mechanism of dynamic regurgitant orifice area variation in functional mitral regurgitation: physiologic insights from the proximal flow convergence technique. *J Am Coll Cardiol* 33:538–545.
36. Levine RA. (2004) Dynamic mitral regurgitation—more than meets the eye. *N Engl J Med* 351:1681–1684.
37. Magne J, Pibarot P, Dagenais F, Hachicha Z, Dumesnil JG, Senechal M. (2007) Preoperative posterior leaflet angle accurately predicts outcome after restrictive mitral valve annuloplasty for ischemic mitral regurgitation. *Circulation* 115:782–791.
38. McCully RB, Enriquez-Sarano M, Tajik AJ, Seward JB. (1994) Overestimation of severity of ischemic/functional mitral regurgitation by color Doppler jet area. *Am J Cardiol* 74: 790–793.
39. Carney EK, Braunwald E, Roberts WC, Aygen M, Morrow AG. (1962) Congenital mitral regurgitation. Clinical, hemodynamic and angiocardiographic findings in nine patients. *Am J Med* 33:223–235.
40. Davachi F, Moller JH, Edwards JE. (1971) Diseases of the mitral valve in infancy. An anatomic analysis of 55 cases. *Circulation* 43:565–579.
41. Carpentier A, Branchini B, Cour JC *et al.* (1976) Congenital malformations of the mitral valve in children. Pathology and surgical treatment. *J Thorac Cardiovasc Surg* 72:854–866.
42. Jones TD, Lingley JR *et al.* (1949) Rheumatic heart disease, with mitral and aortic stenosis. *N Engl J Med* 240:1018–1022.
43. Marijon E, Ou P, Celermajer DS *et al.* (2007) Prevalence of rheumatic heart disease detected by echocardiographic screening. *N Engl J Med* 357:470–476.
44. Messika-Zeitoun D, Serfaty JM, Laissy JP *et al.* (2006) Assessment of the mitral valve area in patients with mitral stenosis by multislice computed tomography. *J Am Coll Cardiol* 48:411–413.

8 The Aortic Root

Fabiana Isabella Gambarin,[1] Massimo Massetti,[2] Roberto Dore,[1]
Eric Saloux,[2] Valentina Favalli[1] & Eloisa Arbustini[1]

[1] *IRCCS Foundation Policlinico San Matteo, Pavia, Italy*
[2] *University Hospital of Caen, Caen, France*

Definition of the Aortic Root

The aortic root is a complex functional unit situated between the left ventricular outflow tract (LVOT) and the ascending aorta. It supports the leaflets of the aortic valve and gives origin to the coronary arteries. The anatomic components that form this functional unit physiologically act as integrated and interdepending structures. The aortic root morphology determines the direction of the flows that are essential for the aortic valve function and coronary perfusion. This chapter illustrates the imaging approach to the aortic root based on current knowledge of the anatomy and physiology, including insights on the aortic valve (see Chapter 4). The physiopathology of the aortic root is illustrated through ultrasound imaging as the key routine tool for the diagnosis and monitoring of aortic root pathology, computerized tomography, and magnetic resonance imaging (MRI).

Anatomy

The aortic root is delineated superiorly by the sinotubular junction or ridge and inferiorly by the ventriculoaortic junction (generally called the "aortic annulus").

The aortic root consists of (Figures 8.1–8.8):

1 the sinotubular ridge/junction,
2 the Valsalva sinuses,
3 the leaflets,
4 the commissures,
5 the interleaflets triangles, and
6 the ventriculoaortic junction.

Revisiting Cardiac Anatomy: A Computed-Tomography-Based Atlas and Reference, 1st edition. Edited by Farhood Saremi, Eloisa Arbustini, Stephen Achenbach and Jagat Narula.

The Sinotubular Junction

The ***sinotubular junction*** or **ridge** forms a circular ring at the level of the attachments of the aortic commissures [1, 2]. The diameter is about 10–15% smaller than that of the ventriculoaortic junction [1]. It lies at the level of the commissural apices. The sinotubular ridge is thicker than that of the adjacent sinuses and separates the aortic root from the tubular portion of the ascending aorta. Since it provides most of the support for the valve cusps at their commissures, its integrity is essential for the correct function of the valve. When the sinotubular ridge is structurally compromised, the aortic valve may be functionally incompetent [2].

Histology. The sinotubular junction is largely made up of elastic fibers, collagen fibers and smooth muscle cells, and it supports the peripheral upper attachments of the valve leaflets.

The Valsalva Sinuses

The *Valsalva sinuses* are expanded portions of the aortic root and make up the external walls of the root. They are named according to the coronary arteries originating from them: right, left, and noncoronary. Although the three sinuses of the root and their leaflets play an identical function, their anatomy differs [1,3]:

- The two coronary sinuses consist mainly of the aortic wall with crescents of ventricular muscle incorporated at the base of each of them; and
- The noncoronary sinus consists exclusively of fibrous wall. In fact, the base of the noncoronary sinus is part of the mitroaortic continuity, which is a feature of the outflow tract of the left ventricle (Figure 8.1).

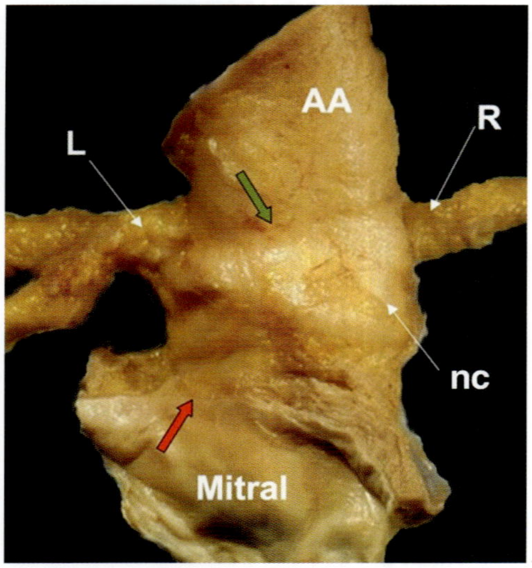

Figure 8.1 External posterior view of the aortic root and first part of the ascending aorta. nc, noncoronary sinus; L, left coronary originating from the left coronary sinus; R, right coronary (the origin is behind the aortic root); the red arrow indicates the mitroaortic continuity; AA, ascending aorta; the green arrow indicates the sinotubular junction.

The base of the left coronary leaflet partially attaches to the septal muscle and partly to the fibrous skeleton of the heart, as well as to the base of the anterior mitral leaflet. The right coronary cusp is attached to both the septal muscle and the membranous septum. The noncoronary leaflet attaches to the membranous septum and then along the fibrous skeleton in continuity with the anterior leaflet of the mitral valve. The posterior aspect of the aortic root (Figure 8.1) is supported by fibrous tissue for approximately 55% of its circumference from the membranous part of the septum to the left trigone. Connective tissue diseases that involve the fibrous skeleton of the heart may stretch the ventriculoaortic junction especially in the region of the noncoronary sinus, which frequently is the first structure that undergoes remodeling in inheritable collagen diseases [4] (Figures 8.9 and 8.10).

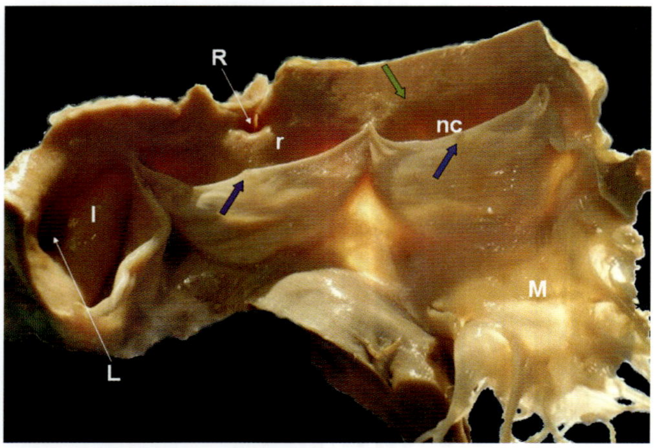

Figure 8.2 The aortic root cut between the noncoronary sinus (nc) and the left coronary sinus (l). In the middle of the free margin of each cusp, there is the Arantius nodulus (blue arrows). Green arrow indicates how the sinotubular ridge appears on the internal face of the root. L, left coronary ostium; M, anterior mitral leaflet; r, right coronary sinus; R, right coronary ostium.

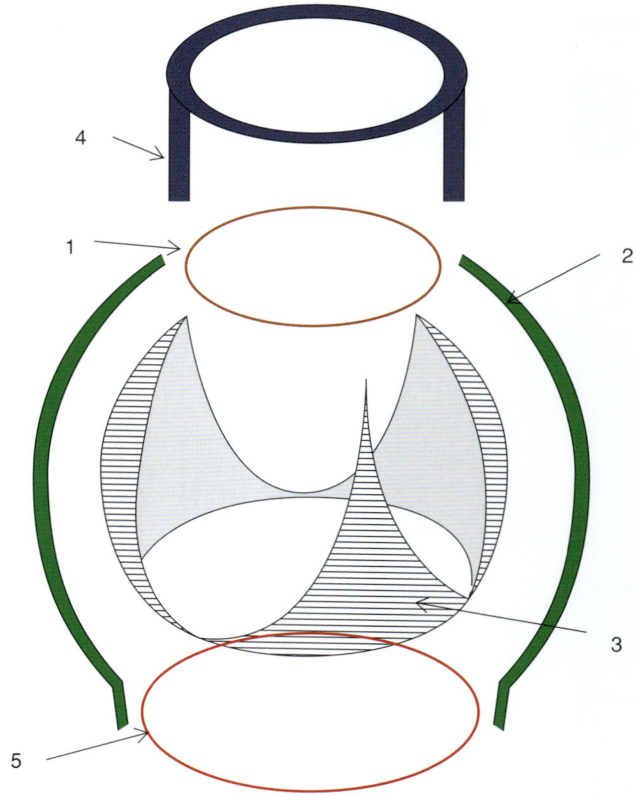

Figure 8.3 Aortic root scheme. Each single component of the aortic root is separately drafted from the others to better show the structure and the geometry of this functional unit. Cusps are not included. (1) The sinotubular junction is a ring that constitutes the boundary from the wall of the Valsalva sinuses into the tubular ascending aorta. The diameter of the sinotubular junction is about 10–15% smaller than the base of the ventriculoaortic junction. (2) The walls of the Valsalva sinuses. (3) The three-coronet shaped ventriculoaortic junction consisting of the three interleaflets triangles. The apices of the triangles insert on the ring of the sinotubular junction, whereas the base of the ventriculoaortic junction corresponds to an ideal ring, which passes through the *nadirs* of the three aortic cusps. The distance between the base and the apex of each interleaflet triangle normally ranges between 12 and 18 mm. (4) The tubular ascending aorta. (5) The virtual ring that constitutes the base of the ventriculoaortic junction, which ideally constitutes the boundary between the left ventricle outflow tract and the aortic root.

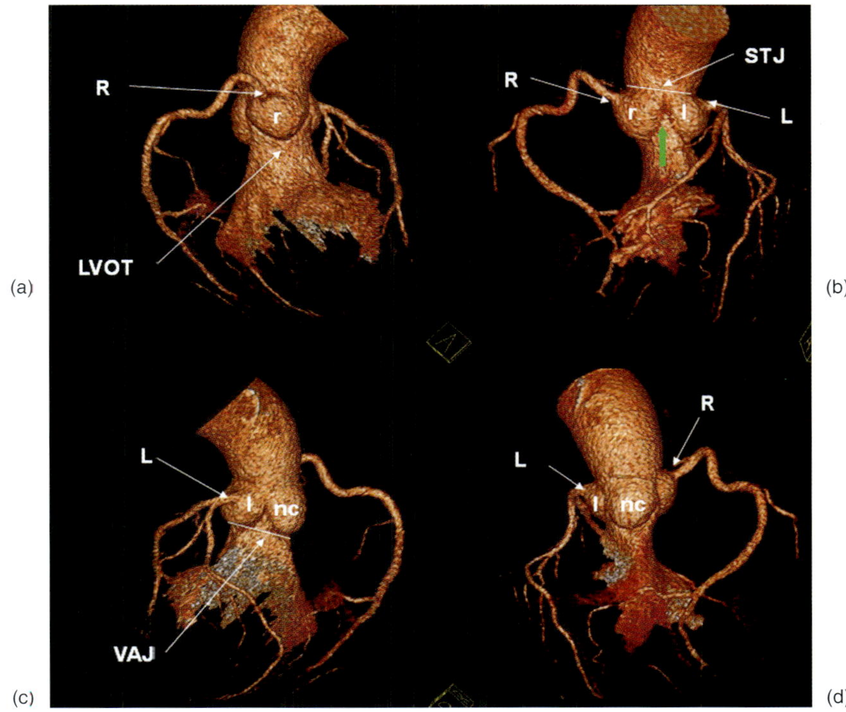

Figure 8.4 Three-dimensional anatomy of the aortic root. Anterior (a), left (b), posterior (c), and right (d) views demonstrate the inside morphology of the left ventricle outflow tract (LVOT) and of the aortic lumen; outflow tract in continuity with the interleaflets triangles (green arrow) interposed between the semilunar aspect of the profile of the parietal attachments of the leaflets. The right (R) and left (L) coronary ostia emerge from the cranial aspect of the Valsava sinuses: right coronary sinus (r), left coronary sinus (l). nc is the noncoronary sinus. The ideal plane through the bases of Valsalva sinuses is defined as annular ring or ventriculoaortic junction. The sinotubular junction (STJ) is smaller than ventriculoaortic junction. Aortic root is located between the ventriculoaortic junction (VAJ) and the sinotubular junction.

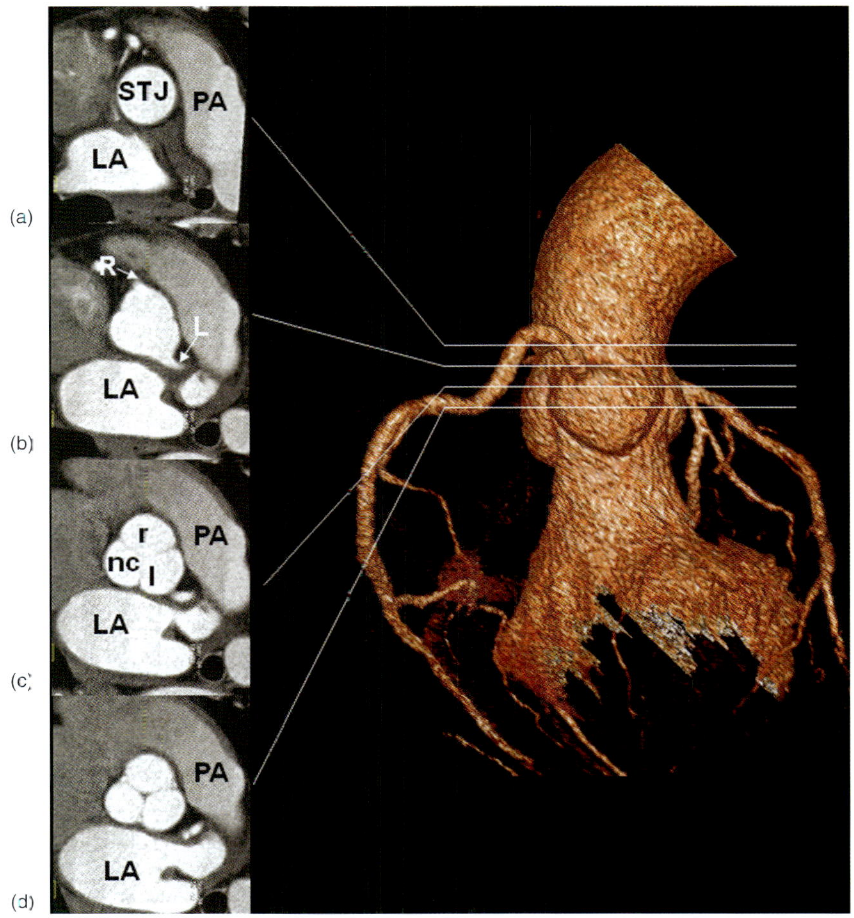

Figure 8.5 Short-axis planes of the aortic root: CT images in mid-diastolic phase. (a) Through sinotubular junction (STJ) where diameter is smaller than tubular aorta and aortic root. (b) Through right (R) and left (L) coronary ostia where parietal insertion of the valve leaflet and the shape of sinuses are evident. (c) Through the free margins of the valve leaflets where noncoronary (nc) left coronary (l), and right coronary (r) sinuses are evident. LA, left atrium; PA, pulmonary artery. (d) Through the coaptation area of the three leaflets.

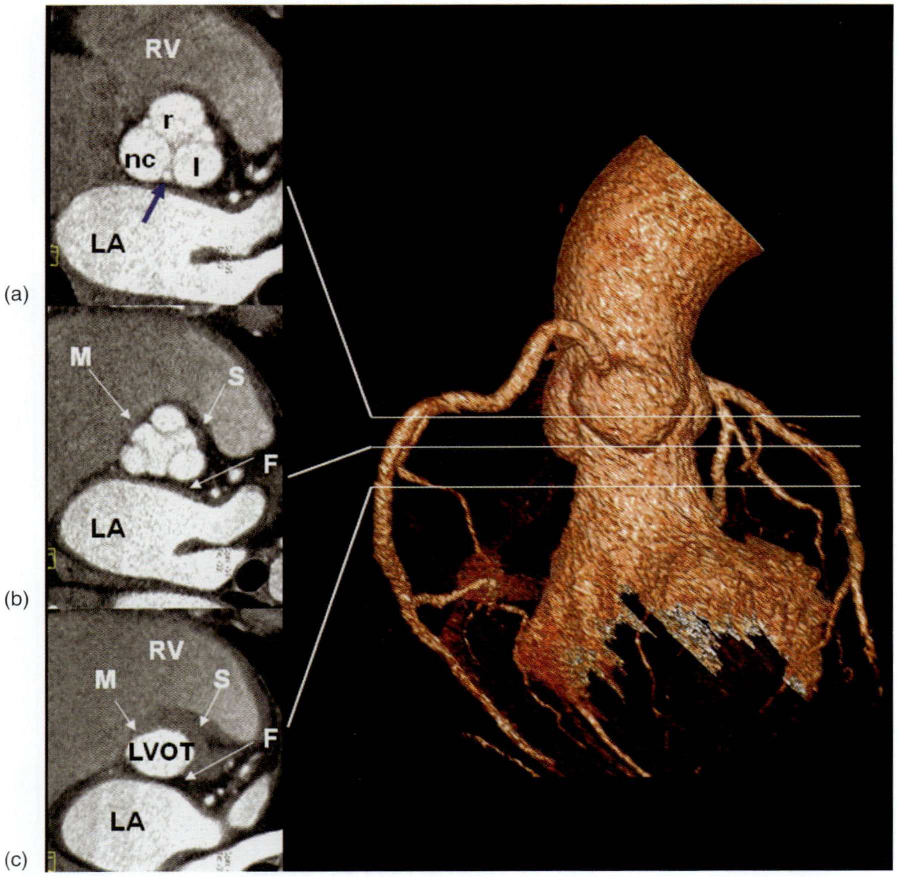

Figure 8.6 Short-axis planes of the aortic root CT images in end-diastolic phase. (a) Through the apices of the interleaflets triangles (blue arrow). (b) Through the base of Valsalva sinuses; the central area between the sinus bases corresponds to the apical segment of outflow tract of the left ventricle; the base of the noncoronary sinus is contiguous to the membranous septum (M) and fibrous skeleton (F). The base of left coronary sinus is partially contiguous to the fibrous skeleton and to the septal muscle (S). (c) Through outflow tract of left ventricle (LVOT) where anterior and left lateral wall correspond to septal muscle, posterior wall corresponds to fibrous skeleton, and right lateral wall to membranous septum. These different wall structures correspond to the elliptical aspect of the axial section of the outflow tract. l, left coronary sinus; LA, left atrium; nc, noncoronary sinus; r, right coronary sinus; RV, right ventricle.

Histology. The structure of the walls of the Valsalva sinuses is similar to that of the aortic wall in terms of composition with elastic lamellae alternated with smooth muscle cell layers and collagen fibers [5].

The Aortic Valve Structure (Semilunar Leaflets and commissures)

The aortic valve consists of three *semilunar leaflets*. The profile of insertion of the leaflets (cusps) is linear and semilunar; the coaptation surface of the leaflets is in the middle between the *nadir* of their insertion and the commissural areas. Each leaflet has a base that contributes to the definition of the ventriculoaortic junction, a "body", and a free margin. The superior aspect ends at the level of the sinotubular junction. Normal aortic leaflets are soft and pliable. When they close, the valve competence depends on the coaptation of the three leaflets (Figures 8.11 and 8.12). At the middle level of each cusp, the coaptation depth is 8–10 mm. The free margin of each cusp shows a central nodule called corpus of Arantius from which the ridges extend to the commissures. Each ridge forms the lower margin of the coaptation surface of the valve. The lunula above each ridge provides the area of coaptation with the corresponding portions of the abutting cusps [2,5]. Each ridge and lunula coaptate to ensure the absence of regurgitation. Fenestrations may recur in the lunulae; in normally coapting valves, fenestrations do not cause regurgitation since they lie, in most cases, above the ridge of closure (Figure 8.13). The aortic leaflets are named in relation to the coronary arteries: left coronary, right coronary, and noncoronary leaflet. The noncoronary leaflet is typically larger than the other two leaflets.

Histology. Aortic leaflets show dense collagen bundles at the level of their semilunar hinge on the arterial wall and of their free margin. The insertion of the apices of the semilunar hinges on the aortic wall corresponds to the apices of the interleaflets triangles (see below). These regions are strongly reinforced with connective fibers and elastic aortic lamellae, thus holding the semilunar leaflets and distributing the tension forces that would otherwise break and distort the leaflets [5] (Figures 8.12 and 8.14). Each cusp consists of three layers: the *fibrosa*, on the aortic side, the *spongiosa* in the middle, and the *ventricularis*

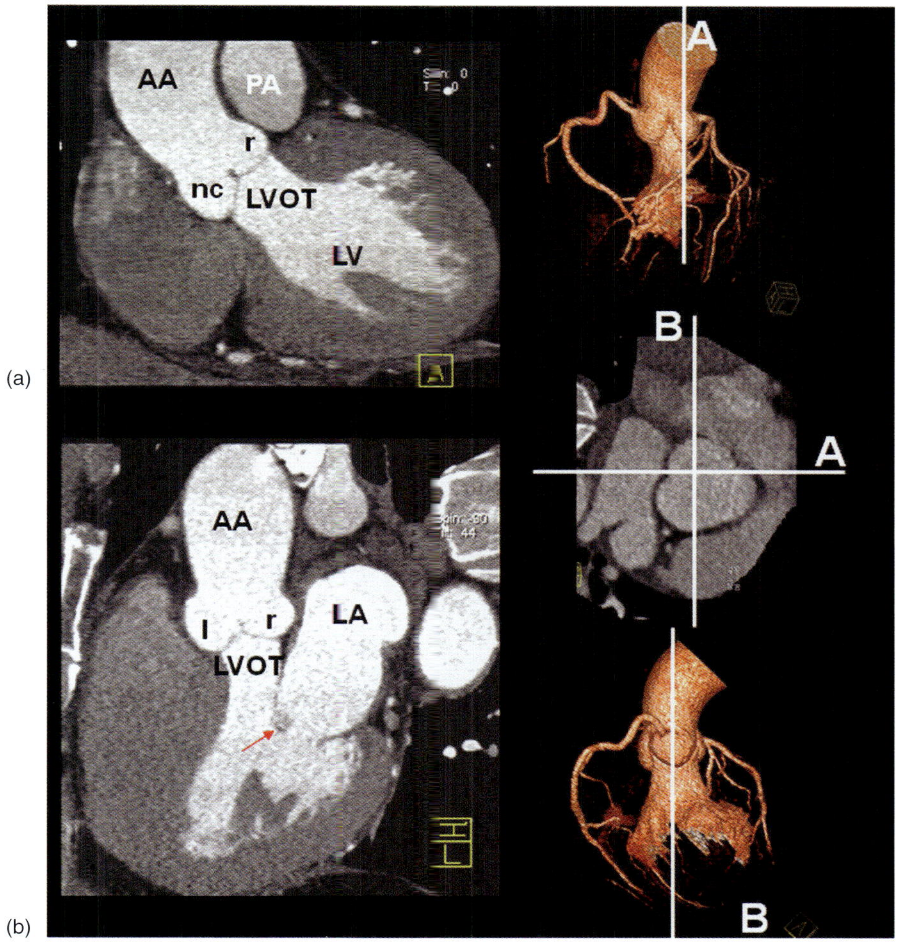

Figure 8.7 Sagittal anatomic planes in CT images. (a) Frontal view in a coronal plane (as seen in axial and three-dimensional reference images on the right side); anatomic continuity from the left ventricle (LV) to outflow tract (LVOT) to coronary sinuses (r, right coronary; nc, noncoronary sinus) and to ascending aorta (AA); PA, pulmonary artery. (b) Lateral view in a sagittal plane demonstrates the right coronary sinus (r) and the left coronary sinus (l); the space between outflow tract and left atrium (LA) corresponds to the fibrous skeleton and to the continuity with the anterior cusp of the mitral valve (red arrow). Both in A and in B planes, the diameter of ventriculoaortic junction (at the bases of the sinuses) is normally larger than the diameter of the sinotubular junction.

in the ventricular site. The *fibrosa* is mostly constituted of collagen fibers, which are primarily arranged in a circumferential direction, from one commissure to the other. These fibers are typically corrugated, thus enabling the leaflet to expand radially up to 50% strain. During diastole, this radial expansion ensures that the three leaflets appose together and seal the orifice, thus preventing regurgitation. The *spongiosa* consists of collagen and elastic fibers, proteoglycans, and mucopolysaccharides that give it a soft consistency. This layer minimizes the friction forces between the *fibrosa* and the *ventricularis* during cusp movements and protects the leaflets from stress-related damage and structural deterioration. Finally, the *ventricularis* mainly consists of elastic fibers, structured in thin sheets, randomly oriented as compared with the highly organized structure of the *fibrosa* [6]. The *ventricularis* provides the tensile recoil necessary to retain the folded and corrugated shape of the *fibrosa*. Elastic fibers produce low but significant tension forces that enable the cusps to maintain the typical retracted and corrugated configuration of the collagen fibers in systole and their typical distended pattern in diastole [7]. In addition to retracting the aortic cusp during systole, the *ventricularis* mechanically contributes to the diastolic cusp stiffness at high transvalvular pressures, thus preventing overdistension of the cusp [6] (Figure 8.15).

The Interleaflets Triangles

The ***interleaflets triangles*** are bordered by insertion of the leaflets and of the leaflet attachments of the aortic sinuses at their base. They are triangular extensions of the LVOT (Figures 8.16 and 8.17).

- The triangle between the left and the right coronary cusps is partly constituted of myocardial tissue,
- The triangle between the right and the noncoronary cusps consists of fibrous tissue and contains the atrioventricular (AV) bundle of the conduction axis, and
- The triangle between the noncoronary and the left cusps is only composed of fibrous tissue.

(a), (b)

(c), (d)

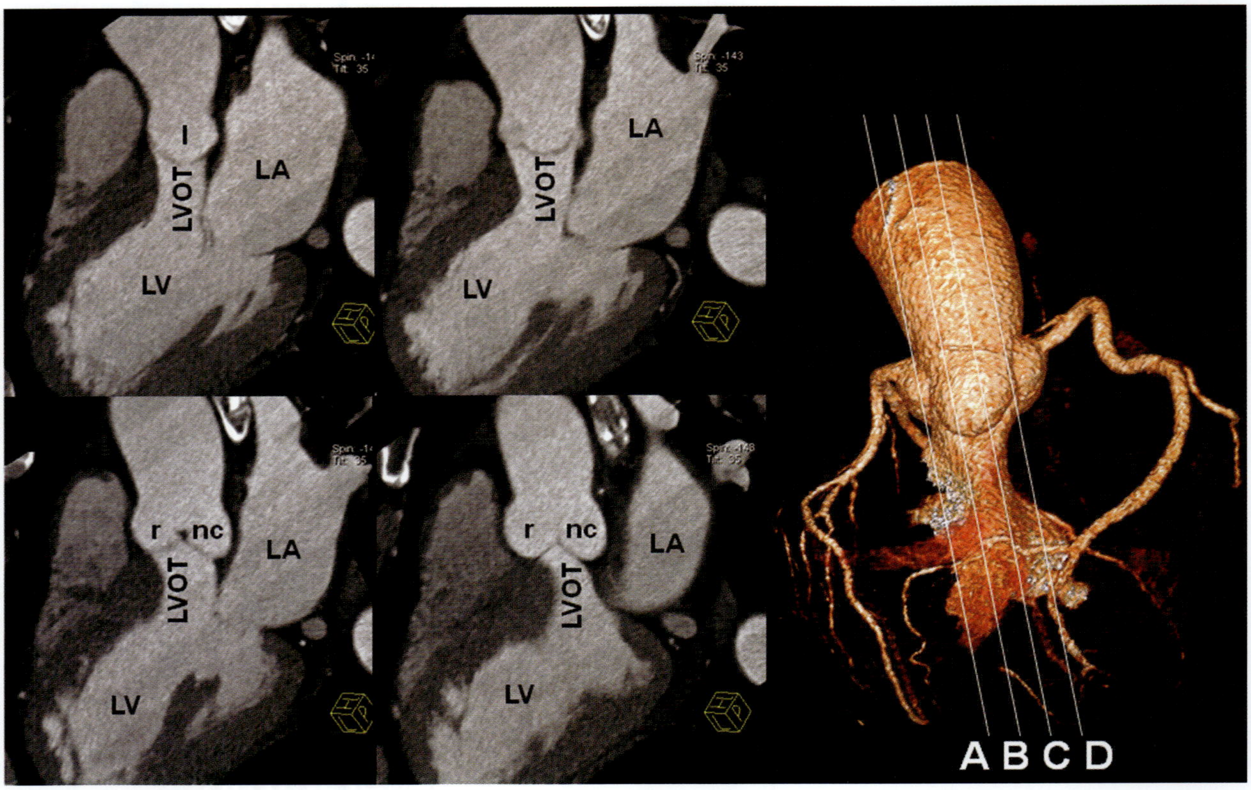

Figure 8.8 Four sagittal sections from left coronary sinus (a) to the interleaflet triangle between right and noncoronary (nc) sinuses (d). Outflow tract of the left ventricle (LVOT) is visualized in relation to left atrium (LA) with the interposed fibrous skeleton in continuity from the noncoronary and left coronary sinuses to the anterior mitral leaflet. l, left coronary sinus; LV, Left Ventricle; r, right coronary sinus.

The AV node and the AV bundle penetrate through the interleaflets triangle between the right and the noncoronary cusps, and this structure should be especially protected during surgery [3].

Histology. At the hinge point of each cusp, dense collagen fibers reinforce the semilunar contour of the cusps' insertion. This reinforcement delineates the border of the three interleaflets triangles and constitutes the fibrous layer of the ventriculoaortic junction. The areas delimited by the collagenous border constitute the "body" of the triangles. They are composed of a thin, circularly oriented layer of collagen fibers and extracellular matrix. In addition, a very thin layer of elastic tissue on the luminal surface is continuous with the elastic layer in the ventricle beneath the endocardium [5].

(a)

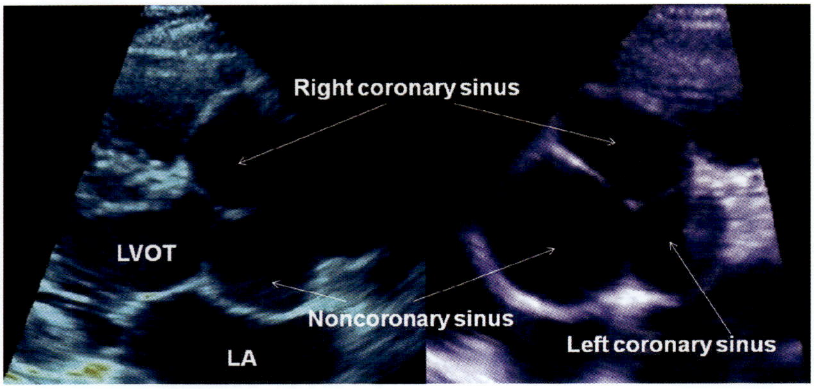

(b)

Figure 8.9 Echocardiography view of a 21-year-old woman with Marfan Syndrome. Severe aortic root dilation with distortion of the geometry at the level of the sinotubular junction. The aortic valve is tricuspid but asymmetric. Part (a) shows parasternal long-axis view. Part (b) shows shot-axis view; the figure shows the larger dimension of the noncoronary Valsalva sinus and the corresponding cusp. The maximum diameter at the level of the Valsalva sinuses is 47 mm. LA, left atrium; LVOT, left ventricle outflow tract.

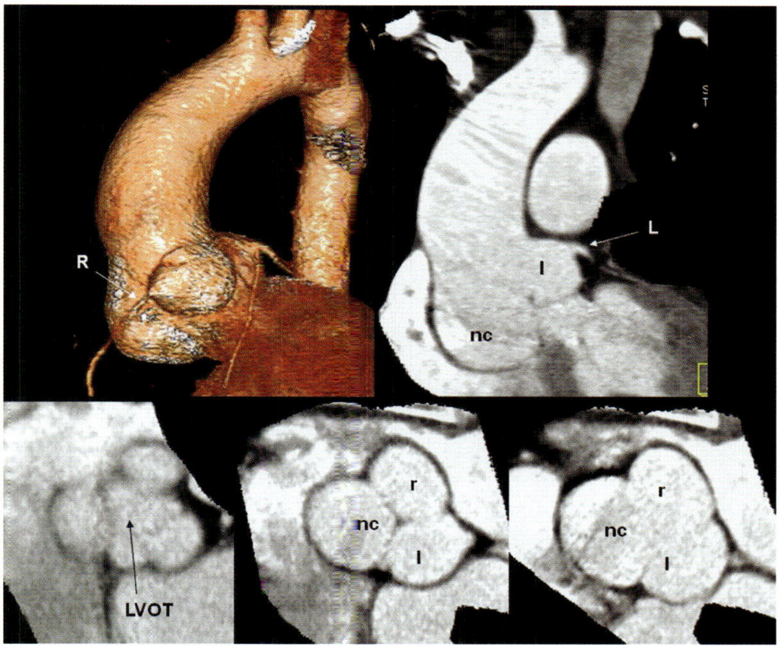

Figure 8.10 Same patient as in Figure 8.9: eccentric dilation of the aortic root. (a) The aortic enlargement involves the root and the proximal tubular segment. (b) Left oblique lateral section: noncoronary sinus is more dilated than the left coronary sinus (l). (c–e) Axial sections through the bases of the sinuses (c), the coaptated leaflets (d) without regurgitation, and through the free margins of the leaflets (e) where the different dilatation of the three sinuses is more evident. L, left coronary artery; LVOT, left ventricular outflow tract; nc, noncoronary sinus; R, right coronary artery; r, right coronary sinus.

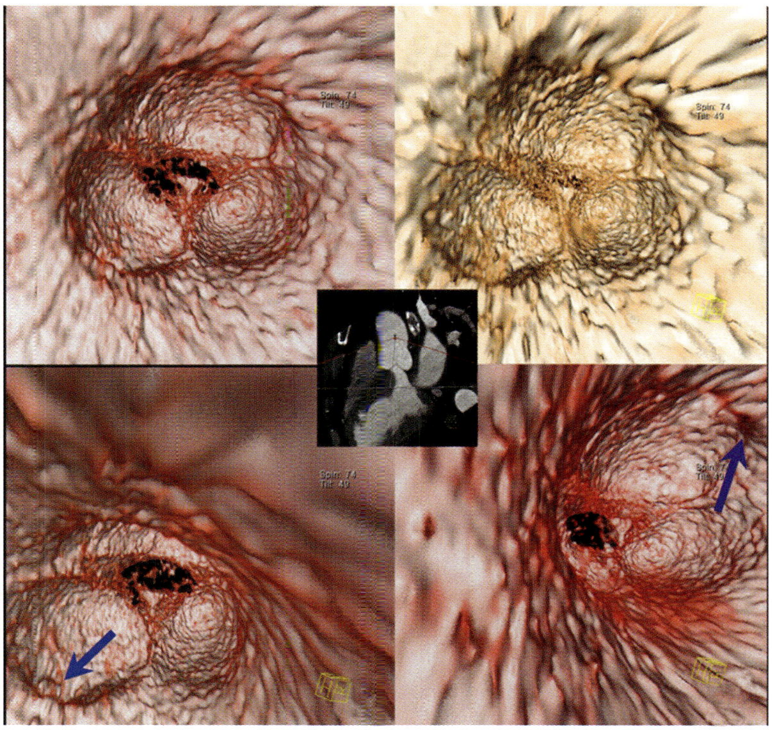

Figure 8.11 Three-dimensional virtual endoscopic view of the aortic root sinuses and leaflets from aortic side. (a) In the area of coaptation, the leaflets are too thin to be visualized, mimicking an open area. (b) The same images as (a), difference is in pixel segmentation demonstrating the complete coaptation of the leaflets. (c) and (d) Oblique endoscopic view of the coronary ostia (arrows). (e) Reference view.

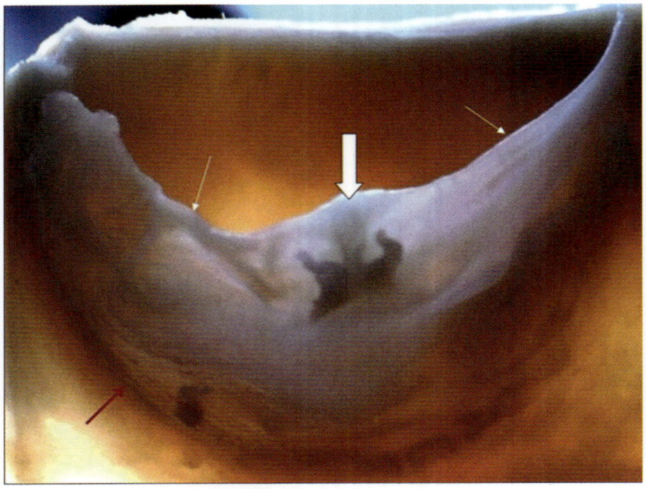

Figure 8.12 The noncoronary cusp. The thick white arrow identifies the Arantius nodulus, thicker than the adjacent *lunulae* (thin white arrows). The thin red arrow indicates the thick collagen bundles that are present along the entire hinge border of each cusp.

The Ventriculoaortic Junction

The *ventriculoaortic junction* (or aortic annulus) is composed of the cusp bases and interleaflets triangles (Figure 8.18); a planar line passing through the *nadir* of the basis of each cusp and through the bases of interleaflets triangles

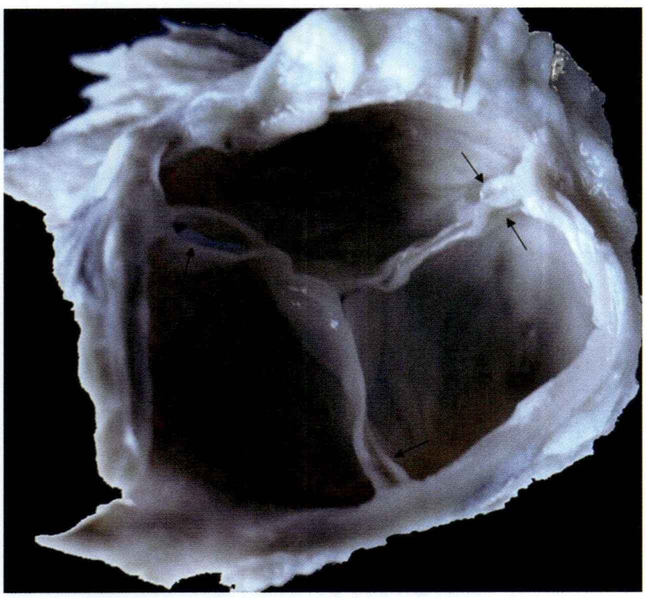

Figure 8.13 The aortic root viewed from the ascending aorta. The coaptation zone between each cusp and the adjacent ones is high to ensure perfect coaptation and absence of regurgitation. In older patients, fenestrations may occur near the commissures, but they are seldom associated to regurgitation, as often fenestrations lie over the lower coaptation margin. Arrows indicate commissures.

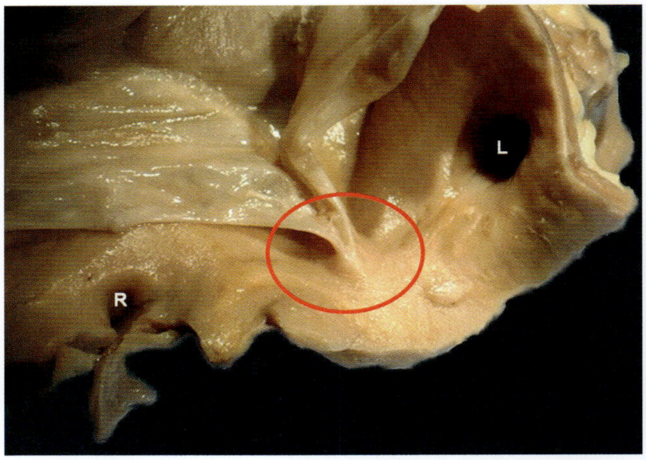

Figure 8.14 The red circle indicates the fibrous reinforcement of the commissure to adequately hold the cusps during diastole distension. (L), left coronary artery's ostium; R, right coronary artery's ostium.

is the ideal ring that is considered the aortic annulus routinely measured by imaging. All structures that are distal to the aorta-ventricular junction are subjected to arterial pressures, whereas all those that are proximal to the attachments are subjected to ventricular pressures [1,3,5].

Histology. Collagen is dense at the hinge point that constitutes the semilunar contour of the leaflet attachment. The three-coronet border, known as annulus fibrosus, is thickest at the *nadir* of the semilunar attachments [3–5].

Functional Anatomy

The aortic root components maintain their proportions over a wide range of sizes. The upper parts of the valve commissures [the apices of the interleaflet triangles (Figures 8.16 and 8.18)] are inserted just below the sinotubular junction at this level, and the diameter of the aortic root is similar to that of the annulus. The length of the base of each leaflet is approximately 1.5 times more than that of its free margin and the height of the leaflets ranges from 12 to 18 mm [1]. The sinuses of Valsalva play an important role in the local hydrodynamic forces that exert their effects on both cup motion and coronary flow; they generate a space behind the open aortic leaflets, preventing closure of the coronary artery orifices. This space favors the generation of "eddy currents" (first described by Leonardo da Vinci) behind the leaflets when these are open [8–10]. Twirling inside the sinuses, the eddy currents prevent the contact of the valve leaflets with the aortic wall and promote smooth valve closure. Although the origin of the eddy currents depends on the shape of sinuses and root, their

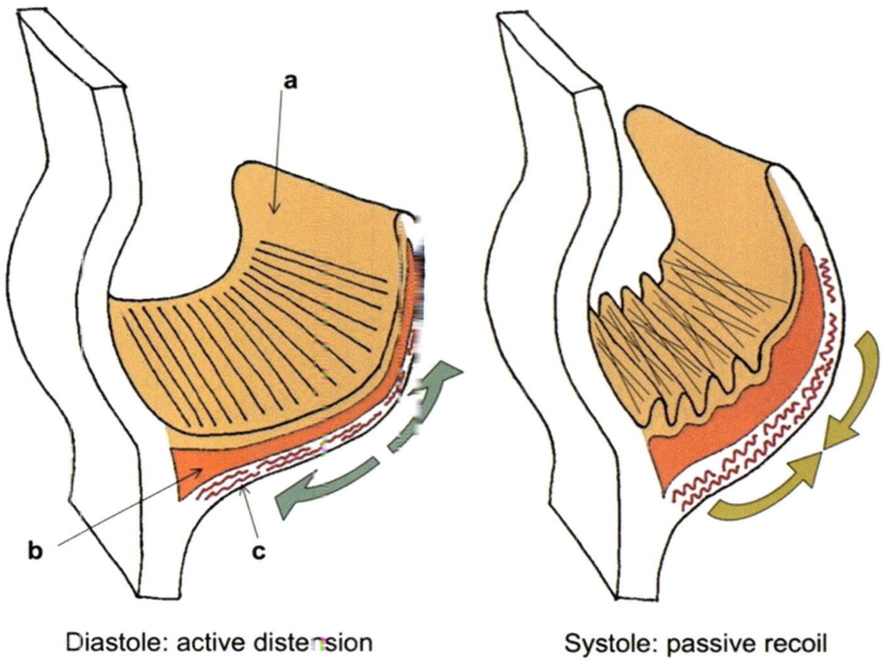

Figure 8.15 The three-layer structure of the aortic cusps contributes to the correct function of the valve. In diastole, the flow generated by the eddy currents actively distends the cusp starting from the portion inserted on the aortic wall and progressing to the free margin. The collagen fibers of the fibrosa (a) are highly organized and contribute to distribute the pressure homogenously over the cusp surface. The elastic fibers of the ventricularis (c) are distended. The spongiosa layer (b) contributes to minimize the friction stress generated by the other two layers. In systole, the passive elastic recoil of the elastic fibers of the ventricularis facilitates the opening of the cusp. The collagen fibers of the fibrosa, not stressed by the distending diastolic pressure, apparently loose the highly orderly distribution seen in diastole.

empowerment depends more on the narrowed sinotubular ridge than on the shape of the sinuses themselves. Early in systole the leaflets move toward the sinuses; vortices generate between the leaflet and the sinus wall. The peripheral *laminae* of the flow in systole encounter the "bottle neck" of the sinotubular junction that forces these *laminae* back down, along the borders of the sinuses, distend the cusp borders at the end of systole, and finally close the cusps during diastole (Figure 8.19). The closure is smooth and synchronous, which prevents leaflet fatigue and optimizes valve mechanics. The dynamic aortic root anatomy, reducing cusp stress and fatigue, prevents structural failure of the valve cusps. The sinuses of Valsalva share with aortic leaflets the diastolic stress during valve closure.

During the cardiac cycle, the aortic root undergoes complex deformation, which consists in the strain of the aortic-ventricular base (putative annulus) and sinotubular junction, aortic root elongation and compression, and shear and torsion deformities [4, 8–11]. The expansion of the root begins at the base during the isovolumic contraction phase, and then progresses to the commissures and ultimately to the sinotubular junction. During the first third of systole, the aortic root gains its maximal expansion, approaching a cylindrical shape. Then its volume decreases in mid-diastole, then it reapproaches a truncated cone shape in end-diastole (Figure 8.20). The 39% increase of the ventriculoaortic junction ring area and the 63% expansion of the apexes of the interleaflets triangles during systole reduce the opposition to ejection, facilitating left ventricular work. This expansion is the proof of the critical role of the elastic properties of the aortic root for the normal mechanics of the ventricular-arterial connection. The maximal stress on the leaflets is concentrated on their insertion at the sinotubular junction and progressively decreases along the border of cusp insertion. During diastole, the stress on the leaflets is almost four times higher than that on the sinuses. If the three sinuses do not uniformly share the stress, the sinus wall would draw inward in diastole. Vice versa, the sinus walls move outward, thus decreasing the stress and wear and tear on the aortic leaflets.

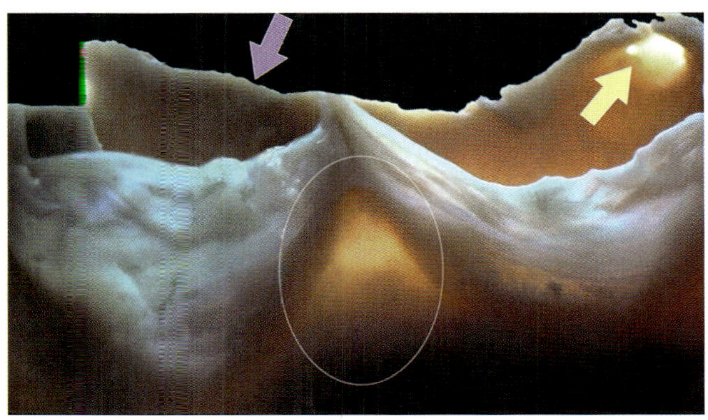

Figure 8.16 The interleaflet triangle between the noncoronary and the left coronary sinuses and cusps (white circle). The interleaflet triangle is thinner than the aortic wall (light violet arrow), reflecting its different structure. The light yellow arrow indicates the left coronary ostium.

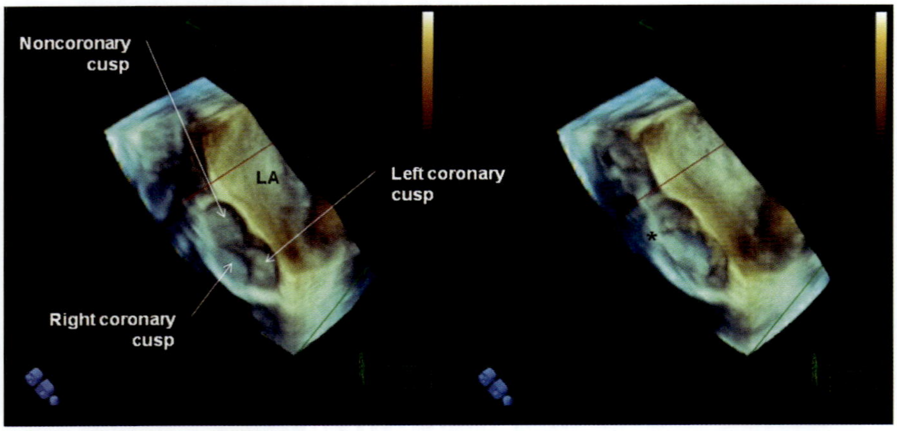

Figure 8.17 Echocardiography three-dimensional image of the aortic valve at the level of the free margin of the aortic cusps. On the left is the diastolic phase; on the right is the systolic phase. When the valve is open (the right panel), the interleaflet triangle between the noncoronary and the right coronary cusps is visible (asterisk).

Pathophysiology of Aortic Root Dysfunction

The correct function of the aortic valve depends on the harmonic morphology and function of all components of the aortic root. Dysfunction of the aortic root is either primary, both acquired and due to heritable connective tissue diseases or it is due to dysfunction of the valve, both stenosis and incompetence. *Valve stenosis* is due to the morphologic changes of the cusps caused by a variety of diseases such as rheumatic disease, congenital cardiac diseases, or calcific degeneration (see Chapter 4). The increased gradient across the aortic root is mostly due to valve stenosis with exceptions of congenital diseases such as supravalvular aortic stenosis (see Chapter 2). Valve stenosis may cause secondary aortic root dilatation and dysfunction.

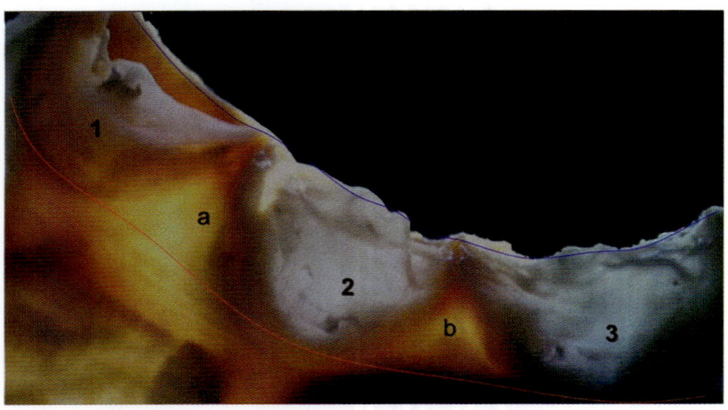

Figure 8.18 The open aortic root. (1) The noncoronary Valsalva sinus and cusp; (2) the left coronary Valsalva sinus and cusp; (3) the right coronary ones. The ventriculoaortic junction is delineated by the semilunar contour of the three cusps and by the ideal line that connects the nadirs of the three cusps (red line). The line that connects the apices of the interleaflets triangles (blue line) identifies the sinotubular junction. (a) and (b) denote interleaflets triangles.

Vice versa, *valve regurgitation* may depend either on the valve or on the dysfunction of each of the nonvalvular components of the aortic root. In a schematic way, the pathophysiology of the aortic valve incompetence may result from failure of each of the six components of the root, either variably combined or as isolated abnormalities of the sinotubular junction or sinuses of Valsalva, or semilunar leaflets or three-coronet shaped ventriculoaortic junction (Table 8.1). Aortic regurgitation may be caused by age-related atherosclerosis and hypertension; infective aortic disease (endocarditis); chronic inflammatory aortic valve disease such as rheumatic disease; heritable connective tissue disease; congenital diseases such as true or false bicuspid aortic valve (BAV); or acquired valve disease (aged aortic valve calcific degeneration leading to mixed steno-insufficient valve). Whatever is the cause of valve insufficiency, once established, all aortic root components enter a vicious circle with corresponding damage and dysfunction, all contributing to worsening the regurgitation.

Morphofunctional Classification of the Aortic Regurgitation

Based on above considerations, the mechanisms that may cause aortic regurgitation in the presence of normal morphology of the aortic cusps are:

1 dilatation of the aortic annulus, generally associated with dilation of the sinuses of Valsalva (known as "annuloaortic ectasia" [4]);
2 isolated single sinus of Valsalva aneurysm affecting the function of a single leaflet;
3 loss of the sinotubular junction shape which assumes a rectilinear and enlarged morphology; and
4 isolated ascending aortic aneurysm (not involving the aortic root) that can stretch the sinotubular junction, valve commissures, and interleaflets triangles.

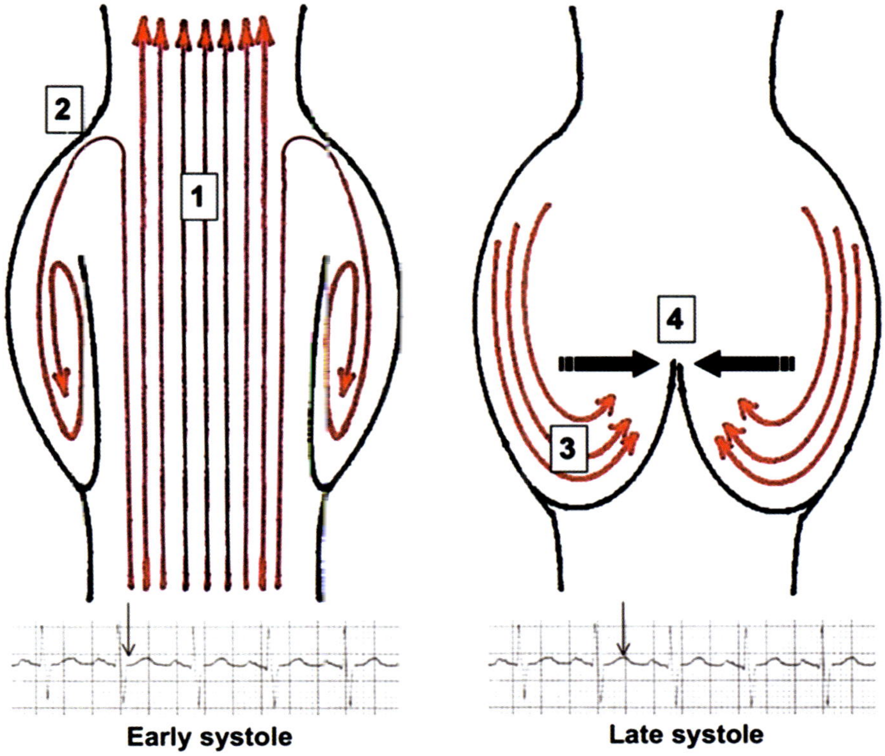

Figure 8.19 The eddy currents and the efficient functioning of the aortic root. (1) Early in systole the flow that is ejected from the left ventricle into the aortic root encounters the bottleneck of the sinotubular junction that is smaller than the ventriculoaortic junction. (2) The peripheral laminae of the ejected blood flow are forced between the wall of the sinuses of Valsalva and the open cusps, thus preventing the contact between the cusps and the aortic wall and allowing the coronary perfusion. (3) In late systole, the vortices caused by the flow introduced between the Valsalva sinuses wall and the aortic cusps begin to distend the cusps facilitating the incoming of the cusps toward the center of the aortic root. (4) Finally, at the end of the systole the free margin of the cusps collate at the center of the aortic root, ensuring the perfect closure of the valve.

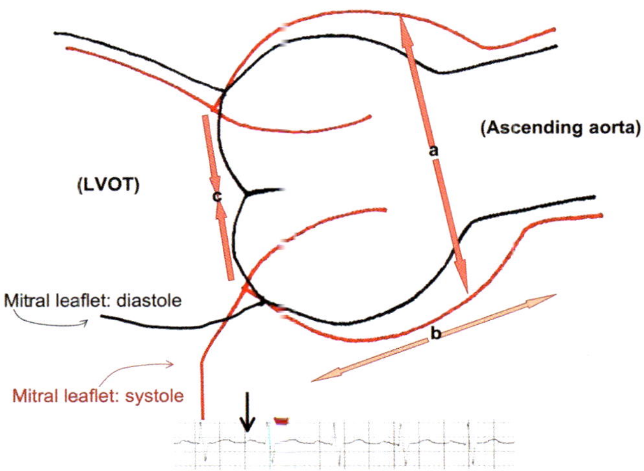

Figure 8.20 The dynamic changes of the aortic root during the cardiac cycle. Black lines identify the aortic root in the last third of the diastole. The aortic root during systole (first third of the cardiac cycle) is identified by the red lines. During systole, the aortic root size increases its dimensions as compared with the diastolic time. Both the root diameter (a) and length (b) increase. The increase of the diameter starts at the level of the valve and then progresses like a wave through the tubular aorta. During the cardiac cycle the basal part of the ventriculoaortic junction acts like the LVOT: when myocardium contracts (c), its diameter mildly decreases rather than increasing. The early diastole (the intermediate third of the cardiac cycle) is the transient phase from the maximal to the minimal dimension of the aortic root. LVOT, left ventricular outflow tract.

Other causes of aortic valve incompetence can be linked to structural abnormalities of the cusps including perforation (Figure 8.26), thickening and retraction of the free margin, and calcification and prolapse (see Chapter 7).

El Khoury and co-workers proposed a simplified functional anatomy classification of the aortic root considering the two main components:

- The functional aortic annulus (FAA) that includes the ventriculoaortic junction, the sinuses of Valsalva, and the sinotubular junction; and
- The three semilunar leaflets [12].

This practical classification provides useful and synthetic information to the surgeon on the cause of aortic insufficiency and possible surgical solutions [12, 13] that may preserve or restore the spatial configuration of the aortic root. Therefore, the two basic mechanisms of aortic regurgitation are FAA dilation and pathology of the leaflets [13] classified as follows:

Type I: normal appearing cusps with FAA dilation

(Ia) ascending aorta dilation (starting at the sinotubular junction) (Figures 8.27 and 8.28)

(Ib) Valsalva sinuses and sinotubular junction dilation (Figure 8.29)

(Ic) FAA dilation

(Id) Cusp perforation (Figure 8.30)

Table 8.1 Major diseases affecting the aortic root

	Aortic root	Ascending aorta	Other arterial districts
Acquired aortic diseases			
Hypertensive		+++	Cranial
Atherosclerotic	++ (valve)	+++	Coronary, cranial, lower limbs
Rheumatic	+++ (valve)		
Infective	+++ (valve)		
Genetic aortic diseases			
Marfan syndrome (Figures 8.21 and 8.22)	+++	+	Rare cranial aneurysms
Loeys Dietz syndrome (Figures 8.23–8.25)	++	++	All arterial districts
Thoracic aortic aneurysm and dissection (TAAD)	+	+++	Thoracic descending aorta
Bicuspid aortic valve	+	+++	
Other rare syndromes (EDS IV, arterial tortuosity syndrome)	+	+	All arterial districts may be dramatically involved

Type II: Cusp prolapse: excess of cusp tissue or commissural disruption (Figure 8.31)

Type III: cusp retraction and thickening (Figure 8.32)

Type I lesions

Type Ia lesions are caused mainly by atherosclerotic and/or hypertensive damage of the aortic wall and are often associated with dilation and degeneration of the tubular ascending aorta and the aortic arch.

Type Ib lesions typically recur in case of degeneration of the media layer of the aortic wall, as in heritable collagen diseases (e.g., Marfan syndrome and Marfan-like syndromes).

The *type Ic lesion* is typical of more complex pathologies such as BAV or associated to mitral valve or coronary

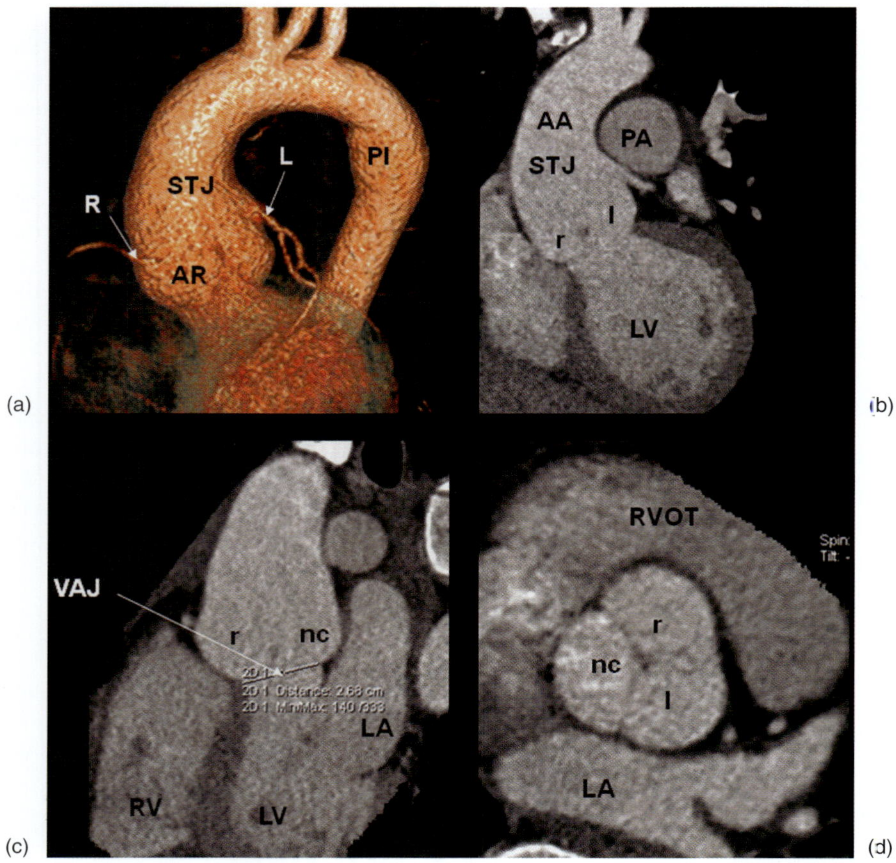

Figure 8.21 Dilation of proximal ascending aorta in a 21-year-old woman with Marfan syndrome at the end of pregnancy. Diastolic CT images. (a) Three-dimensional left oblique lateral view; dilated aortic root (AR) and dilated postisthmic segment (PI); L, left coronary artery; R, right coronary artery. (b) Frontal coronal section; left (l) and right (r) coronary sinuses; the dilation of the aortic root involves also sinotubular junction (STJ) and proximal tubular segment of the ascending aorta (AA); PA, pulmonary artery; LV, left ventricle. (c) Lateral sagittal section; noncoronary (nc) sinuses; the ventriculoaortic junction (VAJ) does not show dilatation; LA, left atrium; RV, right ventricle. (d) Axial plane of leaflets with complete coaptation without regurgitation. RVOT, Right Ventricular Outflow tract.

(a), (b)

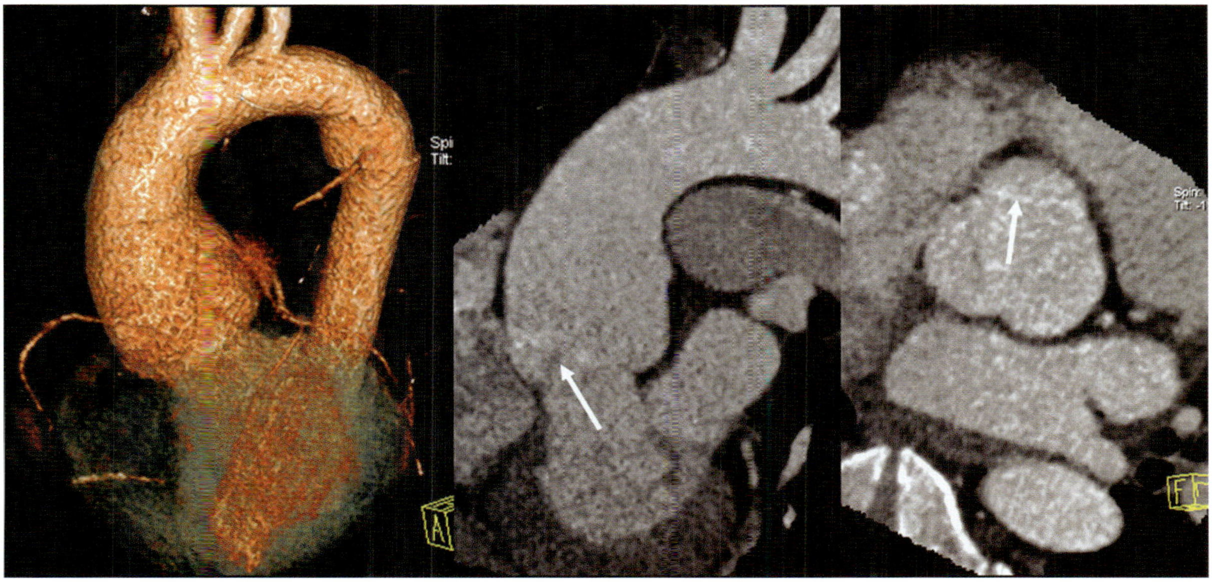

(c)

Figure 8.22 The same patient as Figure 8.24, systolic images. (a) Three-dimensional view of the aortic root. In (b) (left oblique lateral view) and (c) (axial section), the systolic feature of leaflets is visible (arrows).

(a), (b)

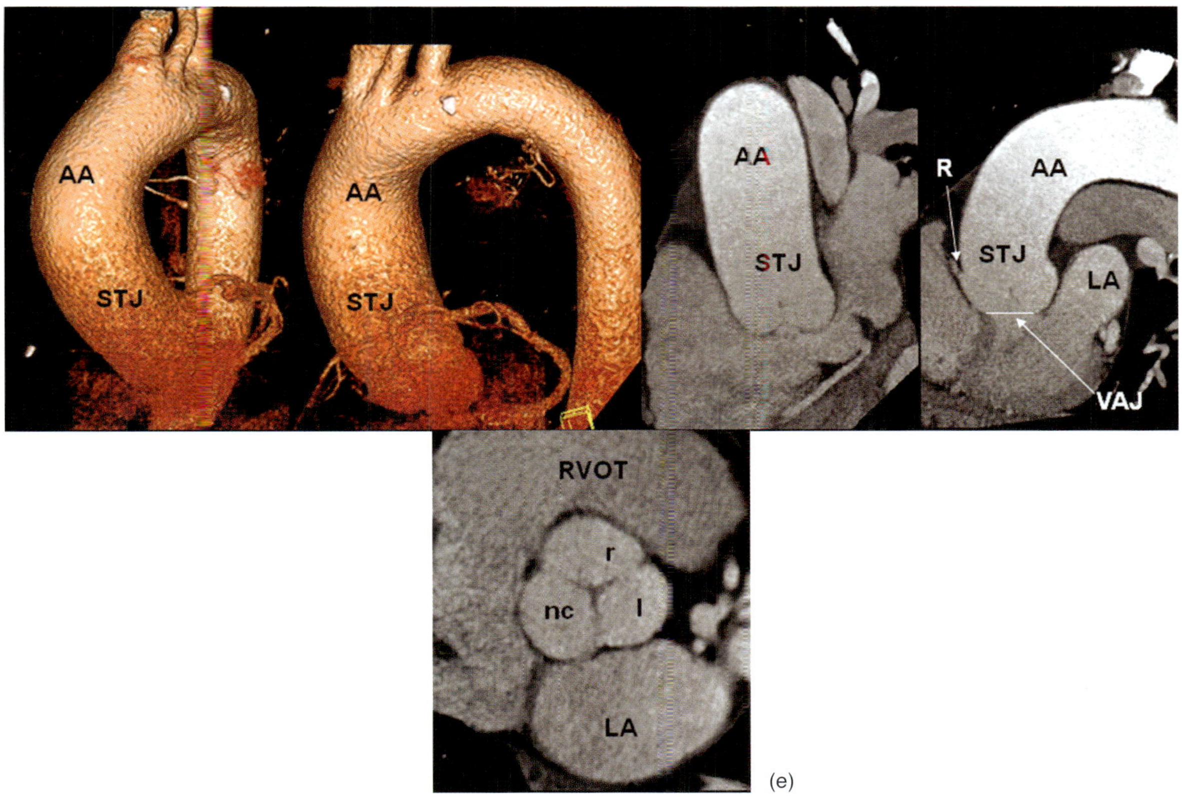

(c), (d)

(e)

Figure 8.23 Tubular dilation of the whole ascending aorta in a 57-year-old woman affected by Loeys Dietz type II syndrome. In three-dimensional images (a, b), the severity and extension of the dilatation as well as the loss of the geometry of the sinotubular junction (STJ) are immediately apparent. Frontal (c) and left oblique lateral section (d) demonstrates the normal dimension of ventriculoaortic junction (VAJ). Axial section (e) reveals the complete coaptation of leaflets without regurgitation. AA, ascending aorta; l, left coronary sinus; nc, noncoronary sinus; R, right coronary; r, right coronary sinus; RVOT, right ventricular outflow tract.

(a) (b)

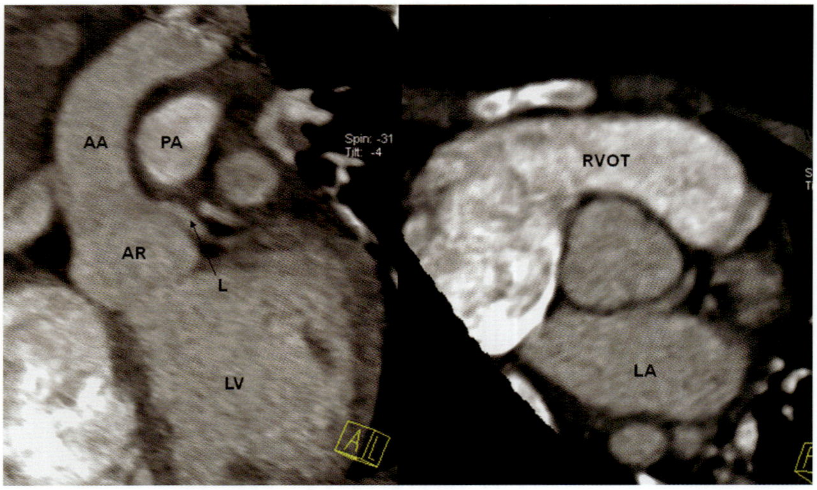

Figure 8.24 Aortic root dilation in a 13-month-old female affected by Loeys Dietz type I syndrome. (a) Coronal section; the dilatation involves only the aortic root (AR). (b) Axial section; symmetric Valsalva sinuses. AA, ascending aorta; L, left coronary artery; LA, left atrium; LV, left ventricle; PA, pulmonary artery; RVOT, right ventricular outflow tract.

artery diseases. The isolated dilation of the ventriculoaortic junction occurs almost exclusively in association with aortic root and sinotubular junction dilation [14].

Type Id lesions are mostly due to infective disease such as endocarditis with perforation of the body of the cusp.

Type II lesions can be either isolated or associated with dilation of the sinuses of Valsalva or of the sinotubular junction with detachment of the apices of the interleaflets triangles (e.g., the commissures) or with leaflet prolapse due to aortic root dissection. Isolated right cusp prolapse can be caused by subaortic ventricular septal defect (Laubry-Pezzi syndrome) [15]. The prolapse of the cusps can be further divided into three groups [16]: (1) cusp flail, when a complete eversion of a cusp in the LVOT is present; (2) whole cusp prolapse, when both the free edge and the entire body of a cusp overrides the plane of the aortic annulus into the LVOT; and (3) partial cusp prolapse, when the distal part of a cusp is prolabing into the LVOT.

Type III lesions are typical of rheumatic disease or degenerative calcific valve degeneration, mostly in the elderly.

Valve Calcification

Valve calcification (Figures 8.33 and 8.34) is classified according to the extent and localization of the calcium deposits [16]. In all imaging evaluations of the aortic root (echocardiography, CT scan, and nuclear magnetic imaging), aortic valve calcification should be graded/classified as follows:

- Grade 1: absence of calcification,
- Grade 2: isolated small calcification spots,
- Grade 3: bigger calcification spots interfering with cusps motion, and
- Grade 4: extensive calcification of all cusps with restricted cusp motion.

For calcifications of $\leq$ grade 3, the localization of the calcium deposits should be specified.

(a), (b) (c)

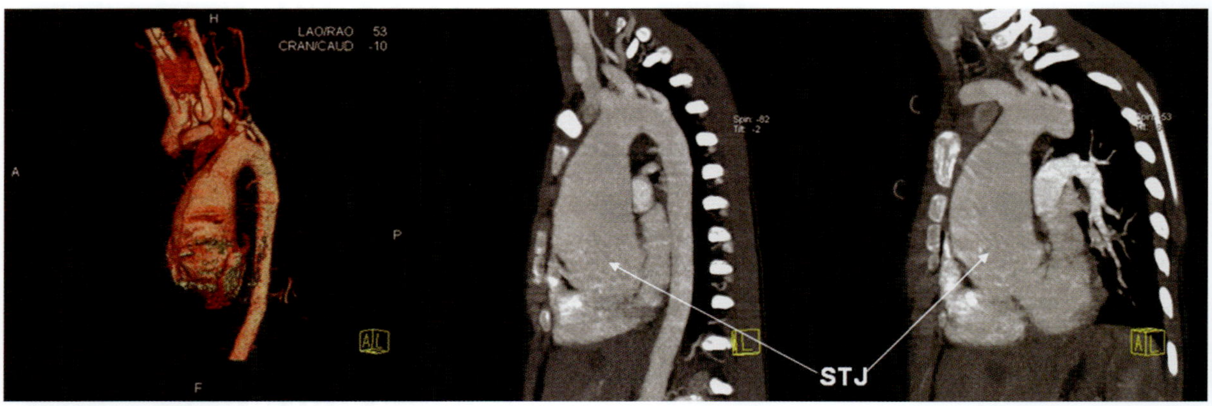

Figure 8.25 Male adult patient affected by Loeys Dietz type II syndrome. The severe dilation of the aortic root and the loss of the sinotubular junction (STJ) are evident. (a) Three-dimensional reconstruction of aortic root, ascending aorta, and aortic arch with tortuous supra-aortic vessels. (b, c) Sagittal views.

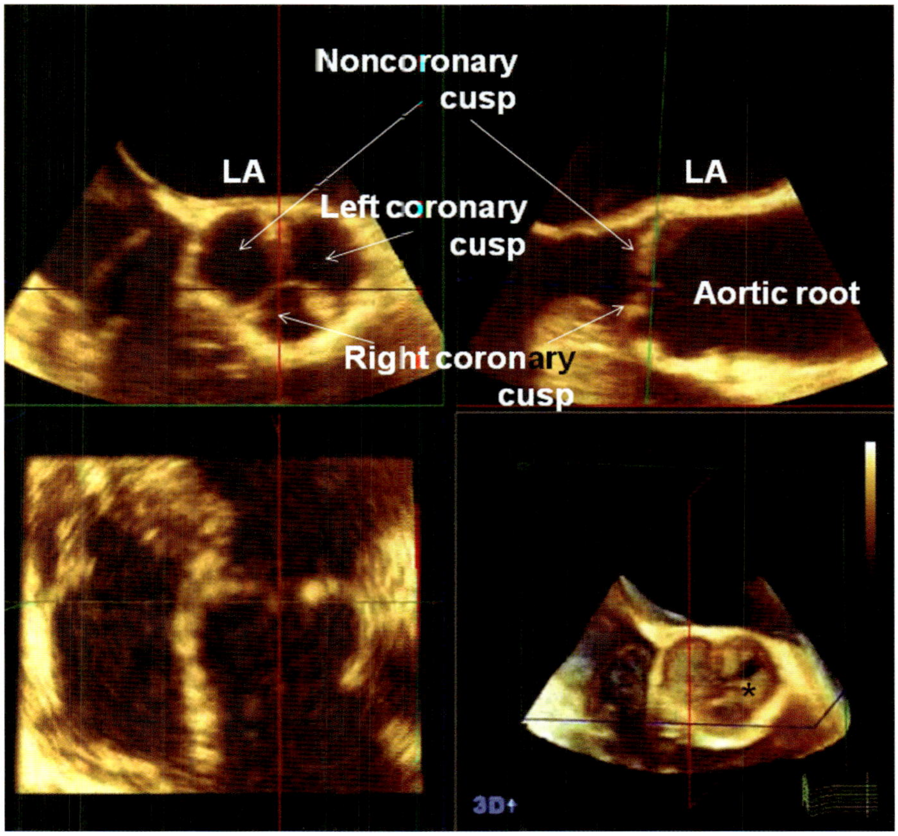

Figure 8.26 Echocardiographic view of aortic regurgitation type Id with perforation of the left coronary cusp. The three-dimensional reconstruction identifies the size of the perforation (asterisk) and the existing relation between the perforated and integer cusps. The colored lines (red, green, and blue) are the reference planes for the three-dimensional reconstruction (see right lower image). LA, left atrium.

Bicuspid Aortic Valve

BAV (Figures 8.35–8.41) exerts strain effects that involve the aortic root and the ascending aorta, starting from the sinotubular junction, thus entering the group of diseases that affect the aortic root. In BAV, the dilation of the ascending aorta is common: up to 50–70% of adult patients without significant BAV dysfunction show aortic dilatation [17] that typically involves both aortic root and ascending aorta and can extend to the aortic arch in patients aged over 40 years [18]. The progression of the aortic root dilation is about 0.5 mm per year, while the ascending aorta rate of growth is up to 1 mm per year [17, 19], irrespective of the BAV function. The dilatation of the ascending aorta and aortic root is an early process that can start in childhood [20]. Patients with normal functioning BAV may present intrinsic aortic wall abnormalities with significantly reduced aortic elasticity [21], which is associated both with the severity of aortic regurgitation and with the degree of left ventricular hypertrophy secondary to the valve disease. A common pathogenetic defect probably underlies both valve malformation and aortic wall weakness [22]. The association of BAV with ascending aorta dilatation could be due to structural weakness of the aortic

(a)

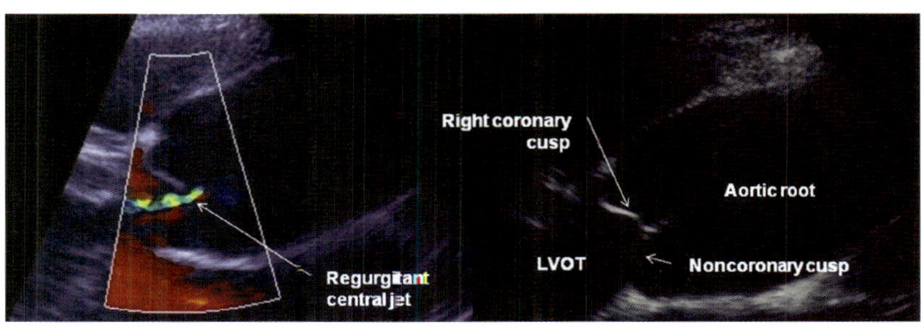

(b)

Figure 8.27 Functional classification of aortic regurgitation: echocardiographic parasternal long-axis view. (a) The application of the Color Doppler mode shows a mild aortic regurgitation. The jet is central. (b) The shape of the aortic root with dilation and loss of the physiologic geometry of the sinotubular junction configure the type Ia aortic regurgitation. LVOT, left ventricular outflow tract.

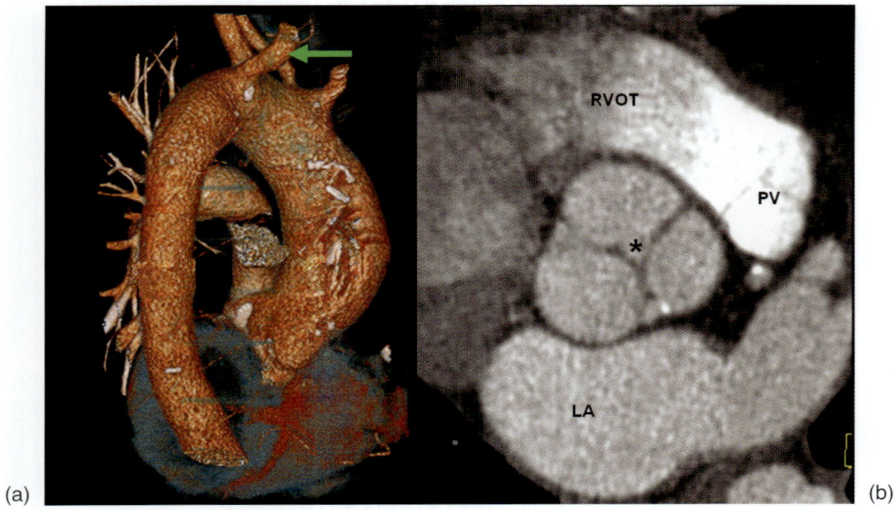

Figure 8.28 Tubular junction and tubular aneurysm with type Ia aortic regurgitation in adult male patient. (a) Three-dimensional left oblique lateral view: prevalence of the proximal tubular dilatation. Green arrow: aberrant right subclavian artery. (b) Axial section of the Valsalva sinuses demonstrates incomplete coaptation of the leaflets in the central area (asterisk). LA, left atrium; PV, pulmonary valve; RVOT, right ventricular outflow tract.

wall of possible genetic origin [23,24]. Moreover, the aortic root dilation can be worsened when hemodynamic factors, such as high velocity and turbulent flow downstream to stenosis, add mechanical stress on the aortic wall [21].

Contribution of the Different Imaging Tools for the Evaluation of the Aortic Root

Echocardiography

Echocardiography is the pivotal imaging tool for the diagnosis and monitoring of the pathology of the aortic root. Echo should provide information on each component of the aortic root and facilitate combined observations in final conclusive diagnosis.

Current echocardiographic study of the aortic root should provide morphologic and hemodynamic information on the valve as a whole and on each single leaflet, diameters of the valve annulus, of the root at the mid-Valsalva sinus level, and sinotubular junction (Figure 8.42). Additional routine information includes the diameter of the ascending aorta, the arch, thoracic, and descending and abdominal aorta.

The physiopathologic approach to the aortic root imaging should take into account the possibility that aortic valve dysfunction results from aortic root disease and dysfunction and *vice versa* that aortic root pathology is due to the aortic valve disease and dysfunction. While it is true that each type of aortic valve dysfunction reflects an aortic root disease, the opposite condition may not be true and the pathology of the aortic root may exist in the presence of normally functioning aortic valves.

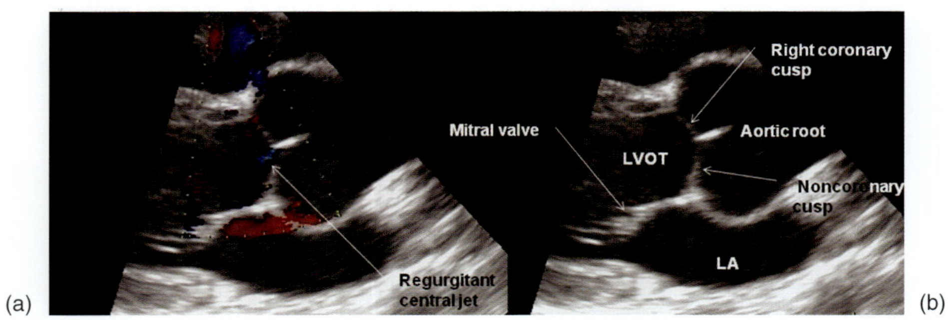

Figure 8.29 Functional classification of aortic regurgitation: echocardiographic parasternal long-axis view. (a) The application of the Color Doppler mode shows a mild aortic regurgitation. The jet is central. (b) The aortic root is dilated at the level of the Valsalva sinuses; the physiologic geometry of the sinotubular junction is maintained and the diameter of the ventriculoaortic junction is normal. This is a type Ib aortic regurgitation. LA, left atrium; LVOT, left ventricular outflow tract.

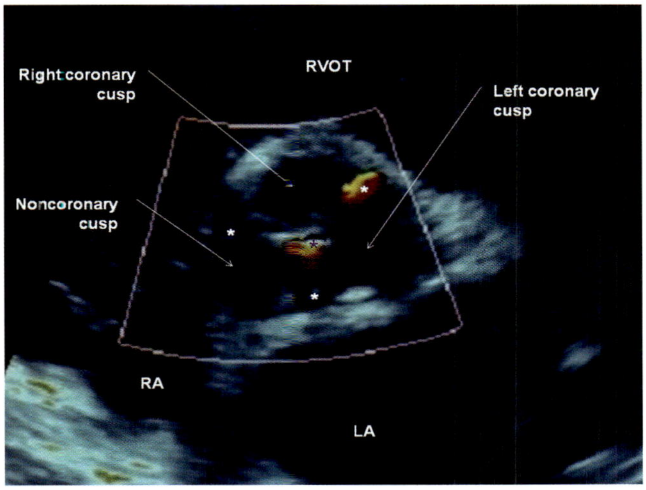

Figure 8.30 Functional classification of aortic regurgitation: echocardiographic parasternal short-axis view. The application of the Color Doppler mode shows a mild aortic regurgitation, consisting of four very mild origins of the regurgitation: three originate at the level of each commissural apex (white asterisks), the fourth (violet) is central. The three small regurgitation jets corresponding to the apices of the commissures take origin from fenestrations of the free margins of the cusps. The aortic root at the level of the Valsalva sinuses is not dilated. This is a type Id aortic regurgitation. LA, left atrium; RA, right atrium; RVOT, right ventricular outflow tract.

An optimal echocardiographic study of the aortic valve dysfunction should delineate the precise grade of severity of the disease, address the indication to surgical correction and timing, and provide preoperative data supporting the preoperative choice of the surgical technique. Best preoperative diagnostic workup may benefit from joint echocardiographist and surgeon evaluation: this could save time during interventions and support the decision of surgical techniques, tailored to each single case, and contribute to prevent perioperative and postoperative complications thus decreasing the risk of reinterventions [16, 25].

Transthoracic Echocardiography

The M-mode study of the aortic root should be performed with the cursor (probe) perpendicular to the long axis of the ascending aorta at the level of the sinuses of Valsalva (Figure 8.43). The aortic root should be measured using leading edge methodology (outer-inner layer) [26], i.e., from the anterior portion of the anterior aortic wall to the inner or anterior boundary of the posterior aortic wall, in an area in which at least two aortic cusps are visualized; this minimizes the angulations error. The aortic root should be measured at end-diastole at the onset of the first rapid deflection of the QRS complex of the ECG.

The two-dimensional echocardiography shows the entire aortic root and provides the best view to measure the aortic diameters (Figures 8.44 and 8.45) [27]. The ascending aorta should be measured in parasternal long-axis view at the levels that are significantly associated with aortic root dilation and aortic regurgitation in morphologically normal aortic valves [28, 29]: (1) aortic annulus, which is echocardiographically defined as the hinge points of the aortic cusps; (2) sinuses of Valsalva; (3) sinotubular junction; (4) proximal ascending aorta (Figure 8.42). Aortic root should also be measured in the short-axis view at the level of the valve leaflets [27] to better evaluate the symmetry of the sinuses of Valsalva. In heritable collagen diseases, the sinuses of Valsalva may be asymmetric with single cusp larger than the others both in tricuspid aortic valves and in true or functional bicuspid valves (Figures 8.9, 8.35–8.37 and 8.41).

The measurements should be given both as absolute values and according to age and body size (body surface area as determined by height and weight according

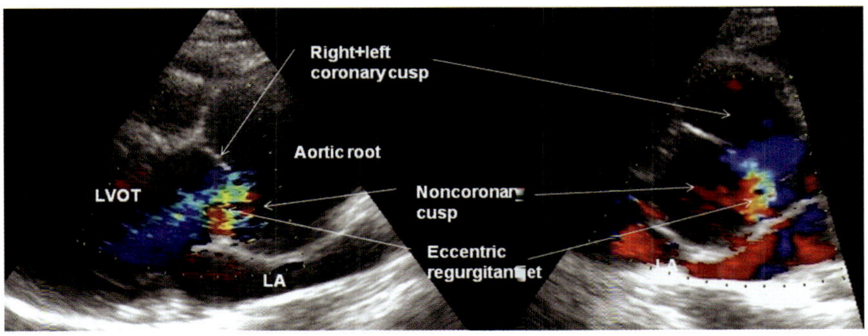

Figure 8.31 Functional classification of aortic regurgitation: echocardiographic parasternal long-axis view (a) and short-axis view (b). The application of the Color Doppler mode shows a moderate aortic regurgitation, with eccentric jet directed posteriorly against the anterior mitral leaflet. As shown in (b), the origin of the regurgitation jet in this functional bicuspid valve is between the noncoronary and the right coronary cusp due to prolapse of the free margin of the right cusp. This is a type II aortic regurgitation. The aortic root diameter is 49 mm. LA, left atrium; LVOT, left ventricular outflow tract.

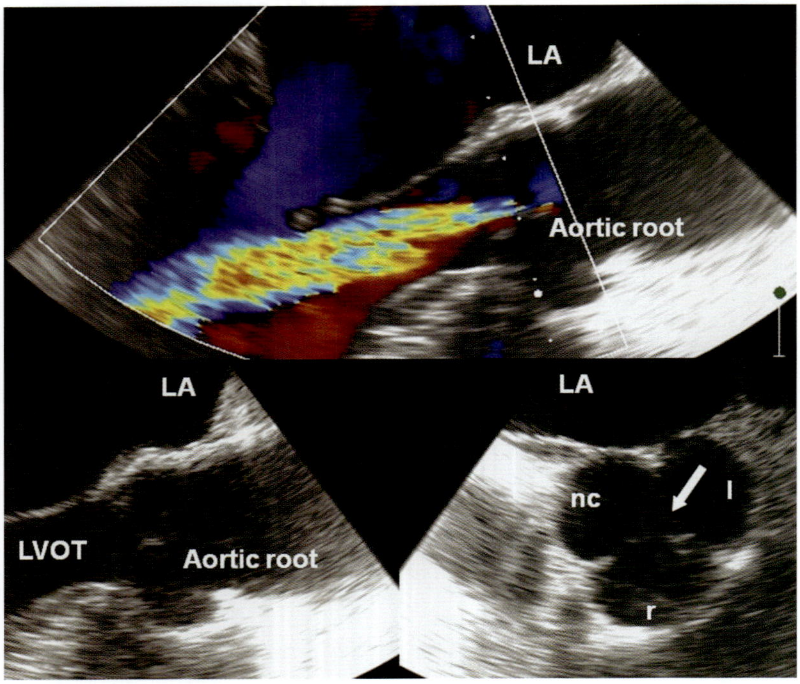

(a) (b) (c)

Figure 8.32 Functional classification of aortic regurgitation: transesophageal view. (a) The application of the Color Doppler mode shows a moderate aortic regurgitation. The jet is central. (b, c) Long-axis and short-axis views, respectively, showing the rheumatic remodeling of the valve with thickening of the cusps and retraction. The cusps retraction is evident in (c) (thick white arrow), with central lack of coaptation of the cusps. The abnormal cusps morphology configures a type III aortic regurgitation. The diameter of the aortic root is normal; the rheumatic disease also affects the sinotubular junction, which is remodeled and thickened. l, left coronary sinus; LA, left atrium; LVOT, left ventricular outflow tract; nc, noncoronary sinus; r, right coronary sinus.

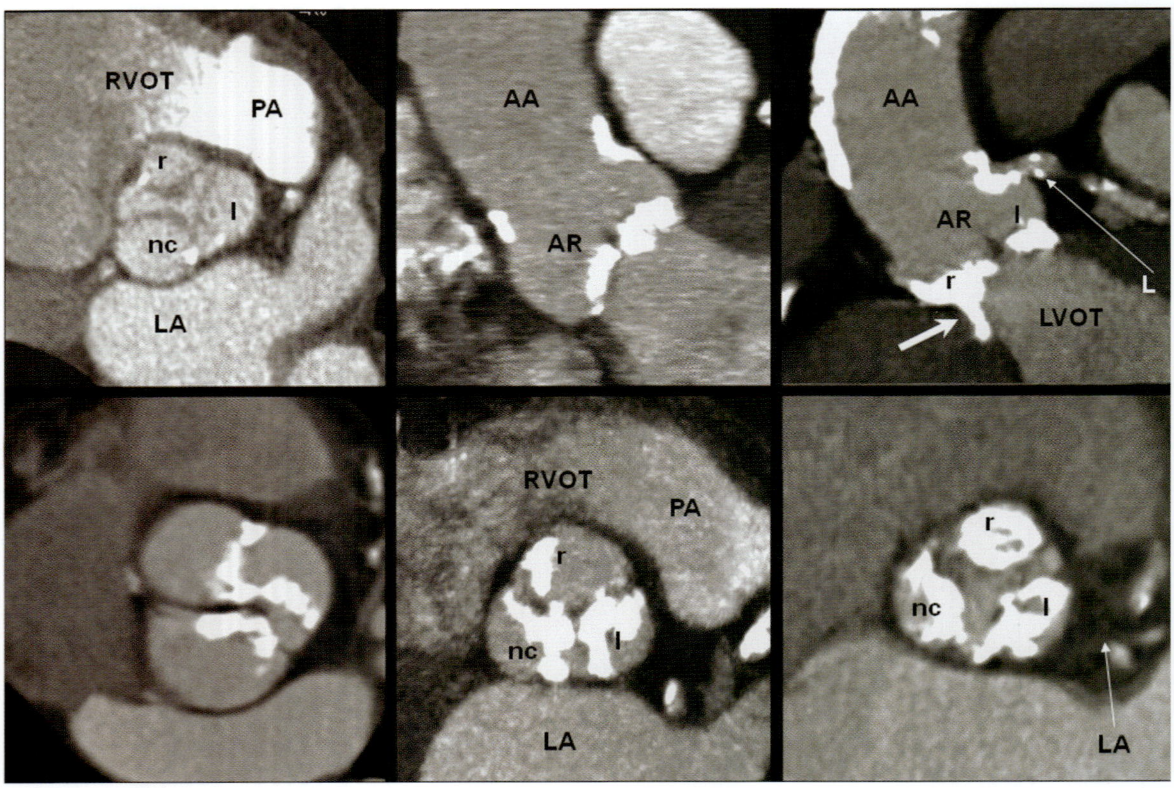

(a), (c) (e) (b), (d) (f)

Figure 8.33 Calcifications of aortic valve. (a) Grade 2: Tubular aortic aneurysm in a 78-year-old man. (b) Grade 3: 71-year-old man with aortic stenosis. (c, d) Grade 4: 79-year-old woman with aortic stenosis. (e–f) Grade 4: 70-year-old man with heavy aortic stenosis; extension of the right coronary sinus calcification to the distal wall of the outflow tract of the left ventricle (white arrow). AA, ascending aorta; AR, aortic root; l, left coronary sinus; L, left coronary sinus; LA, left atrium; LVOT, left ventricular outflow tract; nc, noncoronary sinus; PA, pulmonary artery; r, right coronary sinus; RVOT, right ventricular outflow tract.

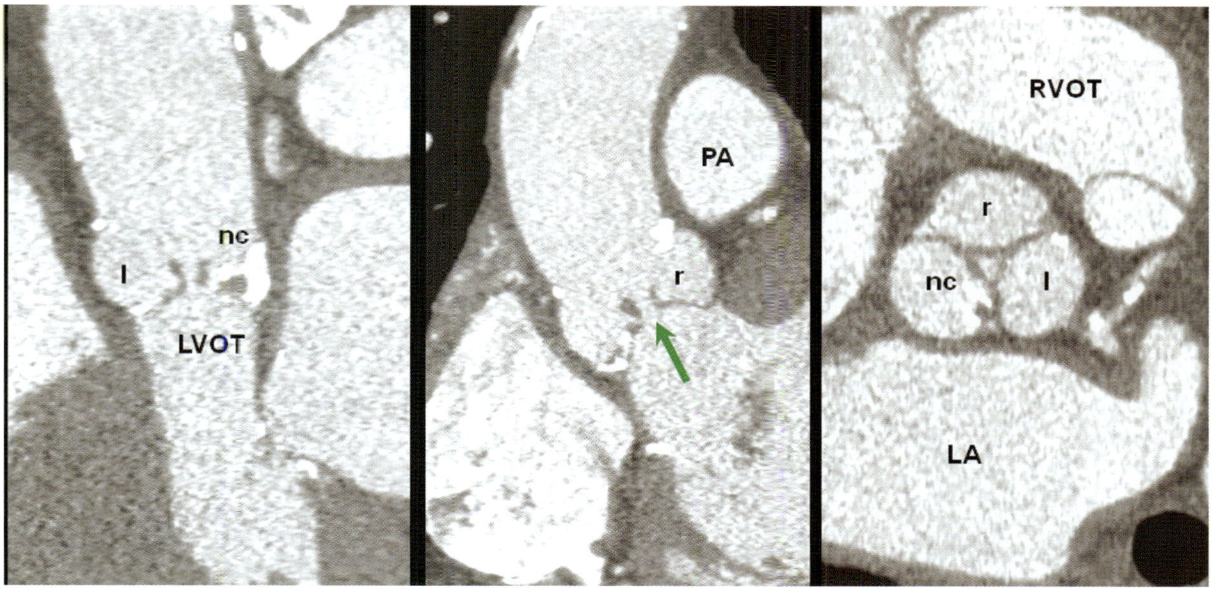

Figure 8.34 Grade 2 aortic calcifications in 87-year- old man with ascending aorta aneurysm and aortic valve regurgitation. The central defect of the coaptation of the leaflets is visible and can be estimated in each image (arrow). l, left coronary sinus; LA, left atrium; LVOT, left ventricular outflow tract; nc, noncoronary sinus; PA, pulmonary artery; r, right coronary sinus; RVOT, right ventricular outflow tract.

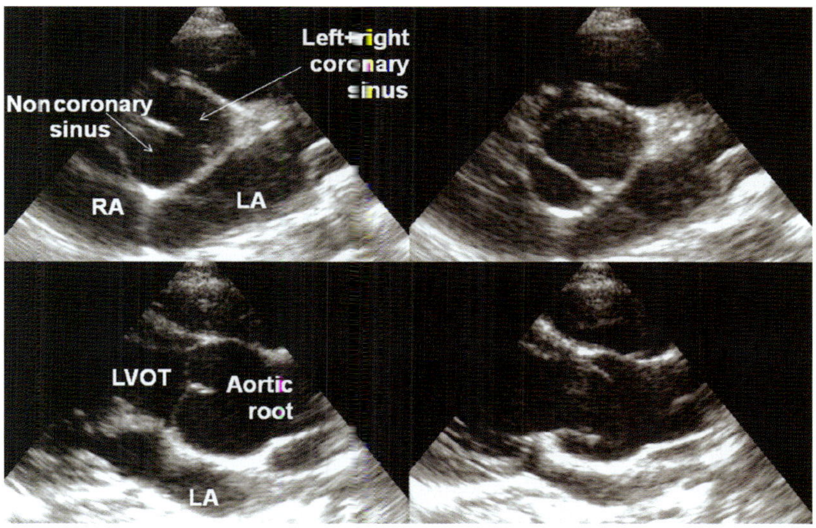

Figure 8.35 True bicuspid aortic valve, parasternal short-axis (a, b diastolic and systolic views) and long-axis views (c, d diastolic and systolic views). In the long-axis projection, the abnormal shape and dilatation of the aortic root is evident at the level of the Valsalva sinuses. In both short and long axes, the Valsalva sinuses are asymmetrical. LA, left atrium; LVOT, left ventricular outflow tract; RA, right atrium.

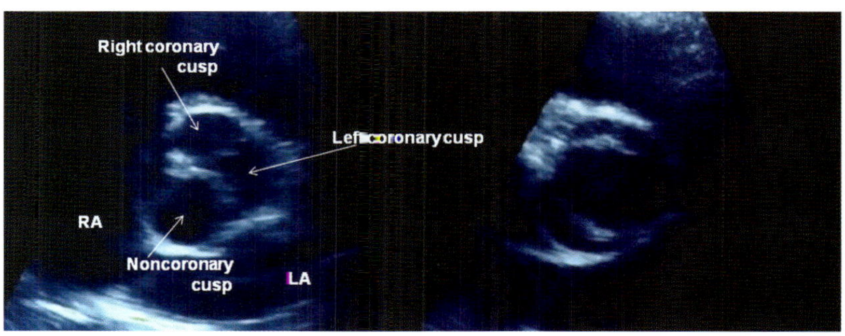

Figure 8.36 Echocardiographic short-axis view of bicuspid aortic valve. The aortic root is dilated at the level of the Valsalva sinuses. In (a) (diastolic view), the fusion *rafe* between the right and left cusps (functional bicuspid aorta) is recognizable. (b) Systolic view. LA, left atrium; RA, right atrium.

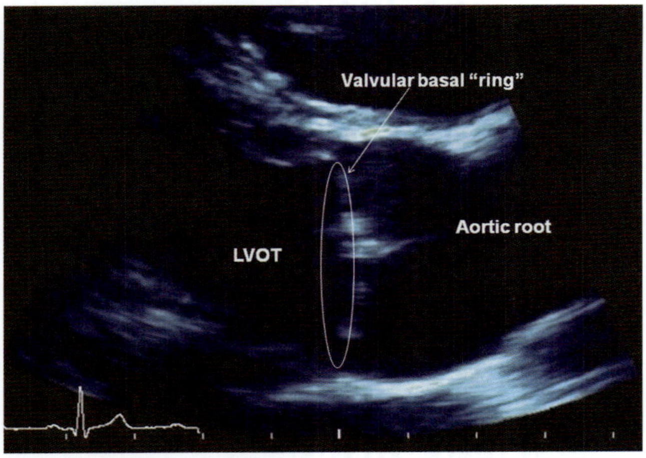

Figure 8.37 Echocardiographic parasternal long-axis view of bicuspid aortic valve. The short-axis (not shown) documented the fusion between two cusps, thus configuring a functional bicuspid aortic valve. Both annulus and Valsalva sinuses are dilated. LVOT, left ventricular outflow tract.

to the Dubois, Mosteller, Gehan, and George or Haycock formula [30–33]); both age and body size are the most important determinants of aortic root size in the general population [28, 34] and they are crucial in the pediatric population.

The diameter of the sinotubular junction measured at the level of the apices of the interleaflets triangles of ≥37 mm has been reported to be highly predictive of aortic valve regurgitation due to aortic root abnormality with a sensitivity of 96.7%, a specificity of 88.1%, and a diagnostic accuracy of 91.6% [2]. Experimental models and clinical observations indicate that dilatation of the sinotubular junction is a major determinant of functional aortic regurgitation [35]. The dilatation of the aortic root may occur not only in severe and moderate aortic regurgitation but also in mild ones. The supra-aortic ridge stands out as the level mostly involved in the dilation with a significantly higher rate of dilation in moderate and severe aortic regurgitation than in mild regurgitation [2, 29].

In the normal population, the aortic root growth rate is 0.008 cm per year in men and 0.009 cm per year in women [34]. The growth is faster in patients with aortic regurgitation. In mild regurgitation, the growth rate is prominent at the level of the tubular ascending aorta, whereas in severe regurgitation, the dilation is more uniform in all segments of the aortic root and this mechanism can contribute to worsening the aortic regurgitation [29].

The extent of the regurgitation is assessed through the integration of Doppler parameters with higher accuracy (up to 98%) as compared with angiography [36, 37]. These parameters include dimensions of the regurgitation flow

(a), (b)

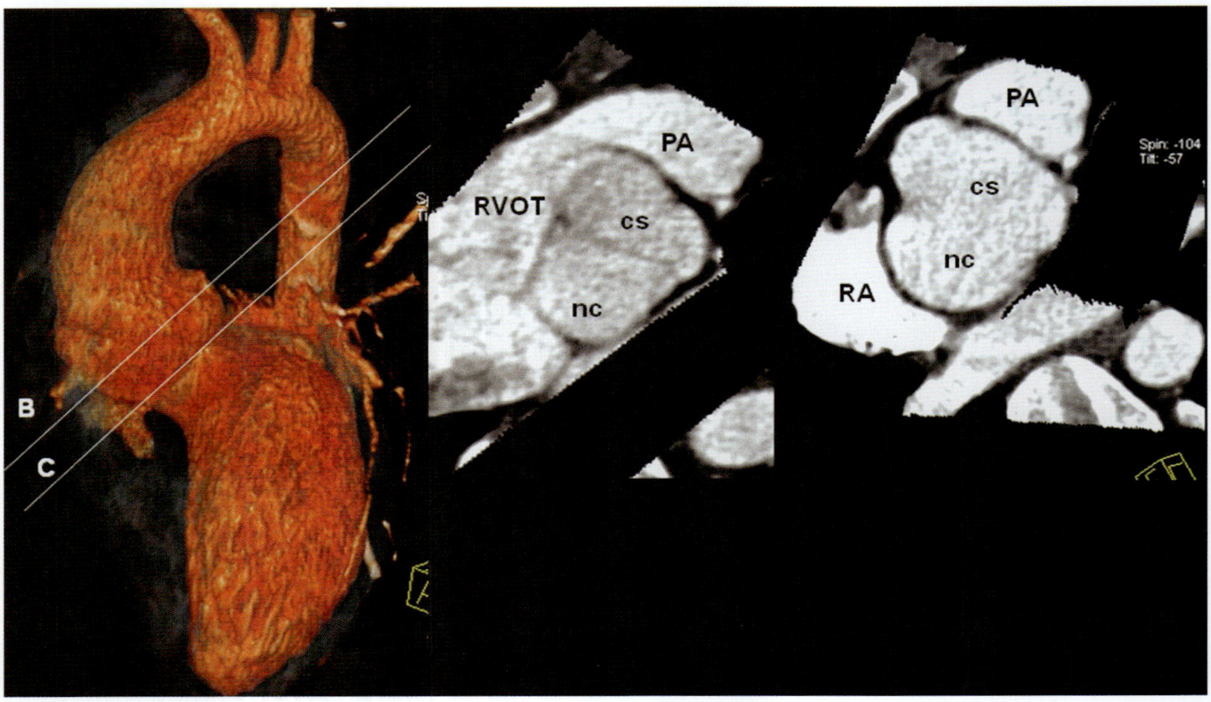

(c)

Figure 8.38 Dilatation of aortic root in a 14-year-old girl with Marfan syndrome. (b, c) B and C are axial sections perpendicular to long axis on aortic root evaluated in three-dimensional image (a); bicuspid aortic valve in telediastolic phase. Two leaflets coapt one another and delimitate laterally the apices of interleaflets triangles; noncoronary sinus (nc) has semilunar shape; and coronary sinus (cs) has bilobated shape. PA, pulmonary artery; RA, right atrium; RVOT, right ventricular outflow tract.

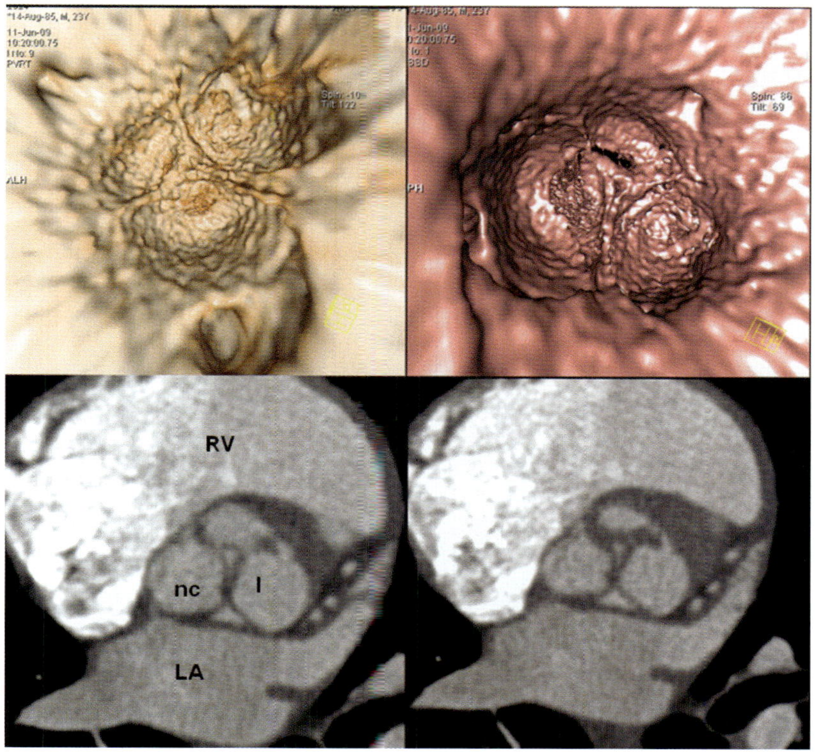

Figure 8.39 A 23-year-old man with ascending aortic dilatation and type Ia valve regurgitation. In three-dimensional virtual endoscopic view (a,b) and in axial section, right coronary sinus is abnormal and hypoplastic. On echocardiographic examination, it mimicked a bicuspid valve. In (c) and (d), central defect of leaflets coaptation is evident. l, left coronary sinus; LA, left atrium; nc, noncoronary sinus; RV, right ventricle.

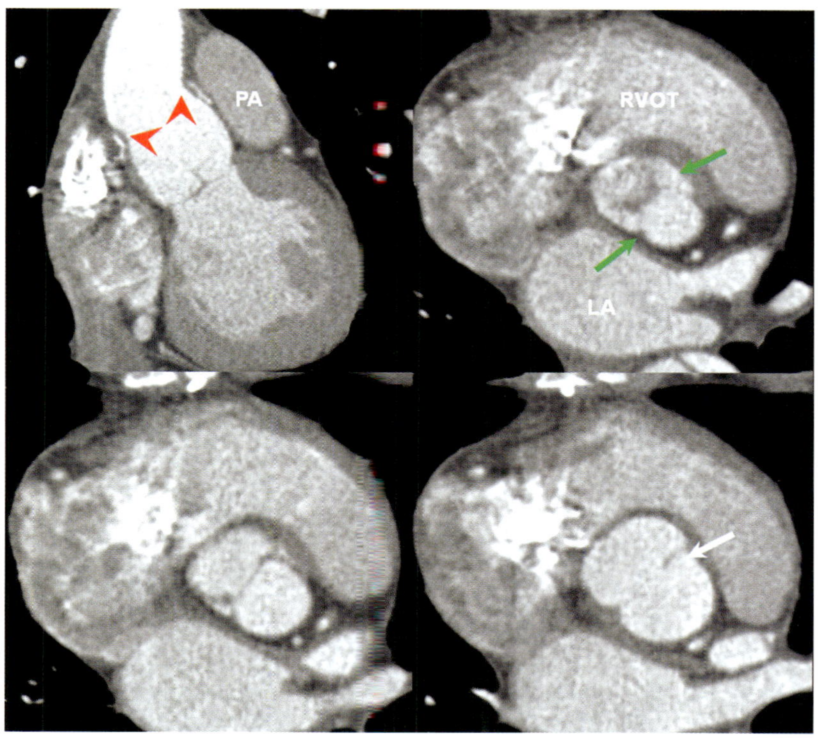

Figure 8.40 Aortic bicuspid valve in a 35-year-old man. (a) Surgical suture at the sinotubular junction level (red arrowhead); dilatation of ventriculoaortic junction. (b) The two interleaflets triangles (green arrows): the anterior triangle corresponds to the septal muscle whereas the posterior triangle corresponds to fibrous skeleton. (c, d) The right and left coronary sinuses are morphologically and dimensionally symmetric. White arrow indicates the commissure. LA, left atrium; PA, pulmonary artery; RVOT, right ventricular outflow tract.

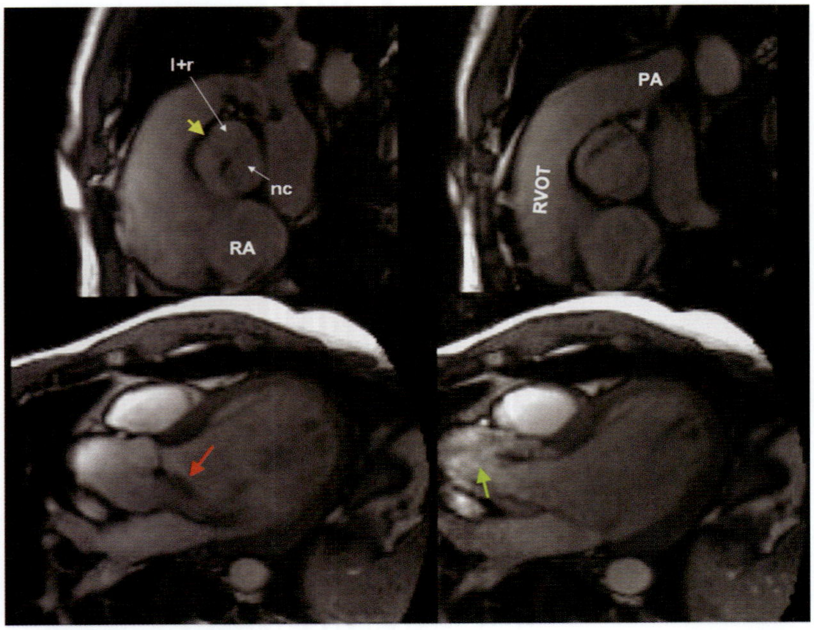

Figure 8.41 Cine MRI sequence in a patient with bicuspid aortic valve. (a, b) Short-axis view, diastolic and systolic time, respectively; (c, d) long-axis view, diastolic and systolic time, respectively. The yellow arrow indicates the fusion *rafe* between the right and left coronary cusp, thus defining a functional bicuspid valve. The red arrow indicates the aortic valve regurgitation: eccentric jet directed against the anterior mitral leaflet. The green arrow indicates the turbulent systolic jet across the valve. The aortic root is dilated. l, left coronary sinus; MRI, magnetic resonance imaging; nc, noncoronary sinus; PA, pulmonary artery; r, right coronary sinus; RA, right atrium; RVOT, right ventricular outflow tract.

in the LVOT by Color Doppler [38], the pressure at half time of the diastolic aortoventricular gradient [39] and the evaluation of reverse flow in both thoracic [40] and abdominal [41] aorta.

Transesophageal Echocardiography

Transesophageal (TEE) provides a highly accurate anatomic assessment of all types of aortic regurgitation lesions. The functional anatomy of aortic regurgitation as assessed by TEE is strongly and independently predictive of valve reparability and postoperative outcome [16]. The TEE evaluation of the aortic valve provides high-quality evaluation of the valve leaflets and aortic root in both short- (20–30°) and long-axis views (90–120°). TEE can further provide information on (1) the coaptation height, which is defined as the maximum distance between the first point of protodiastolic coaptation of the leaflet tips and the annulus plane corresponding to the basal insertion of the leaflets; and (2) the tented area, which is defined as the maximum area subtending the ventricular surface of the leaflets as far as the annular plane [42].

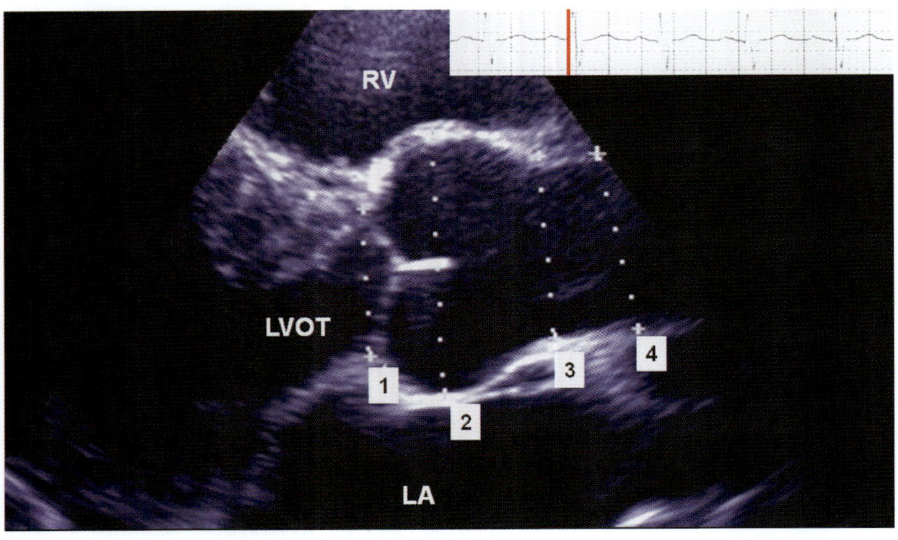

Figure 8.42 Echocardiographic measurement of the aortic root dimensions. The measurements should be taken in the diastolic phase, corresponding to the initial Q wave on the reference EKG (red line on the EKG strip in the upper right part of the picture). Dotted lines indicate the measured diameters according to the Roman method. (1) Ventriculoaortic junction; (2) Valsalva sinuses; (3) sinotubular junction; and (4) ascending aorta (about 4 cm from the valvular plane). The diameters should be traced perpendicular to the long axis of the aortic root. LA, left atrium; LVOT, left ventricular outflow tract; RV, right ventricle.

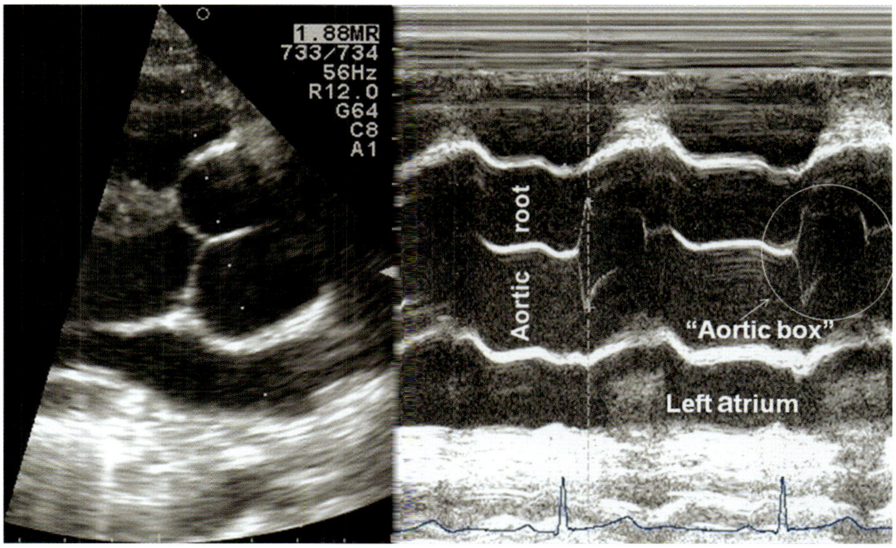

Figure 8.43 Echocardiography. M-mode registration of the aortic root. On the left, the B-mode view with the dotted line (the cursor) that constitutes the reference for the M-mode visualization. On the right, the M-mode visualization. The cursor must be perpendicular to the long axis of the ascending aorta, and it should intersect the aortic root at the level of the Valsalva sinuses.

Other measurements overlap with transthoracic echocardiography (TTE) and include the diameter of the annulus, the Valsalva sinuses, the sinotubular junction, and the tubular tract. The evaluation of the severity of the aortic regurgitation is based on the same Doppler approach as with TTE, but quality and accuracy of the images are higher. TEE usually grades aortic regurgitation more severely as compared to preoperative TTE, and in about 20% of patients the surgical indication can differ on the basis of the severity grade provided by TEE or TTE [43].

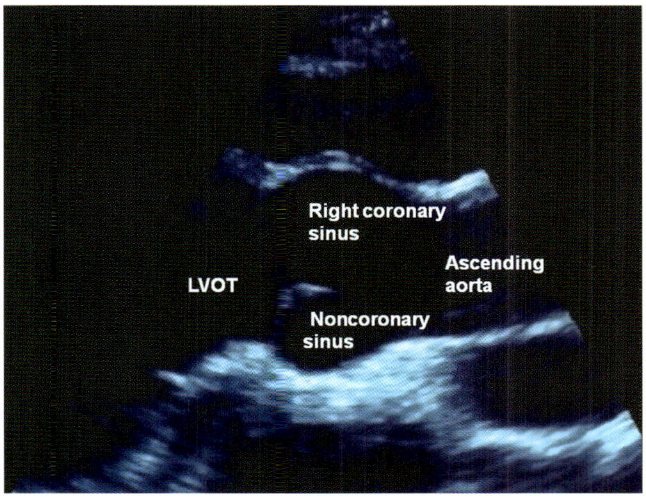

Figure 8.44 Dilation of the aortic root involving both the ventriculoaortic junction and the Valsalva sinuses. The aortic root is asymmetrical, with right coronary sinus larger than the noncoronary one. The diameter of the aortic root at the level of the sinuses of Valsalva is 31 mm, which corresponds to a *z* score of 3.75 in this 12-year-old male patient affected by Marfan syndrome. LVOT, left ventricular outflow tract.

The evaluation of the LVOT is crucial for the precise assessment of aortic valve stenosis severity [44].

The postoperative assessment of the correct function of the mechanical prosthesis and the exclusion of possible complications in the mid- and long-term follow-up is accurately evaluated with TEE. In particular, the follow-up of patients affected by rare and severe heritable disorders that affect the aortic root wall should be performed with both TEE and multidetector computerized tomography (MDCT) because they give complementary information. In fact, MDCT (see below) accurately measures the diameters of the aortic root segments and gives precise information about the presence and the nature of possible masses or hematomas surrounding the vascular prosthesis. TEE detects very early pseudoaneurysms or fissurations that can complicate both early and late postoperative course (Figures 8.46 and 8.47).

Three-Dimensional Echocardiography

Three-dimensional echocardiography shows (in a single image) the whole valve and the aortic root. It ensures the representation of depth without multiple two-dimensional slices or views to analyze the entire valve [45, 46]. The evaluation of the cusps is also accurate: in particular, their thickness is correctly represented as thin as in their real consistence (Figures 8.26 and 8.48).

Moreover, the assessment of the LVOT area through three-dimensional echocardiography provides more accurate values as compared to M-mode-based calculation, and this is mostly due to the imperfect circular area of the LVOT [47].

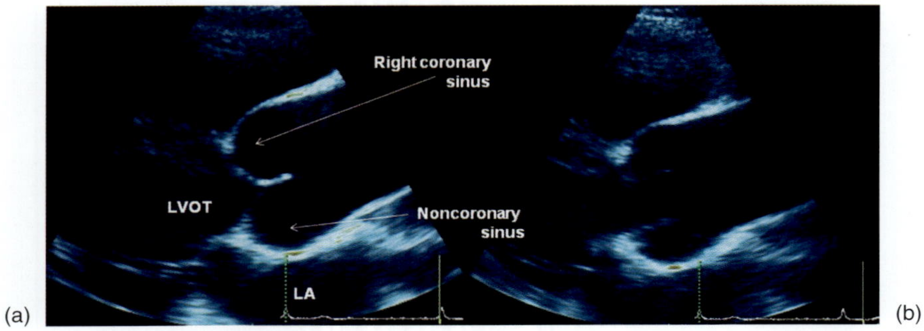

Figure 8.45 Echocardiographic view of aortic root dilation with loss of the physiologic geometry of the sinotubular junction. The aortic root is enlarged both at the level of the Valsalva sinuses and at the level of the sinotubular junction (about 1 cm from the aortic annulus). The ventriculoaortic junction has normal diameter. (a) Diastole. (b) Systole. LA, left atrium; LVOT, left ventricular outflow tract.

Multidetector Computerized Tomography

MDCT measurements of the thoracic aorta should use ECG-gated double-oblique short-axis images for precise measurements. In normal population, the 95% confidence intervals of end-diastolic diameter have been calculated to be 2.5–3.7 cm for the aortic root, 2.1–3.5 cm for the ascending aorta, and 1.7–2.6 cm for the descending thoracic aorta. At end-systole, aortic diameters are greater than at end-diastole (mean difference 1.9 ± 1.2 mm for ascending and 1.3 ± 1.8 for descending thoracic aorta, $P < 0.001$) [48]. In annuloaortic ectasia with aortic insufficiency, the three aortic cusps are significantly larger than those of control

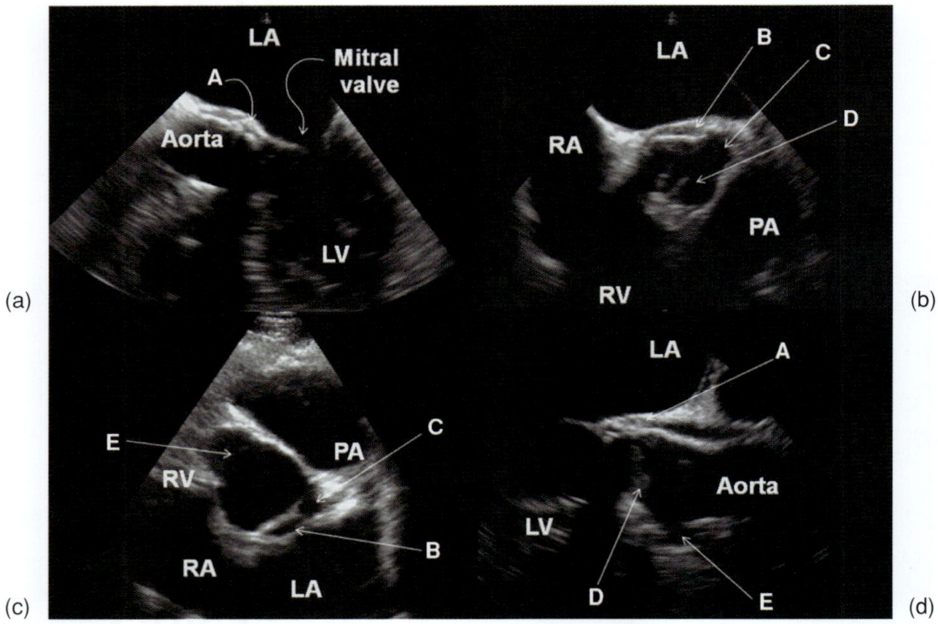

Figure 8.46 Late postoperative complication after surgical correction (Bentall operation) of acute aortic dissection in Loeys Dietz syndrome; the dissection dates back 5 years before this examination. The figure illustrates the early phase of the formation of a pseudoaneurysm surrounding the valve and vascular prostheses with initial fissuration at the level of the mitroaortic continuity. (a) Transesophageal view. (A): the fissuration in the mitroaortic continuity. Part (b) Transesophageal view. (B): the initial detachment at the level of the prosthetic aortic root that involves the left coronary sinus and the left part of the noncoronary sinus. (C) the left coronary ostium which had been reimplanted during the surgical procedure and is now involved in the pseudoaneurysm, as the left coronary originates from the straddle on the flap. (D) the mechanic hemidiscs of the prosthetic valve (c) Transthoracic view, short axis. (B) the same flap seen in (b), which involves the origin of the left coronary artery (C). (E) indicates the reimplanted origin of the right coronary artery, which is complicated by dilatation, without other complications. (d) Transesophageal view. (A) the fissuration in the mitroaortic continuity progresses along the tubular prosthesis for about 4 cm. (D) the closed hemidisc of the prosthetic valve. (E) the origin of the right coronary artery. The Color Doppler analysis (not shown) confirms the presence of flow in (A) and (B) and also confirms the coronary perfusion, both right and left coronary artery. LA, left atrium; LV, left ventricle; PA, pulmonary artery; RA, right atrium; RV, right ventricle.

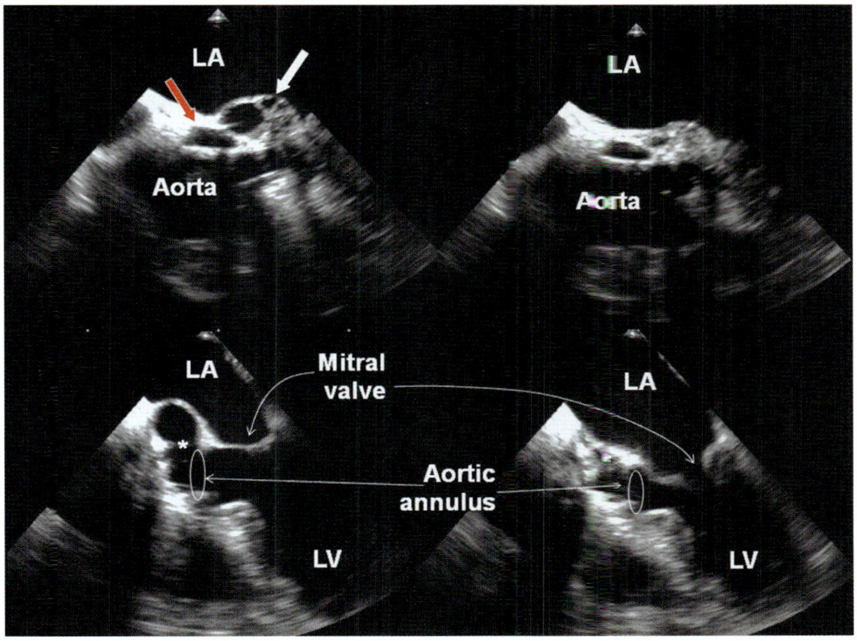

Figure 8.47 Late postoperative complication after surgical correction (Bentall operation) of acute aortic dissection in Loeys Dietz syndrome; the dissection and surgery date back 12 years before this examination. The figure illustrates the advanced phase of the formation of a pseudoaneurysm surrounding the valvular and vascular prostheses with severe involvement of the mitroaortic continuity. (a) and (b) show the systolic time; (b) and (d) show the diastolic one. (a) and (b) transesophageal view shows the large pseudoaneurysm in the context of the mitroaortic continuity (thick white arrow). During systole the pseudoaneurysm inflates to a maximal dimension of 21 mm; it deflates during diastole as it communicates with the LVOT. The thick red arrow shows the pseudoaneurysm surrounding the ascending aorta (c), (d): transesophageal view showing the wide communication between the LVOT and the pseudoaneurysm (asterisk): the orifice is about 6 mm in diameter in systole and it collapses in diastole. LA, left atrium; LV, left ventricle; LVOT, left ventricular outflow tract.

subjects, and the sinotubular junction diameter is larger in systole than in diastole [49].

Quantitative Information

MDCT images provide precise diameters of the ventriculoaortic junction, root at the level of Valsalva sinuses, sinotubular junction, ascending aorta and of the aorta at all levels of its length (Figure 8.49). Any preoperative decision on aortic root, both aneurysms and dissections, is taken on the basis of MDCT angiography.

Qualitative Information

These data include cusp morphology, symmetry of the Valsalva sinuses and related measures, and linear or tortuous course and collaterals, including coronary arteries and calcifications of both valve and root components.

Magnetic Resonance Imaging

MRI does not administer radiations and does not require iodinated contrast procedure. Patients who cannot tolerate intravenous iodated procedure for MDCT can be alternatively evaluated with MRI. Therefore in elective conditions, this tool is preferable to MDCT angiography, especially in children. For adult patients who do not suffer claustrophobia, the length of the procedure does not represent a limitation. A single cine magnetic resonance is sufficient for evaluation of the thoracic aorta, including the aortic root; frequently, however, more information are needed on the entire vascular tree and this implies more MRI procedures (cranial, thoracic, and abdominal districts). In children, the presence of the anesthesiologist is compulsory, as is for MDCT angiography, which is, however shorter and requires only a few minutes of sedation.

Advantages of MDCT angiography and magnetic resonance as compared to echocardiography include: more precise measurements of the diameters of the vessels, identification of calcium in terms of site of deposition and extension. In patients who suffer type A dissection both MRI and CT techniques can add information on top of those provided by echocardiography, on the exact location of the dissection flap, direction of the dissection, true and false lumen size, thrombosis of the false lumen,

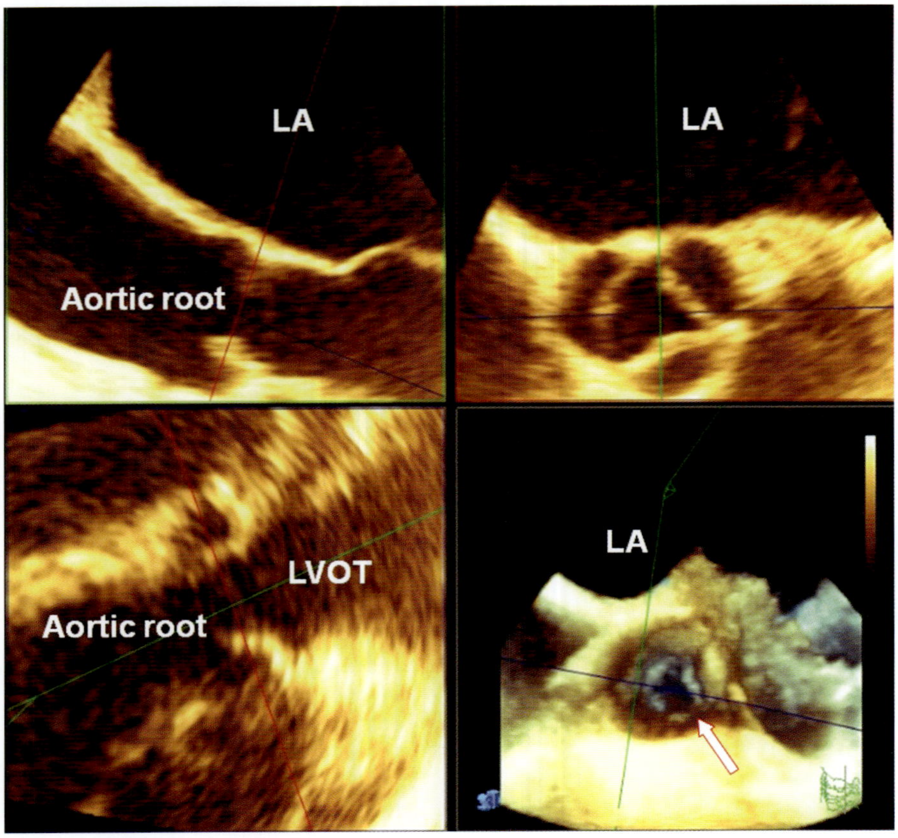

Figure 8.48 Three-dimensional echocardiography (transesophageal approach). The three-dimensional reconstruction documents the structural changes of the rheumatic valve with cusps retraction and deformation (thick white arrow). The aortic root is normal. LA, left atrium; LVOT, left ventricular outflow tract.

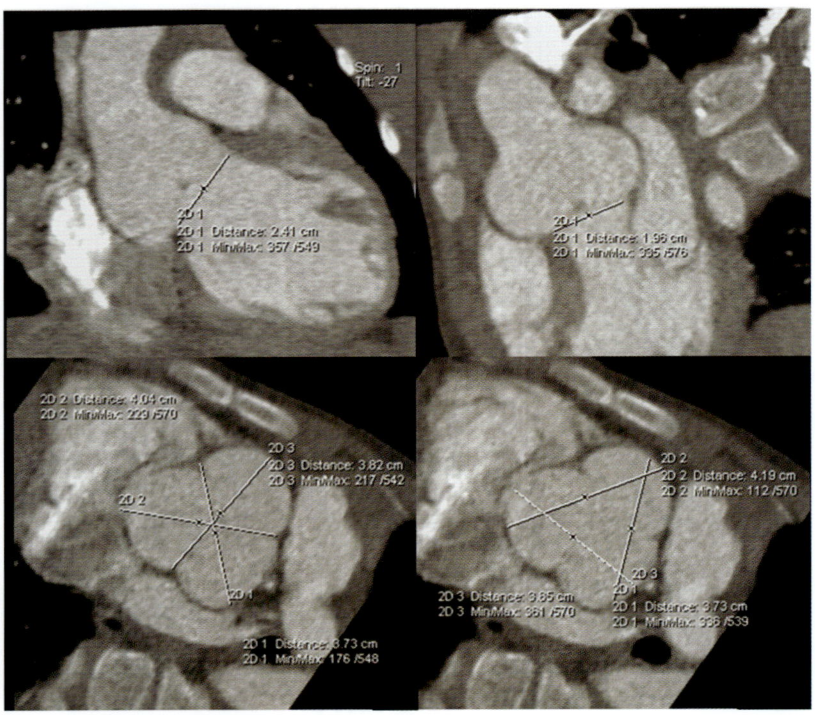

Figure 8.49 Annular-sinusal dilatation in a 4-year-old girl with Marfan syndrome. Coronal (a) and sagittal (b) sections: eccentric expansion of the annular region and enlarged aortic root with normal sinotubular junction. (c, d) Measurement modalities of the aortic root diameters by "commissure to sinus" (c) or by "sinus to sinus" (d).

pressure conditions in the true relative to the false lumen, fenestrations and perfusion of the false lumen.

Surgical Implications

During the past 25 years, the aortic root surgery impressively progressed and introduced the possibility of preserving the native valve leaflets when repairing aortic insufficiency due to aortic root dysfunction. The traditional Bentall technique with substitution of the aortic valve with a mechanical prosthesis has obvious hemodynamic and clinical implications both for the prosthetic body and for the anticoagulation therapy. The valve-sparing root replacement (VSRR) procedures are progressively increasing in both children and adults as they generate a "paraphysiologic" aortic root and maintain the native aortic valve leaflets that are less prone to deterioration as compared to biological prostheses [1, 4, 9]. In children in particular, VSRR procedures show a favorable long-term outcome [50]. The postoperative evaluation of surgical results and monitoring are based on imaging techniques of the aortic root including echocardiography, MDCT angiography, and magnetic resonance.

The exhaustive comprehension and visualization of the pathophysiologic mechanisms and related effects is taken into consideration in the decision making before surgery for deciding best repair technique [25]. The current multidisciplinary and collaborative approach involves surgeon, cardiologists, and radiologists. The two novel issues challenging these multidisciplinary teams are the *preventive* surgery of (1) aortic root dissection without valve regurgitation and of (2) both dilation of the root and aortic regurgitation due to the root pathology, prolapse or defects of the cusps, or both. Dilation of the aortic root can be corrected by subcommissural plication, remodeling of the root or mobilization of the valve with subsequent reimplantation within a vascular graft. Only a correct preoperative imaging study providing the anatomical and functional data on the underlying disease gives surgeon all necessary information that may support the choice of the most appropriate surgical technique.

In case of aortic valve replacement with a bioprosthetic valve, the to-date choice includes both stented and stentless prosthesis [51], which may need single suture or two-line sutures. The clear preoperative anatomy is crucial for decisions. While the implantation of a stented prosthesis transforms the scalloped native "ring" in a planar ring, a single-suture stentless valve is implanted following the three-coronet profile of the bases of the valve cusps on the aortic wall. Two-line sutures stentless prostheses are implanted following the planar ring for the inflow suture, and the three-coronet profile for the outflow suture. Therefore, two measurements are required to determine the correct stentless prosthesis: (1) the diameter of the ideal planar ring (inflow suture) and (2) the diameter of the sinotubular junction (outflow suture) that should be 10–15% smaller than the first one. If the sinotubular junction is larger than the "planar" annulus, then the stentless valve can be positioned only after surgical reduction of the sinotubular junction. Preoperative imaging should provide this information.

The type of aortic root surgery procedure is determined on the preexisting degree of dilatation. For remodeling and valve reimplantation, good mid- and long-term results have been reported (10-year free from reoperation approximately 90%). In bicuspid anatomy, the frequently observed cusp prolapse can be corrected using plicating suture on the free cusp margins, excision and reapproximation of cusp tissue, or patch implantation into perforation or fenestrations. The decision on the type of valve remodeling technique is facilitated by information provided by the preoperative imaging: (a) number and consistency of the cusps, (b) geometrical relationship between the anatomic subunits that form the aortic root, and (c) underlying disease that causes the dysfunction (the approach in repairing an atherosclerotic aortic root is different from that of heritable collagen diseases).

Conclusions

Echocardiography techniques flanked by magnetic resonance and computerized tomography are the major players in diagnosing, monitoring, and decision making for best surgery in aortic root pathology. Best imaging of the aortic root is largely contributing to expanding the surgical techniques to a wider spectrum of choices tailored to the patient's exact anatomy and pathophysiology, rather than to standard identical procedures. Skill and expertise of the operators, both imaging and surgery, provide the basis for a novel more physiological approach to the management of the aortic root diseases.

References

1. Underwood MJ, El Khoury G, Deronck D, Glineur D, Dion R. (2000) The aortic root: structure, function, and surgical reconstruction. *Heart* 83:376–380.
2. Guiney TE, Davies MJ, Parker DJ, Leech GJ, Leatham A. (1987) The aetiology and course of isolated severe aortic regurgitation: a clinical, pathological, and echocardiographic study. *Heart* 58:358–368.
3. Anderson RH. (2006) The surgical anatomy of the aortic root. *Multimedia Manual of Cardiothoracic Surgery* (MMCTS). doi:10.1510/mmcts.2006.002527.

4. Feindel CM, David TE. (2004) Aortic valve sparing operations: basic concepts. *Int J Cardiol* 97(Suppl 1):61–66.
5. Sutton JP 3rd, Ho SY, Anderson RH. (1995) The forgotten interleaflet triangles: a review of the surgical anatomy of the aortic valve. *Ann Thorac Surg* 59:419–427.
6. Sacks MS, Smith DB, Hiester ED. (1998) The aortic valve microstructure: effects of transvalvular pressure. *J Biomed Mater Res* 41:131–141.
7. Vesely I. (1998) The role of elastin in aortic valve mechanics. *J Biomech* 31:115–123.
8. Maselli D, Montalto A, Santise G, Minardi G, Manzara C, Musumeci F. (2005) A normogram to anticipate dimension of neo-sinuses of Valsalva in valve-sparing aortic operations. *Eur J Cardiothorac Surg* 27:831–835.
9. Hopkins RA. (2003) Aortic valve leaflet sparing and salvage surgery: evolution of techniques for aortic root reconstruction. *Eur J Cardiothorac Surg* 24:886–897.
10. Robicsek F. (1991) Leonardo da Vinci and the sinuses of Valsalva. *Ann Thorac Surg* 52:328–335.
11. Kunzelman KS, Grande KJ, David TE, Cochran RP, Verrier ED. (1994) Aortic root and valve relationships. Impact on surgical repair. *J Thorac Cardiovasc Surg* 107:162–170.
12. Jeanmart H, de Kerchove L, Glineur D *et al.* (2007) Aortic valve repair: the functional approach to leaflet prolapse and valve-sparing surgery. *Ann Thorac Surg* 83:S746–S751.
13. El Khoury G, Glineur D, Rubay J *et al.* (2005) Functional classification of aortic root/valve abnormalities and their correlation with etiologies and surgical procedures. *Curr Opin Cardiol* 20:115–121.
14. Silver MA, Roberts WC. (1985) Detailed anatomy of the normally functioning aortic valve in hearts of normal and increased weight. *Am J Cardiol* 55:454–461.
15. Perrin A, Aerichide N, Gravier J, Cahen P, Froment R. (1962) Interventricular communications with aortic insufficiency (Laubry-Pezzi syndrome). *Arch Mal Coeur Vaiss* 55:289–310.
16. de Waroux JB, Pouleur AC, Goffinet C *et al.* (2007) Functional anatomy of aortic regurgitation: accuracy, prediction of surgical repairability, and outcome implications of transesophageal echocardiography. *Circulation* 116(11 Suppl): I264–I269.
17. Ferencik M, Pape LA. (2003) Changes in size of ascending aorta and aortic valve function with time in patients with congenitally bicuspid aortic valves. *Am J Cardiol* 92:43–46.
18. Cecconi M, Manfrin M, Moraca A *et al.* (2005) Aortic dimensions in patients with bicuspid aortic valve without significant valve dysfunction. *Am J Cardiol* 95:292–294.
19. Dore A, Brochu MC, Baril JF, Guertin MC, Mercier LA. (2003) Progressive dilation of the diameter of the aortic root in adults with a bicuspid aortic valve. *Cardiol Young* 13:526–531.
20. Beroukhim RS, Kruzick TL, Taylor AL, Gao D, Yetman AT. (2006) Progression of aortic dilation in children with a functionally normal bicuspid aortic valve. *Am J Cardiol* 98:828–830.
21. Grotenhuis HB, Ottenkamp J, Westenberg JJ *et al.* (2007) Reduced aortic elasticity and dilatation are associated with aortic regurgitation and left ventricular hypertrophy in nonstenotic bicuspid aortic valve patients. *J Am Coll Cardiol* 49: 1660–1665.
22. Keane MG, Wiegers SE, Plappert T, Pochettino A, Bavaria JE, Sutton MG (2000). Bicuspid aortic valves are associated with aortic dilatation out of proportion to coexistent valvular lesions. *Circulation* 102(19 Suppl 3):III35–III39.
23. Fedak PW, Verma S, David TE, Leask RL, Weisel RD, Butany J. (2002) Clinical and pathophysiological implications of a bicuspid aortic valve. *Circulation* 106:900–904.
24. Cecconi M, Nistri S, Quarti A *et al.* (2006) Aortic dilatation in patients with bicuspid aortic valve. *J Cardiovasc Med (Hagerstown)* 7:11–20.
25. Germing A, Mügge A. (2009) What the cardiac surgeon needs to know prior to aortic valve surgery: impact of echocardiography. *Eur J Cardiothorac Surg.* 35(6):960–964.
26. Sahn DJ, DeMaria A, Kisslo J, Weyman A. (1978) Recommendations regarding quantitation in M-mode echocardiography: results of a survey of echocardiographic measurements. *Circulation* 58:1072–1083.
27. Roman MJ, Devereux RB, Kramer-Fox R, O'Loughlin J. (1989) Two-dimensional echocardiographic aortic root dimensions in normal children and adults. *Am J Cardiol* 64:507–512.
28. Roman MJ, Devereux RB, Niles NW *et al.* (1987) Aortic root dilatation as a cause of isolated, severe aortic regurgitation. Prevalence, clinical and echocardiographic patterns, and relation to left ventricular hypertrophy and function. *Ann Intern Med* 106:800–807.
29. Padial LR, Oliver A, Sagie A, Weyman AE, King ME, Levine RA.(1997) Two-dimensional echocardiographic assessment of the progression of aortic root size in 127 patients with chronic aortic regurgitation: role of the supraaortic ridge and relation to the progression of the lesion. *Am Heart J* 134: 814–821.
30. Du Bois D, Du Bois EF. (1989) A formula to estimate the approximate surface area if height and weight be known. 1916. *Nutrition* 5(5):303–311.
31. Mosteller RD. (1987) Simplified calculation of body-surface area. *N Engl J Med* 317:1098.
32. Haycock GB, Schwartz GJ, Wisotsky DH. (1978) Geometric method for measuring body surface area: a height-weight formula validated in infants, children, and adults. *J Pediatr* 93:62–66.
33. Gehan EA, George SL. (1970) Estimation of human body surface area from height and weight. *Cancer Chemother Rep* 54:225–235.
34. Vasan RS, Larson MG, Levy D. (1995) Determinants of echocardiographic aortic root size. The Framingham Heart Study. *Circulation* 91:734–740.
35. Furukawa K, Ohteki H, Cao ZL *et al.* (1999) Does dilatation of the sinotubular junction cause aortic regurgitation? *Ann Thorac Surg* 68:949–953.
36. Zarauza J, Ares M, Vílchez FG *et al.* (1998) An integrated approach to the quantification of aortic regurgitation by Doppler echocardiography. *Am Heart J* 136:1030–1041.
37. Evangelista A, del Castillo HG, Calvo F *et al.* (2000) Strategy for optimal aortic regurgitation quantification by Doppler echocardiography: agreement among different methods. *Am Heart J* 139:773–781.
38. Perry GJ, Helmcke F, Nanda NC, Byard C, Soto B. (1987) Evaluation of aortic insufficiency by Doppler color flow mapping. *J Am Coll Cardiol* 9:952–959.

39. Pye M, Rae AP, Hutton I, Cobbe SM. (1990) Quantification of aortic regurgitation using continuous and pulsed wave Doppler echocardiography. *Int J Cardiol* 27:101–106.
40. Tribouilloy C, Avinée P, Shen WF, Rey JL, Slama M, Lesbre JP (1991) End diastolic flow velocity just beneath the aortic isthmus assessed by pulsed Doppler echocardiography: a new predictor of the aortic regurgitant fraction. *Br Heart J* 65:37–40.
41. Mitani M, Tamai J, Miyatake K. (1994) Consequence of diseases in aorta on evaluation of aortic regurgitation by aortic flow velocity profiles. *Angiology* 45:613–619.
42. La Canna G, Maisano F, De Michele L *et al.* (2009) Determinants of the degree of functional aortic regurgitation in patients with anatomically normal aortic valve and ascending thoracic aorta aneurysm. Transoesophageal Doppler echocardiography study. *Heart* 95:130–136.
43. Neuman YM, Brasch AV, Sobal S *et al.* (2003) Comparison of transthoracic and intraoperative transesophageal color flow Doppler assessment of mitral and aortic regurgitation. *Cardiology* 99:145–152.
44. Leye M, Brochet E, Lepage L *et al.* (2009) Size-adjusted left ventricular outflow tract diameter reference values: a safeguard for the evaluation of the severity of aortic stenosis. *J Am Soc Echocardiogr* 22(5):445–451.
45. Houck RC, Cooke JE, Gill EA. (2006) Live 3D echocardiography: a replacement for traditional 2D echocardiography? *AJR Am J Roentgenol* 187:1092–1106.
46. Vogel M, Ho SY, Anderson RH. (1995) Comparison of three dimensional echocardiographic findings with anatomical specimens of various congenitally malformed hearts. *Br Heart J* 73:566–570.
47. Khaw AV, von Bardeleben RS, Strasser C *et al.* (2008) Direct measurement of left ventricular outflow tract by transthoracic real-time 3D-echocardiography increases accuracy in assessment of aortic valve stenosis. *Int J Cardiol.* In press.
48. Lin FY, Devereux RB, Roman MJ *et al.* (2008) Assessment of the thoracic aorta by multidetector computed tomography: age- and sex-specific reference values in adults without evident cardiovascular disease. *J Cardiovasc Comput Tomogr* 2:298–308.
49. Kazui T, Kim H, Tsuboi J, Yoshioka K, Okabayashi H, Kawazoe K. (2008) Perioperative dynamic morphological changes of the aortic annulus during aortic root remodeling with aortic annuloplasty at systolic and diastolic phases. *J Heart Valve Dis* 17:366–370.
50. Lausberg H, Schäfers HJ. (2004) Recent progress in heart valve surgery: innovation or evolution? *Minerva Cardioangiol* 52:243–254.
51. Dapunt OE, Easo J, Hölzl PP *et al.* (2008) Stentless full root bioprosthesis in surgery for complex aortic valve-ascending aortic disease: a single center experience of over 300 patients. *Eur J Cardiothorac Surg* 33:554–559.

9 Coronary Anatomy for Interventionalists

Stephan Achenbach

University of Erlangen, Erlangen, Germany

Introduction

Detailed knowledge of coronary artery anatomy as well as a feeling for spatial relationships between various coronary arteries, their side, veins, and surrounding structures is essential to interpret invasive coronary angiography and to perform coronary artery interventions. Computed tomography (CT), when performed with state-of-the-art equipment and after adequate patient preparation, provides high-resolution, three-dimensional datasets that allow to display the anatomy of the heart and the coronary arteries in great detail (see Figure 9.1). Three-dimensional renderings as obtained by CT clearly visualize the epicardial course of the coronary arteries. However, some issues need to be takes into account. CT reconstructions, even though they closely resemble actual gross anatomy, do not perfectly reflect reality. Spatial resolution of cardiac CT is approximately 0.5 mm so that very fine details may be lost. Images are usually acquired and displayed in diastole to minimize cardiac motion, but to some extent, motion artifacts may be present and lead to a subtle distortion of images. Finally, the three-dimensional reconstructions use a certain threshold for display—only structures above a certain CT attenuation (density) are visualized. Usually, the three-dimensional reconstructions will show the contrast-enhanced blood pool: contrast agent is injected intravenously for data acquisition and the cardiac chambers, as well as the lumen of the great vessels and coronary arteries filled with blood are displayed. To some extent, left ventricular myocardium—which saturates with contrast during the examination—may also be visible. However, other structures, such as pericardial fat and fluid, or the pericardium itself, as well as the walls of the great vessels and coronary arteries are not visible in most three-dimensional reconstructions. Coronary veins also fill more slowly with contrast than arteries do and are not fully visible on most CT images. For the display of coronary artery anatomy, all of this may be of advantage, since the thresholding provides a clear view of the coronary vessels. The very proximal course of the coronary arteries is covered by superimposed structures such as the pulmonary artery and the atrial appendages. Manual "segmentation" allows to remove these structures from the three-dimensional reconstructions and to display all segments of the coronary arteries (see Figure 9.1).

Revisiting Cardiac Anatomy: A Computed-Tomography-Based Atlas and Reference, 1st edition. Edited by Farhood Saremi, Eloisa Arbustini, Stephen Achenbach and Jagat Narula.

Normal Coronary Anatomy

Normally, two coronary arteries are present, one originating from the right coronary sinus and one from the left coronary (Figures 9.2–9.4) sinus.

The left coronary artery originates from the middle portion of the left anterior sinus of Valsalva—usually with a single ostium, thus forming a left main trunk. The left main coronary artery divides into a left anterior descending coronary artery and a left circumflex coronary artery (note that these are not called "branches" but much rather "arteries" [1], while further, secondary ramifications of the left coronary arteries are called "branches"). In some instances, the left main coronary artery gives rise to an "intermediate branch" that originates between the left anterior descending coronary artery and the left circumflex coronary artery.

The left anterior descending coronary artery travels in the anterior interventricular groove toward the apex of the heart and usually terminates within 2 cm before or after the apex. It gives rise to septal branches, or "septal perforators," and to diagonal branches, of which typically between one and three will exist. Occasionally, a large diagonal branch may be of equal size to the left anterior

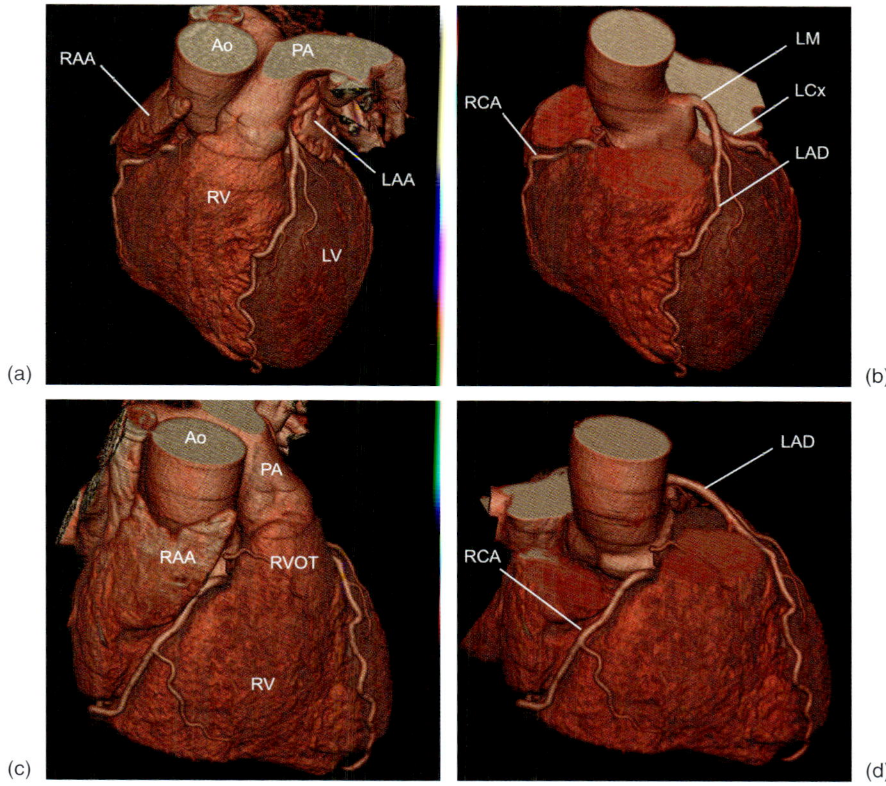

Figure 9.1 Three-dimensional visualization of the heart as obtained by contrast-enhanced computed tomography. (a) View of the anterior face of the heart. (b) By manual segmentation of the computed tomography images, parts of the right ventricular outflow tract, pulmonary artery, as well as the left and right atrial appendage have been removed. Now, the entire course of the left main and left anterior descending coronary arteries can be seen. (c) View of the right lateral face of the heart. (d) By manual segmentation, parts of the right ventricular outflow tract, the pulmonary artery, as well as the right atrial appendage have been removed. Now, the left anterior descending coronary artery and the proximal two thirds of the right coronary artery can be seen. Ao, aorta; LAA, left atrial appendage; LAD, left anterior descending coronary artery; LCx, left circumflex coronary artery; LM, left main coronary artery; LV, left ventricle; PA, pulmonary artery; RAA, right atrial appendage; RCA, right coronary artery; RV, right ventricle; RVOT, right ventricular outflow tract.

descending coronary artery itself or it may be even larger. While it is usually assumed that septal branches arise only from the left anterior descending coronary artery itself, they may occasionally also arise from the proximal segment of a large first diagonal branch [2]. The left anterior descending coronary artery frequently has small branches that are directed toward the free wall of the right ventricle. They may become more prominent when collateral circuits develop ("Vieussen's circle" when in the proximal part of the left anterior descending coronary artery) [1].

The left circumflex coronary artery arises from the left main coronary artery and then travels posteriorly and inferiorly, under the left atrial appendage, to reach the left atrioventricular (AV) groove, between the left ventricle and left atrium, in close proximity to the mitral valve. The further course of the left circumflex coronary artery is highly variable. The left circumflex coronary artery, by definition, runs in the AV groove. It usually sends at least one branch over the lateral wall of the left ventricle. This branch or these branches are called "obtuse marginal branches" and may be larger than the circumflex coronary artery, or even represent the end branch of the left circumflex coronary artery. A posterolateral branch is called present when there is a branch extending to the posterolateral surface of the left ventricle. It can be a division of an obtuse marginal branch, and it can also constitute the end branch of the left circumflex system. Finally, in some cases the left circumflex coronary artery may terminate in a posterior descending artery that runs in the posterior interventricular groove. The left circumflex coronary artery can give rise to a sinoatrial nodal branch and to "atrial circumflex" branches, which run across the left atrium.

The right coronary artery originates from the right sinus of Valsalva (with a somewhat variable position of the ostium in this sinus). The artery then travels within epicardial fat into and along the right AV groove. In the majority of cases, the right coronary artery will travel as a large vessel around the right margin of the heart and toward the posterior interventricular groove, where, at the crux of the heart, it bifurcates into two branches. The posterior descending branch (often incorrectly called "PDA—posterior descending *artery*") travels in the posterior interventricular groove toward the apex of the heart, but normally not beyond it. The right posterolateral branch courses across the posterolateral wall of the left ventricle, toward the apex, in a direction roughly parallel to the obtuse marginal branches of the left circumflex coronary artery. This branch or these branches are usually small, but may be larger than the posterior descending branch of the right coronary artery.

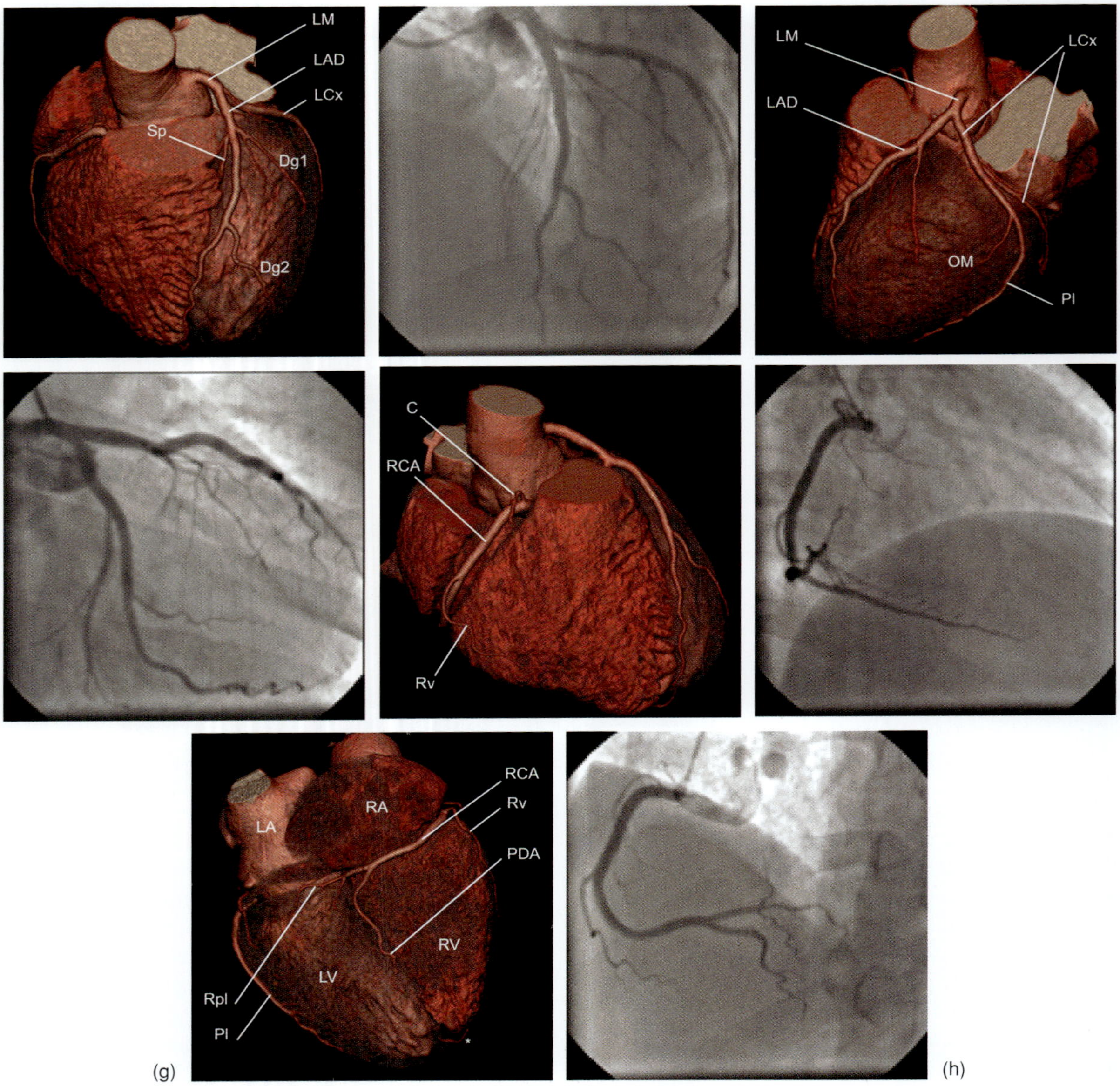

Figure 9.2 Three-dimensional anatomy of the coronary arteries. (a) Anatomy of the left anterior descending coronary artery on the anterior surface of the heart. (b) Corresponding invasive coronary angiogram to (a). (c) Anatomy of the left circumflex coronary artery. (d) Corresponding invasive coronary angiogram to (c) (note that the projection is not oriented the same way as (c)). (e) Anatomy of the proximal right coronary artery seen from a right lateral view. (f) Corresponding invasive coronary angiogram to (e). (g) Anatomy of the distal right coronary artery on the inferior face of the heart. (h) Corresponding invasive coronary angiogram to (g) (note that the projection is not oriented the same way as (g)). C, conus branch of the right coronary artery; Dg1, first diagonal branch; Dg2, second diagonal branch; LA, left atrium; LAD, left anterior descending coronary artery, LCx, left circumflex coronary artery; LM, left main coronary artery; LV, left ventricle; OM, obtuse marginal branch, PDA, posterior descending branch; Pl, posterolateral branch of the left circumflex coronary artery; RA, right atrium; RCA, right coronary artery; Rpl, posterolateral branch of the right coronary artery; Rv, right ventricular branch; RV, right ventricle; Sp, septal branch.

Coronary Dominance

Usually, the left anterior descending coronary artery supplies approximately 50% of the left ventricular muscle mass, the left circumflex coronary artery supplies about 25% of the left ventricular myocardium, and the right coronary artery supplies the remaining 25% [2]. Roughly 85–90% of hearts will be of a "right dominant" type where the right coronary artery reaches and crosses

(a), (b) (c)

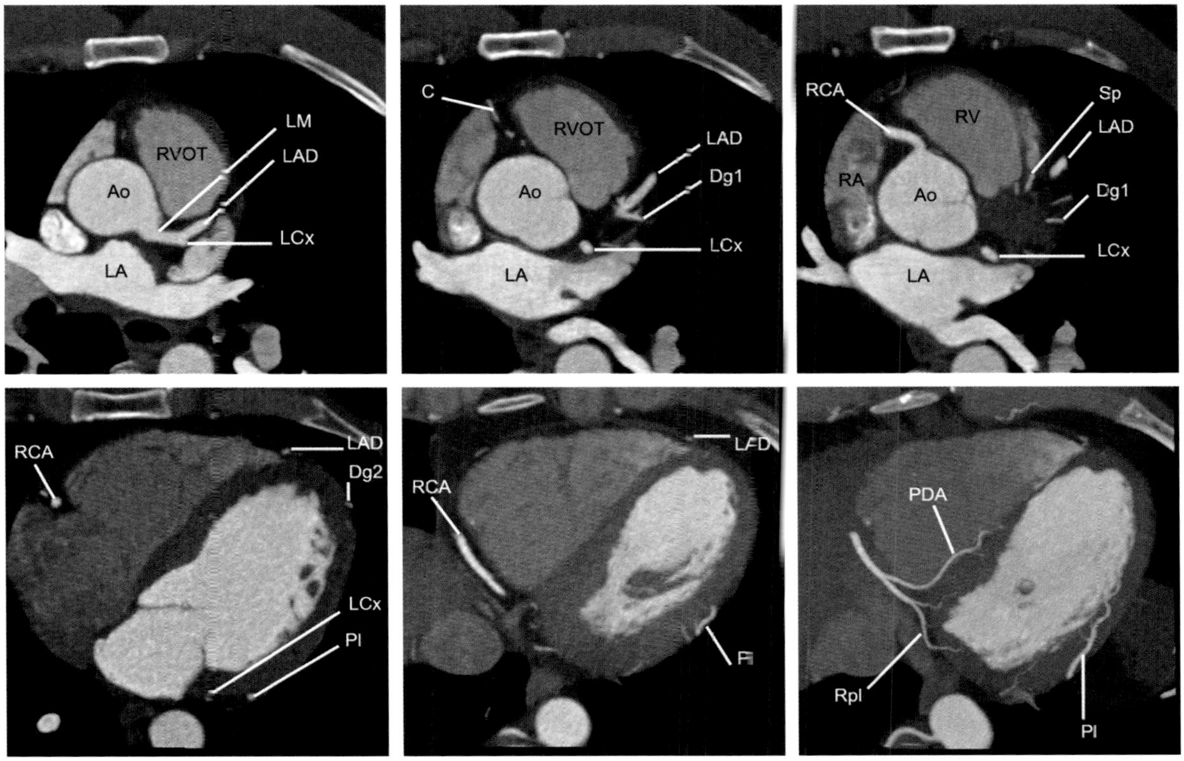

(d), (e) (f)

Figure 9.3 Transaxial (horizontal) cross sections obtained by computed tomography (here: Dual Source CT) that shows details of coronary and cardiac anatomy. By convention, CT images are displayed as if looking up from the patient's feet so that the patient's left side is at the right side of the image. Images are acquired after injection of contrast agent so that cavities filled with blood are displayed in bright gray. (a) Transaxial image at the level of the left main coronary artery. The left main coronary artery can be seen leaving the aorta. It divides into the left anterior descending coronary artery and the left circumflex coronary artery. (b) Transaxial image a few millimeters below the level of image (a). The left anterior descending coronary artery can be seen coursing toward the left ventricular apex, while the left circumflex artery is directed toward the left atrioventricular groove. The conus branch of the right coronary artery can be appreciated. (c) Transaxial image at the level of the right coronary artery ostium. (d) Transaxial image at a mid-ventricular level. The left anterior descending coronary artery travels in the anterior interventricular sulcus, the left circumflex coronary artery in the left atrioventricular groove (while a larger posterolateral branch has left the atrioventricular groove and courses over the lateral wall of the left ventricle), and the right coronary artery is embedded in the right atrioventricular groove. (e) Basal level of the left ventricle. The distal right coronary artery follows a horizontal course. (f) This image shows the end branches of the right coronary artery. Ao, aorta; C, conus branch; Dg1, first diagonal branch; Dg2, second diagonal branch; LA, left atrium; LAD, left anterior descending coronary artery; LCx, left circumflex artery; LM, left main coronary artery; PDA, posterior descending branch; Pl, posterolateral branch of the left circumflex coronary artery; RA, right atrium; RCA, right coronary artery; Rpl, posterolateral branch of the right coronary artery; RV, right ventricle; RVOT, right ventricular outflow tract; Sp, septal branch.

the posterior interventricular groove and supplies the posterior descending branch as well as posterolateral branches to the left ventricle [3–5] (Figure 9.4). In about 8% of cases, the left circumflex coronary artery crosses into the posterior interventricular groove and supplies the posterior descending branch ("left dominant" coronary circulation). In a "codominant pattern," the right coronary artery supplies the posterior descending branch, but all posterolateral branches of the left ventricle stem from the left circumflex artery. This is found in 2–8% of cases. The definitions used for "right dominance," "left dominance," and "codominance" vary slightly, but right dominance is always present in approximately 80–90% of patients [3–5].

Coronary Artery Segments

Several classifications exist as to the exact nomenclature and numbering of coronary artery segments. The substantial variability of coronary anatomy between individuals contributes to the difficulty of assigning unambiguous segment names and numbers as well as creating a classification scheme that is sufficiently accurate and practical at the same time. The American College of Cardiology and American Heart Association Guidelines for Invasive Coronary Angiography propose a classification system that consists of 29 segments [6] (see Table 9.1).

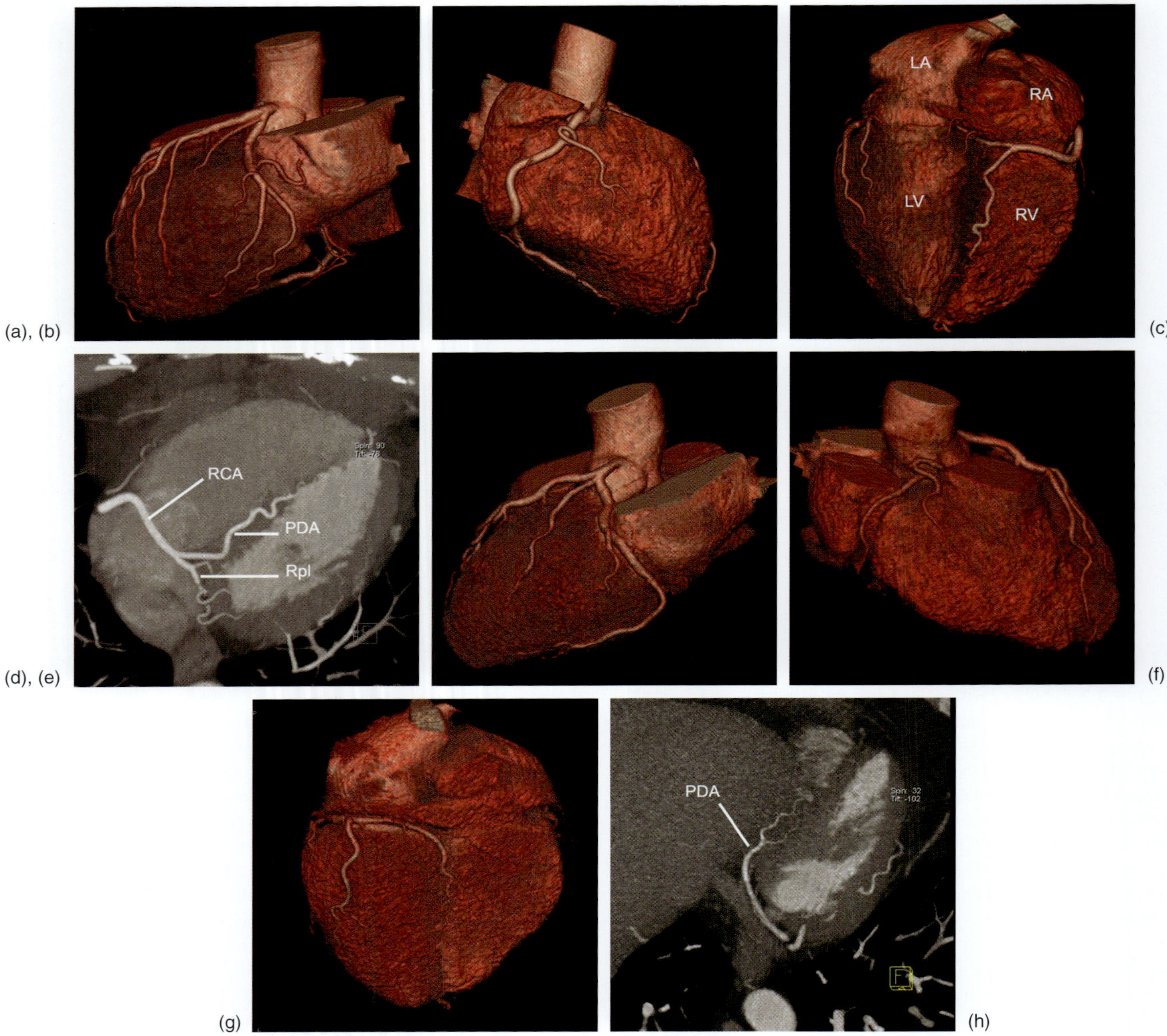

Figure 9.4 Comparison of right dominant and left dominant coronary artery distribution. Images (a–d) show a case of right dominance; images (e–h) show a case of left dominance. (a) Right dominance. Three-dimensional reconstruction view of the left lateral wall. The end branches of the left circumflex coronary artery do not reach beyond the posterolateral wall. (b, c) Three-dimensional reconstructions that show the course of the right coronary artery. The right coronary artery divides into a posterior descending branch and a right posterolateral branch. (d) Two-dimensional image that shows the end branches of the right coronary artery (view from below). (e) Left dominance. View of the left lateral wall showing a large left circumflex coronary artery. (f) Small right coronary artery. (g) View of the inferior wall, which demonstrates that the posterior descending coronary artery originates from the left circumflex artery. LA, left atrium, LV, left ventricle; PDA, posterior descending branch; RA, right atrium; RCA, right coronary artery; Rpl, right posterolateral branch; RV, right ventricle.

For practical purposes of reporting coronary angiography findings—whether invasive or noninvasive, simplified models that base on an Ad Hoc Committee Report of the American Heart Association published in 1975 [7] are often used (see Table 9.2). The model has some limitations, such as the difficulty of dealing with the tremendous variability of left circumflex coronary artery branching patters. Also, the initial model described only 15 segments. It did not include the right posterolateral branch, which is almost always present, and it uses the same segment number (segment 6) for the first diagonal branch and the intermediate branch, if present. For this reason, various

Table 9.1 Classification system for coronary artery segments [6]

Right coronary artery (RCA)		Left main /left anterior descending coronary artery (LAD)		Left circumflex coronary artery (LCx)	
1	Proximal RCA	11	Left main coronary artery	18	Proximal LCx
2	Mid-RCA	12	Proximal LAD	19	Distal LCx
3	Distal RCA	13	Mid-LAD	20	First obtuse marginal
4	Right posterior descending branch (if from RCA)	14	Distal LAD	21	Second obtuse marginal
5	Right posterior atrioventricular branch	15	First Diagonal	22	Third obtuse marginal
6	First right posterolateral branch (if from RCA)	16	Second Diagonal	23	LCx atrioventricular groove continuation segment
7	Second right posterolateral branch (if from RCA)	17	LAD septal perforators	24	First left posterolateral branch (if from LCx)
8	Third right posterolateral branch (if from RCA)	28	Ramus intermedius	25	Second left posterolateral branch (if from LCx)
9	Posterior descending septal branches (if from RCA)	29	Third diagonal	26	Third left posterolateral branch (if from LCx)
10	Acute marginal segment (s			27	Left posterior descending branch (if from LCx)

Table 9.2 Definition of coronary artery segments according to a report of the Ad Hoc Committee for Grading of Coronary Artery Disease, Council on Cardiovascular Surgery, American Heart Association [7]

Right coronary artery (RCA)		
1	Proximal	RCA from ostium to one half the distance to the acute margin of the heart. Note: The distal portion of this coronary segment may coincide with origin of one of the large right ventricular branches.
2	Mid	RCA from end of the above segment to acute margin of the heart. Note: Distal portion of this segment usually (but not always) coincides with origin of the acute marginal branch.
3	Distal	RCA running among the posterior right atrioventricular groove from the acute margin of heart to the origin of the posterior descending branch. Note: In the "predominant" left coronary pattern (posterior descending from the left circumflex), this segment may be very small.
4	Posterior descending	Posterior descending branch, when present.
Main left coronary artery (LCA)		
5	Main left	LCA extends from the ostium of LCA through bifurcation into left anterior descending and left circumflex branches.
Left Anterior descending artery (LAD)		
6	Proximal	LAD proximal to and including origin of first major septal perforator branch.
7	Mid	LAD immediately distal to origin of first major septal perforator branch and extending to the point where LAD forms an angle (RAO view) and often but not always coinciding or close to the origin of second diagonal branch (D_2). If this angle or branch is not identifiable, this segments ends at one half the distance from the first major septal perforator branch to apex of heart.
8	Apical	Terminal portion of LAD running along interventricular sulcus, beginning with the end of previous segment, and usually extending beyond apex.
9	First diagonal	First diagonal (D_1): The largest, and usually the first, diagonal branch having its origin from proximal segment of LAD. Occasionally, this can be a separate branch off main LCA.
10	Second diagonal	Second diagonal (D_2): The second diagonal branch, which often has its origin at the "angle" of LAD, descending when visualized in RAO projection.
Left Circumflex coronary artery (CIRC)		
11	Proximal	Main stem of circumflex branch from its origin off main LCA to an including origin of obtuse marginal branch
12	Obtuse marginal (OM)	The largest branch of the circumflex running in general area of obtuse margin of heart.
13	Distal	The stem of the circumflex distal to origin of obtuse marginal branch and running along or close to posterior left atrioventricular groove. Caliber of this portion may be small.
14	Posterolateral (PL)	Posterolateral branch of circumflex distributing to posterolateral surface of left ventricle, almost always smaller in caliber than obtuse marginal. May be absent or may be a division of obtuse marginal branch.
15	Posterior descending (PD)	Posterior descending, when present as a branch of the circumflex.

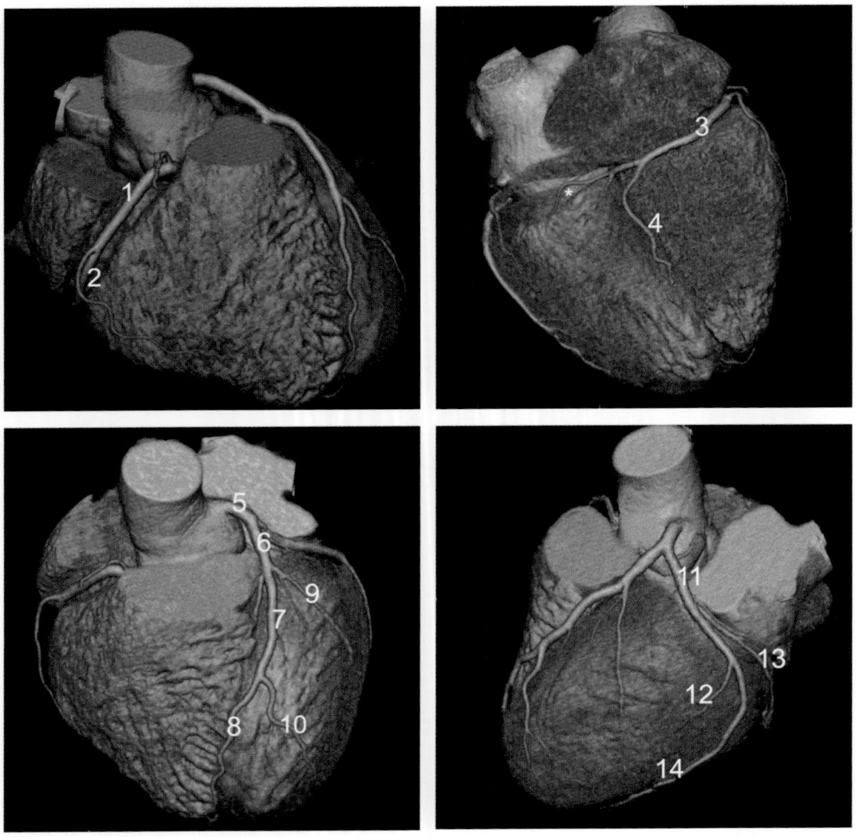

Figure 9.5 Simplified model of coronary artery segments according to [7]. Segments 1–4 belong to the right coronary artery. The asterisk (*) indicates the right posterolateral branch, which is sometimes assigned the number 16. Segment 5 represents the right coronary artery, numbers 6–10 designate segments of the left anterior descending coronary artery, and segments 11–14 designate branches of the left circumflex artery. Segment 15 would be the posterior descending branch of the left circumflex coronary artery which is not present in cases of right dominant coronary circulation.

modifications of the model have been used to describe coronary anatomy. Often, the right posterolateral branch is added as "segment 16," and a separate segment is assigned to the intermediate branch. Also, some of the definitions of the original report are not carried over to daily practice. For example, the original model defines the end of the "proximal" left anterior descending coronary artery by the first *septal* branch. In daily practice, the origin of the first *diagonal* branch is usually considered to represent the border between the proximal and mid-left anterior descending coronary artery—and in fact, if the diagonal branch is very proximal, many angiographers will extend the "proximal" segment even beyond the first diagonal (see Table 9.2 and Figure 9.5).

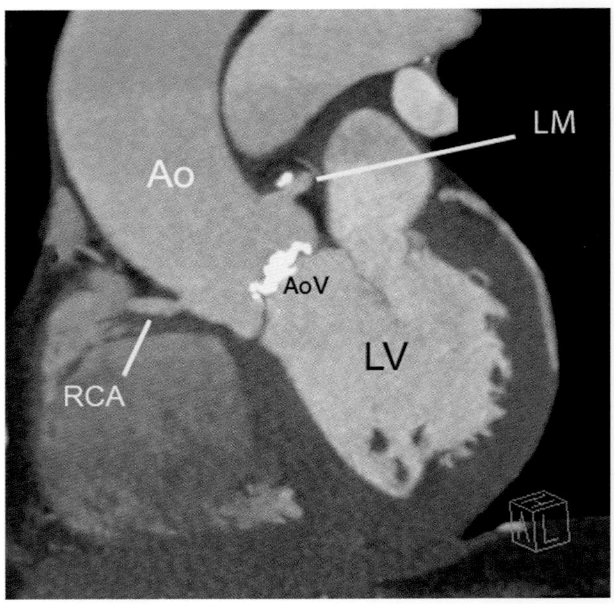

Figure 9.6 Origin of the coronary arteries from the aortic root. Here the aortic valve is calcified. The distance of the right coronary ostium from the plane of the aortic valve is larger than the distance of the left main coronary artery to the aortic valve plane. Ao, aorta; AoV, aortic valve; LM, left main coronary artery; LV, left ventricle; RCA, right coronary artery.

Origin of the Coronary Arteries from the Aortic Root

The coronary ostia are usually localized in the middle of the aortic sinuses, just above the upper free margin of the aortic valve leaflets (when in the open position), and just below the sinotubular junction. In invasive angiography, the right coronary ostium is usually perceived to be closer to the aortic valve plane than the left coronary ostium. However, this is not true and the impression is based on the fact that the aortic valve has an oblique position (see Figure 9.6). In careful measurements of aortic root anatomy, it has been shown that the mean distance of the right coronary ostium from the aortic annulus was 17 ± 3 mm, while the distance of the left coronary ostium from the aortic annulus was 14 ± 3 mm [8].

Since abnormalities of origin are possible, it is important to note that coronary arteries are named for the territory that they perfuse and not for their site of origin. A coronary artery that arises from the right sinus of Valsalva but then gives rise to a left anterior descending coronary artery and a left circumflex coronary artery is not called a "right coronary artery" but much rather a left main coronary artery with an ectopic origin [1].

Details of Coronary Anatomy

Left Main Coronary Artery

The left main coronary artery will in most cases arise from the left sinus of Valsalva and, after a distance between 2 and 20 mm, divides into the left anterior descending coronary artery and the left circumflex coronary artery (see Figure 9.7a, b). Often, an intermediate branch (or "Ramus intermedius") arises exactly between the left anterior descending coronary artery and the left circumflex coronary artery (see Figure 9.7c, d). The left main coronary artery and its branches are often oriented almost exactly in the horizontal plane—which is straightforward to be visualized by CT, but impossible to exactly achieve in invasive angiography (it would require to perform fluoroscopy

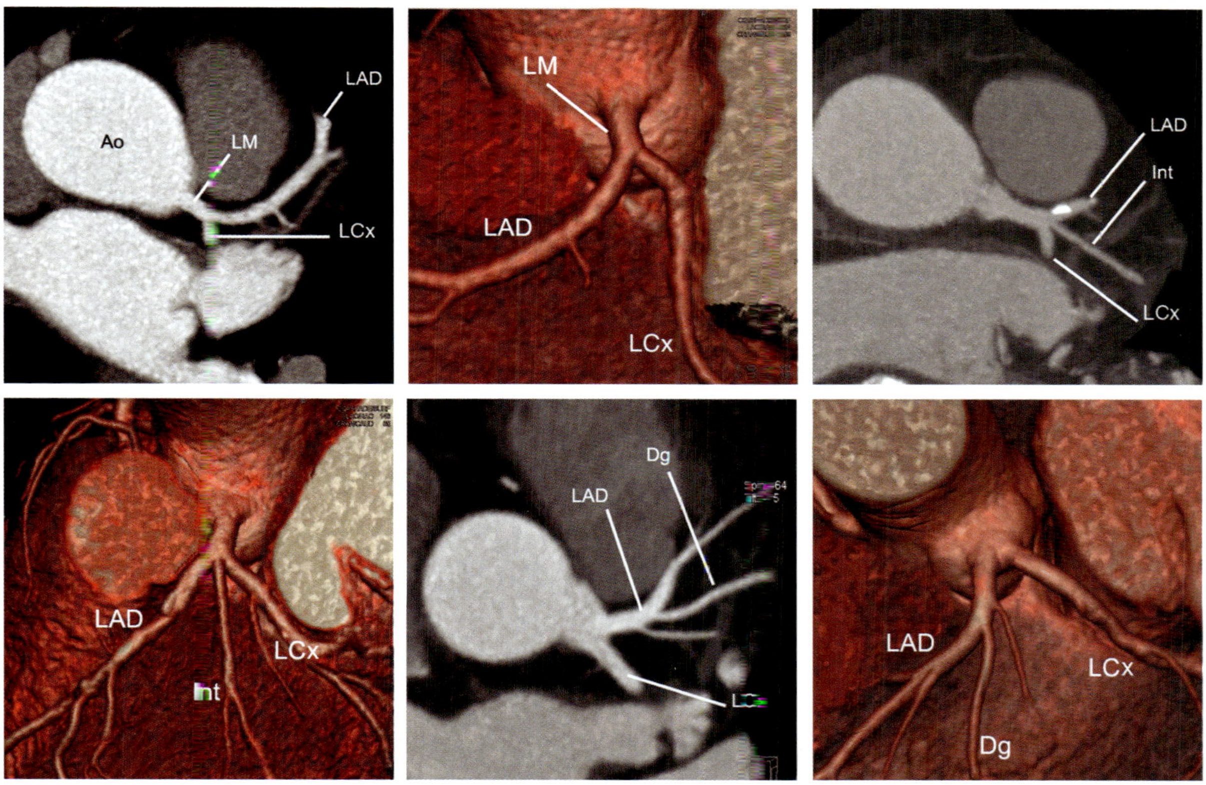

Figure 9.7 Variants of left main coronary anatomy. By convention in computed tomography, the two-dimensional images show the anatomy from below (as if looking up from the feet). (a, b) Normal left main coronary artery that has a bifurcation into a left anterior descending coronary artery and a left circumflex coronary artery. (c, d) Trifurcation of the left main coronary artery into a left anterior descending coronary artery, left circumflex coronary artery, and intermediate branch. (e, f) Absent left main coronary artery. The left anterior descending coronary artery and the left circumflex coronary artery have separate ostia from the aortic root. Ao, aorta; Dg, diagonal branch; Int, intermediate branch; LAD, left anterior descending artery; LCx, left circumflex coronary artery; LM, left main coronary artery.

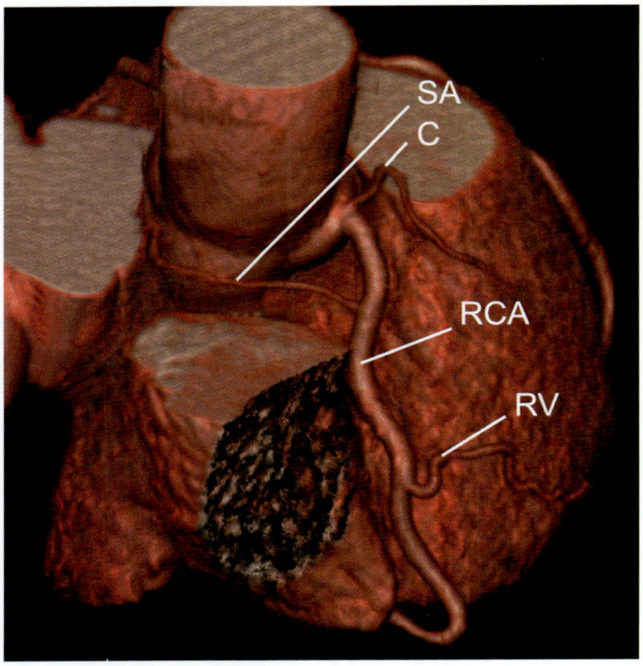

Figure 9.8 Anatomy of the right coronary artery. The proximal right coronary artery gives rise to the conus branch, which is directed toward the right ventricular outflow tract and to the sinoatrial nodal branch, which is directed toward the sinus node, in the region where the superior vena cava enters the right atrium. C, conus branch; RCA, right coronary artery; RV, right ventricular branch; SA, sinoatrial nodal branch.

directly from the feet or head). Therefore, "trifurcations" of the left main coronary artery are sometimes assumed in invasive angiography because of overlap of proximal vessel segments when, in fact, a very proximal diagonal branch arises from the left anterior descending coronary artery or a very proximal obtuse marginal branch arises from the left circumflex coronary artery.

The left main coronary artery can be absent. In this case, the left anterior descending coronary artery and the left circumflex coronary artery arise from two separate or one joint ostium (see Figure 9.7e, f). This situation is considered a variant, but not an abnormality of the coronary arteries.

Conus Branch

The conus branch usually arises from the proximal right coronary artery. It can also originate from a joint ostium with the right coronary artery or, with a separate ostium, directly from the aorta. The conus branch courses upwardly and to the left, toward the right ventricular outflow tract (see Figures 9.8 and 9.9).

Sinoatrial Nodal Branch

The sinoatrial nodal branch travels toward the region where the superior vena cava enters the right atrium. This is where the sinus node is situated. In approximately two thirds of cases, the sinoatrial nodal artery arises from the right coronary artery—usually within 40 mm from its ostium (Figure 9.10). Origin from the left circumflex coronary artery is found in one third of cases—either from the proximal left circumflex or from the mid- or distal circumflex, in which case the sinoatrial nodal branch travels around the ostium of the left atrial appendage and across the roof of the left atrium. Origin from the left circumflex coronary artery is not tied to left dominance of the coronary artery system (Saremi): A dual vessel supply of the sinoatrial node, both from the right and from the left circumflex coronary artery, is possible [9]. For more details on the anatomy of the sinoatrial nodal branch, see Chapter 11.

AV nodal Branch

In the majority of cases, the small AV nodal artery arises from the distal right coronary artery (Figure 9.11). It typically originates from the right posterolateral branch, often

(a) 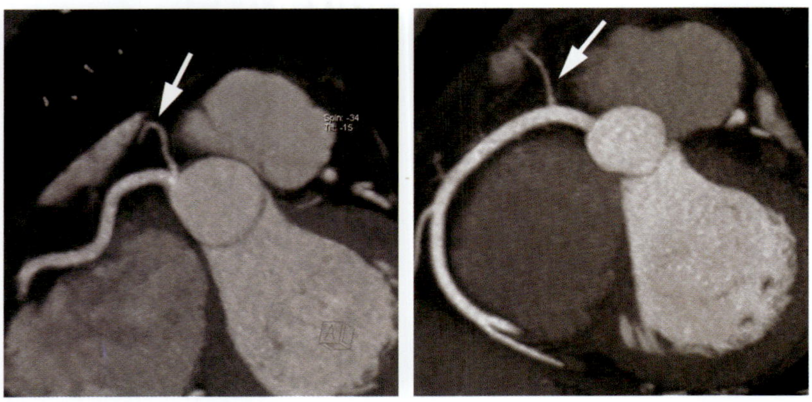 (b)

Figure 9.9 Origin of the conus branch (arrow). (a) The conus branch can arise from the right coronary artery ostium (or, in infrequent cases, directly from the aorta). (b) Alternatively, the conus branch can arise from the proximal right coronary artery.

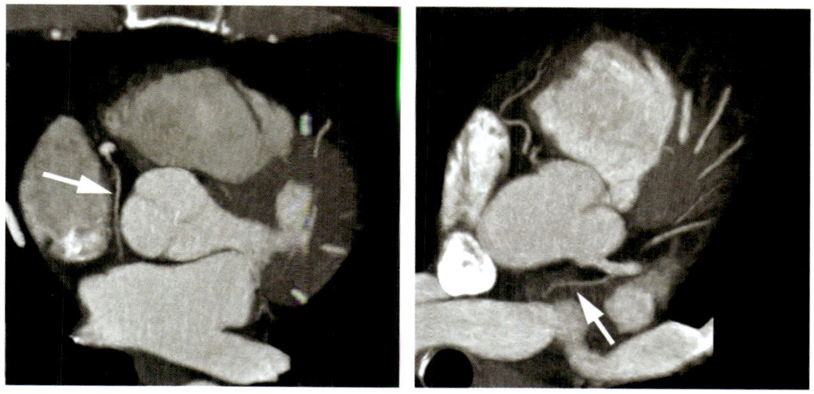

(a) (b)

Figure 9.10 Anatomy of the sinoatrial nodal artery (arrow). (a) In most cases, the sinoatrial nodal branch will arise from the proximal right coronary artery. (b) Alternatively, the sinoatrial nodal branch can arise from the left circumflex coronary artery. This is not correlated to left dominance.

from an upward vessel loop, and enters the septum from the inferior face of the heart. In approximately 10% of cases, the AV nodal artery originates from a dominant left circumflex coronary artery. Dual blood supply of the AV node, both from the right coronary artery and from the left circumflex coronary artery, is possible [9].

Myocardial Bridging

Myocardial bridging is defined as a segment of a major epicardial coronary artery that has an intramural course through the myocardium beneath a muscle bridge [10,11]. The segment of the coronary artery that has an intramyocardial course is called the "tunneled" segment. In autopsy studies, bridging is very frequent (up to 80% of hearts), and it affects mainly the mid-left anterior descending coronary artery (although the right coronary artery and left circumflex can also be affected, see Figures 9.12 and 9.13). In invasive angiography, bridging is seen as a systolic compression of the tunneled segment, and this is much less frequent than autopsy (or CT) evidence of a muscle bridge. The estimated frequency in invasive angiography is between 1.5 and 16% [10]. Even though in some cases, myocardial bridging may be connected to symptoms or even sudden death, it is generally a benign condition and follow-up studies of patients with bridging have not demonstrated an impaired prognosis [10,11]. Interestingly, the arterial segment proximal to the myocardial bridge frequently shows atherosclerosis, while the tunneled segment itself is typically spared.

Especially in association with myocardial bridging, the left anterior descending coronary artery often has an extremely close anatomic relationship to the right ventricle (see Figure 9.12). This may be the reason why perforation of the left anterior descending coronary artery into the right ventricle has been reported in context with stenting within a myocardial bridge, and right ventricular rupture is a complication with surgical dissection of the overlying myocardium as treatment for symptomatic bridging [10,11].

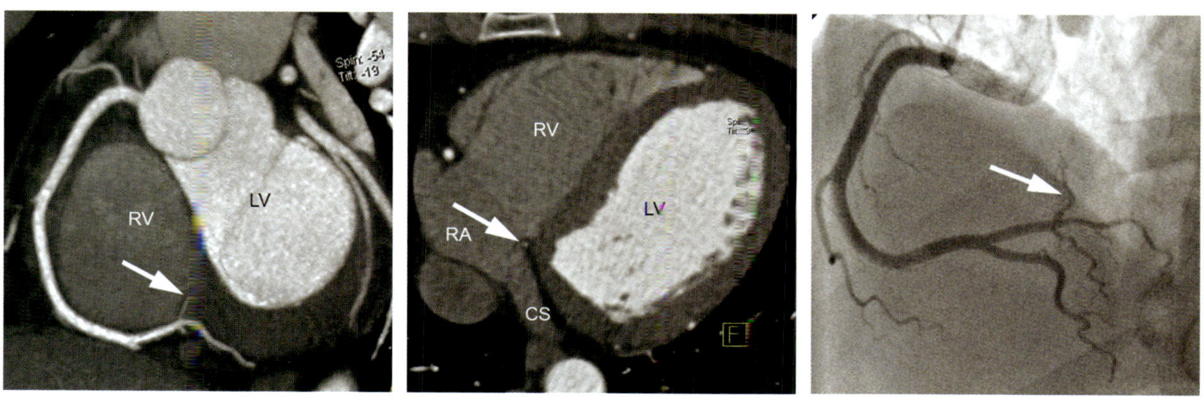

(a), (b) (c)

Figure 9.11 Anatomy of the atrioventricular (AV) nodal branch. (a) The AV nodal branch (arrow) arises from the distal right coronary artery and penetrates the interventricular septum. (b) Transaxial image that shows a cross section of the AV nodal branch (arrow). (c) Corresponding right coronary angiogram. Arrow point to the AV nodal artery. CS, coronary sinus; LV, left ventricle; RA, right atrium; RV, right ventricle

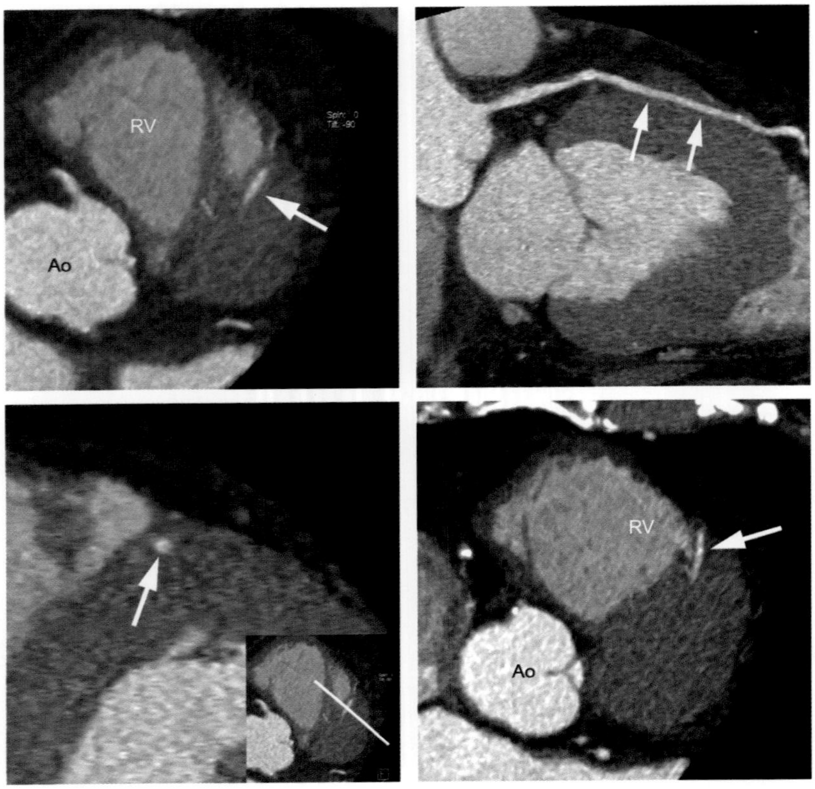

(a) (b) (c) (d)

Figure 9.12 Myocardial bridging of the left anterior descending coronary artery. (a) This transaxial image shows the left anterior descending coronary artery (arrow) entirely surrounded by myocardium. (b) In a longitudinal view, the left anterior descending coronary artery (arrow) can be seen to tunnel through the left ventricular wall. (c) A cross-sectional view of the left anterior descending coronary artery also demonstrates that the vessel (arrow) is completely surrounded by myocardium. (d) Note the very close anatomic relationship of the left anterior descending coronary artery (arrow) to the cavity of the right ventricle. Ao, aorta; RV, right ventricle.

Anomalous Coronary Arteries

Congenital anomalies of the coronary arteries occur in 0.6–1.3% of the general population [12]. The most frequent variant, next to absence of the left main coronary artery with separate ostia of the left anterior descending coronary artery and the left circumflex coronary artery, is an anomalous origin of the left circumflex coronary artery from the right coronary cusp or proximal right coronary artery, with a subsequent course dorsal to and below the aortic root to the left AV sulcus—this anomaly is completely benign (except in the context of Valvular surgery where the artery may be injured or compressed by prosthetic valves, see Figure 9.14). The left anterior descending coronary artery and the left main coronary artery may also originate from the right sinus of Valsalva (see Figures 9.15 and 9.16). In this case, a course dorsal to the aorta (retroaortic, similar to an abnormal circumflex) as well as a course anterior to the pulmonary artery (see Figure 9.15) is considered benign. If the anomalous vessel that arises from the right coronary cusp passes between the aorta and pulmonary artery (so-called interarterial course, see Figure 9.16), it is assumed

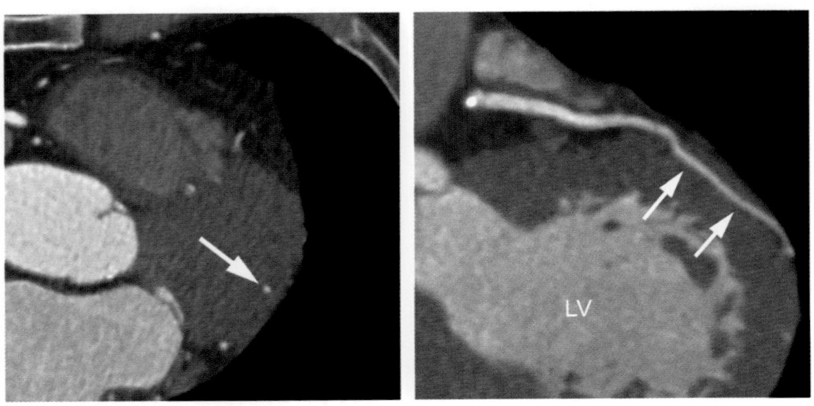

(a) (b)

Figure 9.13 Myocardial bridging can also occur in other vessel segments, here an obtuse marginal branch. (a) Cross-sectional image that shows the obtuse marginal branch of the left circumflex coronary artery (arrow) completely surrounded by myocardium. (b) Longitudinal reconstruction that shows the segment of the obtuse marginal branch that tunnels through the myocardium (arrows). LV, Left ventricle.

(a), (b)
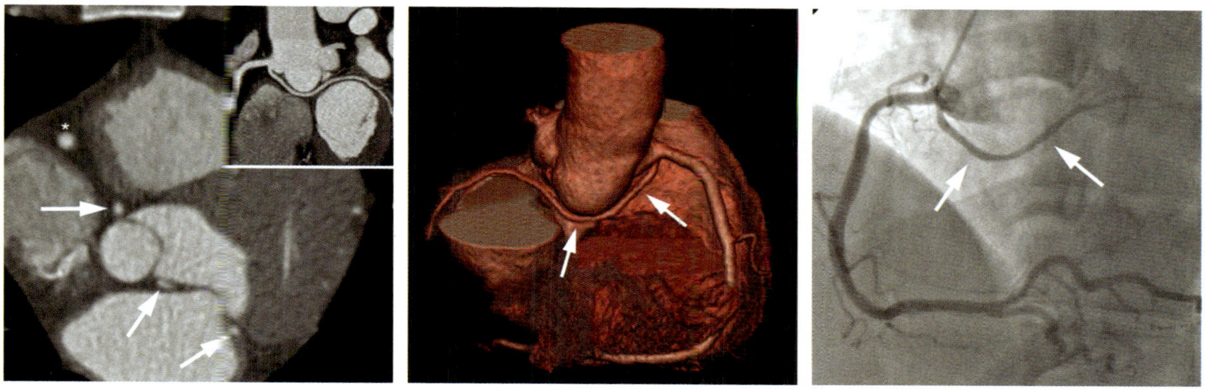
(c)

Figure 9.14 Anomalous origin of the left circumflex coronary artery from the right sinus of Valsalva. (a) Transaxial cross-sectional image that shows sections of the anomalous left circumflex artery as it passes below and posterior to the aortic root from the right sinus of Valsalva to the left atrioventricular groove. (b) Three-dimensional reconstruction that shows the heart from a posterior view and displays the course of the anomalous coronary artery (arrows). Large sections of the left and right atrium have been removed to allow visualization of the anomalous left circumflex coronary artery. (c) Invasive coronary angiography of the same patient (arrows, anomalous left circumflex coronary artery).

that ischemia may be caused either by vessel compression or by distortion of the ostium so that the interarterial course of a left coronary artery is considered a potentially malignant coronary anomaly. When the anomalous artery has a deeper course, below the pulmonary valve and embedded in the interventricular septum, it is usually considered benign ("Transseptal course," see Figure 9.17) [12]. There is a bit of controversy whether an anomalous right coronary artery that originates from the left coronary cusp and follows an interarterial course between the aorta and pulmonary artery also constitutes a malignant anomaly (see Figure 9.18). The relatively high frequency of this anomaly, along with the fact that the reported cases of fatal complications are rare, suggests that this may be a relatively benign condition, especially when ischemia has not been demonstrated [13, 14]. However, divergent opinions do exist. It has also been suggested that the most important factor that determines whether an anomalous artery is potentially dangerous or not is an intramural course of the very proximal segment (within the aortic wall, leading to slit-like distortion of the ostium) [15].

The anomalous origin of a coronary artery—typically the left main artery—from the pulmonary artery is possible and usually leads to symptoms in childhood. This rare situation is termed ALCAPA (anomalous left coronary artery from the pulmonary artery) or "Bland-White-Garland syndrome." Collaterals develop between the orthotopic contralateral artery and the artery that is connected to the pulmonary artery, so that a left-to-right shunt is present (arterial blood from the normal coronary artery flows via collaterals into the anomalous vessel and from there into the pulmonary artery).

Small fistulas from the coronary arteries to the pulmonary artery are not infrequent (see Figure 9.19), they

(a), (b)
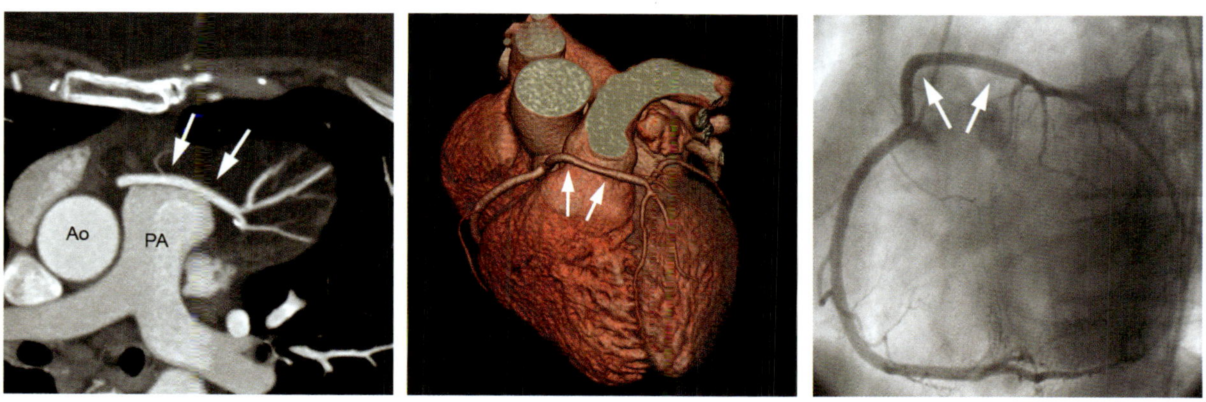

(c)

Figure 9.15 Anomalous origin of the left main coronary artery from the right coronary ostium with a course anterior to the pulmonary artery. (a) Transaxial cross-sectional image that shows the anomalous left main coronary artery passing anterior to the pulmonary artery. (b) Three-dimensional reconstruction that shows the heart from an anterior view and displays the course of the anomalous coronary artery (arrows). (c) Invasive coronary angiography of the same patient (arrows, anomalous left main coronary artery). Ao, aorta; PA, pulmonary artery.

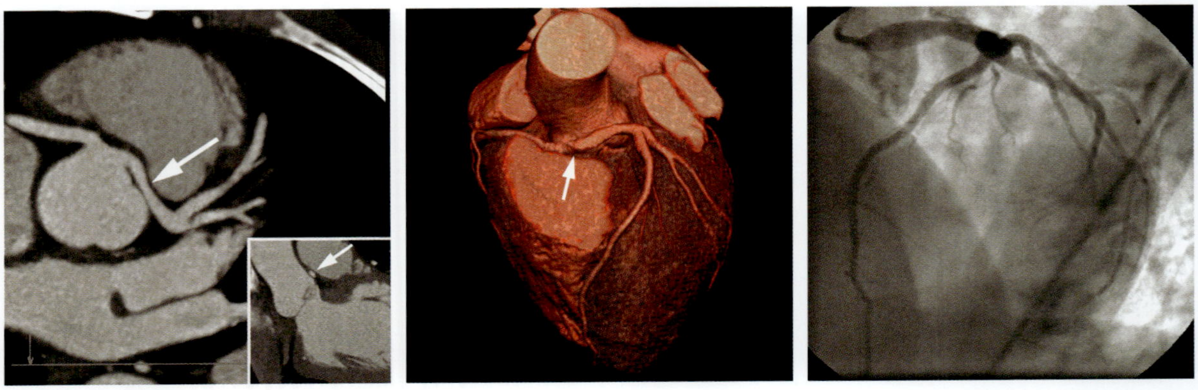

Figure 9.16 Anomalous origin of the left main coronary artery from the right coronary ostium with a course between the aorta and the pulmonary artery ("interarterial course"). (a) Transaxial cross-sectional image that shows the anomalous left main coronary artery (arrow) passing between the aorta and the pulmonary artery. The insert visualizes the position of the left main coronary artery between the aortic root and the pulmonary artery (arrow). (b) Three-dimensional reconstruction that shows the heart from an anterior view and displays the course of the anomalous coronary artery (arrow). The right ventricular outflow tract and pulmonary artery have been removed. (c) Invasive coronary angiography of the same patient.

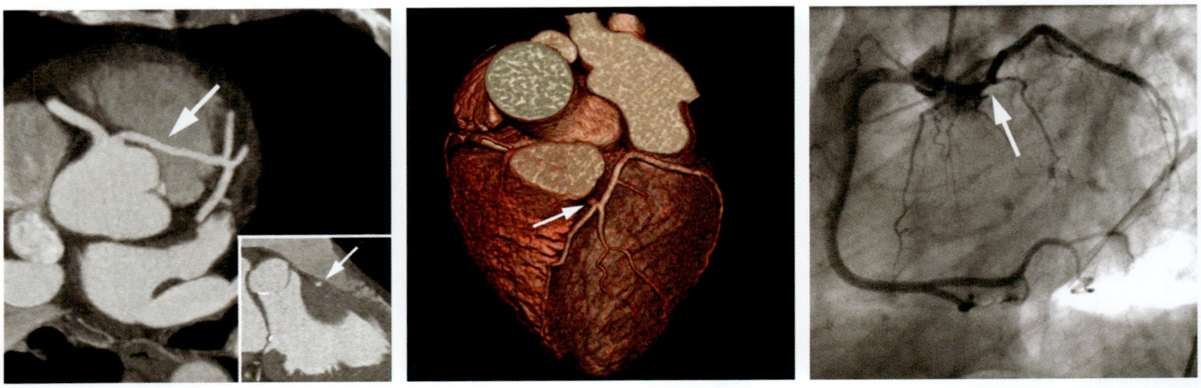

Figure 9.17 Anomalous origin of the left main coronary artery from the right coronary ostium with a course below pulmonary artery ("transseptal course"). (a) Transaxial cross-sectional image that shows the anomalous left main coronary artery (arrow) passing below the pulmonary artery. The insert visualizes the position of the left main coronary artery in the septum, and not immediately between the aorta and the pulmonary artery (arrow). (b) Three-dimensional reconstruction that shows the left main coronary artery surfacing in the left interventricular sulcus (arrow) after it passes through the septum and below the pulmonary valve. Parts of the pulmonary artery and left atrium have been removed. (c) Invasive coronary angiography of the same patient (arrow, anomalous vessel)

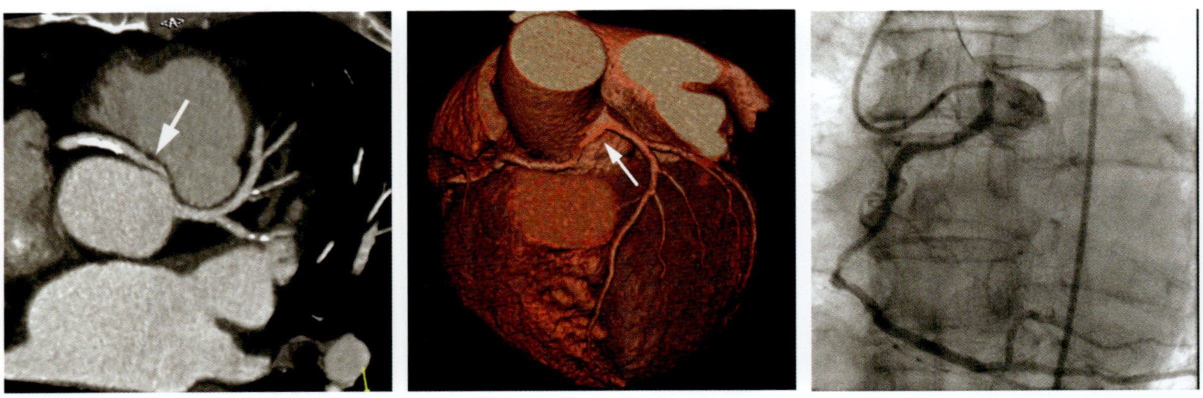

Figure 9.18 Anomalous origin of the right coronary artery from the left sinus of Valsalva with a course between the aorta and pulmonary artery ("interarterial course"). (a) Transaxial cross-sectional image that shows the anomalous right coronary artery (arrow) passing between the aorta and pulmonary artery. Note the slit-like ostium of the right coronary artery. (b) Three-dimensional reconstruction that shows the course of the anomalous vessel (arrow). Parts of the pulmonary artery and left atrium have been removed. (c) Invasive angiogram of the right coronary artery in the same patient.

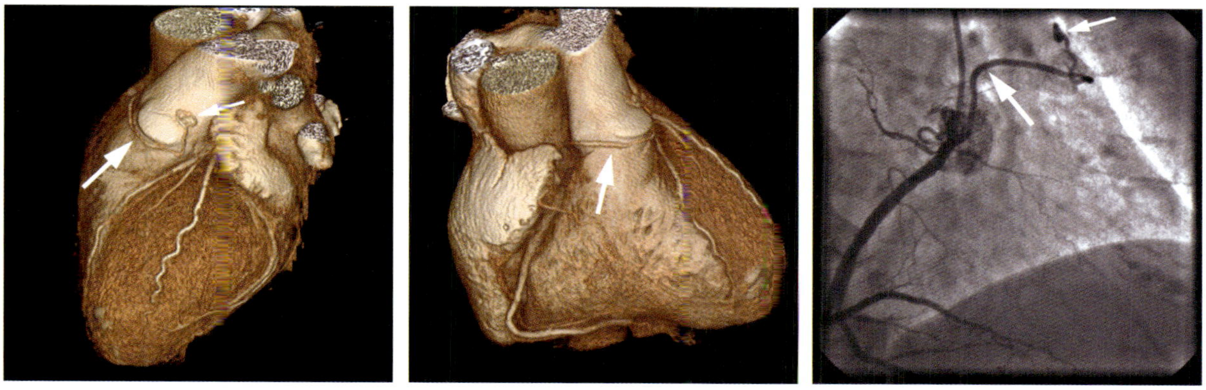

(a), (b) (c)

Figure 9.19 Coronary artery fistula from the proximal right coronary artery to the pulmonary artery. (a, b) Three-dimensional reconstructions that display the course of the small fistula (arrows). (c) Invasive coronary angiogram (arrows, fistula from the right coronary artery to pulmonary artery).

lack hemodynamic significance. Occasionally, large fistula may occur between a coronary artery and a cardiac chamber or the coronary sinus. These may be hemodynamically relevant if a large shunt volume occurs.

Coronary Atherosclerosis

Coronary atherosclerosis is frequent in Western societies. Much more frequent than focal, severe stenoses of the coronary arteries (which typically cause chest pain or shortness of breath on exertion) are deposits of atherosclerotic plaque that are not associated with a relevant luminal stenosis—and may therefore not be detectable on invasive coronary angiography (see Figure 9.20).

Coronary Artery Bypass Grafts

Most commonly, veins from the lower extremity or the internal mammary artery are used to create coronary artery bypass grafts (see Figure 9.21). Venous grafts typically

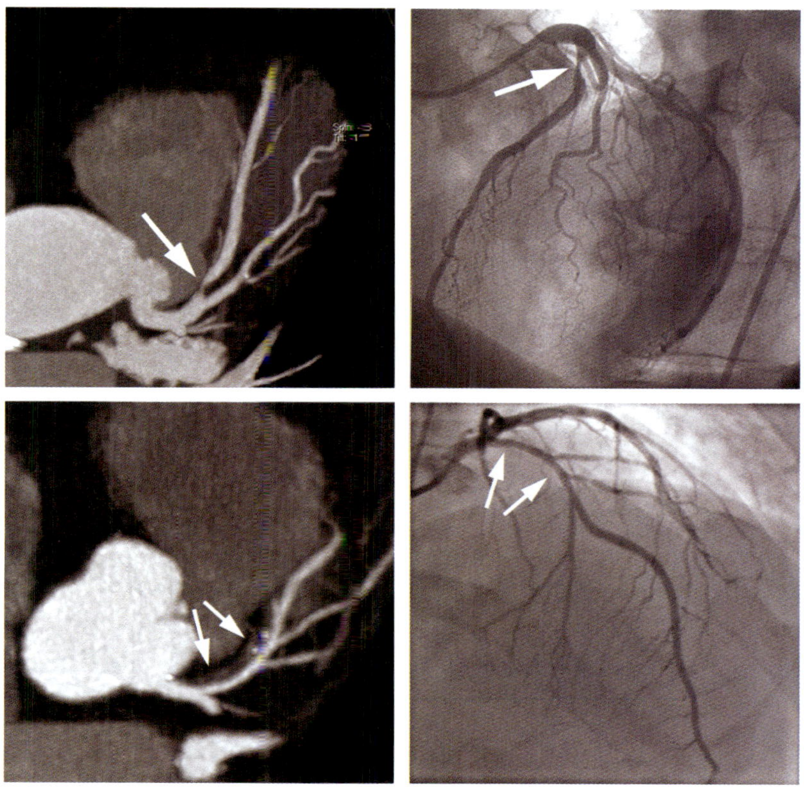

(a) (b) (c) (d)

Figure 9.20 Manifestations of coronary artery disease. Even large amounts of coronary atherosclerotic plaque are not necessarily tied to the presence of a high-grade coronary artery stenosis. (a, b) Severe stenosis of the left anterior descending coronary artery, immediately distal to a large diagonal branch (arrow). (c, d) Pronounced coronary atherosclerotic plaque, but absence of a significant luminal stenosis in the proximal left anterior descending coronary artery (arrows).

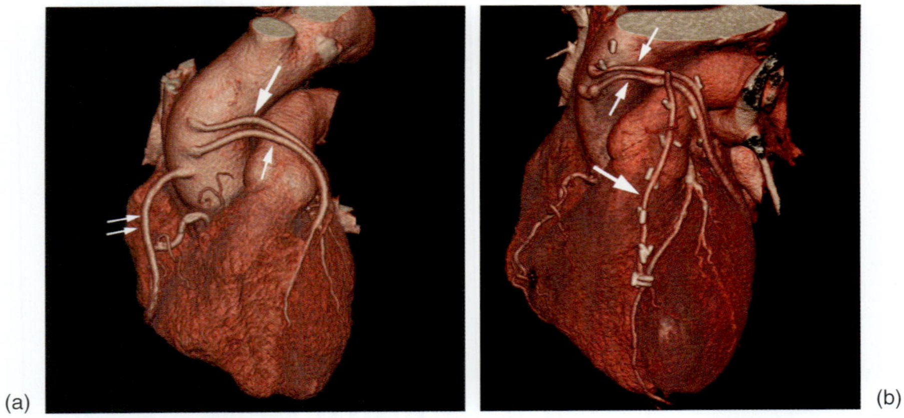

Figure 9.21 Anatomy of coronary artery bypass grafts. (a) Typical anatomy of venous grafts from the aorta to the coronary arteries. The topmost graft (large arrow) is the graft to the left circumflex coronary artery territory. Below follows a venous graft to the left anterior descending coronary artery (small arrow). The lowest aorta anastomosis is that of the bypass graft to the right coronary artery (double arrows). (b) Normal anatomy of a patient who has received not only venous but also an arterial bypass graft. Next to the two vein grafts—both to the left circumflex territory (small arrows)—an internal mammary artery bypass graft to the left anterior descending coronary artery is present (large arrows). It is accompanied by numerous metal clips that are used to ligate side branches.

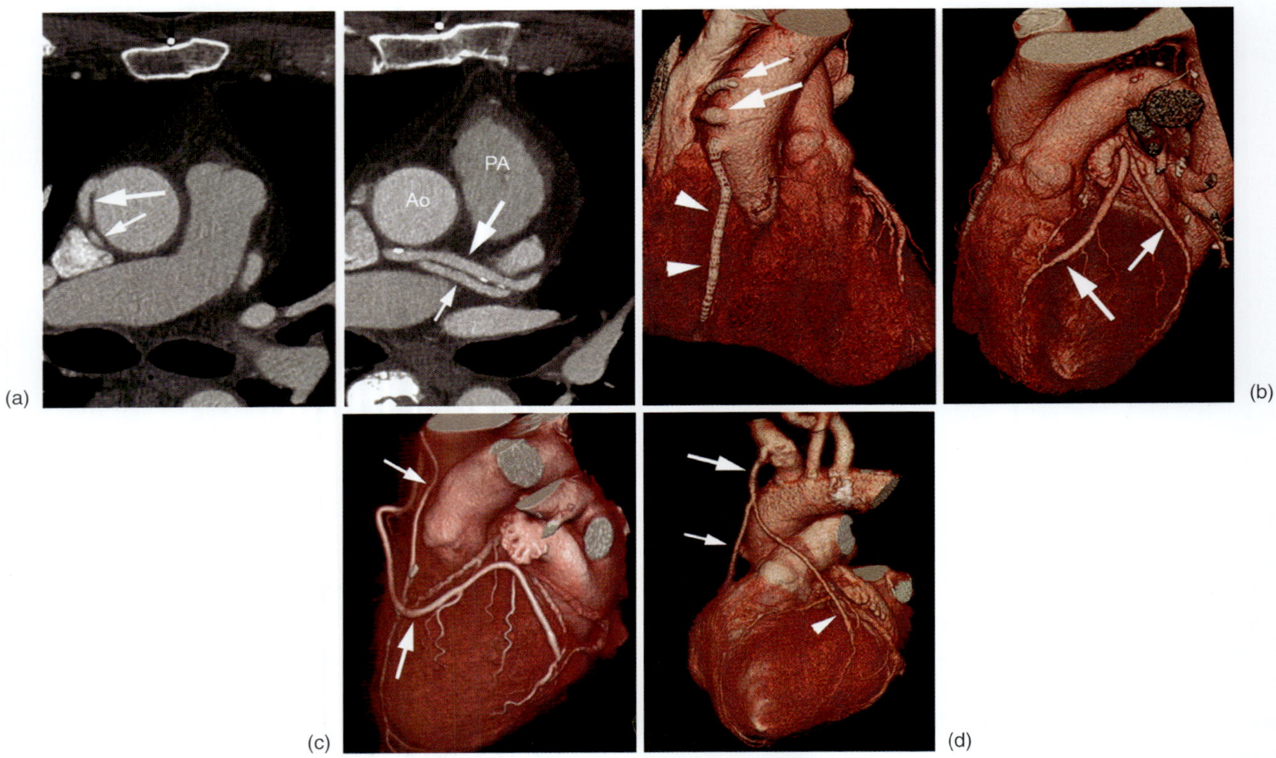

Figure 9.22 Variants of the anatomy of coronary artery bypass grafts. (a, b) In some cases, venous coronary artery bypass grafts may follow a course through the transverse sinus, posterior to the aorta. Here, two vein grafts to the left anterior descending coronary artery (large arrow) and to an obtuse marginal branch of the left circumflex coronary artery take a course posterior to the aorta. The arrowheads point at a vein graft to the right coronary artery that carries multiple stents. (c) "Jump Grafts," which have several anastomoses to the native coronary arteries, are not infrequent. Here, the vein graft (large arrow) has a side-to-side anastomosis to a diagonal branch as well as an end-to-side anastomosis to the posterolateral branch of the left circumflex coronary artery. (d) In rare instances, the proximal anastomosis may to the brachiocephalic artery. Here, because of severe ascending aortic calcification, the proximal anastomosis of this vein graft (large arrow) was placed to the brachiocephalic artery. Also, this is a "Y"-shaped graft with peripheral anastomoses to an intermediate branch (arrowhead) and the right coronary artery (small arrow). Ao, Aorta; PA, Pulmonary artery.

(a), (b)

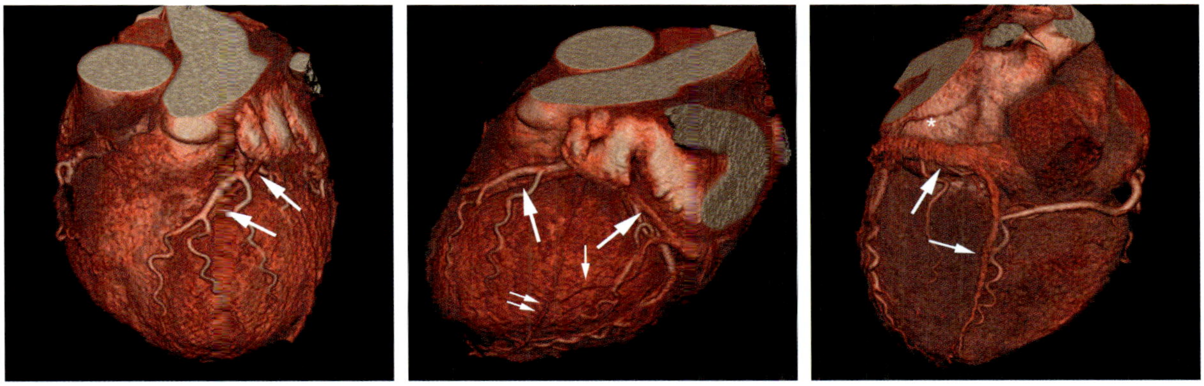

(c)

Figure 9.23 Anatomy of the coronary veins. The coronary veins do not fill with contrast agent whereas the arteries do in coronary computed tomography (CT) angiography. Therefore, they are more difficult to visualize. (a) View of the anterior face of the heart. The great cardiac vein can be seen, it has a course parallel to the left anterior descending coronary artery (arrows). (b) In this view of the lateral wall, the great cardiac vein can be seen parallel to the left anterior descending coronary artery and to the left circumflex coronary artery (large arrows). The small arrow points at the marginal vein of the left ventricle. (Note the double arrows that point at the phrenic vein, which indicates the position of the pericardiophrenic bundle that contains the phrenic nerve). (c) In this inferior view of the heart, the coronary sinus can be seen. It receives the middle cardiac vein (small arrow) just before it enters the right atrium. The asterisk (*) indicates the small oblique vein of the left atrium ("oblique vein of Marshall").

have separate aortic anastomoses in the ascending aorta. To avoid bypass grafts crossing over each other, the topmost graft will typically go to the left circumflex region, while grafts to the diagonal branch and left anterior descending coronary artery usually have their anastomoses a little but further below. Finally, the anastomoses closest to the aortic valve will in most cases belong to grafts that supply the right coronary artery. If the internal mammary artery is used as a bypass graft, the proximal vessel segment is usually left in place (and thus originates from the subclavian artery). However, internal mammary arteries (and other arteries such as the radial artery) may be used as free transplants and thus originate from the aorta.

In some cases, bypass grafts may follow a retroaortic course through the transverse sinus (see Figure 9.22). Often, a bypass graft may have anastomoses to more than one distal coronary artery (so-called jump grafts). Y-shaped grafts are also possible. Especially in cases of severe aortic calcification, the proximal anastomosis may be placed in the subclavian artery or brachiocephalic trunk.

Coronary Veins

Venous anatomy of the heart (see Figure 9.23) is even more variable than the anatomy of the coronary arteries. Approximately 80% of venous blood return is achieved via the coronary veins on the epicardial surface of the heart. Twenty percent of venous return occurs via the Thebesian veins (venae cordis minimae), which drain directly into the cardiac chambers. In addition, several small "anterior cardiac veins" drain blood directly into the right atrium. The major epicardial coronary vein is the great cardiac vein, which runs along the left anterior descending coronary artery. Close to the left main bifurcation, it enters the left AV groove and runs parallel to the left circumflex coronary artery. The left marginal vein and the posterior vein of the left ventricle enter the great cardiac vein, which is then referred to as the "coronary sinus." The coronary sinus enters the right atrium. Immediately before the ostium, the middle cardiac vein (which has a course parallel to the posterior descending artery) and the small cardiac vein (which runs parallel to the right coronary artery) also enter the coronary sinus. For more detail on coronary venous anatomy, see Chapter 11.

References

1. Angelini P, Villason S, Chan AV, Diez JG. (1999) Normal and anomalous coronary arteries in humans. In Angelini P (ed.) *Coronary Artery Anomalies*. Lippincott Williams & Wilkins, Baltimore, MD, pp. 27–79.
2. King SB, Douglas JS. (1985) Normal coronary anatomy. In King SB, Douglas JS (eds) *Coronary Arteriography and Angioplasty*. McGraw-Hill, New York, pp. 10–31.
3. Goldberg A, Southern DA, Galbraith PD *et al.* (2007) Coronary dominance and prognosis of patients with acute coronary syndrome. *Am Heart J* 154:1116–1122.
4. Gorlin R. (1976) Coronary anatomy. *Major Probl Intern Med* 11:40–58.
5. Patel S. (2008) Normal and anomalous anatomy of the coronary arteries. *Semin Roentgenol* 43(2):100–112.

6. ACC/AHA Guidelines for Coronary Angiography (1999) A Report of the American College of Cardiology/American Heart Association Task Force on Practice Guidelines (Committee on Coronary Angiography). Developed in Collaboration with the Society for Cardiac Angiography and Interventions. *J Am Coll Cardiol* 33:1756–1824
7. Austen WG, Edwards JE, Frye RI *et al.* (1975). A Reporting System on Patients Evaluated for Coronary Artery Disease. Report of the Ad Hoc Committee for Grading of Coronary Artery Disease, Council on Cardiovascular Surgery, American Heart Association. *Circulation* 51; 4 Suppl: 5–40.
8. Tops LF, Wood DA, Delgado V *et al* (2008) Noninvasive evaluation of the aortic root with multislice computed tomography: implications for transcatheter aortic valve replacement. *J Am Coll Cardiol Img* 1321–1339.
9. Saremi F, Abolhoda A, Ashikyan O *et al.* (2008). Arterial blood supply to sinuatrial and atrioventricular nodes: Imaging with multidetector CT. *Radiology* 246:99–107.
10. Alegria JR, Herrmann J, Holmes DR *et al.* (2005). Myocardial bridging. *Eur Heart J* 26:1159–1168.
11. Möhlenkamp S, Hort W, Ge J, Erbel R. (2002) Update on myocardial bridging. *Circulation* 106:2616–2622.
12. Rapp AH, Hillis D. (2001). Clinical consequences of anomalous coronary arteries. *Coron Artery Dis* 12:617–616.
13. Mirchandani S, Phoon CKL. (2005) Management of anomalous coronary arteries from the contralateral sinus. *Int J Cardiol* 102:383–389.
14. Gersony WM. (2007) Management of anomalous coronary artery from the contralateral coronary sinus. *J Am Coll Cardiol* 50:2083–2084.
15. Angelini P. (2002) Coronary artery anomalies—current clinical issues. *Tex Heart Inst J* 29:271–278.

10 Coronary Anatomy for Surgeons

Farhood Saremi,[1] Amir Abolhoda[1] & Gustavo Abuin[2]

[1] *University of California Irvine, UCI Medical Center, Irvine, CA, USA*
[2] *Instituto de neurobiología, Buenos Aires, Argentina*

Introduction

Surgical anatomy of the coronary circulation has been extensively reviewed in several previously published textbooks and articles [1–3]. However, a definite compilation of high-resolution multidetector CT (MDCT) images of coronary vessels relevant to surgical interventions, especially as pertaining to coronary artery bypass grafting, does not exist. In this chapter, divided in three separate sections, we present: (1) a brief description of the normal coronary arteries, (2) common anatomic variants of the main coronary arteries, and (3) the anatomy of coronary artery bypass grafts (CABGs) as depicted by cardiac MDCT. A complete review of the coronary anatomy relevant to interventionalists has been presented in Chapter 3. For coronary veins please refer to Chapter 9.

Normal Coronary Arteries

The right and left main (LM) coronary arteries are the first branches of the aortic root, arising from the right and left aortic sinuses of Valsalva, respectively. There are normally three individual sinuses of Valsalva, representing the widest segment of the aortic root (see Chapter 1, Figure 1.52), each spanning from the respective portion of the aortic valve annulus to the junction of the sinus and the tubular portions of the ascending aorta, namely, the sinotubular junction. With the exception of a typically short LM artery traveling within the transverse pericardial sinus and above the dome of the left atrium, all the major coronary arteries including the right coronary artery (RCA) follow an epicardial course along an either atrioventricular (AV) or interventricular groove.

The RCA originates perpendicular to the right aortic sinus. In contrast, the LM coronary artery meets the surface of the left coronary sinus at a 45° angle (Figure 10.1).

However, because of oblique orientation of the heart in the thorax, the long axis of the LM is usually parallel to transverse plane of the thorax.

High takeoff of the RCA orifice above the sinus aorta is not uncommon, and therefore, this vessel can be prone to inadvertent injury during surgical procedures near aortic root (Figure 10.1). In contrast, high takeoff of the LM artery above the left coronary sinus is uncommon [1]. Because of the oblique plane of the aortic valve, the orifice of the LM is superior and posterior to that of the RCA [3].

Right Coronary Artery

The RCA enters the right AV groove fat pad and travels in a remarkably constant course until its major first division at the crux into the posterior descending artery (PDA) and the posterolateral (PL) branches (right dominant coronary circulation) (see Chapter 3, Figure 3.3). The PDA travels in the posterior interventricular groove toward the apex and can give rise to several inferior septal perforators supplying the posterior third of the interventricular septum. One or several PL branches supply the diaphragmatic surface of the left ventricle.

Left Coronary Artery

The LM coronary artery arises from the left sinus aorta and travels a short distance (5–15 mm) within the transverse pericardial sinus, behind the main pulmonary trunk, before dividing into its two major branch vessels, the left anterior descending (LAD) and the left circumflex (LCx) coronary arteries (see Chapter 3, Figure 3.7). In one third of cases the LM divides into three or more branches with an

Revisiting Cardiac Anatomy: A Computed-Tomography-Based Atlas and Reference, 1st edition. Edited by Farhood Saremi, Eloisa Arbustini, Stephen Achenbach and Jagat Narula.

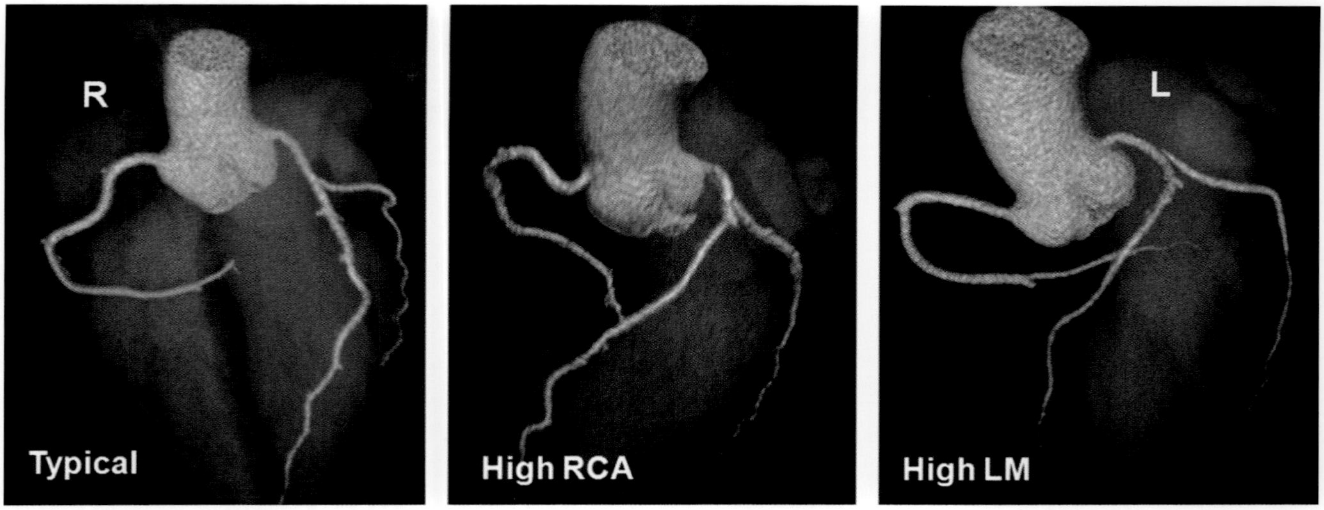

Figure 10.1 Normal anatomic variants of the origin of the right and left coronary arteries from their sinuses. The orifices of the coronary arteries are usually in the upper third of the sinuses of Valsalva but below the sinotubular junction. High takeoff above the sinotubular junction is more common for the RCA than the LM. L, left; LM, left main; R, right; RCA, right coronary artery.

average angle of 85° [4]. A positive correlation between the length of the LM and the angle of division of its terminal branches is shown with the longest LMs having the largest angle of division [4]. The LAD emerges to the left of the pulmonary trunk and enters the epicardial adipose tissue overlying the anterior interventricular groove, heading toward the apex and frequently curving around the apex onto the posterior interventricular groove (see Chapter 3, Figure 3.4). Along its long course, LAD gives off three to five septal perforators feeding the anterior two thirds of the interventricular septum (Figure 10.2), as well as two to six diagonal branches to the anterolateral wall of the left ventricle. The first diagonal generally is the largest and may arise from the bifurcation of the LM stem (also known as the ramus intermedius artery) [3] (see Chapter 3, Figure 3.7). The LCx enters the left AV groove, emerging anterior to the base of the left atrial appendage, and stays within the AV groove in close proximity to the coronary sinus. From its epicardial course, LCx gives off several obtuse marginal (OM) branches supplying the PL aspect of the left ventricle including the posteromedial papillary muscle. In the left dominant coronary circulation, LCx terminates by giving rise to the PDA (see Chapter 3, Figure 3.4).

Blood Supply of the Cardiac Conduction System

Cardiac MDCT provides excellent anatomic characterization of the origin, course, and variability of the vessels supplying blood to myocardial conduction tissue, including the sinoatrial node (SAN) and the atrioventricular node (AVN) [5]. The anatomic course and variants of these vessels are described in Chapter 9. SAN artery arises from

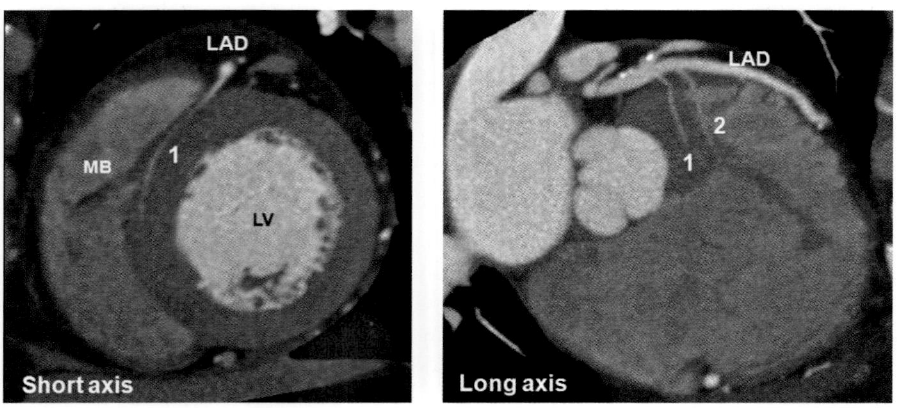

Figure 10.2 Septal perforating arteries of the left anterior descending artery (LAD). These vessels originate at a right angle from the LAD and travel on the right side of the interventricular septum. The first septal artery [1] is usually the largest and varies in length from 2 to 5 cm. The inferior branches of the first septal perforator are directed toward the moderator band (MB) and supply the anterior papillary muscle of the tricuspid valve. Its superior branches supply the right bundle branch and the bundle of His. (1, 2) Short-axis and long-axis views of the heart. LV, left ventricle.

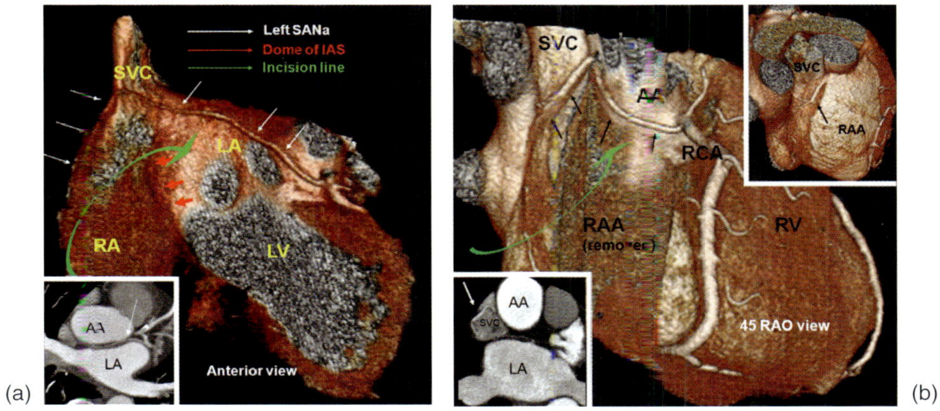

Figure 10.3 Sculptured three-dimensional reconstruction views with corresponding axial images demonstrate precaval SAN artery arising (a) from LCx (white arrows) and (b) from right coronary artery (RCA) (black arrows). Information regarding the termination of the SAN artery may be important when planning a superior transseptal approach in mitral valve surgery. The approximate incision line from the right atrium toward the dome of the left atrium superior to interatrial groove (IAS) is below the level of the course of SAN artery (SANa) in precaval variant in which the artery is terminating anterior to the SVC. This variant exists in 45% of patients. In this variant the risk of injury to the vessel is negligible if the incision is made with caution. AA, ascending aorta; LA, left atrium; LV, left ventricle; RA; right atrium; RAA, right atrial appendage; RAO, right anterior oblique; RV, right ventricle; SVC, superior vena cava.

either the proximal RCA (60–70%) or the proximal LCx artery (30–40%) (Figure 10.3). In <1% of human hearts, the SAN artery may originate directly from the right coronary sinus (Figure 10.15), descending aorta (Figure 10.4), or distal RCA (Figure 10.5). Pre-surgical knowledge of these anatomic variants can be important.

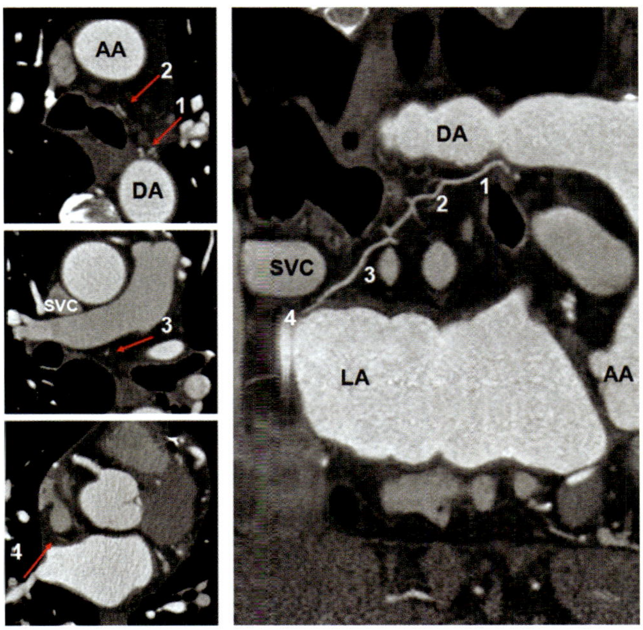

Figure 10.4 Direct origin of the sinoatrial node artery from the medial wall of the descending aorta (DA). Following it origin (1) from the DA, the SAN artery travels (from left to right) in the epicardial fat along the transverse sinus (2 and 3) and then posterior aspect of the SVC (4) toward the SA node in the lateral margin of the SVC. AA, ascending aorta; DA, descending aorta; LA, left atrium; SVC, superior vena cava.

Patients who have undergone left atrial surgery, such as atrial fibrillation ablation surgery, often exhibit postoperative disturbances in sinus node function, which may possibly be related to SAN artery damage [6,7]. However, this condition is usually transient without clinically troublesome manifestations [8,9]. Potential sources of damage to the SAN artery are incisions near the superior cavoatrial junction, incisions through the dome of left atrium, and incisions through the superior border of interatrial septum (Figure 10.15, see also Chapter 9).

Information regarding the termination of the SAN artery may be important when planning a superior transseptal approach in mitral valve surgery [6,7] (Figures 10.3 and 10.16, see also Chapter 9). The SAN artery crosses the superior posterior border of the interatrial septum in 54% of hearts. MDCT data have shown that the terminal SAN artery travels closer to the superior aspect of the interatrial septum in selected groups when the artery is moving behind the cava (47%) [4]). Such anatomy predisposes the SAN artery to injury during a superior transseptal approach to the mitral valve [10].

Another important variant of the SAN artery with surgical importance is the existence of a left SAN artery with an S-shaped course arising from the proximal LCx, seen in 8% of the hearts studied by Nerantzis *et al.* [11]. This artery is larger than the normal SAN artery, and supplies blood to almost the whole left atrium, a large part of the interatrial septum and right atrium, as well as part of the sinus and the AV nodal areas. The superb resolution of MDCT provides definitive localization of this artery

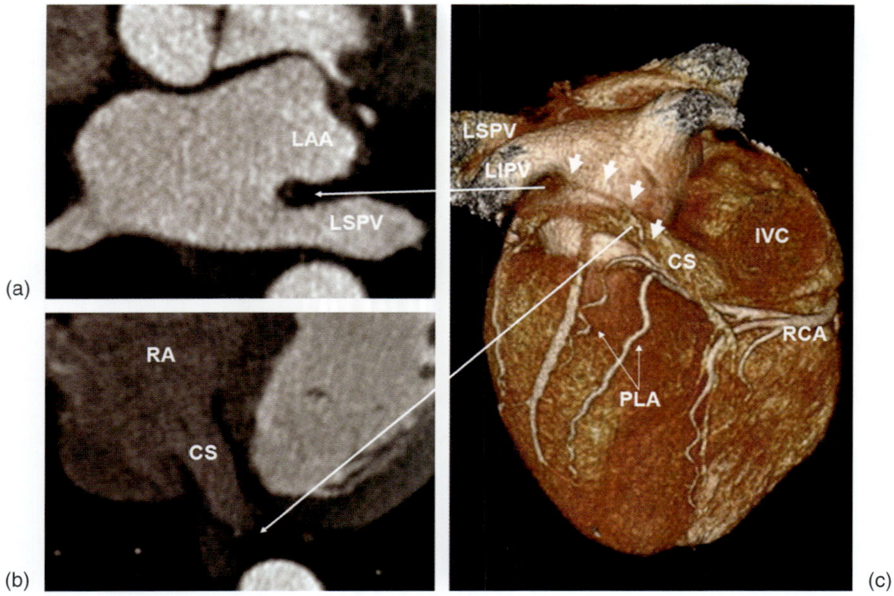

Figure 10.5 The S-shaped SAN artery arising from the distal RCA (arrows). Axial images at the level of the left atrial appendage (a) and the coronary sinus (b) as well as a three-dimensional posterior view of the heart (c) are shown. This rare variant originates from the terminal branches of a dominant right coronary artery (RCA), posterior to the coronary sinus (CS) as shown in (b) and (c), then traveled along the posterolateral wall of the left atrium toward the groove between the left atrial appendage (LAA) and the left superior pulmonary vein (LSPV). IVC, inferior vena cava; LIPV, left inferior pulmonary vein; PLA, posterolateral artery; RA, right atrium. (Reprinted from Saremi *et al.* [12] with permission.)

where it passes in the sulcus between the left superior pulmonary vein and the left atrial appendage [12] (Figure 10.49; see also Chapter 9, Figure 9.5). In this location, the artery is susceptible to injury during catheter or surgical ablation procedures on the left atrium.

The major blood supply to the AVN is the AVN artery [13,14] (Figure 10.6). According to Anderson and Murphy

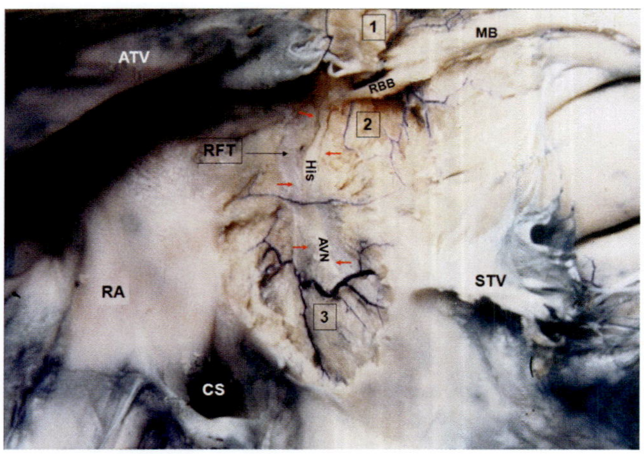

Figure 10.6 View of the right atrium (RA). The AV node (AVN), penetrating His bundle (His), and AV node artery (3) are exposed. Red arrows demarcate the conduction system. The AVN artery is the main supplier of the AVN. Branches of the first left septal artery extends to the right bundle branch (RBB) and moderator band (MB) (1). Distal branches of the right superior septal artery nourish the His bundle (2). ATV, anterior leaflet of the tricuspid valve; CS, coronary sinus; MB, moderator band; RA, right atrium; RFT, right fibrous trigone; STV, septal leaflet of the tricuspid valve.

[14], the vessel supplies the AVN in 90% of hearts but terminates before reaching the node in 10%. Alternative sources of arterial supply to the AV conducting pathway include the first septal perforating artery; the descending septal artery; and anterior atrial branches, including the Kugel anastomotic artery [14,15].

The Kugel anastomotic artery was first described by Kugel [16,17] as a large atrial artery (arteria anastomotica auricularis magna). This artery is an uncommon but sometimes important collateral between the proximal LCx or RCA (3%) and whatever artery supplying the crux of the heart (distal RCA or distal LCx) (Figure 10.7 and 10.8). It passes anterior to the mitral valve ring, coursing in the lower interatrial septum and may anastomose with the AVN artery. The right Kugel anastomotic artery [17] may be a continuum of right superior septal [18,19] or a branch of SAN artery or conus branch (Figure 10.9).

It is difficult to see these anastomotic arteries using conventional angiography. However, most MDCT studies of coronary arteries are able to show these vessels [4] (Figure 10.9). Since both Kugel arteries originate from the beginning of the coronary trunks, they have to be taken into consideration in many surgical procedures involving the aortic root [18]. The clinical significance of these atrial collateral vessels is a matter of debate, and their importance might primarily be their potential as a source of collateral circulation in the event of acquired obstruction in the vessel(s) with which they connect.

First septal perforating artery is a branch of left LAD artery supplying basal septum with branches to conduction system including His bundle and proximal bundle

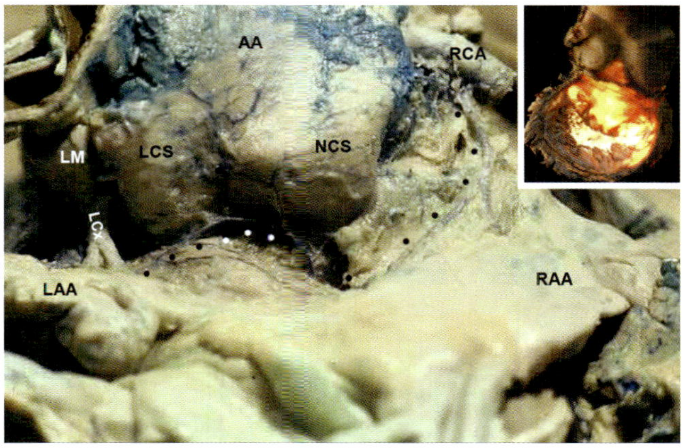

Figure 10.7 Kugel artery (black and white dots) is part of the atrial anastomotic network connecting the proximal right coronary artery (RCA) or left circumflex (LCx) artery to the distal RCA or LCx through the interatrial septum. In the right panel of the photo is shown the aorta, the mitral valve without the atria for better orientation. AA, ascending aorta; LAA, left atrial appendage; LCS, left coronary sinus; LM, left main artery; NCS, noncoronary sinus; RAA, right atrial appendage.

branches [20] (Figure 10.10). It is not a primary arterial source to AV node. However, its terminal branches can connect with the right superior septal artery (Figure 10.11). Complete heart block is a common complication of alcohol septal ablation for the treatment of hypertrophic obstructive cardiomyopathy [21].

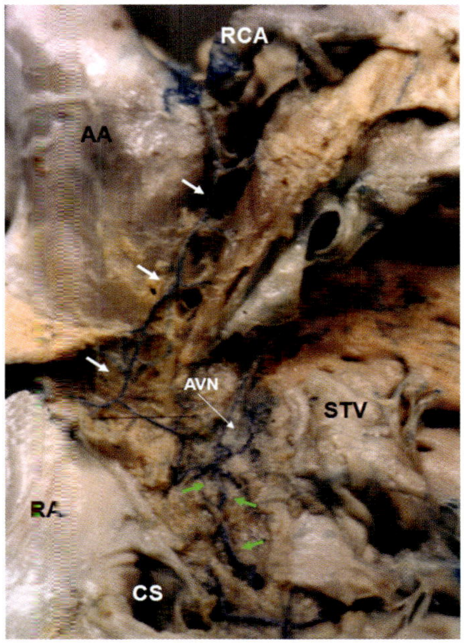

Figure 10.8 Right superior septal artery (right Kugel) originates from the proximal right coronary artery (RCA) or directly from the right coronary cusp. It then penetrates into the interatrial septum (white arrows) near the aortic root. From this point, the artery extends toward the atrioventricular node (AVN) where it may anastomose with branches of the AVN artery (green arrows). During aortic root surgery (i.e., Bental procedure), the vessel can be injured during mobilization of the coronary ostia or at the time of anastomosis of the ascending aorta to the prosthesis. AA, ascending aorta; CS, coronary sinus; RA, right atrium; STV, septal leaflet of the tricuspid valve.

(a), (b)

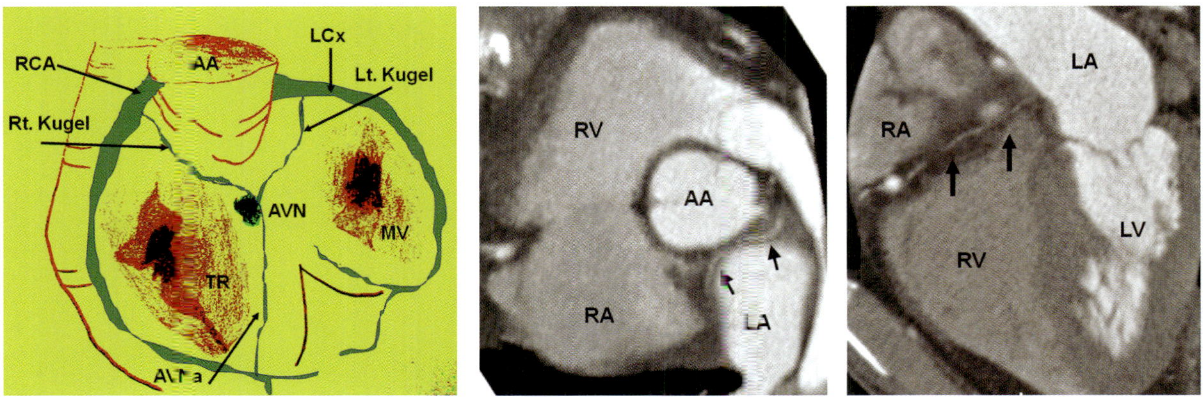

(c)

Figure 10.9 (a) Schematic representation of posterior view at CT of heart demonstrates atrial vessel supply to AVN, including right (Rt. Kugel) and left (Lt. Kugel) Kugel anastomotic arteries and atrioventricular nodal artery (AVNa). (b) Tilted short-axis and (c) four-chamber views show accessory branches to AVN area. In (b), left Kugel anastomotic artery arising from proximal LCx artery (black arrows) is evident. In (c), right Kugel anastomotic artery is shown originating from proximal RCA (black arrows). Kugel anastomotic arteries travel through epicardial fat in the atrioventricular groove, extending along the side of aorta and then behind it, and reach the interatrial septum near its junction with the interventricular septum. AA, ascending aorta; LA, left atrium; LV, left ventricle; MV, mitral valve; RA, right atrium; RCA, right coronary artery; RV, right ventricle; TR, tricuspid valve. (Reprinted with permission from Saremi *et al.* [5].)

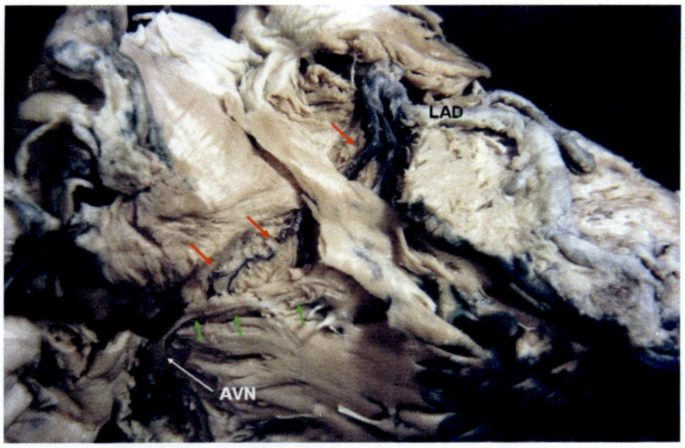

Figure 10.10 Anatomic course of the first septal artery (red arrows) is shown. It originates at the junction of the proximal and mid-parts of the left anterior descending (LAD) artery perpendicular to the vessel. It travels into the interventricular septum for 3–5 cm (white arrows). Its terminal branches nourish the penetrating His bundle and the right bundle branch (green arrows). AVN, atrioventricular node.

Anatomic Variants of the Coronary Arteries

Congenital anomalies of the coronary arteries are uncommon findings in healthy individuals, incidentally discovered in approximately 0.3–1.0% of the general population [22–25]. Although conventional angiography has been the primary modality for identification and characterization of the coronary abnormalities in the past, high-resolution MCDT allows accurate, noninvasive, and possibly superior anatomic delineation of the ostial origin and course of certain anomalous coronary vessels [23].

LAD Variants

It is not uncommon for the LAD to wrap around the apex to feed the distal portion of the posterior interventricular groove. Rarely, it extends along the entire length of the posterior groove to replace the PDA (Figure 10.12).

True dual LAD is rare (<1%) and should be differentiated from a diagonal or ramus traveling parallel to the LAD [24, 26]. Different variants of dual LAD have been described in Ref. [26]. In the most common type, the dual LAD can be recognized by an early bifurcation of the proximal LAD (the LAD proper). Of the resulting two vessels, one is too short to reach the apex; this "short LAD" stays in the anterior interventricular groove. The other, the "long LAD," initially runs parallel to the short LAD and then reenters the anterior interventricular groove before reaching the apex (Figure 10.12). Only few cases of dual LAD arteries with origin of each anomalous vessel from a different sinus of Valsalva have been published [26–29]. The

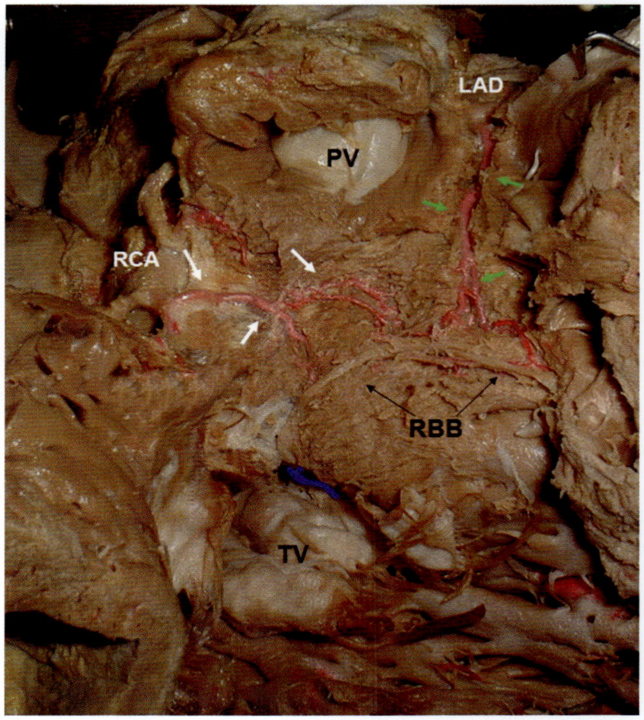

Figure 10.11 Arterial supply of the right bundle branch (RBB) by terminal branches of the right superior septal artery (white arrows) and the first septal branch (green arrows) of the left anterior descending (LAD) artery. The right superior septal artery branch frequently originates from the proximal 2 cm of the right coronary artery (RCA) and nourishes the crista supraventricularis, part of the superior portion of the interventricular septum, the right and left bundle branches, and the His bundle. This vessel can be sacrificed during a Bentall procedure (aortic valve replacement, ascending aorta replacement, and reinsertion of coronary ostia). This vessel may also play a role in the development of atrioventricular (AV) block after acute occlusion of the RCA at its origin. However, most of these patients recover to sinus rhythm. This is explained by the rich collateral circulation that supplies the AV conduction axis, particularly the AV node. Occlusion of the first left septal artery can cause complete heart block. The blue vessel represents the AVN artery. PV, pulmonary valve; TV, tricuspid valve.

presence of this congenital coronary anomaly can potentially have clinical implications on coronary revascularization procedures (Figure 10.13). Familiarity with dual LAD variants can help the surgeon avoid incorrect coronary bypass construction [30]. If both short and long LADs are severely stenosed, grafts to both the vessels may be needed.

Myocardial Bridging

Intramyocardial course of a coronary artery represents an inborn anomaly with a high prevalence in autopsy series [31] (Figure 10.13). It is shown in 3.5–30% of MDCT series [32, 33]. The most common location involves the mid-LAD. Involvement of other coronary arteries such as RCA,

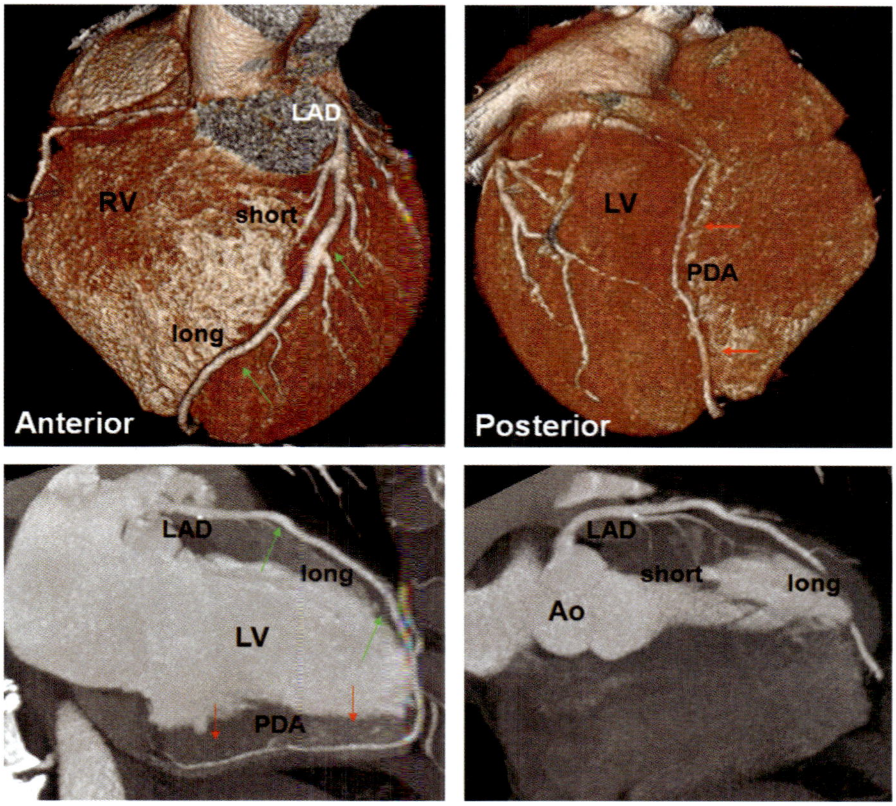

Figure 10.12 Dual LAD continues as the PDA. Anterior and posterior three-dimensional views and long-axis images of an asymptomatic patient demonstrate a dual left anterior descending (LAD) artery. The "short" LAD give rise to small septal perforators and the "long" LAD gives off multiple diagonal branches. Following a course on the left side of the interventricular groove, the long LAD turns medially into the interventricular groove, wraps around the apex, and continues its long journey as a PDA in the posterior interventricular groove. Note that RCA is small and branches of obtuse marginal artery (from the left circumflex artery) supply the posterolateral wall of the left ventricle. Ao, aorta; LV, left ventricle; PDA, posterior descending artery; RV, right ventricle.

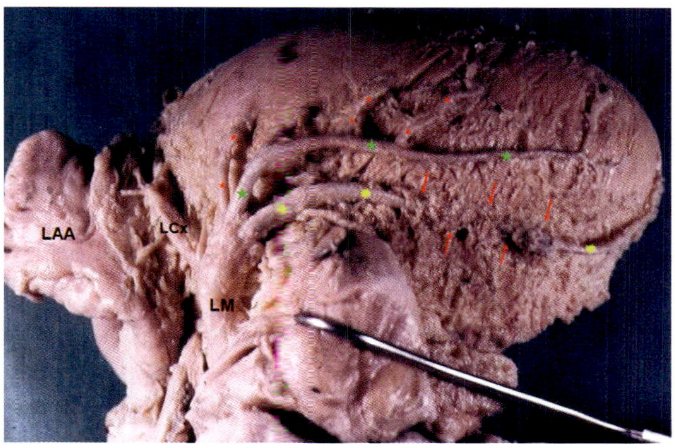

Figure 10.13 Intramyocardial LAD and dual anatomic course anterior view of a heart specimen showing myocardial bridging (red arrow) over a 3 cm length of the mid-portion of the LAD. This photograph shows an uncommon anatomic variant (dual LAD system), with the main LAD (yellow asterisks) giving rise to the septal perforators and continuing to the left ventricular apex along the anterior interventricular groove, and a large anterolateral branch (green stars), running parallel to the primary LAD and giving rise to all of the diagonal branches (red stars) to the anterolateral wall of the left ventricle. A cardiac surgeon may mistaken this large "second LAD" for the primary LAD in course of construction of distal anastomosis. The left circumflex artery (LCx) and a large left main (LM) trunk are shown. LAA, left atrial appendage.

first diagonal, second diagonal, ramus, and the marginal branches of the LCx artery is less common [32, 33]. Most patients are asymptomatic. An intramyocardial LAD coronary artery is particularly troublesome during a coronary artery bypass operation, and inadvertent intracavitary entry is a possibility during coronary exposure [34, 35](Figure 10.14).

Aberrant Origin

Multiple orifices arising from the right aortic sinus is the most common finding with approximately 50% of hearts having two separate orifices within this sinus [1]. The second orifice is frequently a conus artery and of little surgical significance. Rarely, the right SAN artery or the right superior septal artery can directly originate from the right aortic sinus (Figure 10.15). Multiple orifices arising from the left sinus are rare. Anomalous origin from posterior sinus is very rare in humans; however, examples are seen in patients with transposition of great vessels [1].

High takeoff of origins of either right or LM coronary artery above the sinotubular junction (STJ) have been reported in 6% of adult hearts and rarely has surgical significance [36]. It is more common on the right side (Figure 10.1). Knowledge of such anomaly should result in slight

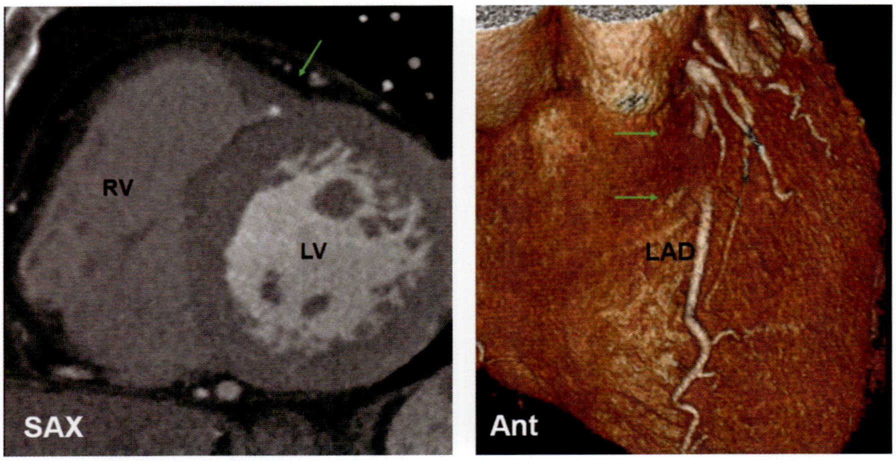

Figure 10.14 Myocardial bridge (green arrow) covering the proximal left anterior descending artery (LAD). Note that in the tunneled segment the LAD has almost penetrated into the right ventricle (RV). Ant, anterior view; LV, left ventricle; SAX, short-axis view.

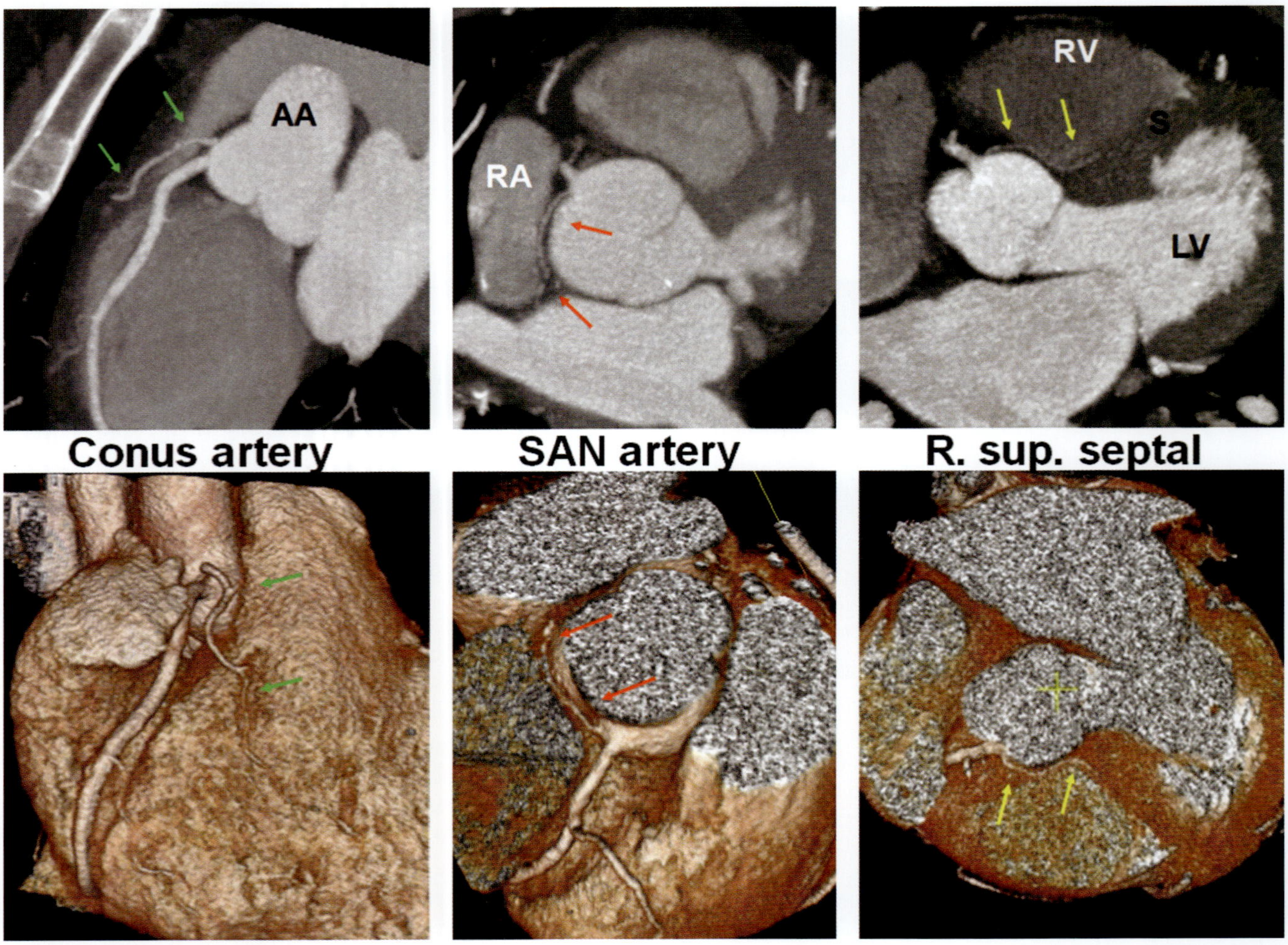

Figure 10.15 Multiple orifices in the right coronary sinus are common (50%). Direct origin of the conus artery is the most common variant (green arrows). Direct origin of the sinoartial node (SAN) artery (red arrows) can be seen in 1% of CT coronary studies. Direct origin of the right (R) superior (sup) septal artery (yellow arrows) from the right coronary sinus s less common. This artery penetrates into the superior part of the interventricular septum (S). AA, ascending aorta; LV, left ventricle; RA, right atrium; RV, right ventricle.

modification of the location and course of aortic incision for aortic valve replacement to avoid main coronary artery injury; also, in performing major aortic root reconstructions requiring main coronary artery button reimplantation, surgeon should be mindful of such high takeoff coronary ostia. Finally, high takeoff coronary ostia may pose a difficulty for an interventional cardiologist attempting selective intubation of the vessel during a diagnostic or therapeutic coronary angiography.

Translocation of the LCx from the right coronary sinus is the most common form of anomalous origin of coronary arteries. It may originate directly from the right sinus or as a branch of the RCA (Figure 10.14, see also Chapter 3). The clinical significance of this anomaly is a matter of controversy [22, 25]. Anomalous origin of the right or LM coronary artery from the contralateral sinus of Valsalva, although often asymptomatic, can present with ischemic symptoms and even sudden death and occasionally require surgical correction. The proximal portion of the anomalous vessel often exits the aorta at an acute angle and may travel in an interarterial course (between the aortic root and the pulmonary trunk), potentially resulting in exercise-induced malperfusion [22,37] (Figure 10.16).

Single coronary anomalies are one of the rarest varieties, with incidence of absence of LM coronary ostium at 0.05–0.4% of this selected population [38,39].

In patients with absence of the left coronary ostium, there are four variations in the initial course of the LAD arising from the RCA: anterior, interarterial, septal, and rarely posterior (retroaortic) [1,40]. In the anterior

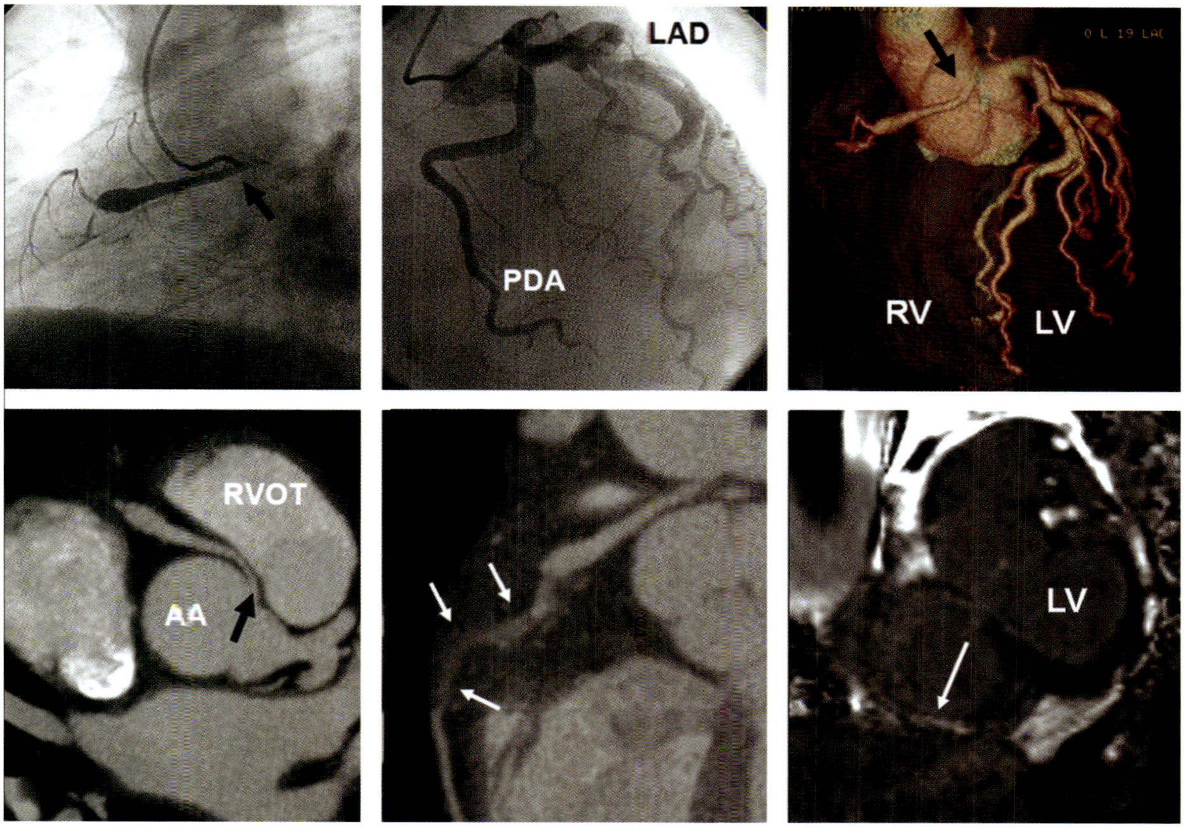

(a), (b) (c) (d), (e) (f)

Figure 10.16 Isolated right ventricular infarction due to anomalous origin of right coronary artery (RCA). In the upper panel, there are left anterior oblique view of the RCA (a) and right anterior oblique view of the left coronary system (b) on coronary angiography. Part (a) demonstrates the proximally occluded RCA, and part (b) shows the large ectatic left coronary artery. Note that the large left coronary system including a dominant left circumflex artery gives rise to the posterior descending artery (PDA). Three-dimensional volume-rendered reconstruction of the coronary vessels (c) corresponding to the same projection obtained by coronary catheterization and axial MDCT image at the level of the RCA origin (d) show anomalous origin of the RCA above the anterior commissure of the ascending aorta is shown. The proximal RCA appears funnel-shaped and compressed between ascending aorta (AA) and right ventricle outflow tract (RVOT) with a short intramural segment at the origin (black arrows). It is occluded approximately 25 mm from its orifice. Curved reconstruction image (e) shows the thrombosed segment of the RCA (small white arrows). A linear filling defect is seen within the thrombosed segment surrounded by contrast that may represent clot. Short-axis image of delayed contrast enhanced MR (f) shows hyperenhancement of the inferior wall of the right ventricle at the basal level. LAD, left anterior descending artery; LV, left ventricle; RV, right ventricle.

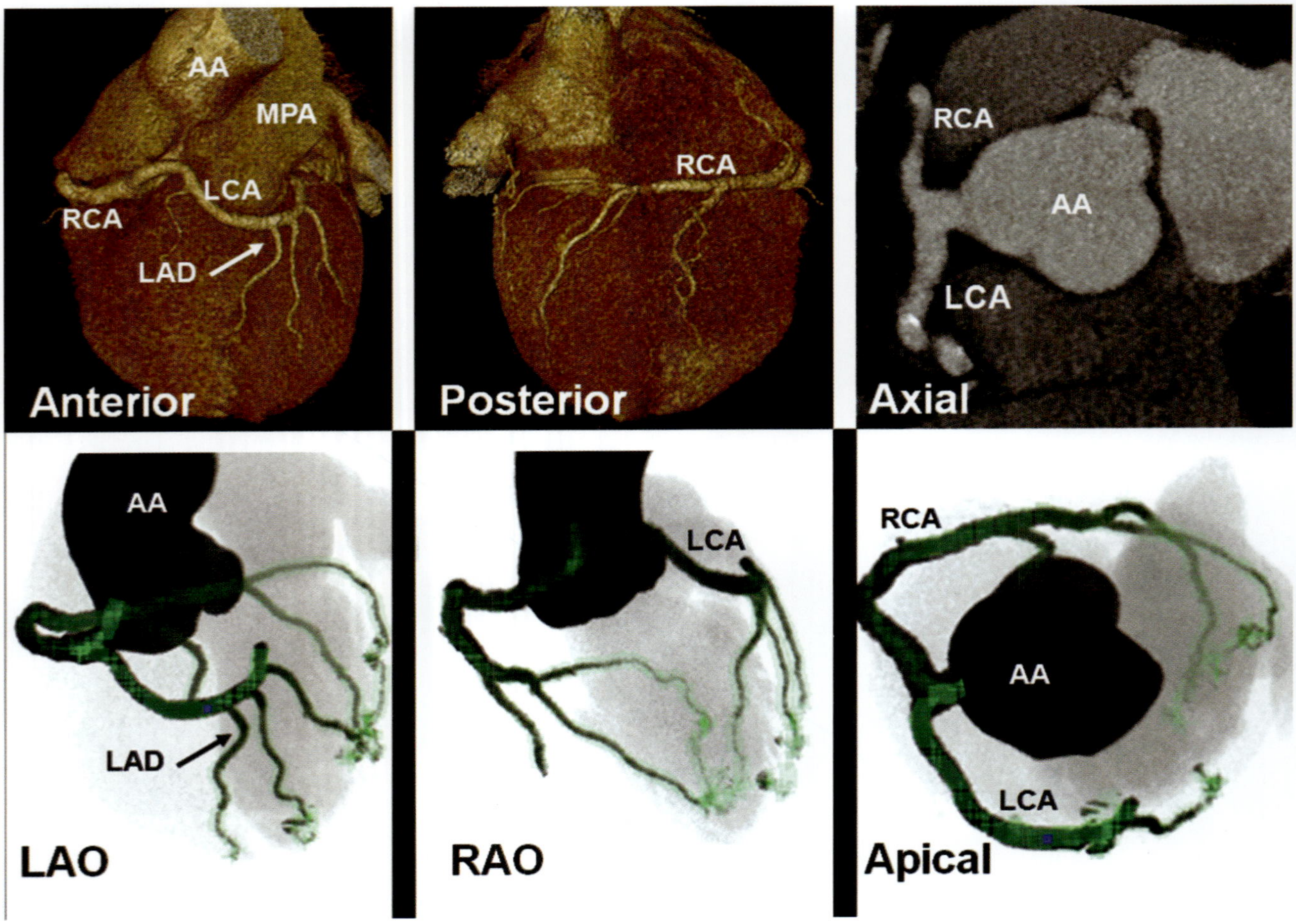

Figure 10.17 Coronary CT angiography demonstrates a single coronary artery arising from the right coronary cusp bifurcating into the right coronary artery (RCA) and left coronary artery (LCA). The RCA is the dominant artery. The LCA passes anterior to the MPA (anterior type). The left circumflex artery is a continuation of the LCA in the atrioventricular groove, and the LAD is a branch of the LCA. Three-dimensional volume rendered, and axial images are shown in the upper row and maximum intensity angiographic projections in the lower row. AA, ascending aorta; LAD, left anterior descending artery; LAO, left anterior oblique; MPA, main pulmonary artery; RAO, right anterior oblique. (Reprinted with permission, Kempf and Saremi [41].)

variant, the most common of the three, the LAD courses anterior to the right ventricular infundibulum (Figure 10.17), and in the septal variant, within the ventricular septum beneath the right ventricular infundibulum [41]. The interarterial type can be life-threatening, but the septal type is a largely benign variant (Figure 10.18).

Anomalous pulmonary origin of the coronaries is one of the most serious congenital anomalies, presenting almost invariably with symptoms in infancy and early childhood [22]. The most common variant is the emergence of the LM coronary artery from the pulmonary trunk. Aortic reimplantation is the preferred surgical technique followed by ligation and bypass of the anomalous artery in the remaining patients.

Aberrant Termination

Another rare congenital anomaly commonly requiring surgical intervention is fistulous termination of a right or left coronary artery (0.1–0.2%) into a cardiac chamber, the pulmonary trunk, the coronary sinus, or a central vein such as the superior vena cava [22,42] (Figure 10.19). The pulmonary artery is the most dominant drainage site and

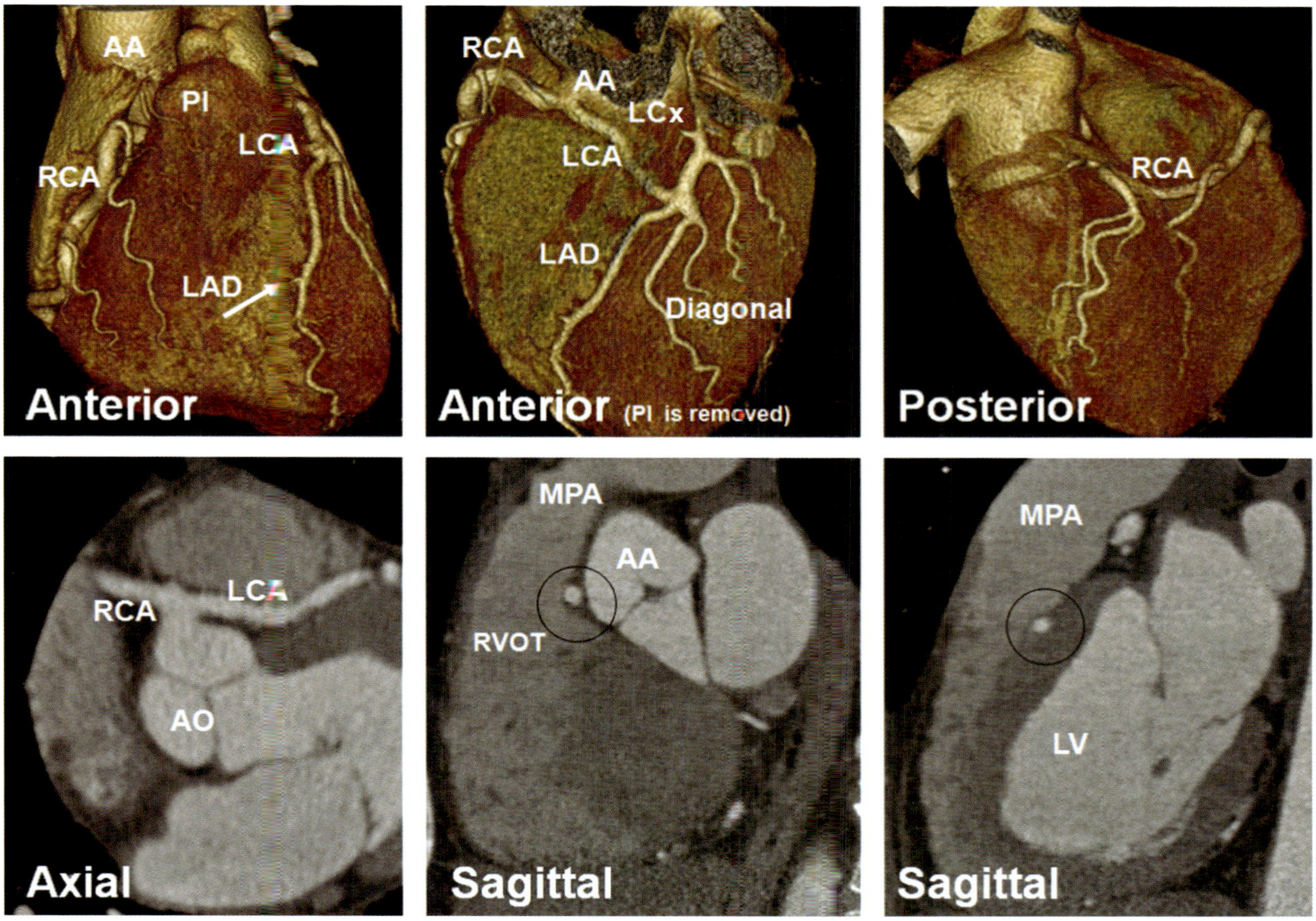

Figure 10.18 Coronary CT angiography demonstrates a single coronary trunk arising from the right coronary cusp (septal variant). Shortly after its takeoff, the trunk bifurcates into the RCA and LCA. The RCA is again the dominant artery. The left coronary artery demonstrates abnormal course between the pulmonary infundibulum (PI) and AA and then within the infundibular septum (circles) before trifurcating into the LAD, diagonal (ramus), and the LCx. The LCx artery is continuation of the LCA in the atrioventricular groove, and the LAD is a branch of the LCA. Diagonal branches are evident. Three-dimensional volume-rendered images are shown in the upper row and axial and sagittal projections in the lower row. AA, ascending aorta; Ao, aorta; LAD, left anterior descending artery; LCA, left coronary artery; LCx, left circumflex artery; LV, left ventricle; MPA, main pulmonary artery; RCA, right coronary artery; RVOT, right ventricular outflow tract. (Reprinted with permission, Kempf and Saremi [41].)

is usually asymptomatic (Figure 10.19, see also Chapter 3). In surgical candidates, the most common corrective technique is internal closure of the fistula.

CT Imaging of Coronary Bypass Grafts

CABG surgery is one of the most commonly performed surgical procedures. Surgical indications for CABG include, but not limited to, significant (≥50%) LM coronary artery stenosis, LM equivalent disease [critical stenoses of ostial LAD and ostial LCx coronary arteries], and severe three-vessel coronary artery disease [43–46]. Coronary CT angiography (CTA), using MDCT with electrocardiographic gating, has a promising role in diagnostic imaging of CABG conduits both for postoperative graft surveillance and in preoperative planning for redo-surgery [47–49].

Anatomy of Patent Grafts

In order to accurately describe the MDCT anatomy of a coronary artery bypass conduit, a corollary to surgical

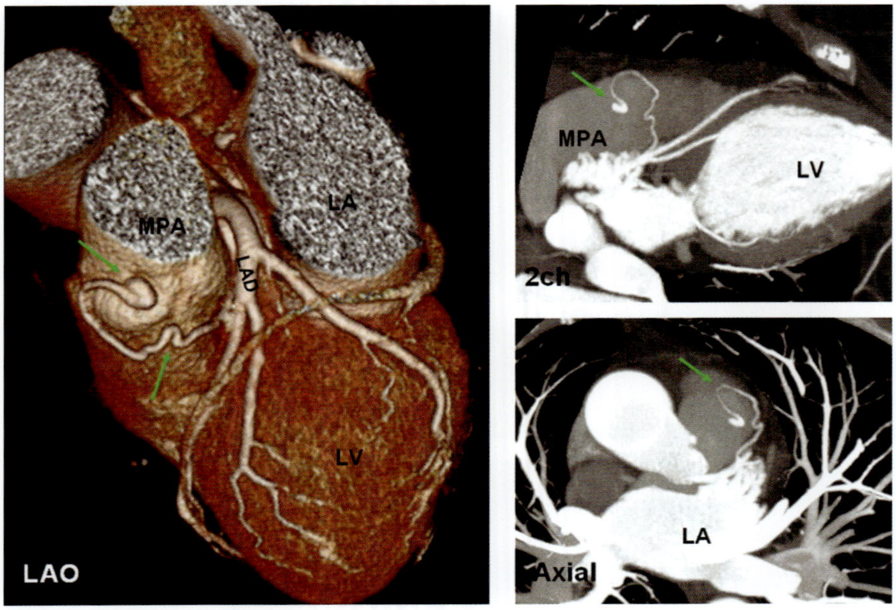

Figure 10.19 Fistulous communication (green arrows) of the proximal left anterior descending artery (LAD) with the main pulmonary artery (MPA) in a 75-year-old asymptomatic female. 2ch, two-chamber view; LA, left atrium; LAO, left anterior oblique view; LV, left ventricle.

descriptions and intraoperative photographs is essential. There are two types of coronary bypass grafts: arterial and venous (Figure 10.20). As a rule, arterial grafts are smaller in caliber than venous grafts [49, 50]. The most frequent arterial conduit, utilized in greater than 90% of all CABG procedures, is the left internal mammary artery (LIMA). This conduit is primarily used to bypass LAD and/or a major diagonal branch of LAD. In order of decreasing frequency, the other arterial grafts are the right internal mammary artery (RIMA), free radial artery, right gastroepiploic artery, and inferior epigastric artery. Although the internal mammary arterial grafts, i.e., both LIMA and RIMA, have far superior long-term patency in comparison to the vein conduits, vein grafts have been shown to have equivalent patency to other arterial grafts [43,51]. Ease of harvest and its ready availability makes the greater saphenous vein (GSV) the most commonly employed conduit in surgical revascularization procedures.

A free vein or arterial graft is usually divided into three imaging segments: the origin or proximal anastomosis of

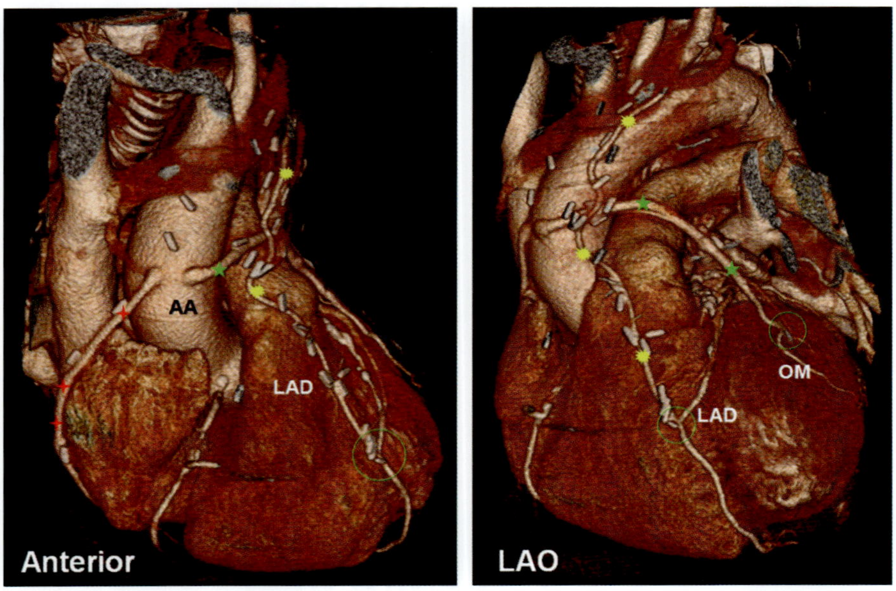

Figure 10.20 Anterior and left anterior oblique (LAO) views of a three-dimensional volume-rendered image shows the typical appearances of right (arrow) and left (solid arrowhead) saphenous vein grafts (SVG) sutured to the anterior wall of ascending aorta (AA). The left SVG is attached to the obtuse marginal (OM) artery distally (green stars). The distal anastomosis of the right SVG (red stars) to the posterior descending artery is not shown. There is also a left internal mammary artery (LIMA) graft (yellow asterisks), which is connected to the left anterior descending (LAD) artery.

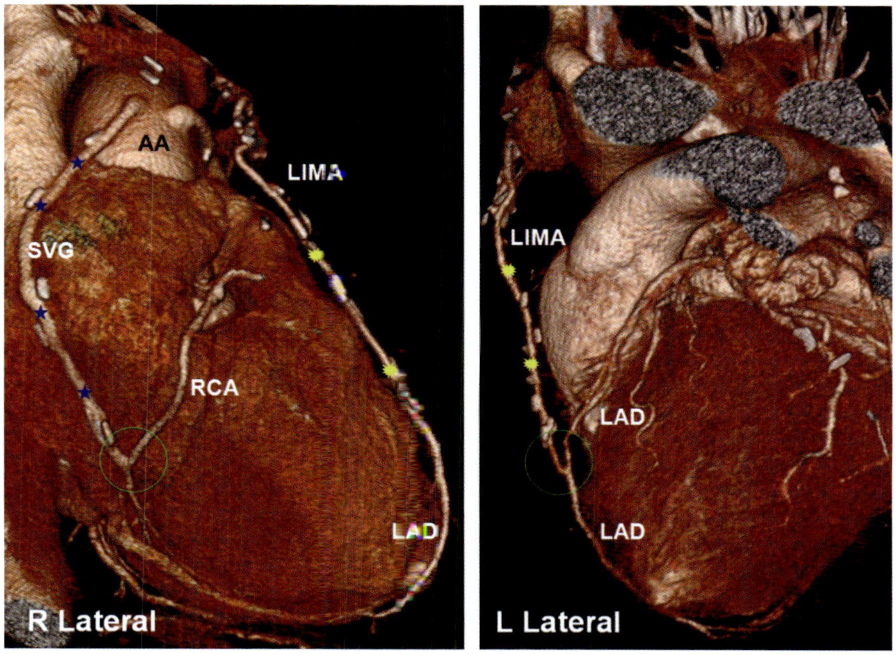

Figure 10.21 Three-dimensional volume-rendered images show the typical appearances end-to-side anastomosis (green circles). The right (R) lateral view shows a saphenous vein graft (SVG) arising from the right side of the ascending aorta (AA). A right-sided SVG is usually attached either to the lower aspect or to the right side of the ascending aorta. The graft (blue stars) passes over the terminal groove and acute margin of the right ventricle to anastome with distal right coronary artery (RCA). The left (L) lateral view demonstrates end-to-side anastomosis of the left internal mammary artery (LIMA) (yellow asterisks) with the left anterior descending (LAD) artery.

the graft to the ascending aorta, the body of the graft, and the single (or sequential) distal anastomosis(es) (Figure 10.21). During the CTA evaluation of bypass grafts, the proximal anastomosis is usually better visualized than the distal anastomosis. In cases in which the distal anastomosis is not well evaluated, the bypass graft is usually considered patent as long as contrast is evident within the graft lumen.

Surgical clips are used routinely to occlude branch vessels of the LIMA, and metallic artifact may limit full CT assessment of arterial graft in some instances. Typically, there are few surgical clips accompanying venous bypass grafts, lessening streak artifacts that may limit graft evaluation (Figure 10.20).

Vein Grafts

A cardiac surgeon's almost exclusive choice of vein conduit in performing a CABG operation is the reverse (GSV) harvested as a free graft from either lower extremity. This conduit is primarily utilized for revascularization of non-LAD coronary artery territories; these include distal RCA and its terminal branch vessels, PDA and posterior left ventricle (PLV), OM branches of LCx, and diagonal branches of LAD. After construction of a distal end to side anastomosis between the vein graft and the epicardial coronary artery target, the vein graft is attached to the corresponding side of the mid-portion of the ascending aorta, few centimeters above the sinotubular junction, to create an obtuse angle, kink-free proximal anastomosis. A left-sided GSV is connected to the left side of the ascending aorta, with the graft reaching the aorta draping over the left atrial appendage and the main pulmonary artery. An OM graft typically lies in the superior portion of the oblique sinus of the pericardial sac and attached to the ascending aorta in the most cephalad position (Figure 10.20). A diagonal vein graft courses over the main pulmonary trunk, passing underneath the envisioned internal mammary graft, and is commonly attached to the ascending aorta proximal to the OM vein graft (Figure 10.22). A right-sided saphenous vein graft (SVG) emerges from the obtuse angle of the right heart, overlying the free wall of right atrium, passing anterior and medial to the cavoatrial junction to be attached to the greater curvature of the right aspect of the ascending aorta (Figures 10.20 and 10.21). A free GSV graft is sometimes utilized to revascularize LAD (Figure 10.22). On occasions, a single GSV is utilized for distal anatomoses in sequential fashion to two or more coronary targets using end-to-side and side-to-side configurations, respectively.

Arterial Grafts

Left Internal Mammary Artery

Pedicled LIMA is the most valuable and durable conduit utilized in a routine CABG procedure (Figures 10.20–10.23). Pedicled LIMA is left attached to the proximal

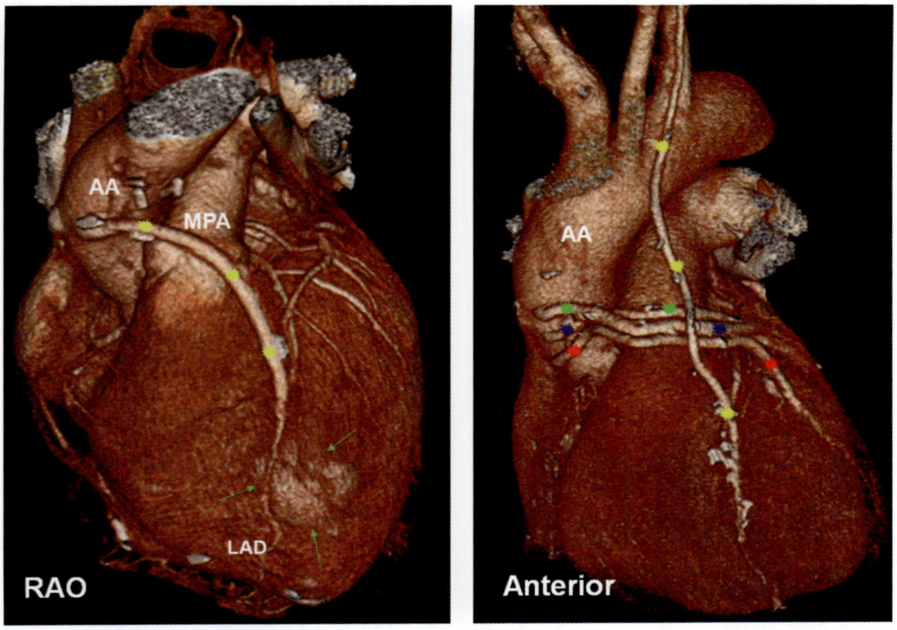

Figure 10.22 Coronary CT angiography (CTA) in two different patients. The right anterior oblique (RAO) view in a 61-year-old patient with history of myocardial infarction. A venous graft (yellow asterisks) is used to revascularize the left anterior descending (LAD) artery distribution. An aneurysm related to prior myocardial infarction is seen adjacent to LAD (between green arrows). The anterior view of CTA in a different patient shows sequential order of venous graft attachments to the anterior wall of the ascending aorta (AA) (green, blue, and red asterisks). There is also a patent left internal mammary artery (LIMA) graft (yellow asterisks) to LAD. MPA, main pulmonary artery.

subclavian artery after ligation of its segmental intercostal branches and is distal detachment from the chest wall by division of its terminal branches, namely, the musculophrenic and the superior epigastric arteries. This graft is typically utilized to bypass to the mid-portion of the LAD; occasionally, LIMA is also utilized to bypass a large diagonal vessel either as an independent graft or in sequential fashion in addition to LAD.

Following construction of a tension-free LIMA to mid-LAD end-to-side anastomosis, a pericardial cradle is created by incising the left side of the pericardial reflection overlying the pulmonary trunk with careful attention to avoid injury to nearby left phrenic nerve (Figure 10.24). This cradle houses the mammary graft deep within the pericardial sac, medial to the hilum of the left lung, in order to avoid axial tension and ventral displacement of the pedicle. Excessive length or foreshortened pedicle should be avoided. If there is documented or suspected proximal left subclavian artery stenosis, or a pedicled LIMA is too short to reach the coronary target, the mammary graft can

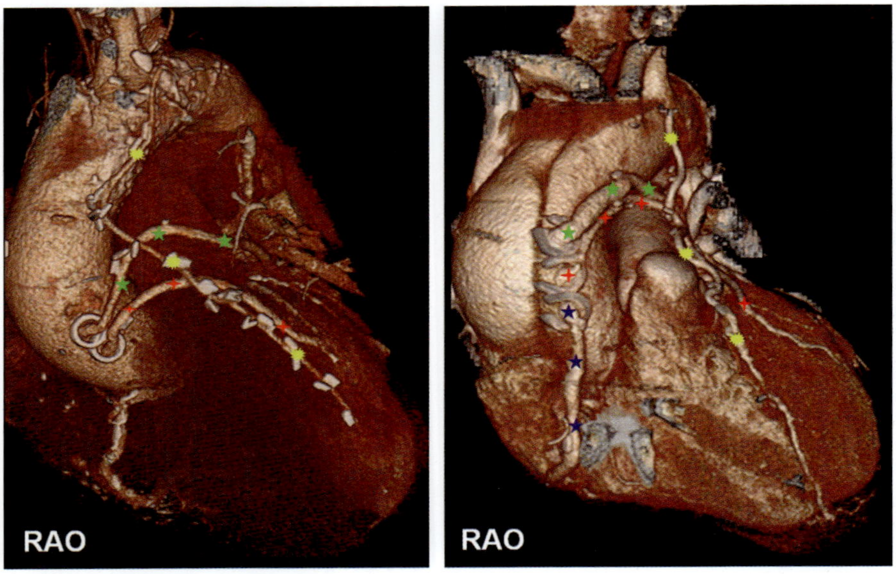

Figure 10.23 Right anterior oblique (RAO) views of coronary CT angiography (CTA) in two different patients. Suturing the graft is a critical part of the CABG procedure and requires application of a clamp on the aorta, thereby increasing the risk of stroke and other embolic complications. The recent development of a mechanical aortovenous connector allows quicker attachment of venous grafts to the aorta without use of aortic clamps or sutures. Green stars, obtuse marginal venous graft; yellow asterisks, left internal mammary artery graft; red stars, diagonal venous graft; blue stars, right coronary venous graft; CABG, coronary artery bypass graft.

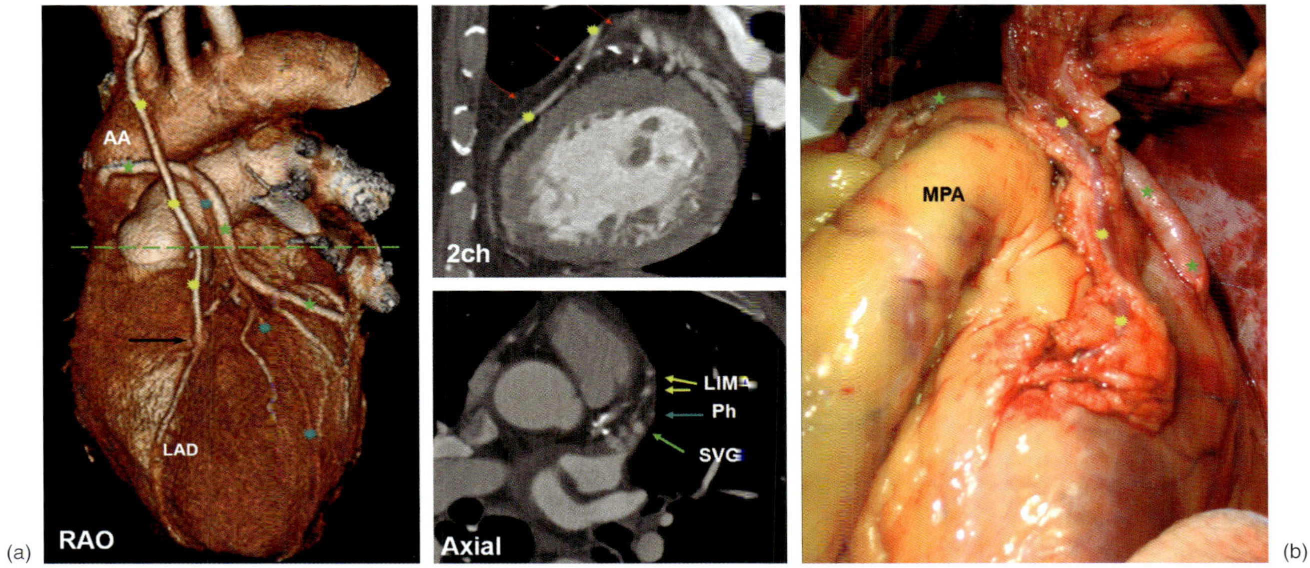

Figure 10.24 Anatomic course of an in situ left internal mammary graft (LIMA) is shown. (a) LIMA graft (yellow asterisks) is left pedicled to the proximal subclavian artery. LIMA to mid-LAD anastomosis is shown in three-dimensional right anterior oblique (RAO) view (long black arrow). Careful attention is needed to avoid injury to the left phrenic nerve during creation of a pericardial cradle. The site of pericardial entrance of the LIMA is shown by broken green line on the three-dimensional image and by red arrows on two-chamber view (2ch). Note close apposition of the phrenic neurovascular bundle (Ph) (blue asterisks) to the LIMA and saphenous vein graft (SVG) (green stars). (b) The anterior view of the heart at the time of CABG surgery. Pedicled LIMA (yellow asterisks) is shown passing anterior to the saphenous vein graft (green stars). AA, ascending aorta; CABG, coronary artery bypass graft; MPA, main pulmonary artery.

be detached proximally and used as a free graft in a similar fashion as described for the vein conduits.

Right Internal Mammary Artery

On occasions, surgeons utilize both RIMA and LIMA conduits, especially in younger patients, for near total or total arterial revascularization [52–54]. A pedicled RIMA graft is prepared in a similar manner as LIMA and will be directed to the chosen coronary target in a tension-free fashion. Three most common pedicled RIMA constructs are RIMA coursing via right aspect of the pericardial sac to distal RCA, RIMA coursing via transverse pericardial sinus to ramus intermedius or high-OM branch of LCx (Figure 10.25), or RIMA coursing anterior to ascending aorta to mid-LAD (Figure 10.26). RIMA can also be used as a free graft.

Radial Artery

Utilization of free radial artery graft as a CABG conduit is dependent on surgeon preference or lack of availability of a suitable vein conduit [55]. Initial attempts at using radial artery grafts were complicated by frequent graft closure. However, with recent improvements in atraumatic surgical harvesting and with use of postoperative calcium channel blockers to overcome graft spasm, the radial artery is currently regarded as a valid arterial graft option. As with a RIMA graft, the radial artery may be used as a free or composite graft with the goal of providing greater arterial revascularization (Figure 10.27). Patency rates are similar but perhaps slightly superior to GSV grafts [55].

Early Graft Patency

Mainstay of postoperative surveillance for patency of CABG grafts (arterial or venous conduits) has been invasive arterial angiography. Certainly, in patients with clinically overt symptoms of myocardial ischemia shortly following a CABG procedure, urgent coronary angiography and possible percutaneous coronary intervention should remain the mainstay of diagnosis and therapy. However, in those hemodynamically stable patients with minor or atypical postoperative symptomatology and inconclusive signs of myocardial ischemia or infarction, noninvasive MDCT imaging of the coronary conduits can be quite useful and informative. GSV is less resistant to spasm than its arterial counterparts. However, vein conduits are more prone to surgical trauma, both during harvest and grafting procedures, and thus in general more prone to early

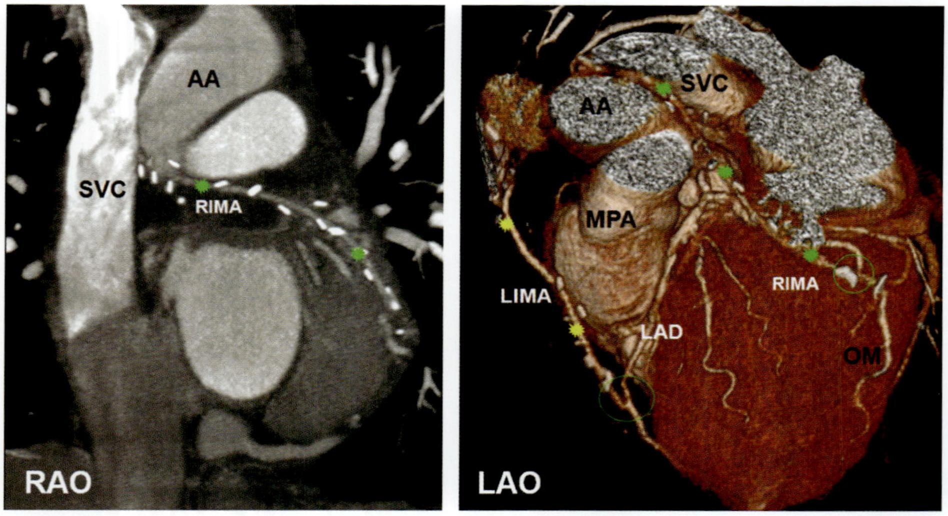

Figure 10.25 Right anterior oblique (RAO) and volume-rendered left anterior oblique (LAO) reconstructions of a coronary CT angiography demonstrate a right internal mammary artery (RIMA) graft anastomosed to the obtuse marginal (OM) artery and a left internal mammary artery (LIMA) (yellow asterisks) graft anastomosed to the left anterior descending (LAD) artery. RIMA may also be used in a variety of ways. As an in situ graft (in this case), the RIMA remains attached to the right subclavian artery proximally and anastomoses with the target coronary artery distally (green asterisks). When grafted to the left-sided coronary system, the RIMA will often pass through the transverse sinus, since this has been shown to result in higher patency rates. Alternatively, the right IMA may be removed from the subclavian artery and used as a free or composite graft. AA, ascending aorta; MPA, main pulmonary artery; SVC, superior vena cava.

graft closure. Also, early intimal hyperplasia at both proximal and distal anastomotic sites and poor distal coronary runoff can contribute to early vein graft failure [56, 57]. It has been reported that up to 10% of vein conduits are occluded by the end of the first postoperative year [58,59]. Majority of these subclinical or clinically "silent" closures can be accurately detected by MDCT (Figure 10.28).

Late Graft Patency

The major cause of late vein or nonmammary arterial CABG conduit closure or stenosis is either development of occlusive atherosclerosis of the graft or progressive atherosclerosis of the native coronary runoff vasculature. Although, currently, repeat cardiac catheterization and

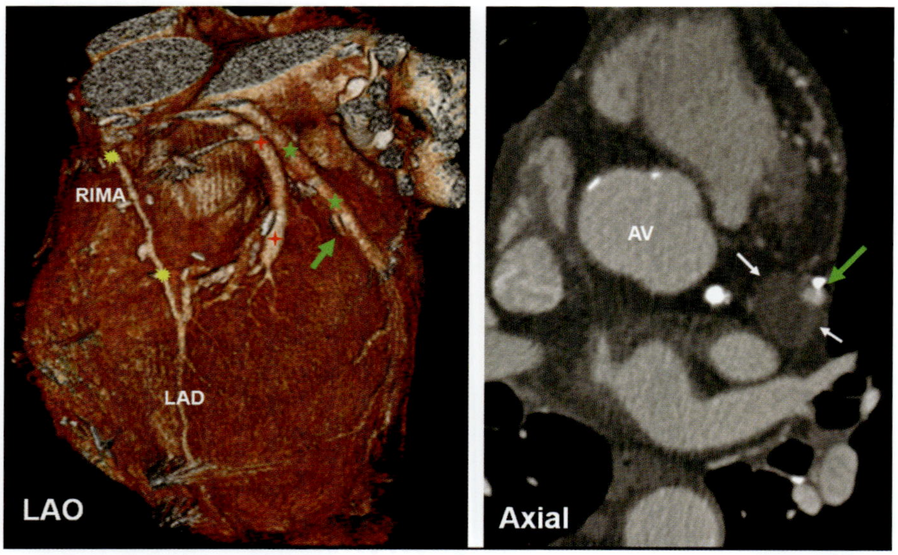

Figure 10.26 Coronary CT angiography in a 79-year-old man shows a patent right internal mammary artery (RIMA, yellow asterisks) that is anastomosed to the left anterior descending (LAD) artery. RIMA has passed anterior to the right ventricular outflow tract before reaching the LAD. The left anterior oblique (LAO) view of the heart also demonstrates two venous grafts (green and red stars) that appear patent. However, axial image at the level of aortic valve (AV) shows a large thrombosed aneurysm (white arrows) medial to the obtuse marginal venous graft (green arrow).

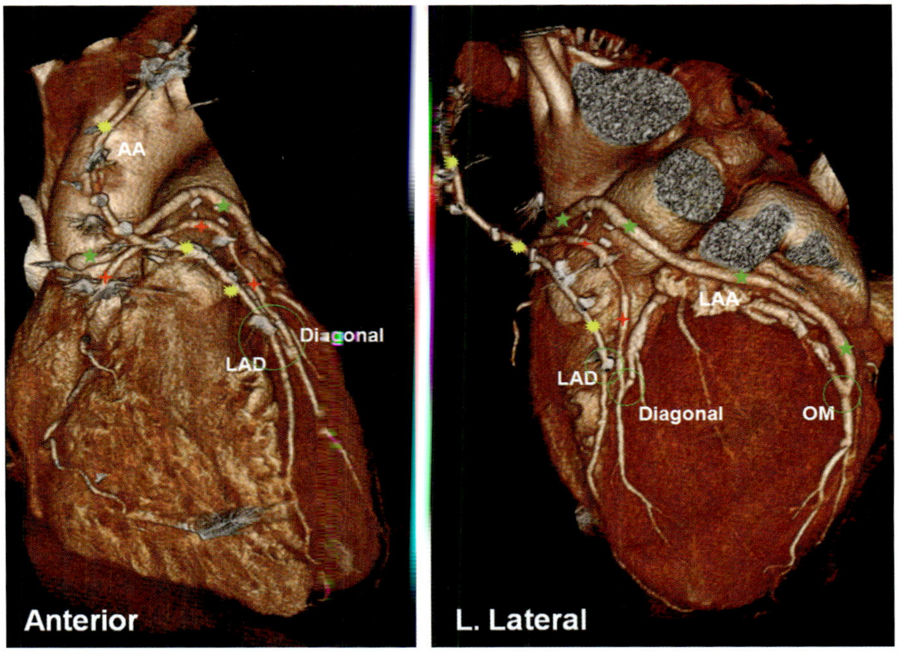

Figure 10.27 Anterior and left lateral views of a three-dimensional volume rendered coronary CT angiography (CTA) after CABG demonstrates three patent grafts. Obtuse marginal (OM) venous graft (Green stars) graft typically travels above the left atrial appendage (LAA) to reach the aortopulmonary window. A free radial graft (red stars) is anastomosed to the anterior wall of the ascending aorta (AA) and to the diagonal artery (end to side). Diagonal graft courses over the main pulmonary trunk and underneath the left internal mammary graft (yellow asterisks) and is commonly attached to the ascending aorta proximal to the OM venous graft. Green circles denote the location of coronary anastomoses. Note the difference in caliber between the arterial and venous grafts. CABG, coronary artery bypass graft; LAD, left anterior descending artery.

coronary angiography are considered the gold standards in the evaluation of remotely constructed bypass conduits, MDCT can produce equal information regarding conduit patency and thus negate the need for repeat angiography in this group of patients (Figures 10.29 and 10.30).

Preoperative Imaging in Redo-Surgery

Another area of great interest in utilization of MDCT for imaging of coronary bypass grafts is in preoperative evaluation of the patients undergoing noncardiac or noncoronary valvular operations with history of a remote prior

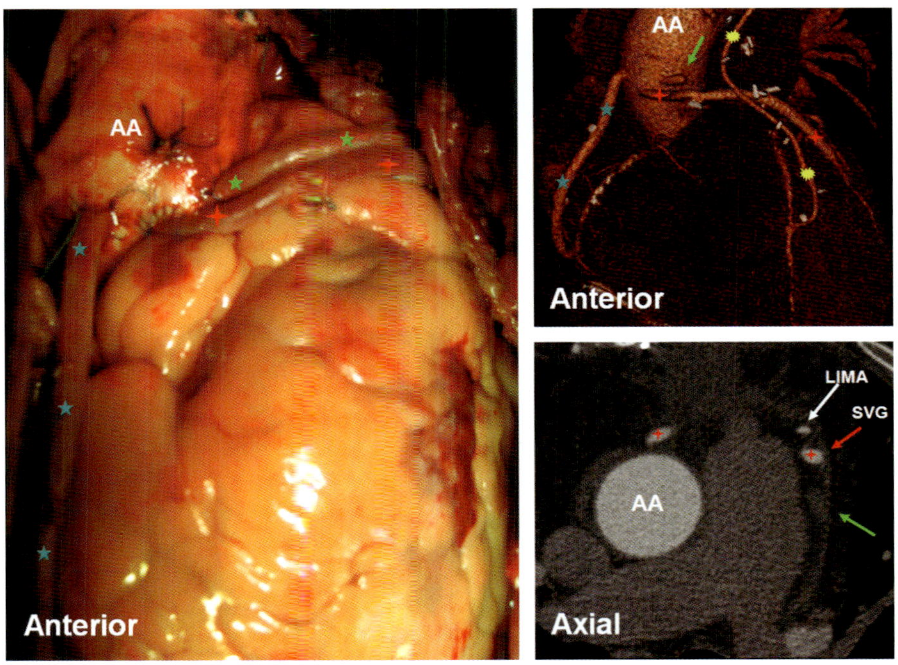

Figure 10.28 The anterior view of the heart at the time of CABG surgery and before construction of the pedicled left internal mammary artery (LIMA) anastomosis. Aortic anastomoses of saphenous vein grafts (SVG) to the right coronary (blue stars), obtuse marginal (green stars), and diagonal arteries (red stars) are shown. Anterior three-dimensional and axial images of coronary CT angiography (CTA) obtained one day after operation shows thrombosed obtuse marginal vein graft (green arrows). The origin of the graft from ascending aorta (AA) is seen on three-dimensional image (green arrow). Diagonal venous graft (yellow stars) and LIMA (yellow asterisks) remain patent. CABG, coronary artery bypass graft.

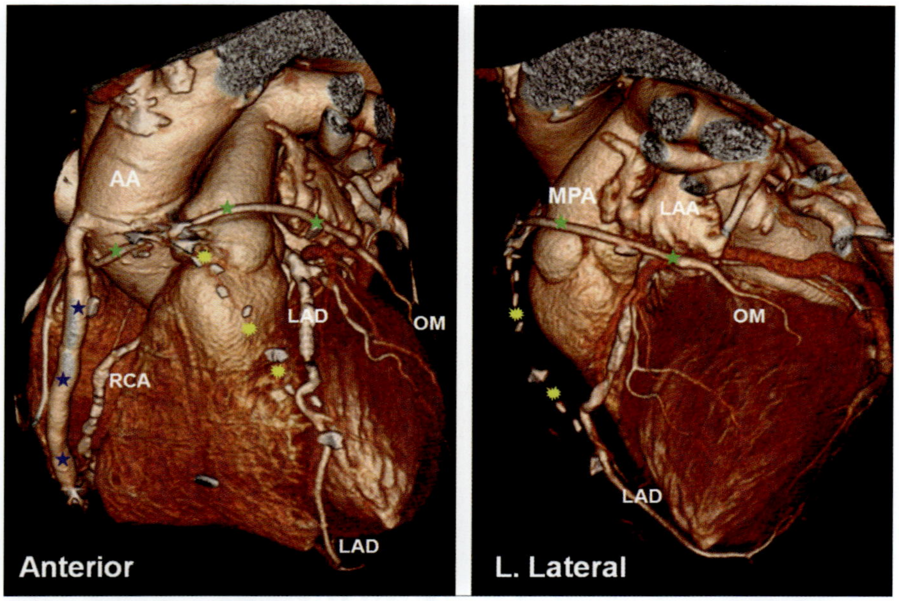

Figure 10.29 Anterior and left (L) lateral views of a three-dimensional volume-rendered coronary CT angiography. MDCT can produce important information regarding the number, anatomic course, and patency of coronary bypass grafts. The right-sided venous graft (blue stars) emerges from the acute margin of the right heart, passing over the free wall of right atrium, to be attached to right anterior wall of the ascending aorta (AA). The obtuse marginal (OM) venous graft is shown (green stars) traveling anterior to the ascending aorta (AA) and main pulmonary artery (MPA), and inferior to the left atrial appendage (LAA) before connecting to the OM artery. The study shows complete occlusion of the left internal mammary artery (LIMA) (yellow asterisks). LAD, left anterior descending artery; RCA, right coronary artery.

CABG procedure [60,61]. Again, traditionally, repeat cardiac catheterization and coronary angiography have been considered the gold standards in evaluation of remotely constructed bypass conduits; however, MDCT may provide equal information regarding conduit patency and thus negate the need for repeat angiography in this group of patients [62] (Figures 10.29 and 10.30).

Furthermore, and perhaps more importantly, MDCT provides superior anatomic detail regarding relationship of the live conduits to the surrounding intrathoracic structure. An important example of the latter advantage is the usefulness of MDCT in delineation of the relationship of a live LIMA graft to the inner table of the sternum, which may result in a major modification of the surgical approach and strategy during sternal reentry [63] (Figure 10.31).

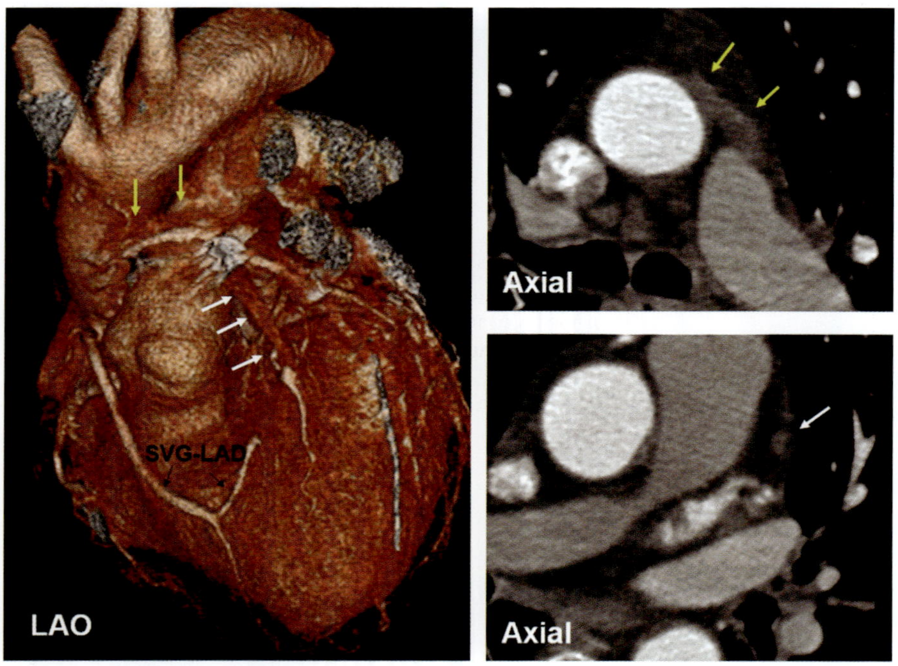

Figure 10.30 Coronary CT angiography is performed in a 73-year-old woman complaining of chest pain. Saphenous vein graft to left anterior descending (SVG-LAD) anastomosis is patent. However, venous grafts to the obtuse marginal artery (yellow arrows) and diagonal artery (white arrows) are occluded. LAO, left anterior oblique view.

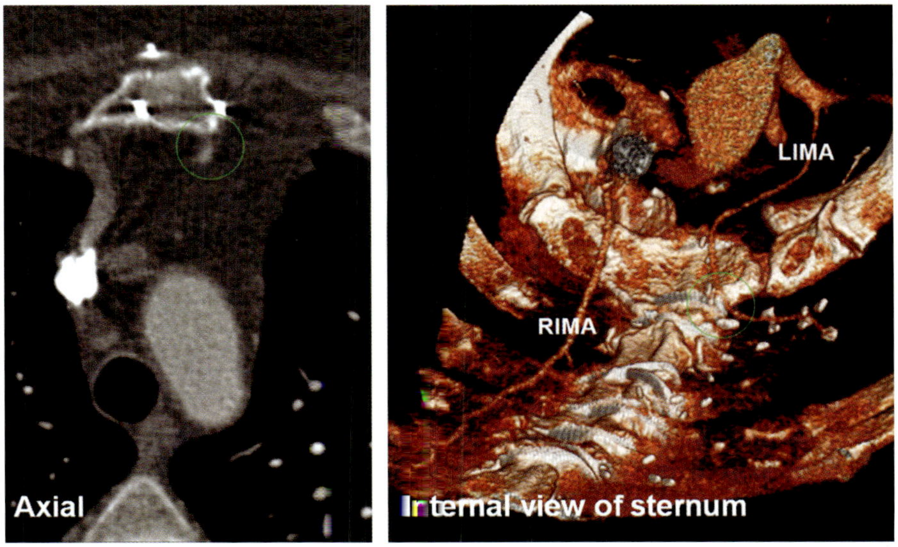

Figure 10.31 Close approximation of left internal mammary artery (LIMA) graft to the posterior wall of sternum (green circle). This may results in a modification of the surgical approach and strategy during sternal reentry. Normal right internal mammary artery (RIMA) is shown. Note, sternal wires from previous surgery on the axial image.

References

1. McAlpine WA. (1975) *Heart and Coronary Arteries: An Anatomical Atlas for Clinical diagnosis, Radiological Investigation, and Surgical Treatment*. Springer-Verlag, New York, pp. 133–178.
2. Wilcox BR, Cook AC, Anderson RH. (2005) *Surgical Anatomy of Heart* (3rd edition). Cambridge University Press, New York, pp. 83–98.
3. Mill MR, Wilcox BR, Anderson RH. (2003) Surgical anatomy of the heart. In Cohn LH. Edmunds LH Jr (eds) *Cardiac Surgery in the Adult*. McGraw-Hill, New York, pp. 31–52.
4. Reig J, Petit M. (2004) Main trunk of the left coronary artery: anatomic study of the parameters of clinical interest. *Clin Anat* 17(1):6–13.
5. Saremi F, Abolhoda A, Ashikyan O *et al.* (2008) Arterial supply to sinuatrial and atrioventricular nodes: imaging with multidetector CT. *Radiology* 246(1):99–107.
6. Kumar N, Saad E, Prabhakar G, De Vol E, Duran CM. (1995) Extended transseptal versus conventional left atriotomy: early postoperative study. *Ann Thorac Surg* 60(2):426–430.
7. Guiraudon GM, Ofiesh JG, Kaushik R. (1991) Extended vertical transatrial septal approach to the mitral valve. *Ann Thorac Surg* 52:1058–1062.
8. Takeshita M, Furuse A, Kotsuka Y, Kubota H. (1997) Sinus node function after mitral valve surgery via the transseptal superior approach. *Eur J Cardiothorac Surg* 12(3):341–344.
9. Misawa Y, Fuse K, Kawahito K, Saito T, Konishi H. (1999) Conduction disturbances after superior septal approach for mitral valve repair. *Ann Thorac Surg* 68(4):1262–1264.
10. Berdajs D, Patonay L, Turina MI. (2003) The clinical anatomy of the sinus node artery. *Ann Thorac Surg* 76:732–735.
11. Nerantzis C, Avgoustakis D. (1980) An S-shaped atrial artery supplying the sinus node area. An anatomical study. *Chest* 78(2):274–278.
12. Saremi F, Channual S, Abolhoda A *et al.* (2008) MDCT of the S-shaped sinoatrial node artery. *AJR Am J Roentgenol* 190(6):1569–1575.
13. Sow ML, Ndoye JM, Lo EA. (2000) The artery of the atrioventricular node: an anatomic study based on 38 injection-dissections. *Surg Radiol Anat* 22(2):93–96.
14. Anderson KR, Murphy JG. (1983) The atrio-ventricular node artery in the human heart. *Angiology* 34(11):711–716.
15. Abuin G, Nieponice A. (1998) New findings on the origin of the blood supply to the atrioventricular node. Clinical and surgical significance. *Tex Heart Inst J* 25:113–117.
16. Kugel MA. (1927) Anatomical studies on the coronary arteries and their branches. I. Arteria anastomotica auricularis magna. *Am Heart J* 3:260–270.
17. Nerantzis CE, Marianou SK, Koulouris SN, Agapitos EB, Papaioannou JA, Vlahos LJ. (2004) Kugel's artery: an anatomical and angiographic study using a new technique. *Tex Heart Inst J* 31:267–270.
18. Abuin G, Nieponice A, Martinez S, Fernando C. (2000) The role of atrial vessels in aortic root and mitral valve operations. *Ann Thorac Surg* 70:1234–1237.
19. von Ludinghausen M, Ohmachi N. (2001) Right superior septal artery with normal right coronary and ectopic early aortic origin: A contribution to the vascular supply of the interventricular septum of the human heart. *N Clin Anat* 14:312–319.
20. Singh M, Edwards WD, Holmes DR Jr, Tajil AJ, Nishimura RA. (2001) Anatomy of the first septal perforating artery: a study with implications for ablation therapy for hypertrophic cardiomyopathy. *Mayo Clin Proc* 76:799–802.
21. Nagueh SF, Ommen SR, Lakkis NM *et al.* (2001) Comparison of ethanol septal reduction therapy with surgical myectomy for the treatment of hypertrophic obstructive cardiomyopathy. *J Am Coll Cardiol* 38(6):1701–1706.
22. Reul RM, Cooley DA, Hallman GL, Reul GJ. (2002) Surgical treatment of coronary artery anomalies: report of a 371/2

year experience at the Texas Heart Institute. *Tex Heart Inst J* 29:299–307.
23. Kim SY, Seo JB, Do KH *et al.* (2006) Coronary artery anomalies: classification and ECG-gated multi-detector row CT findings with angiographic correlation. *RadioGraphics* 26:317–334.
24. Baltaxe HA, Wixson D. (1977) The incidence of congenital anomalies of the coronary arteries in the adult population. *Radiology* 122:47–52.
25. Vilallonga RJ. (2004) Anatomical variations in the coronary arteries. II. Less prevalent variations: coronary anomalies. *Eur J Anat* 8(1):39–53
26. Spindola-Franco H, Grose R, Solomon N. (1983) Dual left anterior descending coronary artery: angiographic description of important variants and surgical implications. *Am Heart J* 105:445–455.
27. Bittner V, Nath HP, Cohen M, Soto B. (1989) Dual connection of the left anterior descending coronary artery to the left and right coronary arteries. *Cath Cardiovasc Diagn* 16:168–172.
28. Topaz O, Vetrovec GW, Wheeler T, Holdaway BK. (1999) Dual anterior interventricular arteries. *Clin Anat* 12(3):153–158.
29. Agarwal PP, Kazerooni EA. (2008) Dual left anterior descending coronary artery: CT findings. *AJR Am J Roentgenol* 191(6):1698–1701.
30. Sajja LR, Farooqi A, Shaik MS, Yarlagadda RB, Baruah DK, Pothineni RB. (2000) Dual left anterior descending coronary artery: surgical revascularization in 4 patients. *Tex Heart Inst J* 27(3):292–296.
31. Möhlenkamp S, Hort W, Ge J, Erbel R. (2002) Update on myocardial bridging. *Circulation* 106:2616–2622.
32. Konen E, Goitein O, Sternik L, Eshet Y, Shemesh J, Di Segni E. (2007) The prevalence and anatomical patterns of intramuscular coronary arteries: a coronary computed tomography angiographic study. *J Am Coll Cardiol* 49(5):587–593.
33. Kantarci M, Duran C, Durur I *et al.* (2006) Detection of myocardial bridging with ECG-gated MDCT and multiplanar reconstruction. *AJR Am J Roentgenol* 186(6 Suppl 2):S391–S394.
34. Vianna CB, Gonzalez MM, Jatene FB, Gama MN, Timerman S, Cesar LA. (2007) Myocardial bridging causing transmural ischemia. Successful coronary artery bypass surgery. *Int J Cardiol* 115; 1: e49–e51.
35. Pratt JW, Michler RE, Pala J, Brown DA. (1999) Minimally invasive coronary artery bypass grafting for myocardial muscle bridging. *Heart Surg Forum* 2(3):250–253.
36. Vlodaver Z, Neufeld HN, Edwards JE. (1972) Pathology of coronary disease. *Semin Roentgenol* 7:376–394.
37. Saremi F, Gurudevan SV, Harrison AT. (2009) Isolated right ventricular infarction owing to anomalous origin of right coronary artery: role of MR and CT in diagnosis. *J Thorac Imaging* 24(1):34–37.
38. Click RL, Holmes DR Jr, Vliestra RE *et al.* (1989) Anomalous coronary arteries: location, degree of atherosclerosis and effect on survival—a report from the coronary artery surgery study. *J Am Coll Cardiol* 13:531–537.
39. Desmet W, Vanhaecke J, Vrolix M *et al.* (1992) Isolated single coronary artery: a review of 50000 consecutive coronary angiographies. *Eur Heart J* 13:1637–1640.
40. Tuncer C, Batyraliev T, Yilmaz R *et al.* (2006) Origin and distribution anomalies of the left anterior descending artery in 70850 adult patients: multicenter data collection. *Cathet Cardiovasc Inverv* 68(4):574–585.
41. Kempf A, Saremi F. (2008) Diagnosis of variants of single right coronary trunk using 64 multidetector computed tomography. *J Radiol Case Rep* 2(5):19–22.
42. Kamiya H, Yasuda T, Nagamine H *et al.* (2002) Surgical treatment of congenital coronary artery fistulas: 27 years' experience and a review of the literature. *J Card Surg* 17(2):173–177.
43. Bourassa MG, Fisher LD, Campeau L *et al.* (1985) Long-term fate of bypass grafts: The Coronary Artery Surgery Study (CASS) and Montreal Heart Institute experiences. *Circulation* 72(6 Pt 2):V71–V78.
44. Campeau L, Lesperance J, Corbara F *et al.* (1978) Aorto coronary saphenous vein bypass graft changes 5 to 7 years after surgery. *Circulation* 58(3 Pt 2):I170–I175.
45. Cameron A, Davis KB, Green G, Schaff HV. (1996) Coronary bypass surgery with internal-thoracic-artery grafts; effects on survival over a 15-year period. *N Engl J Med* 334:216–219.
46. Eagle KA, Guyton RA, Davidoff R *et al.* (2004) ACC/AHA 2004 guideline update for coronary artery bypass graft surgery: A report of the American College of Cardiology/American Heart Association Task Force on Practice Guidelines (Committee to Update the 1999 Guidelines for Coronary Artery Bypass Graft Surgery). *Circulation* 110:e340–e437.
47. Nieman K, Pattynama PM, Rensing BJ *et al.* (2003) Evaluation of patients after coronary artery bypass surgery: CT angiographic assessment of grafts and coronary arteries. *Radiology* 229:749–756.
48. Chiurlia E, Menozzi M, Ratti C *et al.* (2005) Follow-up of coronary artery bypass graft patency by multislice computed tomography. *Am J Cardiol* 95:1094–1097.
49. Meyer TS, Martinoff S, Hadamitzky M *et al.* (2007) Improved noninvasive assessment of coronary artery bypass grafts with 64-slice computed tomographic angiography in an unselected patient population. *J Am Coll Cardiol* 49:946–950.
50. Frazier AA, Qureshi F, Read KM *et al.* (2005) Coronary artery bypass grafts: Assessment with multidetector CT in the early and late postoperative settings. *RadioGraphics* 25:881–896.
51. Marano R, Liguori C, Rinaldi P *et al.* (2007) Coronary artery bypass grafts and MDCT imaging: What to know and what to look for. *Eur Radiol* 17:3166–3178.
52. Loop FD, Lytle BW, Cosgrove DM *et al.* (1986) Influence of the internal-mammary-artery graft on 10-year survival and other cardiac events. *N Engl J Med* 314:1–6.
53. Ura M, Sakata R, Nakayama Y *et al.* (1998) Long-term patency rate of right internal thoracic artery bypass via the transverse sinus. *Circulation* 98:2043–2048.
54. Pick AW, Orszulak TA, Anderson BJ, Schaff HV. (1997) Single versus bilateral internal mammary artery grafts: 10-year outcome analysis. *Ann Thorac Surg* 64:599–605.
55. Possati G, Gaudino M, Prati F *et al.* (2003) Long-term results of the radial artery used for myocardial revascularization. *Circulation* 108:1350–1354.
56. Cox JL, Chiasson DA, Gotlieb AI. (1991) Stranger in a strange land: the pathogenesis of saphenous vein graft stenosis with emphasis on structural and functional differences between veins and arteries. *Prog Cardiovasc Dis* 34(1):45–68.

57. Motwani JG, Topol EJ. (1998) Aortocoronary saphenous vein graft disease: pathogenesis, predisposition, and prevention. *Circulation* 97:916–931.
58. Shah PJ, Gordon I, Fuller J *et al.* (2003) Factors affecting saphenous vein graft patency: clinical and angiographic study in 1402 symptomatic patients operated on between 1977 and 1999. *J Thorac Cardiovasc Surg* 126:1972–1977.
59. Fitzgibbon GM, Kafka HP, Keon WJ, Hooper GD, Burton JR. (1996) Coronary bypass graft fate and patient outcome: angiographic follow-up of 5065 grafts related to survival and reoperation in 1388 patients during 25 years. *J Am Coll Cardiol* 28:616–626.
60. Barner HB. (2008) Operative treatment of coronary atherosclerosis. *Ann Thorac Surg* 85:1473–1482.
61. Cremer J, Teebken OE, Simon A, Hutzelmann A, Heller M, Haverich A. (1998) Thoracic computed tomography prior to redo coronary surgery. *Euro J Cardiothorac Surg* 13:650–654.
62. Kamdar AR, Meadows TA, Roselli EE *et al.* (2008) Multidetector computed tomographic angiography in planning of reoperative cardiothoracic surgery. *Ann Thorac Surg* 85:1239–1245
63. Follis FM, Pett SB, Miller KB, Wong RS, Temes RT, Wernly JA. (1999) Catastrophic hemorrhage on sternal reentry: still a dreaded complication? *Ann Thorac Surg* 68:2215–2219.

11 Anatomy for Electrophysiologic Interventions

Farhood Saremi[1] & Damián Sánchez-Quintana[2]

[1] *University of California Irvine, UCI Medical Center, Irvine, CA, USA*
[2] *University of Extremadura, Badajoz, Spain*

Introduction

Catheter ablation of cardiac arrhythmias has rapidly evolved from a highly experimental procedure to a standard form of therapy for various tachyarrhythmias, surpassing pharmacological treatments, and surgical methods [1, 2]. The advances in this field has included (a) the development of techniques of catheter ablation that often requires the precise destruction of minute amounts of arrhythmogenic tissues and (b) techniques of resynchronization therapy that require pacing different parts of the atria as well as the ventricular branches of the coronary venous system [1–3]. Preprocedural knowledge about cardiac anatomy can save time and improve the success rate and safety of the procedure by helping the electrophysiologist choose the appropriate region to perform the ablation. Localization of the anatomic structures of the atria before ablation is usually performed by using fluoroscopy, electroanatomic mapping, and intracardiac echocardiography [4, 5].

With recent technological advancement in multidetector CT (MDCT) scanners, it has been possible to perform a "virtual dissection" of the heart and cardiovascular system [6, 7]. In this chapter, we describe the normal anatomy of the heart landmarks of interest to electrophysiologists, including their relationship to other structures and their anatomic variants. Most radiological images are performed with a 64-slice scanner using standard retrospectively ECG-gated coronary CT angiography protocol.

Revisiting Cardiac Anatomy: A Computed-Tomography-Based Atlas and Reference, 1st edition. Edited by Farhood Saremi, Eloisa Arbustini, Stephen Achenbach and Jagat Narula.

Catheter-Based Ablations

Catheter-based ablation is usually preceded by a diagnostic electrophysiological study (EPS). A diagnostic EPS involves fluoroscopy-guided insertion of multiple catheters via the venous or arterial system to study and record electrical activity from the atria, ventricles, and other specific parts of the conduction system as well as to induce various arrhythmias to find the underlying mechanism. Atrioventricular (AV) conduction is studied by positioning a separate catheter across the tricuspid annulus and recording a His bundle electrogram. To obtain recordings of the left atrium (LA) and sometimes the left ventricle (LV), a catheter is guided into the coronary sinus (CS). Left-sided procedures involving the LA and the LV are performed via a transseptal approach or via a retrograde approach from the femoral or brachial artery (Figure 11.1).

Radiofrequency (RF) current is the most commonly used energy source for cardiac ablation, delivering thermal energy to destroy the tissue [8]. Typical RF lesions are small, usually 3–6 mm in diameter and up to 3 mm deep when a standard catheter tip is used [1, 9]. Old ablation sites with RF may be smaller than acute lesions. Other energy sources that can be used include lasers, microwave, and ultrasound.

The success of catheter ablation varies depending on the type of arrhythmia and the clinical situation. High success (>90%) and low complications (<3%) are seen in ablation procedures for arrhythmias such as AV nodal reentry, accessory pathways, atrial flutter (AFL), idiopathic ventricular tachycardia, and AV node (AVN) or junction ablation. Lower success (<90%) and higher complications (>3%) are seen in ablation procedures for atrial fibrillation (AF), postinfarction ventricular tachycardia [1, 9].

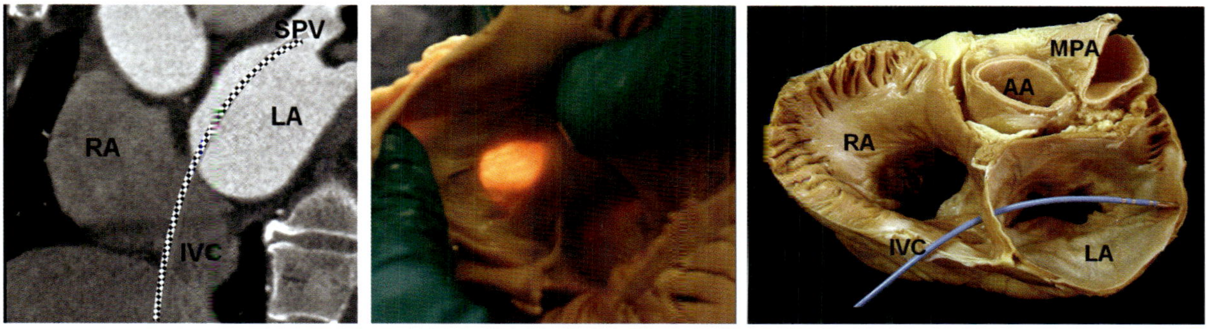

(a), (b) (c)

Figure 11.1 Transseptal intervention is usually performed under fluoroscopic guidance. The oval fossa is probed or a transseptal puncture is made if a patent foramen ovale is absent. This technique is not without complications, which demands precise anatomic characterization of interatrial septum. (a) Short-axis view at the level of inferior vena cava (IVC) demonstrates the location of the oval fossa. The position of a transseptal catheter is shown on the CT image. Transseptal puncture is easier when approached via the IVC. (b) The right atrial view of dissected human heart shows transillumination of thin membranous oval fossa. (c) Short-axis view of dissected human heart showing a probe through the oval fossa going into the left atrium. AA, ascending aorta; LA, left atrium; MPA, main pulmonary artery; RA, right atrium; SPV, superior pulmonary vein.

Tachycardias and Anatomic Considerations for Treatment

Electrocardiographically, tachyarrhythmias are divided based on the width of the QRS complex (Table 11.1).

A variety of tachyarrhythmias can be targeted for percutaneous catheter ablation (Figure 11.2). RF ablation for AVN reentry, isthmus-dependent AFL, and paroxysmal AF is performed almost entirely as an anatomy-based ablation in many centers.

Table 11.1 Narrow QRS complex tachyarrhythmias are generally supraventricular in origin

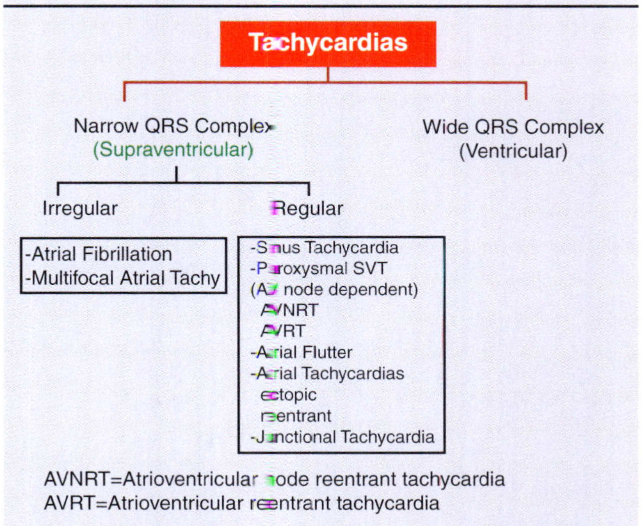

Supraventricular tachycardias (SVT) are defined as any tachycardia in which the atrium including the atrioventricular (AV) node and AV junctional portion are critical to the perpetuation of the tachycardia. The three types of supraventricular tachycardias include AV nodal reentry, atrioventricular reentry, and atrial tachycardia. Generally, atrial flutter and fibrillation are considered to be distinct entities.

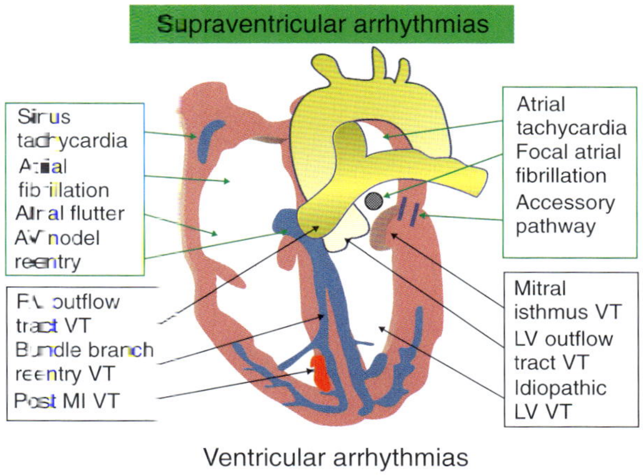

Figure 11.2 Anatomic consideration in the treatment of supraventricular and ventricular arrhythmias. A variety of tachyarrhythmias can be targeted for percutaneous catheter-based ablation, including both atrial and ventricular arrhythmias that are either focal or that utilize reentrant circuits. AV, atrioventricular; LV, left ventricle; MI, myocardial infarction; RV, right ventricle; VT, ventricular tachycardia.

Cardiac Conduction System

The cardiac conduction system consists of the sinoatrial node (SAN), AVN, the penetrating AV bundle (His bundle), the right and left bundle branches, as well as the fascicles and the Purkinje fibers (Figure 11.3). The conduction system is composed of specialized myocytes. Its atrial components, the SAN (subepicardial) and the AVN (subendocardial), are in contact with atrial myocardium [10, 11]. While no morphologically distinct conduction pathway between the SAN and AVN is demonstrable, functional pathways due to geometric arrangement of working muscle fibers could be responsible for conduction between the two structures along certain preferential routes [11,12]. The His bundle penetrates the right fibrous trigone [central fibrous body (CFN)] and runs at the junction of membranous septum with and muscular septum before dividing into the right and left ventricular bundle branches [13]. The His bundle measures 1–2 cm in length. The right bundle branch is a cord-like structure approximately 5 cm in length and 1 mm in diameter, which runs along the septal and moderator bands to reach the anterior papillary muscle. The left bundle branch, in contrast, forms a broad sheet of conduction fibers that divides along the left side of interventricular septum into three indistinct fascicles [14].

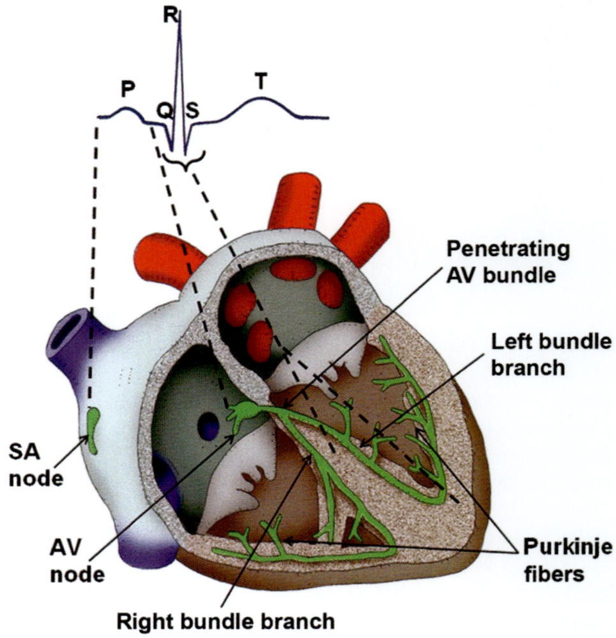

Figure 11.3 Diagrammatic representation of the cardiac conduction system (in green) and the activation sequence on a surface electrocardiogram. The penetrating bundle perforates the insulating tissue plane of the atrioventricular (AV) junction to be the only bridge of muscular continuity between atrial and ventricular myocardium. SA, sinoatrial.

Anatomic Landmarks of the Right Atrium

The right atrium (RA) is the anatomic gateway to the LA and a thorough understanding of its anatomy and anatomic variants is essential. The RA has three components: the appendage, the venous part, and the vestibule [11]. The crista terminalis is a large muscular ridge that separates the smooth walled venous part (sinus venarum) from the trabeculated appendage (Figure 11.4). The right atrial appendage is large and contains multiple pectinate muscles. The sinus venarum is located posterolaterally and receives the systemic [from the superior vena cava (SVC) and inferior vena cava (IVC)] and coronary (via the CS and small Thebesian veins) venous return. The

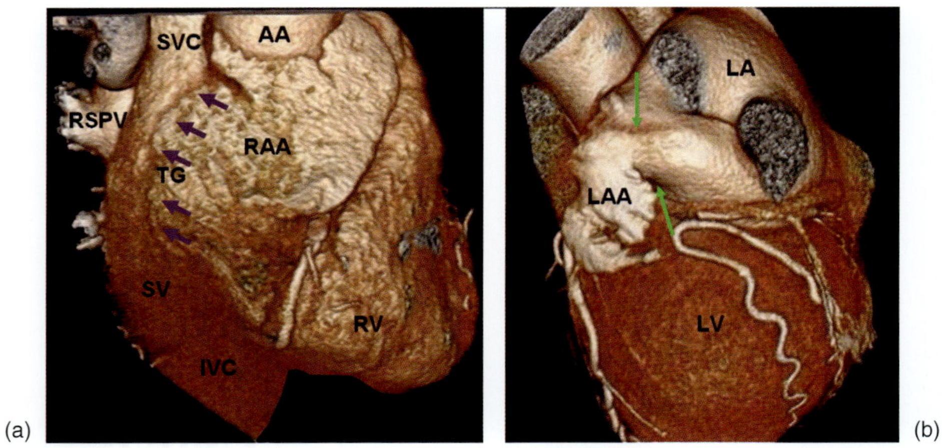

Figure 11.4 Lateral epicardial views of the heart. The dominant feature on the right side (a) is a large triangular-shaped atrial appendage. Usually, a fat-filled groove can be seen along the lateral wall. This is the terminal groove (TG), or sulcus terminalis corresponding to crista terminalis internally. The sinus node is located in this groove, close to the cavoatrial junction. The right superior pulmonary vein (RSPV) passes posterior to the superior vena cava (SVC). The left atrial appendage (b) is characteristically a small-lobulated structure. It is a potential site for deposition of thrombus owing to its tubular shape, trabeculated margin, and narrow junction with the left atrium (arrows in (b)). AA, ascending aorta; IVC, inferior vena cava; LA, left atrium; LAA, left atrial appendage; LV, left ventricle; RAA, right atrial appendage; RSPV, right superior pulmonary vein; RV, right ventricle; SV, sinus venarum; SVC, superior vena cava.

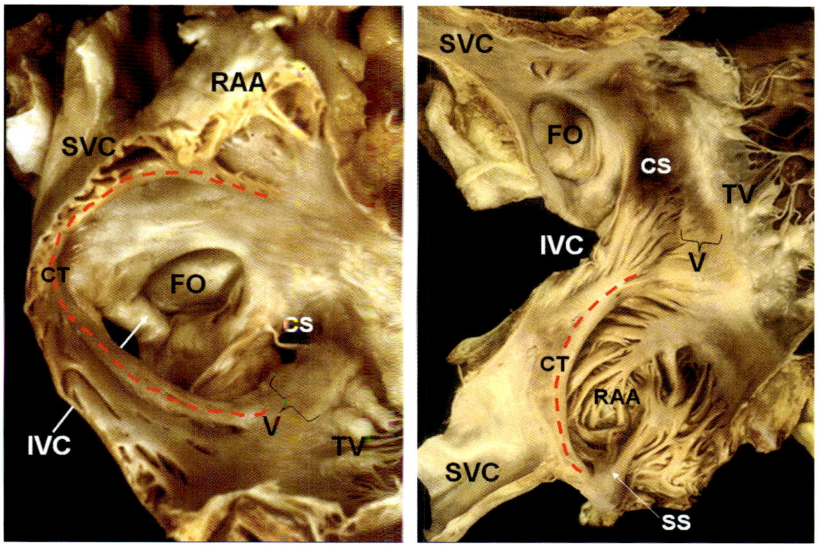

(a) (b)

Figure 11.5 (a) Opened right atrium in simulated right anterior oblique view to show the C-shaped terminal crest (red dotted line). The crest arches anterior to the orifice of the superior vena cava (SVC) and extends to the area of the anterior interatrial groove. Inferiorly, the crest turns in beneath the orifice of the inferior vena cava (IVC), breaking up into a series of trabeculations in the area of the atrial wall. (b) The right atrium opened and the lateral wall deflected so as to display the crest (CT, red line) on the endocardial surface separating the smooth-walled venous component from the trabeculated right atrial appendage (RAA). The "septum spurium" (SS) is the most prominent anterior pectinate muscle arising from the terminal crest (white arrows). CS, coronary sinus; CT, crista terminalis; FO, fossa ovalis; TV, tricuspid valve; V, vestibule (brace).

right atrial vestibule is a smooth muscular wall around the tricuspid orifice and supports the leaflets of the tricuspid valve (TV). The characteristic feature of the vestibule is that it is surrounded by the pectinate muscles of the RA.

Crista Terminalis (Terminal Crest)

The crista terminalis is a C-shaped ridge of muscle formed by the junction of the sinus venosus and primitive RA [12, 15, 16]. The crista terminalis extends from the anteromedial wall on the left side of the entrance of the SVC, passes rightward in front of the venous orifice before descending laterally, curving to the right of the entrance of the IVC to continue as an array of finer bundles that enter the region of the atrial wall recognized as the inferior isthmus or cavotricuspid isthmus (CTI) (Figures 11.5 and 11.6). From the lateral margin of the crest arises a series of muscle bundles known as pectinate muscles that fan out from the crest toward the vestibular portion. One of the anterosuperior bundles is usually more prominent, and it is described as the "septum spurium" or "sagittal muscle bundle," a convenient landmark for dividing the appendage into anteromedial and posterolateral components (Figure 11.5) (also see Figure 1.7 in Chapter 1).

An understanding of the anatomic variant and the normal appearance of a large crista terminalis will minimize the misdiagnosis of this structure (Figures 11.7 and 11.8).

Excess epicardial fat can infiltrate around the RA causing marked thickening of the crista terminalis and interatrial septum (lipomatus hypertrophy of the septum)

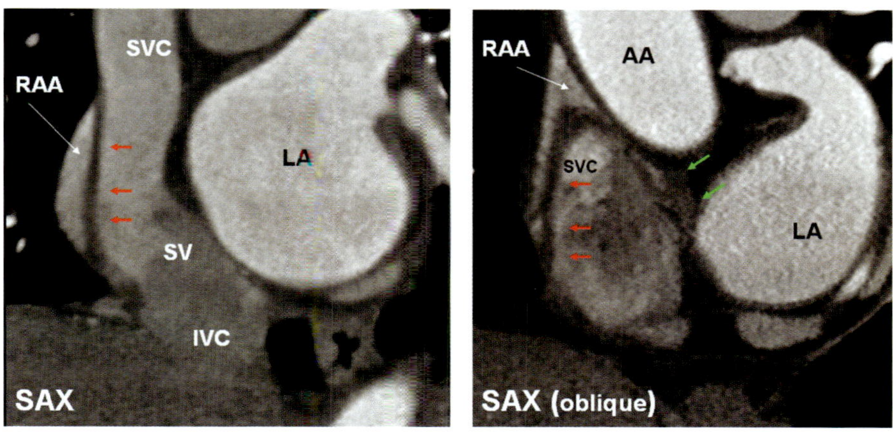

Figure 11.6 Short-axis (SAX) images in two different patients demonstrate the crista terminalis (CT, red arrows) as a dark band between the right atrial appendage (RAA) and the sinus venarum (SV) extending from the superior vena cava (SVC) to the inferior vena cava (IVC). Superiorly, the CT arches anterior to the orifice of the SVC and extends to the area of the anterior interatrial groove and merges with the interatrial bundle, commonly known as Bachmann bundle (green arrows). The inferior border of the CT near the IVC orifice is indistinct and merges with small trabeculations of the inferior portion of cavotricuspid isthmus. AA, ascending aorta; LA, left atrium.

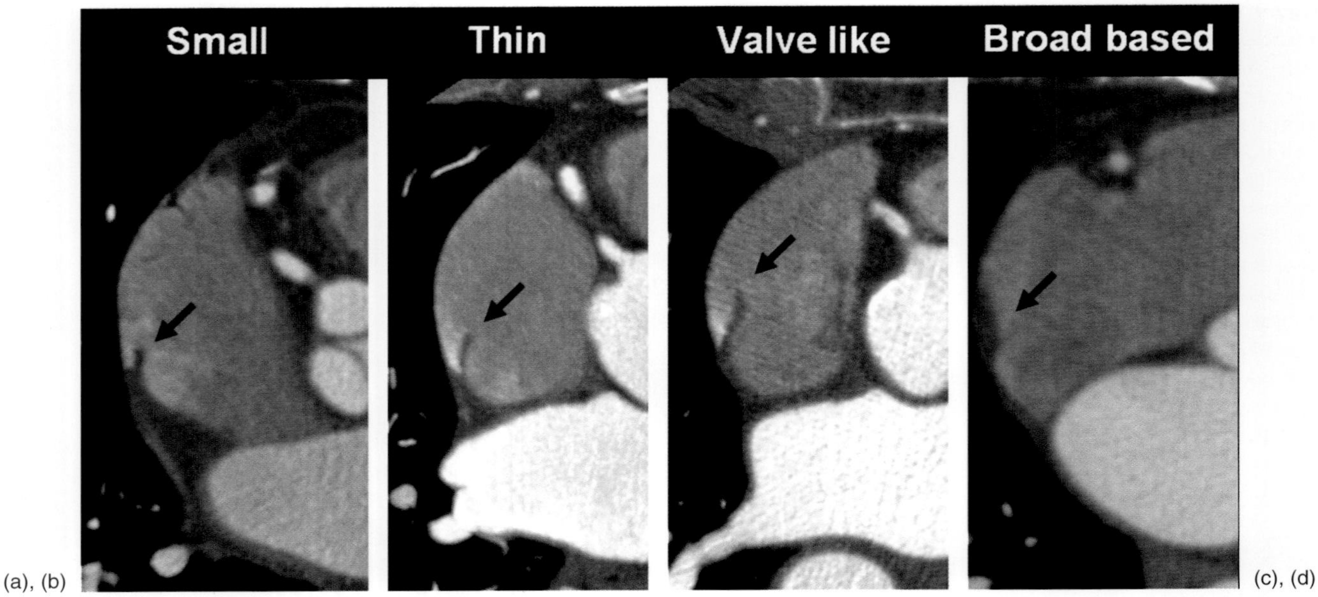

Figure 11.7 The crista terminalis varies in size and extent in different individuals. Axial CT scans show how the crista terminalis (arrowhead) varies in length and thickness, appearing as a small (a), thin (b), valve-like (c), or broad-based (d) structure.

which may mimic a mass (Figures 11.9 and 11.10) [17] or interfere with normal conduction [18, 19]. The crista terminalis is a significant structure in several forms of atrial tachyarrhythmias, and occasionally, it is the target for RF catheter procedures [20, 21]. It is suggested that the thickness of the crista terminalis may lead to the development of typical AFL [20].

SAN and SAN Artery

The SAN is the source of the cardiac impulse. Histologically, it is composed of cells slightly smaller than normal working cells [22–24]. The SA is a subepicardial spindle-shaped structure at superior cavoatrial junction that extends from SVC along crista terminalis toward the IVC [24]. It gradually penetrates musculature of the crest to

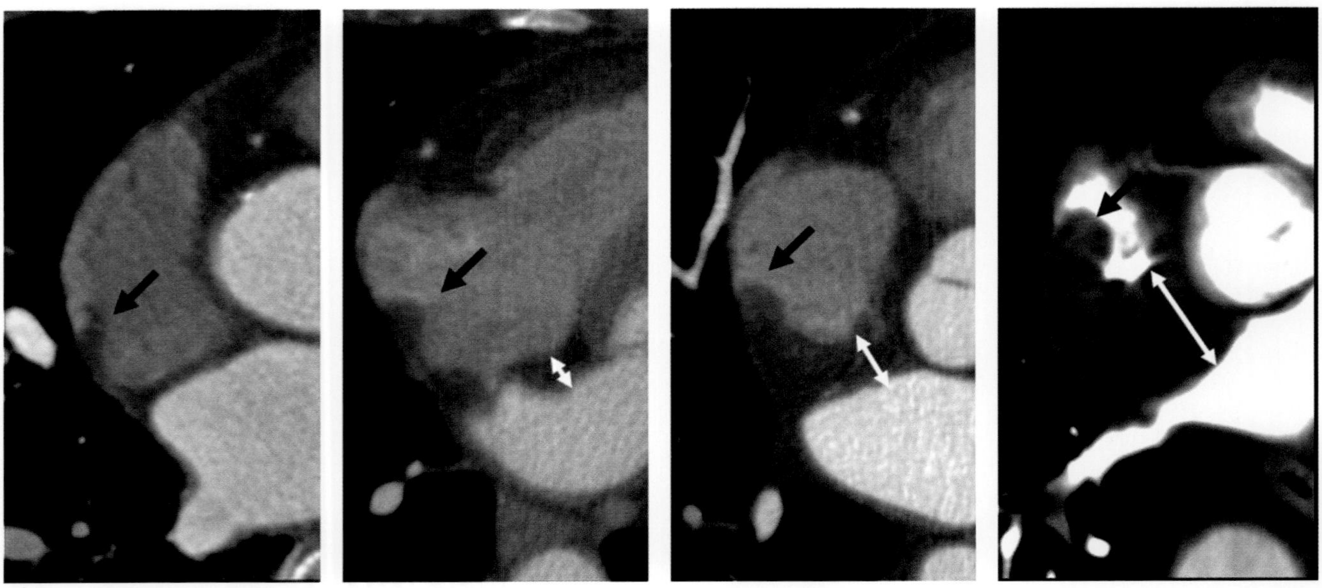

Figure 11.8 Axial CT scans show differing amounts of fat infiltration of the crista terminalis (black arrows) and varying degrees of lipomatous hypertrophy of the septum (double-headed arrow). A large crista terminalis can mimic a mass at echo studies. (Reprinted with permission from Saremi and Krishnan [7].)

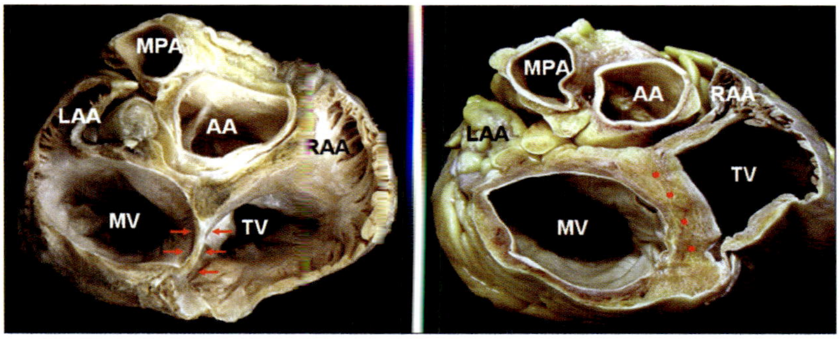

Figure 11.9 Right and left atrioventricular junctions at the ventricular base are displayed with the heart positioned anatomically. The true atrial septum (red arrows in (a)) is limited to the floor of the fossa ovalis, and its immediate muscular rim at the anteroinferior part. The epicardial fat can infiltrate around the interatrial septum the so-called lipomatose septum (b) (red dots). AA, ascending aorta; LAA, left atrial appendage; MPA, main pulmonary artery; MV, mitral valve; RAA, right atrial appendage; TV, tricuspid valve.

rest in the subendocardium. SAN varies in position and length along the crista terminalis. Mean length of the SAN is reported 20 ± 3 mm [16]. Sinus cells are characterized by being clearer and embedded in a dense connective tissue matrix (Figure 11.11). With age, the amount of connective tissue increases with respect to the area occupied by the nodal cells [25] in the periphery of the node; specialized cells are mixed with those of the working myocardium (Figure 11.11). In addition, multiple radiations or extensions interdigitating with the working atrial myocardium have been described. These penetrate intramyocardially into the crest, epicardium, and the SVC [24]. SAN can be localized in axial CT images by locating the SAN artery along the crista terminalis (Figures 11.12 and 11.13).

Modification of the sinus node using RF has been established as a treatment for inappropriate sinus tachycardia [26]. Because of the subepicardial location of SAN, approaching from the endocardial surface requires more RF energy to ablate the sinus node [15]. MDCT can be used to measure the thickness of the crest and demonstrate the approximate location of SAN artery within the nodal tissue. The centrally located nodal artery may provide a cooling effect, reducing the RF damage [15, 24, 26].

The SAN artery is usually, a single branch, arising from the proximal right coronary artery (RCA) (60%) or left circumflex (LCx) artery (40%) [27, 28] (Figure 11.14).

In a recent anatomic study of the conduction system arteries by MDCT, a single SAN artery from the RCA was seen in 66% of patients and from the LCx artery in 28% [29]. A dual blood supply to SAN was seen in 6%: one from the RCA and the other from the LCx artery. Regardless of its artery of origin, the SAN artery usually courses along the anterior interatrial groove (IAG) toward the superior cavoatrial junction (Figure 11.15). At the cavoatrial junction, SAN artery course becomes variable and may circle

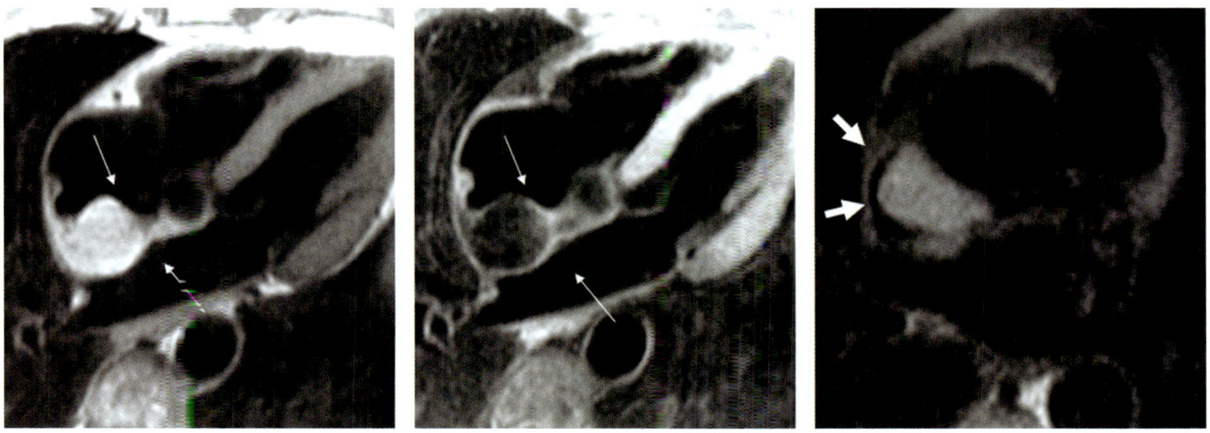

Figure 11.10 Lipomatose hypertrophy of interatrial septum. Axial black blood MR images before (a) and after (b) fat suppression show a large fatty mass in the anatomic region of interatrial septum with approximately 3 × 3 × 3 cm in diameter (arrow). Note complete suppression of the signal of the mass on (b). In addition, the mass causes flow turbulence in the superior vena cava (c) that is narrowed and slit-like, as it empties into the right atrium (thick arrows). At its narrowest point, the SVC measured 2.0 mm in diameter with peak systolic velocity at about 80–100 cm/s on velocity flow mapping (not shown).

(a), (b)

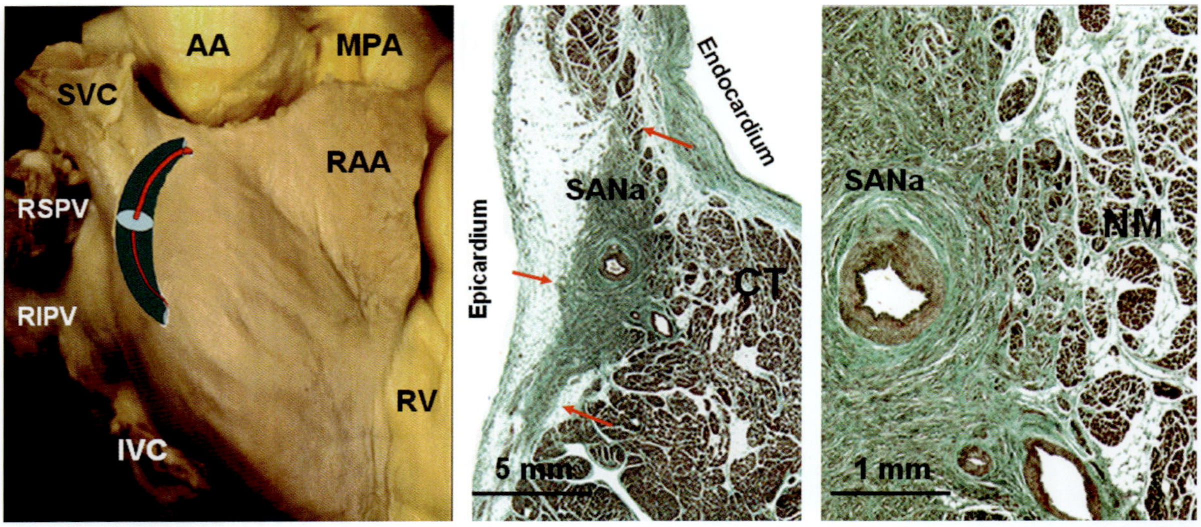

(c)

Figure 11.11 (a) Location of the sinus node (crescent) with a central nodal artery (red line). (b) Histological section of the sinus node body (Masson trichrome stain) within a dense matrix of connective tissue (green color) and showing nodal extensions (arrows) as well as a central position of the nodal artery (NA). Note in (c) the irregular contour of the sinus node intermingled with the neighboring myocardium (NM) without a discrete fibrous border. AA, ascending aorta; Ao, aorta; CT, crista terminalis; IVC, inferior vena cava; MPA, main pulmonary artery; RAA, right atrial appendage; RIPV, right inferior pulmonary vein; RSPV, right superior pulmonary vein; RV, right ventricle; SANa, sinoatrial node artery; SVC, superior vena cava.

either anteriorly (precaval) or posteriorly (retrocaval) to enter the node (Figure 11.16).

Koch's Triangle

Another area of significance to electrophysiologist is the triangle of Koch (Figures 11.17 and 11.18). This triangle is bordered posteriorly by a fibrous extension from the Eustachian valve called the tendon of Todaro [30]. Anterior border is demarcated by the attachment of septal leaflet of the TV. The apex of this triangle corresponds to the CFB of the heart where the His bundle penetrates. The so-called fast pathway corresponds to the area of musculature close to the apex of the triangle of Koch, the anatomic location of AVN. The base of the triangle is the orifice of the CS, and the vestibule of RA immediately anterior to it. This

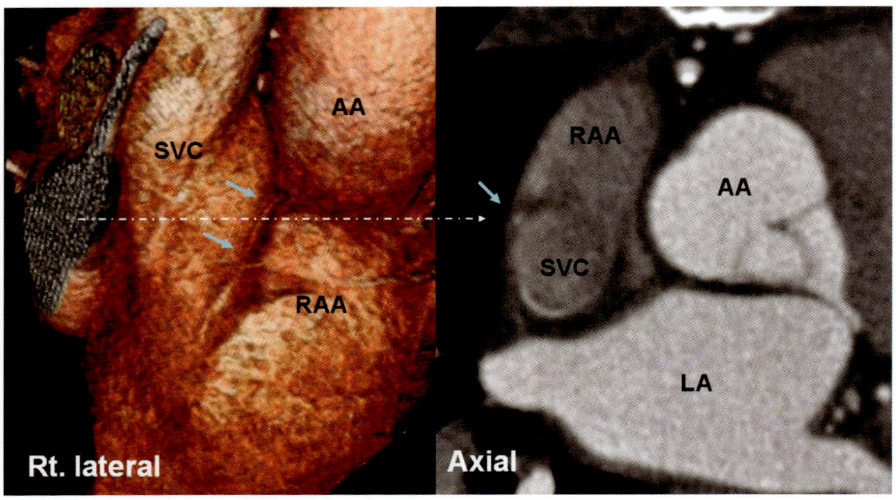

Figure 11.12 Right lateral three-dimensional view of the heart shows the terminal segment of SAN artery (blue arrows) in the sulcus terminalis. Corresponding axial view (long arrow) at the level of SAN demonstrate the central position of the SAN artery within the crista terminalis. The SAN is arranged around the SAN artery. AA, ascending aorta; LA, left atrium; RAA, right atrial appendage; SAN, sinoatrial node; SVC, superior vena cava.

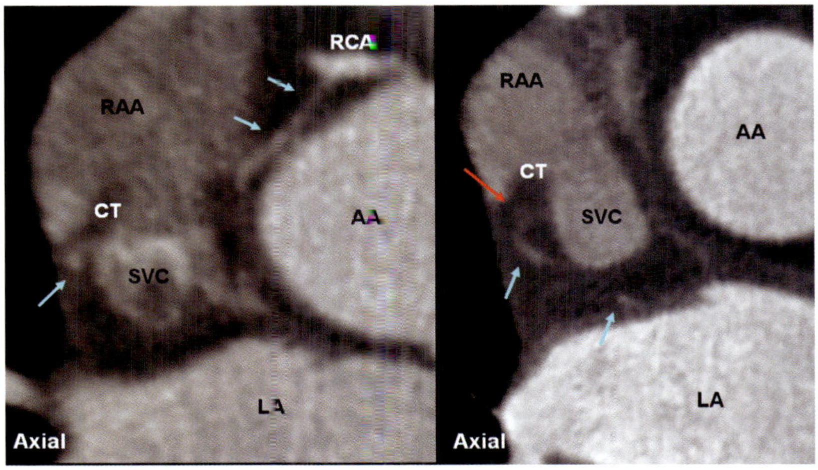

Figure 11.13 Axial images at the level of the superior cavoatrial junction. The SAN is arranged around the SAN artery, which can run centrally inside the node or eccentrically adjacent to it. In the majority of hearts (70%), the SAN artery is located centrally within the node. (a) shows the terminal segment of the SAN artery as a rounded area of enhancement within the crista terminalis (CT) the anatomic location of SAN. (b) Axial image of a different patient again shows the eccentric course of the SAN artery (blue arrows) in relation to the SAN (red arrow). AA, ascending aorta; LA, left atrium; RAA, right atrial appendage; RCA, right coronary artery; SAN, sinoatrial node; SVC, superior vena cava.

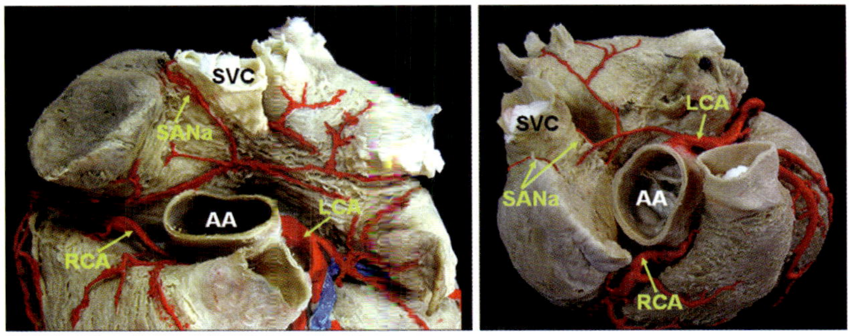

Figure 11.14 Arteries are painted in red. (a) The sinoatrial node artery (SANa) arising from the right coronary artery (RCA) and courses along the anterior interatrial groove toward the superior cavoatrial junction (precaval). (b) Note the SANa arising from the left main coronary artery (LCA) and courses around the SVC=superior vena cava (pericaval) to enter the node. AA, ascending aorta.

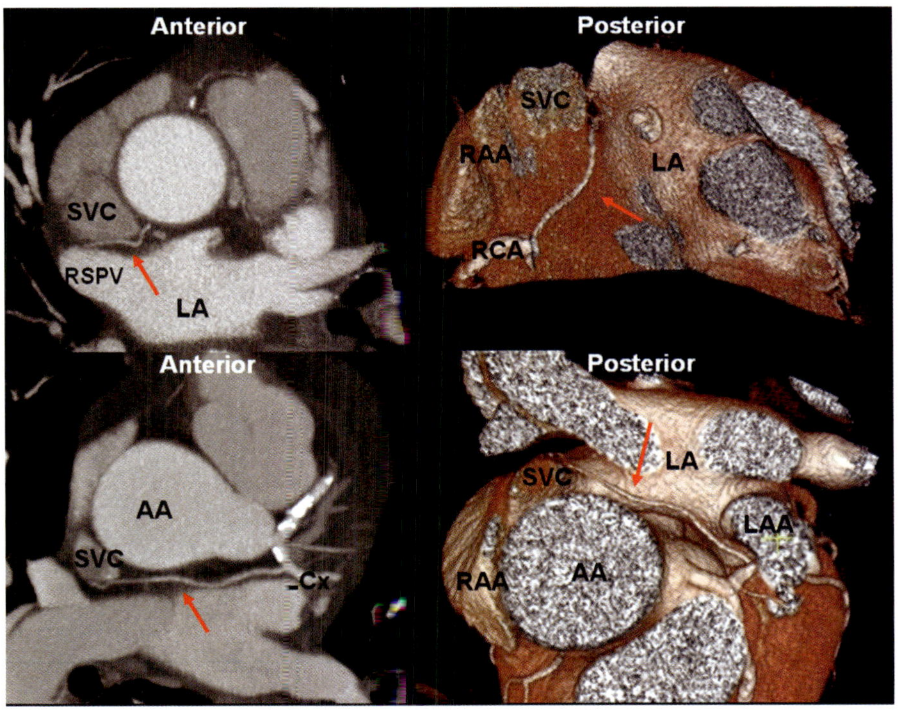

Figure 11.15 Axial images of coronary CT angiogram (left) and the superior views of the sculptured three-dimensional reconstruction of the heart (right) are shown. Straight red arrows point to the retrocaval SAN artery arising from the RCA (upper images) and from the LCx (lower images). In retrocaval variant, the artery is very close to the interatrial groove, posterior wall of the SVC, and right superior pulmonary vein (RSPV). In the transverse sinus, left SAN artery travels very close to the anterior wall of LA (red arrows in lower images) and lefty atrial appendage (LAA). AA, ascending aorta; LA, left atrium; LCx, left circumflex artery; RA, right atrium; RAA, right atrial appendage; RCA, right coronary artery; SVC, superior vena cava. (Reprinted with permission from Saremi *et al.* [29]).

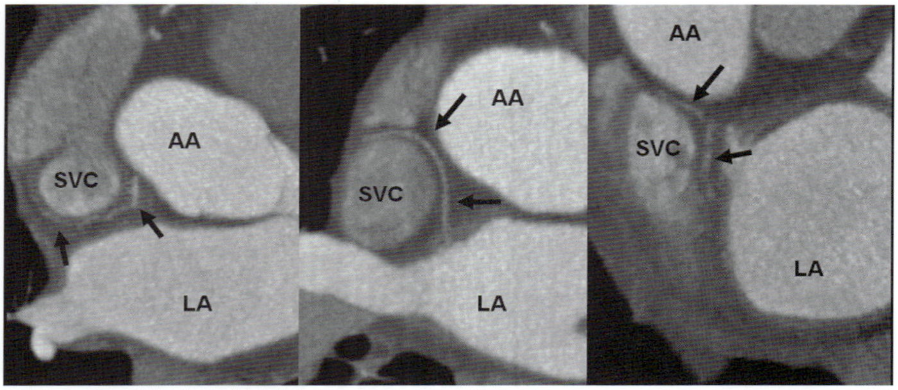

Figure 11.16 Axial images show different modes of termination of the sinoatrial node (SAN) artery (arrows) relative to the SVC. The terminal SAN arteries approach the SAN anterior to the SVC (precaval) 42.5%, posterior to the SVC (retrocaval) in 47.5%, and through multiple branches surrounding the SVC (pericaval) in 10% [29]. AA, ascending aorta; LA, left atrium; SVC, superior vena cava.

part of the vestibule confined between the orifice of the CS and the attachment of the septal leaflet of the TV, often referred to as the septal isthmus, is the area often targeted for ablation of the "slow pathway" in AVNRT [31]. It is also the target for ablation of isthmus-dependent AFL (Figure 11.17). The dimensions of Koch's triangle vary from one individual to another, which is clinically relevant in the case of catheter ablation procedures in this area that are guided largely by anatomic landmarks.

AVN and AVN Artery

The AVN resides at apex of Koch's triangle. AVN consists of a compact portion and an area of transitional cells [31]. The compact portion lies over the CFB (Figure 11.19). The size of the transitional cells is intermediate between those of the AVN and the atrial working cells. They are surrounded by a greater quantity of connective cells than that covering the working cells, but they are not insulated from the adjacent myocardium. Rather, they form a kind of bridge between the working and nodal myocardium and collect electrical information from the atrial walls, transmitting it to the AVN. The AVN continues distally with the His bundle. The penetrating His bundle can readily be distinguished from the compact node at the point where the conduction axis itself becomes completely surrounded by tissues of the CFN and conducts electrical pulses to the ventricles [31]. The transition from AVN to His bundle is close to the apex of the triangle of Koch.

(a), (b)

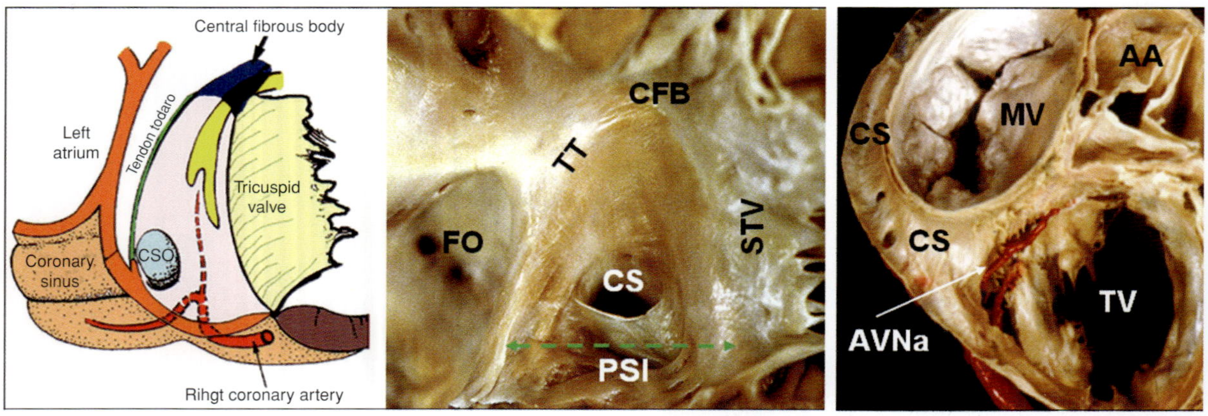

(c)

Figure 11.17 (a) Schematic drawing showing the course of the atrioventricular (AV) nodal artery to the AV node through the triangle of Koch and toward the central fibrous body (CFB). The AV node is colored yellow. (b) Endocardial view of the posterior and septal walls of the right atrium to show the fossa ovalis (FO) and limits of the triangle of Koch, the tendon of Todaro (TT), and the insertion of the septal leaflet of the tricuspid valve (STV). The apex of the triangle is the CFB, and the base is known to electrophysiologists as the paraseptal isthmus (PSI). (c) Basal views showing macroscopically the course of the AV nodal artery (AVNa) across the triangle of Koch. Note the artery at the base of the triangle, the artery runs inferior to the mouth of the coronary sinus and follows a course close to the septal attachment of the tricuspid valve. AA, ascending aorta; CS, coronary sinus; CSO, coronary sinus orifice; MV, mitral valve; TV, tricuspid valve.

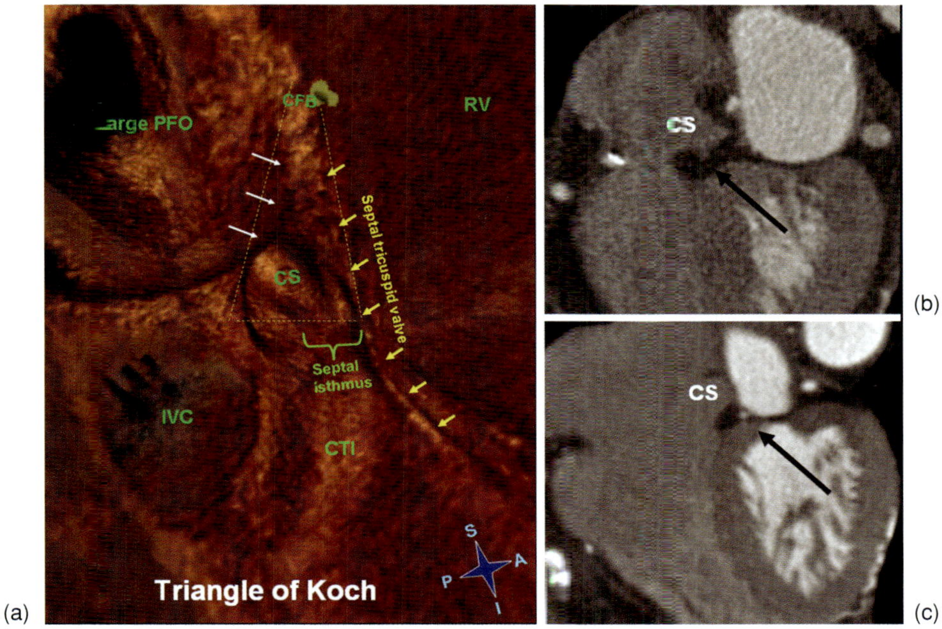

Figure 11.18 Relationship between the atrioventricular (AV) nodal artery and the base of the triangle of Koch (coronary sinus ostium). (a) Endocardial view of the right atrioventricular junction showing the anatomic boundaries of the triangle of Koch. The triangle is oriented with the central fibrous body (CFB) at the apex and is demarcated by the tendon of Todaro posteriorly (white arrows), the hingeline of the septal tricuspid valve (yellow arrows) anteriorly, and the coronary sinus at the base. The septal isthmus (green bracket) is also located at the base of the triangle, connecting the tricuspid annulus to the coronary sinus ostium. (b) and (c) Four-chamber views at the level of CS ostium in two different patients. The black arrows point to AVN artery at the level of septal isthmus. Note variable distances of the AVN artery to the surface of the endocardium. There is a risk of arterial coagulation during ablation procedures when the artery is located in close proximity to the septal wall (b). CS, coronary sinus; CTI, cavotricuspid isthmus; IVC, inferior vena cava; PFO, patent foramen ovale; RV, right ventricle. Orientation: A, anterior; I, inferior; P, posterior; S, superior. (Reprinted with permission from Saremi *et al.* [29]).

The AVN artery originates from the apex of the U turn of distal RCA and penetrates into the base of the posterior interatrial septum (inferior pyramidal space) at the level of crux of the heart in 80–87% of patients [29, 32–34] (Figure 11.20). In the remaining, it originates from the terminal portion of LCx artery (8–13%) or uncommonly from both RCA and LCx (2–10%). The artery provides branches to the posterior interventricular septum, interatrial septum, AVN, and penetrating bundle of His [33].

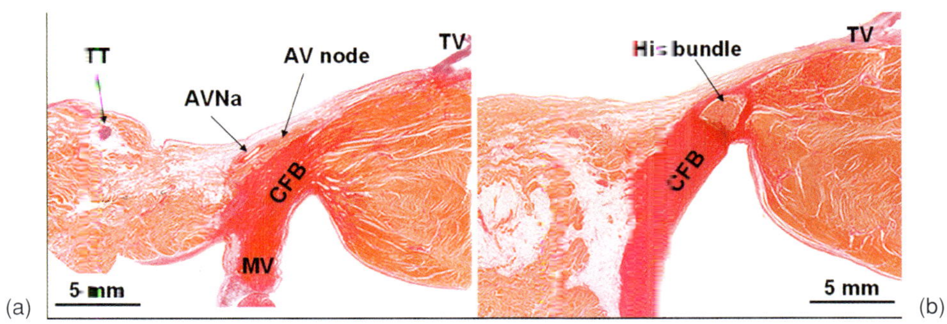

Figure 11.19 Sagittal histological sections through the compact part of the node and penetrating His bundle stained with elastic van Gieson. (a) Note the AV nodal artery (AVNa) in the body AV node, the semioval shape of the compact AV node and the transitional cells in contact with the convex surface of the compact node that lies over the central fibrous body (CFB). Part (b) shows the penetrating bundle of His surrounded by fibrous tissue (red) from the CFB. AV, atrioventricular; MV, mitral valve; TT, tendon of Todaro; TV, tricuspid valve.

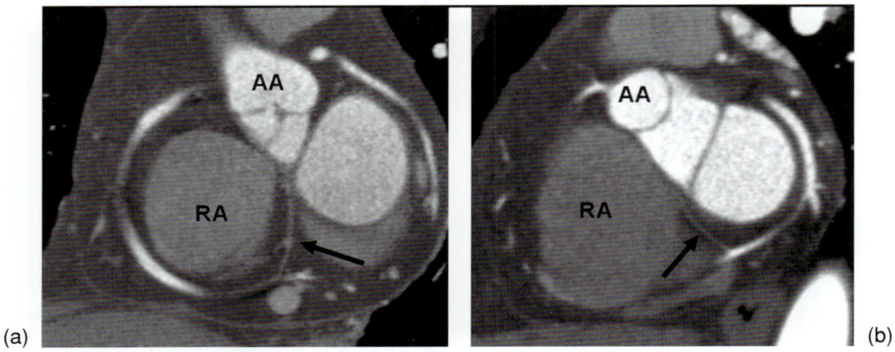

Figure 11.20 Short-axis views of crista terminalis (CT) coronary angiography. Arrows point to right atrioventricular nodal (AVN) artery arising from right coronary artery (RCA) (a) or from left circumflex (LCx) artery (b). AA, ascending aorta; RA, right atrium.

At the level of Koch's triangle, the AVN artery, in some patients, runs just beneath the endocardium near the ostium of the CS and septal isthmus (Figure 11.18). This may explain the possible risk of the AVN artery coagulation during RF ablation in the slow pathway region, although complete AV block is commonly a direct result of tissue injury to AVN [35, 36]. In a study of cadaveric hearts, Sánchez-Quintana *et al.* found that the mean distance of the artery to the endocardial surface at the base of Koch's triangle was 3.5 ± 1.5 mm [36]. Demonstration of this relationship can easily be performed by MDCT scan [29] (Figure 11.18).

CTI and AFL

AFL can be categorized as dependent on the CTI or typical, and nonisthmus dependent or atypical [1]. The commonest type of AFL is isthmus-dependent AFL in which the reentrant circuit is confined to the tricuspid annulus with the wavefront progressing either in a counterclockwise or clockwise direction across the CTI, the area between the IVC and the TV (Figure 11.21).

The CTI is the target of catheter-directed ablation procedures, the treatment of choice for AFL [37, 38]. Autopsies, angiographic, and echocardiographic studies have shown that the anatomy of this structure is highly variable

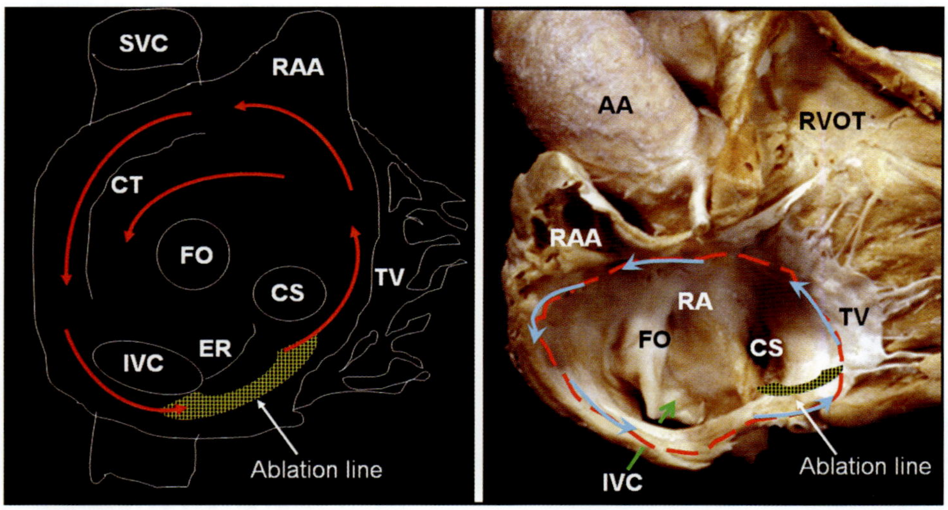

Figure 11.21 Diagrammatic and heart specimen representation of the reentry circuit of the common variety of right atrial flutter (type I). The right atrium (RA) is shown in a right anterior oblique projection. The reentrant circuit (arrows) is confined to the right atrium by the tricuspid valve annulus (TV) and barriers to conduction within the right atrium and circulates in a counterclockwise direction within it (arrows). The shaded area between the tricuspid annulus and the inferior vena cava indicates the critical isthmus of tissue that is targeted for ablation of this type of atrial flutter. AA, ascending aorta; CS, coronary sinus; CT, crista terminalis; ER, Eustachian ridge; FO, fossa ovalis; IVC, inferior vena cava; RAA, right atrial appendage; RVOT, right ventricle outflow tract; SVC, superior vena cava.

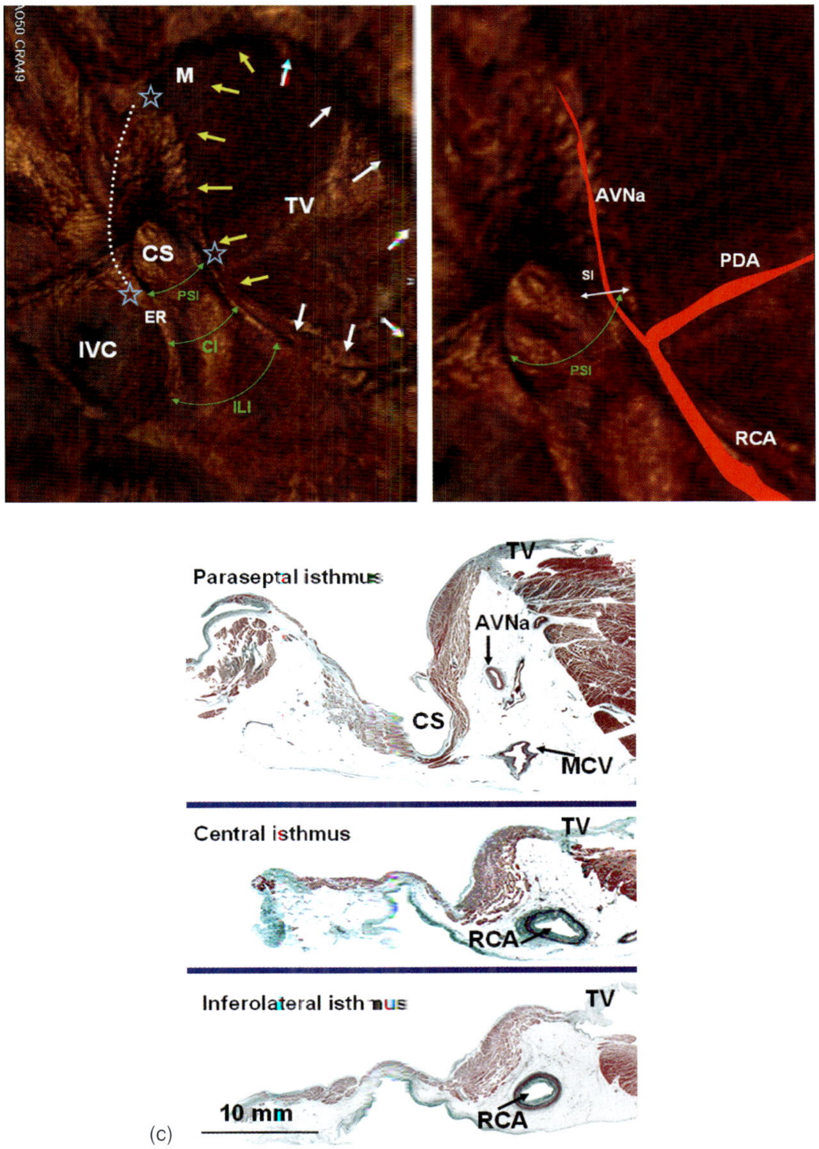

(a) (b) (c)

Figure 11.22 (a) Endocardial view of the right atrioventricular (AV) junction shows the Koch's triangle (demarcated by stars) and right atrial cavotricuspid isthmus (CTI). The CTI lies between the orifice of IVC and septal tricuspid valve (TR). Three levels of CTI are shown (green arrows): inferolateral isthmus (ILI), central isthmus (CI), and paraseptal isthmus (PSI). Central and paraseptal isthmi are common targets for ablation of atrial flutter. The anterior segment of paraseptal isthmus between the coronary sinus (CS) ostium and septal tricuspid valve (yellow arrows) is called septal isthmus (SI). The septal isthmus is often the target for ablation of the "slow pathway" in AV nodal reentrant tachycardia. Koch's triangle is bordered posteriorly by a fibrous extension from the Eustachian valve/ridge (ER) called the tendon of Todaro (white line) and anteriorly by the attachment of septal tricuspid valve (yellow arrows). Paraseptal isthmus forms the base of the Koch's triangle consisting of the ostium of CS (CS) and septal isthmus. In the magnified view of the CTI (b), the anatomic course of the AV nodal artery (AVNa) in relation to the septal isthmus (SI) is shown. The AVNa arises from the penetrating U turn of right coronary artery (RCA) near the takeoff of posterior descending artery (PDA). (c) Sagittal histological sections stained with Masson's trichrome at the level of the three levels of isthmus from a heart specimen that has a dominant RCA. IVC, inferior vena cava; M, membranous septum; MCV, middle cardiac vein; TV, tricuspid valve. (Reprinted with permission from Saremi *et al.* [46].)

[39–41]: patients with a short and straight CTI require fewer RF ablation applications and shorter X-ray exposure [42].

Obstacles such as a large Eustachian ridge/valve (ER), deep sub-Thebesian recess (STR), and other pouchlike recesses may also lead to longer and more difficult ablation sessions [42,43]. Cabrera *et al.* divided the CTI into three parallel levels [39,40]. With the heart in attitudinal orientation, they identified and measured the lengths of three levels of isthmus: paraseptal (24 ± 4 mm), inferior (19 ± 4 mm), and inferolateral (30 ± 3 mm). Paraseptal isthmus forms the base of Koch's triangle. The inferior isthmus also known as the "central isthmus" owing to its location between the other two isthmuses represents the optimal target for ablation, as this is the site where the IVC orifice is closest to the TV insertion (Figure 11.22). It is also shown that most diameters are larger in patients with chronic AFL (larger RA) compared with paroxysmal AFL or control groups [40,44].

The CTI dimension is highly variable (Figure 11.23) Anatomic study with CT scan using image data during different cardiac phases has shown that the CTI is longest at all three parallel levels during mid-ventricular systole [45]. At this phase, the central isthmus length is

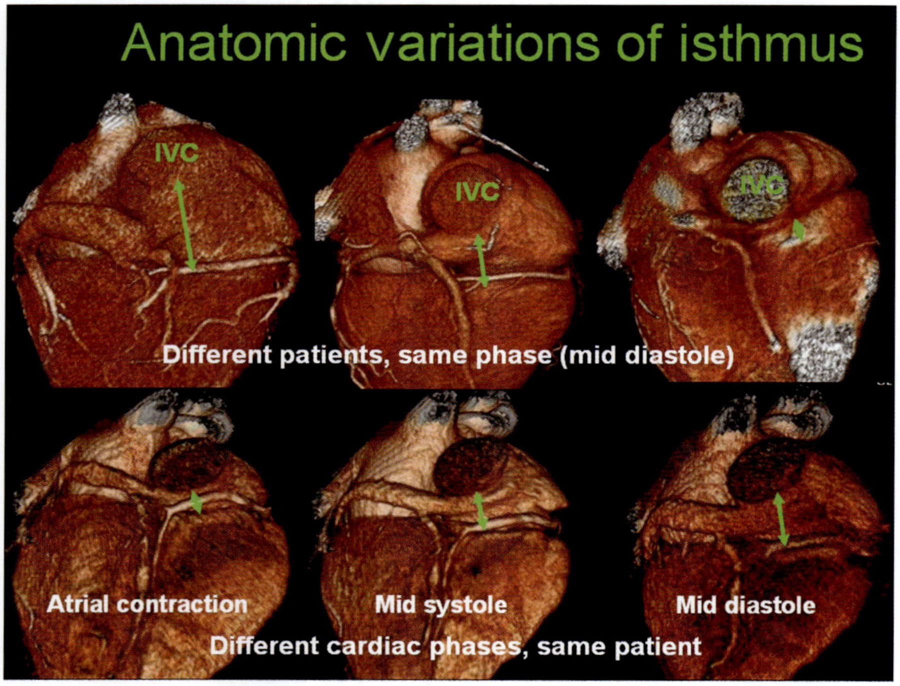

Figure 11.23 Three-dimensional posterior views of the heart. The length of the CTI varies in different individuals (upper row) and different cardiac phases (lower row). Knowledge of these anatomic variants prior to catheter ablation will save time and increases the success rate. CTI, cavotricuspid isthmus; IVC, inferior vena cava. (Reprinted with permission from Saremi *et al.* [45]).

greater than 30 mm in 32% of patients. The CTI varies in size during the cardiac cycle becoming deeper with atrial contraction. The measurements also showed a total of 40% variation in length during one cardiac cycle. In around 28% of population a "hook-shaped" morphology is seen, showing a concave or pouchlike segment posteriorly (at the IVC side) and a flat vestibular part anteriorly (Figure 11.24).

Eustachian Valve/Ridge

Information related to the size of the ER and presence of an enlarged Eustachian valve is important and can be demonstrated with MDCT (Figure 11.25). The free border of the Eustachian valve continues as a tendon of Todaro that runs in the musculature of the Eustachian ridge. A large ER is an anatomic barrier and forms a line of fixed

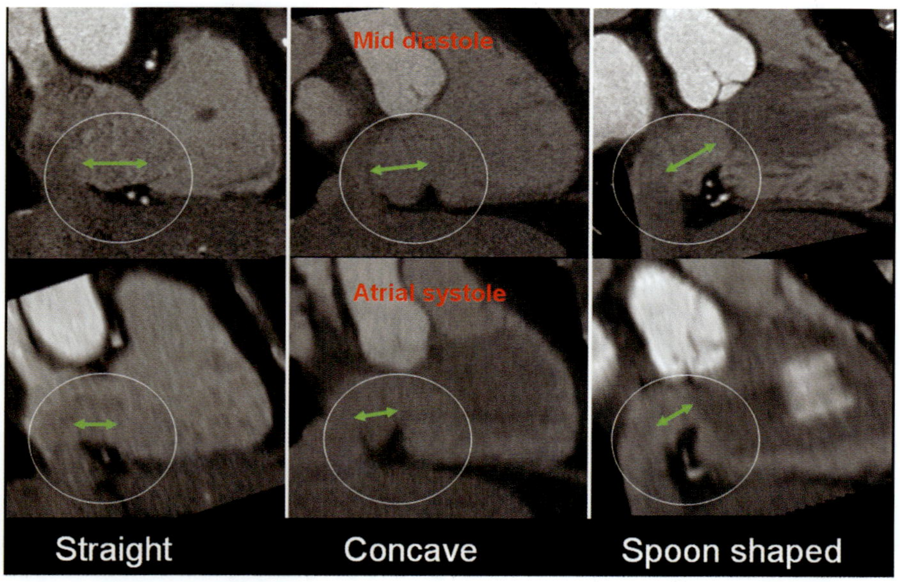

Figure 11.24 Long-axis and two-chamber views of the right heart (right anterior oblique) through the central isthmus of the CTI (green arrows) demonstrate three distinct morphologies: straight, concave/pouchlike, and hook shaped. The profile appearance of the CTI will change in different phases of cardiac cycle particularly with atrial contraction, as it gets deeper and shorter. As shown in the hook-shaped variant, the posterior part of the CTI that is closer to the IVC has nearly disappeared with atrial contraction. Knowledge of these anatomic variants prior to catheter ablation will save time and increases the success rate. CTI, cavotricuspid isthmus; IVC, inferior vena cava.

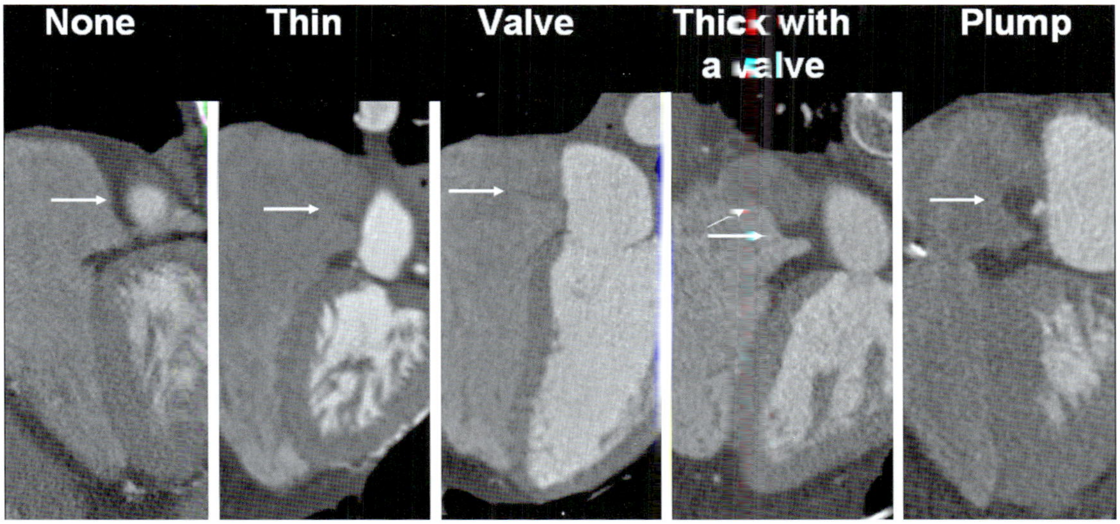

Figure 11.25 Four-chamber images of the heart are the best views to characterize the Eustachian valve/ridge (ER). The ER varies in size and thickness in different individuals. In 26% of patients, a thick ER (>4 mm) can be seen.

conduction block during typical AFL [43,46]. It is demonstrated that in patients with large ER, paraseptal isthmus block can be obtained only after the complete ablation of the enlarged ER [47]. Cabrera *et al.* [39] demonstrated that 26% of their heart specimens had a thickened ER with a mean thickness of 3.2 ± 0.8 mm. A thick ER > 4 mm is seen in 24% of normal population studied with CT scan [45]. Angiographic study by Heidbuchel *et al.* showed an enlarged Eustachian valve in 24% of patients, with consequent increase in number of ablation pulse applications for achievement of successful block [41].

Sub-Thebesian Recess (Sinus of Keith, Sub-Eustachian Sinus)

The presence of a large STR or deep pouches is associated with statistically more RF applications compared with straight isthmus [11,12]. The STR recess is an extension of a pouchlike isthmus under the orifice of the CS (Figures 11.26 and 11.27).

Local RF delivery may be impaired by this structure as an area of limited blood flow results in delayed catheter tip cooling. In one angiographic study of the CTI, this pouch was observed in 47% of patients and had a mean depth of 4.3 ± 2.1 mm (1.5–9.4) [41]. CT scan in normal population has shown a deep STR combined with a pouchlike (>5 mm) central isthmus in 45% of mid-diastolic phase images (Figure 11.28). This finding would be useful in preprocedural planning, where the presence of a large pouch would dictate a central approach to the ablation.

Interatrial Septum

Partitioning the atrial chambers, the true atrial septum is limited to the floor of the fossa ovalis and its immediate muscular rim at the anteroinferior part, which is confluent with the apical part of Koch's triangle. The floor of the fossa ovalis represents the embryonic primary atrial septum (septum primum). On the right side of the septum primum, the major part of the muscular rim (also known as the limbus) is an infolding of the right atrial wall representing the embryonic "septum secundum," and the rim is a characteristic feature of the septal aspect of the right atrial. Epicardial fat fills the groove between the SVC and the right pulmonary veins (PVs), which is also known as IAG or septal raphe and not a true septum [48] (Figures 11.29–11.31). The floor of the fossa is the valve that closes shut against the rim so long as the blood pressure in the LA exceeds that in the RA. For this to happen, the valve has to be large enough to overlap the rim. Closure of the fossa is complete when the valve becomes adherent to the rim. Therefore, inadvertent puncture outside the limited margins (limbus) of the oval fossa during transseptal interventions will perforate the heart, rather than provide access to the LA via the septum. The size of fossa ovalis and its margins may vary greatly. In 25–35% in autopsy studies [49], the seal is incomplete leaving a crevice at the anterosuperior quadrant of the rim that allows a probe to be passed obliquely from the RA (patent foramen ovale, PFO) (Figure 11.29). On the left atrial side, the crevice is marked by the crescentic free edge of the valve. This nonfusion creates the tunnel like PFO

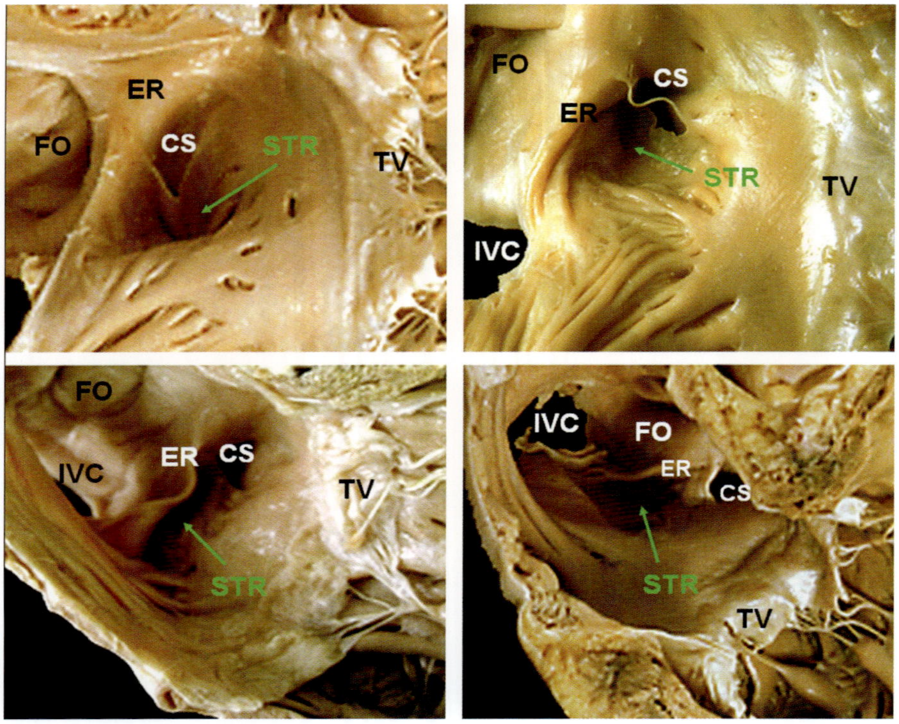

Figure 11.26 Panels show examples of variations in morphology and depth of the sub-Thebesian recess (STR) in different specimens. CS, Coronary sinus; ER, Eustachian ridge; FO, fossa ovalis; IVC, inferior vena cava; TV, tricuspid valve.

orientated in a craniocaudal, dorsoventral, and right-to-left axis.

The probe patent fossa has been linked to multiple clinical events, such as migraines or cryptogenic stroke [50,51]. This has led to the application of percutaneous closure techniques originally developed to treat atrial septal defects [52]. These techniques can have important complications [53], which may be mitigated by precise definition of interatrial septal anatomy. Functional and morphologic characteristics of the PFO are closely related. The floor of the oval fossa varies considerably in dimensions as does the thickness of the muscular rim [54]. Prominent muscular rims are helpful to interventionists to feel a "jump," as the tip of the catheter drops into the flap valve allowing the

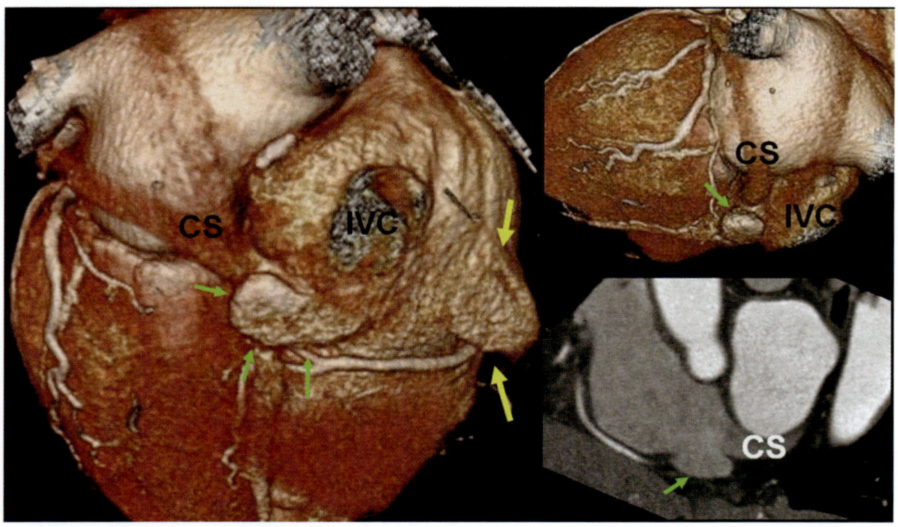

Figure 11.27 Sub-Thebesian recess (STR) is a diverticular extension of cavotricuspid isthmus under coronary sinus (CS). Posterior three-dimensional view and short-axis image at the level of CS demonstrate a relatively large STR (green arrows) inferior to the Thebesian valve. It is anterior to the orifice of the IVC and sub-Thebesian rather than sub-Eustachian. Presence of a large STP may act as an anatomic barrier to access CS or may impair local RF delivery during ablation of isthmus-dependent flutter. A large inferolatral pouch is seen (yellow arrows). IVC, inferior vena cava.

valve to "tent" into the LA when carrying out transseptal punctures. Crossing the "septum" too anteriorly runs the risk of exiting the RA into the transverse pericardial sinus and beyond into the aortic root. The flap valve guarding the oval fossa is usually thin, with a bilaminar crossing arrangement of myofibers and varying amounts of fibrous tissue. In some hearts, it is thinner and aneurysmal in appearance as it herniates into the atrial chambers through the respiratory cycle. Although every PFO has the potential to shunt blood, this potential is much greater in certain morphologies such as with an incompetent valve or atrial septal aneurysm (ASA) [55,56] (Figures 11.32 and 11.33). It is important to know that the presence of a membranous flap valve is not synonymous with a PFO. In a recent anatomic study of interatrial septum with CT scan, a flap valve was seen in 38.3% patients, and out of which, 60% was patent at the entry into the RA (PFO). The length of the flap is important for competency of a PFO tunnel. Short flap length (<6 mm) is usually associated with a shunt through the PFO tunnel [57]. Cardiac views such as short axis (SAX) and four chambers (4ch) perpendicular to the interartrial septum in different phases are required for complete anatomic study of the fossa ovalis including the PFO shunt [57,58] (Figure 11.30).

Anatomic variations of the interatrial septum are common [24]. ASA is defined as a localized bulge (>15 mm) of the interatrial septum that protrudes into the RA or the LA [57]. Anatomically, it is a bulge in the region of septum primum underlying the oval fossa (Figure 11.32). In a CT study, ASA was seen in 4.2% patients, and of these patients, a shunt was seen in 63.6%. ASAs are increasingly being recognized as closely associated with cryptogenic strokes and migraine headaches [59]. A PFO is also as-

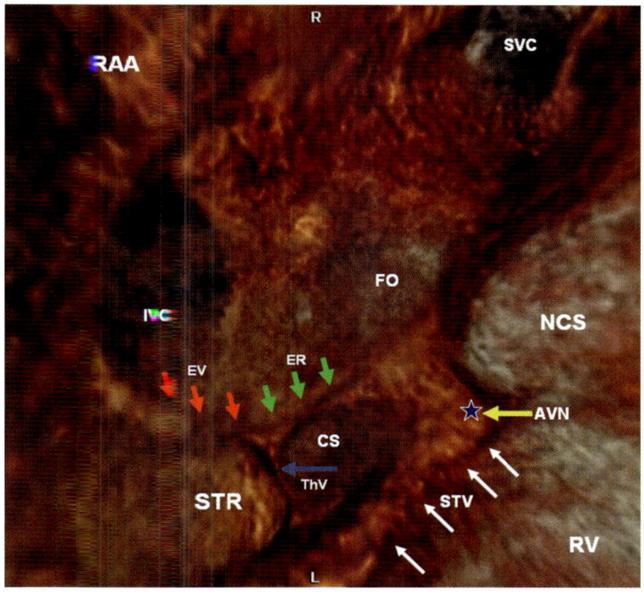

Figure 11.28 Relation of the sub-Thebesian recess (STR) and coronary sinus. Endoscopic view displays the internal aspects of the isthmic region of right atrium and demonstrates the spatial relation of STR with CS and IVC. AVN, anatomic location of the AV node (yellow arrow); CS, coronary sinus; ER, Eustachian ridge (green arrows); EV, Eustachian valve (red arrows); FO, fossa ovalis; IVC, inferior vena cava; NCS, non coronary sinus; RAA, right atrial appendage; RV, right ventricle; STV, septal attachment of the tricuspid valve (white arrows); SVC, superior vena cava; ThV, Thebesian valve (blue arrow). (Reprinted with permission from Saremi and Krishnan [7].)

sociated with the so-called Chiari network, a fenestrated membrane consisting of threads and strands in the RA. It is a congenital remnant of the right valve of the sinus venosus found in 2–3% of the population and may be seen on

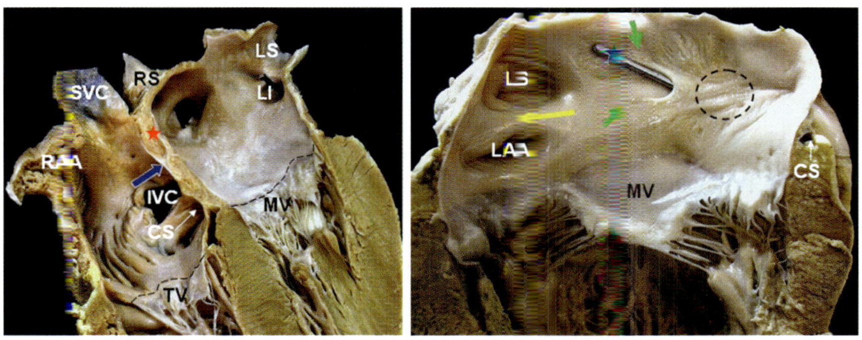

Figure 11.29 (a) Four-chamber section through the heart profiles the atrial septum and displays the valve of the foramen ovale (blue arrow) and the muscular rim on either side. The infolding of the right atrial wall encloses epicardial fat (star). The dotted lines mark the annular attachments of the tricuspid (TV) and mitral (MV) valves. (b) This heart sectioned longitudinally in a plane parallel to that of the atrial septum. The rim of the fossa ovalis on the right atrial side is marked by the black circle. When there is probe patency of the fossa ovalis (star), the left atrium can be accessed from the right atrium through a crevice (between arrows) that is the last part of the valve to be sealed to the rim. The solid yellow arrow indicates the so-called left atrial ridge that is a fold in the atrial wall between the left atrial appendage (LAA) and the left superior (LS) pulmonary vein. In this heart, the course of the coronary sinus (CS) is distant from the mitral valve (MV). CS, coronary sinus; IVC, inferior vena cava; SVC, superior vena cava; LI, LS, RI, RS, left and right inferior and superior pulmonary veins, respectively.

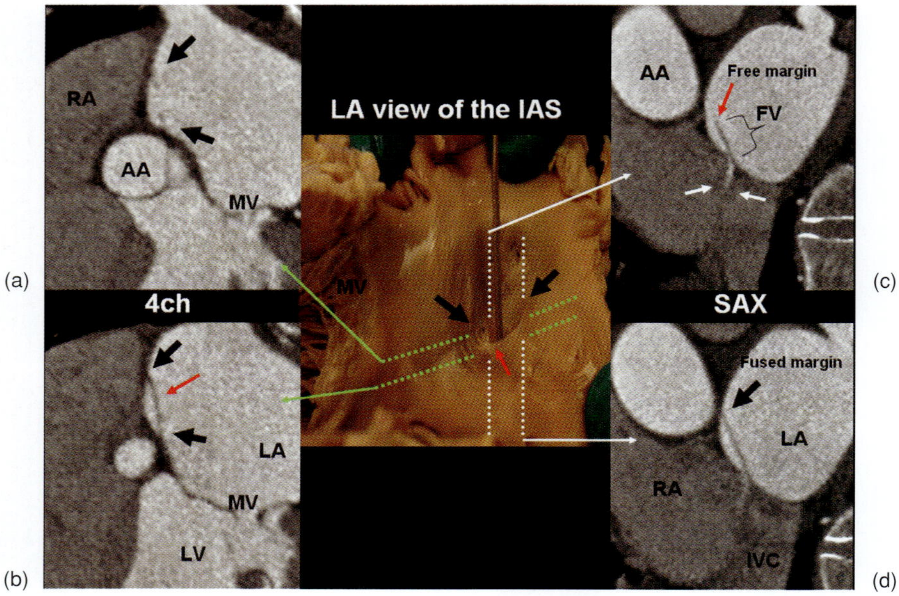

Figure 11.30 Anatomy of the flap valve of the septum primum in patient with patent foramen ovale (PFO) and a left-to-right shunt. The left atrial (LA) view of the interatrial septum (IAS) of a dissected heart is shown in the center. Note a probe is passed into the flap tunnel. Four-chamber (4ch) images of CT angiography are shown on the left side. As shown by the green lines the 4ch slices are passed right above the free margin of the flap valve (a) and through the flap valve (b). Short axis images (SAX) on the right side are obtained through the free margin of the flap valve (c) and through the posterior attachment of the flap valve (d). The SAX slice locations are shown by white lines. Both ends of the flap are fused to the interatrial septum (large black arrows). As shown in this example the fused margins of the flap may reach the left atrial roof but the free margin of the flap valve (FV) remains floating in the left atrial cavity. The length of this free margin varies from patient to patient and may easily let free flow of contrast from left to right (small white arrows) especially when it is too short. The red arrows demarcate the point where the shortest length of the FV was measured from its free margin to the entrance of the PFO tunnel into the right atrium (bracket). AA, ascending aorta; FV, flap valve; IVC, inferior vena cava; LV, left ventricle; MV, mitral valve; RA, right atrium; SAX, short axis. (Reprinted with permission from Saremi F, Channual S, Raney A *et al*. [57]).

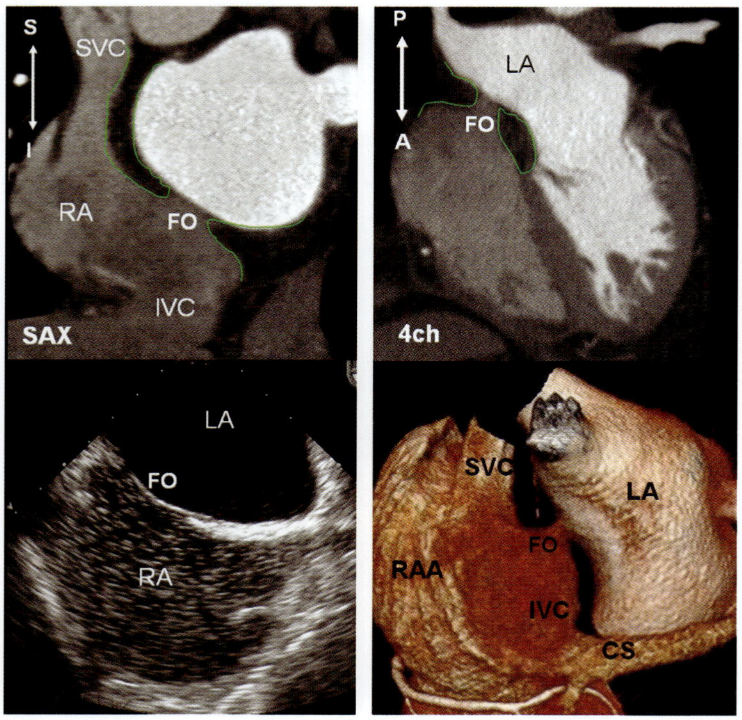

Figure 11.31 Anatomy of the fossa ovalis and associated structures. Short-axis (SAX), four-chamber (4ch), transesophageal echo with bubble, and three-dimensional images from interatrial septum show a completely fused fossa ovalis (FO). A prominent limbus is formed nicely demarcated by thick fatty interatrial groove (green lines). CS, coronary sinus; IVC, inferior vena cava; LA, left atrium; PFO, patent foramen ovale; RA, right atrium; RAA, right atrial appendage; SVC, superior vena cava.

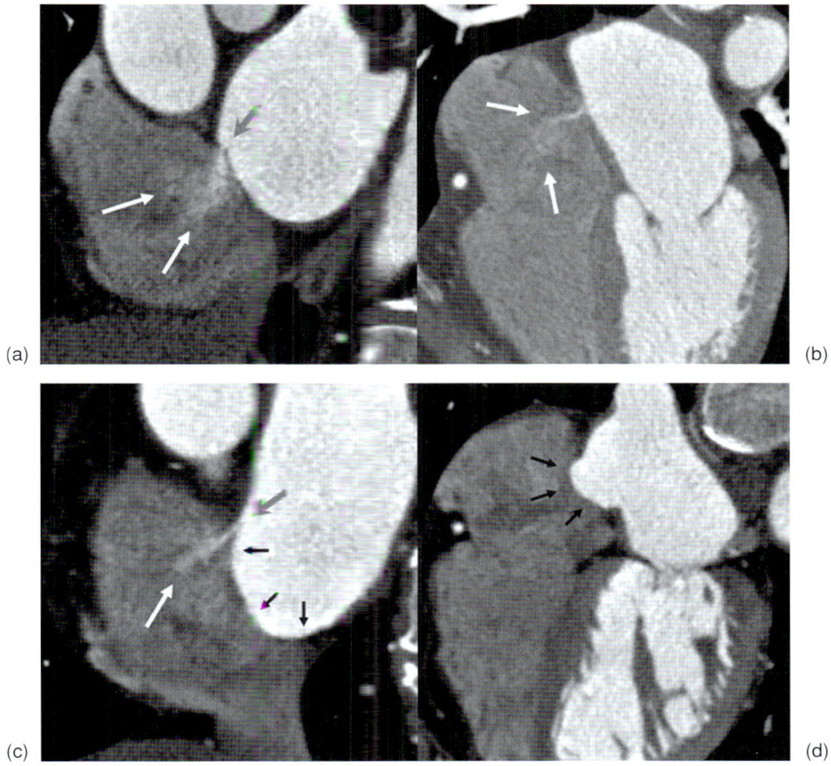

Figure 11.32 Examples of incompetent valves with free flow of contrast through the shunt (white arrows). SAX (a) and four-chamber (4ch) (b) views show grade 3 left-to-right shunt. The free flap valve is too short to cover the superior rim of the septum secundum (gray arrow). SAX (c) and four-chamber (d) views in a patient with atrial septal aneurysm (black arrows) also demonstrates very short PFO tunnel (gray arrow) causing a grade 2 left-to-right shunt (white arrow). Forty-five percent of our patients with ASA had a PFO shunt in which a flap valve <5 mm length was seen.

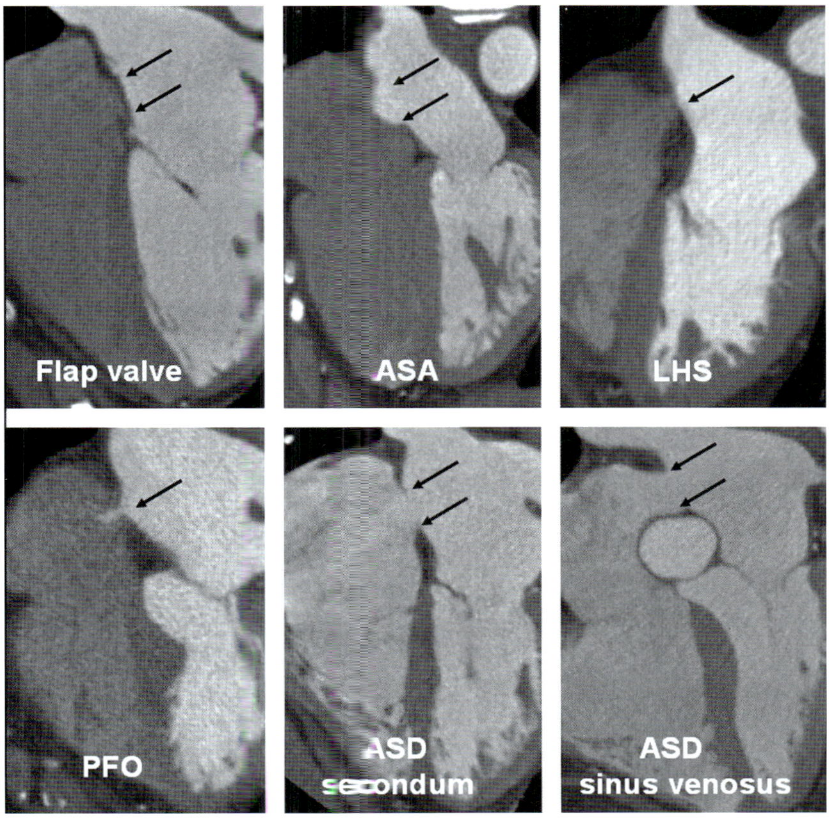

Figure 11.33 Anatomic variations of fossa ovale and interatrial septum. Incidental findings in patients referred for coronary CT angiography. ASA, atrial septal aneurysm; ASD, atrial septal defect; LHS, lipomatose hypertrophy of septum; PFO, patent foramen ovale. (Reprinted with permission from Saremi and Krishnan [7].)

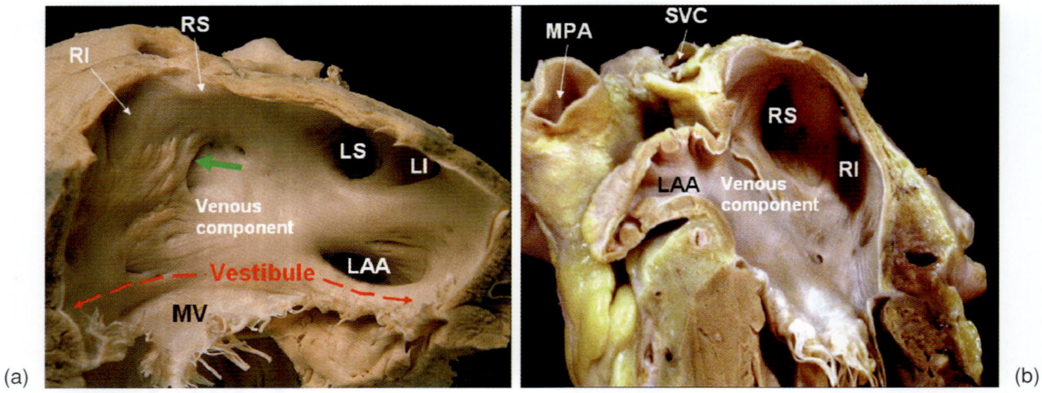

Figure 11.34 (a) Dissection of the posterior wall of the left atrium (LA) close to posterior interatrial groove. The smooth-walled venous component of the LA is the most extensive. The septal aspect of the LA shows the crescentic line of the free edge of the flap valve (green arrow) against the rim of the oval fossa. The orifices of the right superior (RS) and right inferior (RI) pulmonary veins are adjacent to the plane of the septal aspect of the LA. (b) Longitudinal sections through the left atrial appendage (LAA) showing the orifices of the right pulmonary veins. Note the relation of the superior vena cava (SVC) to the right superior (RS) pulmonary vein. LI, left inferior pulmonary vein; LS, left superior pulmonary vein; MPA, main pulmonary artery; MV, mitral valve.

contrast enhanced MDCT images [60]. Prominent Chiari membranes may interfere with interventional procedures by catheter entrapment [61].

Anatomic Landmarks of the LA

The LA is a very important structure for interventional cardiologists where treatment of clinically important issues such as AF, PFO, atrial septal defect, mitral regurgitation, and left atrial thrombus may be approached [62, 63]. As with the RA, the LA possesses a venous component, a vestibule, and an appendage [13, 63]. The pulmonary venous component, with the venous orifices at each corner, is found posteriorly (Figure 11.34). The vestibular component surrounds the mitral orifice. The major part of the LA, including the pulmonary venous component, the vestibule, and the septal component, is smooth walled (Figure 11.34). The left atrial appendage (LAA) is derived from the primitive atrium and has a rough, trabeculated surface. It is a potential site for deposition of thrombus owing to its narrow neck with the LA (Figure 11.4). The atrial appendage of the LA is considerably smaller and tends to have a tubular shape that has one or several bends resembling a little finger (Figure 11.34). The rough zone of the LA is confined mainly to its appendage. A complicated network of fine muscular ridges lines the endocardial aspect. In between the ridges, the wall is parchment thin. The anterior wall just behind the aorta is usually thin and vulnerable to be torn. The superior wall, or dome, is thickest, measuring 3.5–6.5 mm [13].

Pulmonary Veins and AF

AF is the most common sustained cardiac arrhythmia that is characterized by uncoordinated contraction of the atrium. Although different mechanisms of AF exist (Figure 11.35), it is well established that myocardial sleeves (Figure 11.36) of the PVs especially the superior veins are crucial sources of triggers that initiate AF [64, 65]. Cardiac ablation is performed in symptomatic AF that is refractory to at least one Class 1 or 3 antiarrhythmic medications. In the elderly patients, myocardial perforation and thromboembolic complications of the ablation are more prevalent. Furthermore, patients with larger LA size and longer AF duration typically experience a higher incidence of AF recurrence [65].

Techniques for Catheter Ablation of AF

Previously, the most common ablation strategy was electrical isolation of the PVs by creating circumferential ablation lines around the individual or bilateral PV ostia (Figure 11.37). The lines are either guided by fluoroscopy, 3D electroanatomical mapping [66, 67] or intracardiac echocardiography (ICE) [5].

However, the focus of ablation strategies shifted from the PV to the atrial tissue located in the antrum because of the fact that many non-PV trigger points for AF are located in the antrum rather than the PV and that RF delivery may cause PV stenosis [68]. In antrum ablation, the most common sites are the LA "roof" connecting the superior aspects of the left and right upper PV isolation lesions, the region of tissue between the mitral valve and the left inferior PV (the mitral isthmus) [69] (Figure 11.37b).

These techniques result in success rate of >90% with long-term success rate ranging from 60 to 90% in patients with paroxysmal AF but lower rates in those with chronic AF [68,70,71].

Cardiac Autonomic Nervous System and AF

Cardiac ganglia are generally located in the epicardial layer and are surrounded by adipose tissue (Figure 11.35). The largest populations are concentrated along the IAG near the SA (SVC-right PV fat pad) and AVNs (IVC-LA fat pad) [72] (Figures 11.38 and 11.39). Smaller collections are located on the superior and anterior left atrial surfaces, the atrial-appendage–atrial junctions, the base of the great vessels, and the base of the ventricles. Vagal stimulation shortens the atrial effective refractory period that facilitates the initiation and maintenance of AF. Adding LA ganglion plexus to other ablation targets may improve ablation success in patients undergoing circumferential PV ablation for paroxysmal AF [73].

Anatomic Assessment of the Pulmonary Veins

Normal PV anatomy consists of two right-sided and two left-sided PVs with separate ostia. However, from anatomical studies with MDCT, it has been demonstrated that the anatomy of the LA and PVs is commonly variable [74–77] (Figure 11.40).

The PV ostia are ellipsoid with a longer superoinferior dimension. The right superior PV is located close to the SVC or RA, and the right inferior PV projects horizontally.

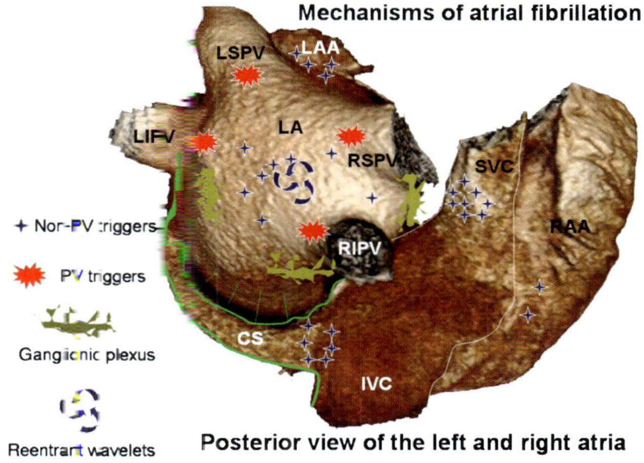

Figure 11.35 Mechanisms of atrial fibrillation. Posterior three-dimensional view of the left and right atria. Four different mechanisms for AF include PV triggers, reentrant wavelets, non-PV triggers, and ganglionic plexus overactivity. The common locations of PV triggers (red stars) and also the common sites of origin of non-PV triggers (blue cross) are shown on the posterior wall of the left atrium (LA). Blue arrows demonstrate reentrant wavelets that play a role in initiating and sustaining AF. Shown in yellow are major locations for autonomic ganglionic plexi on the LA. SVC left atrium and IVC left atrium fad pad contain most of the cardiac autonomic gangli. Bordered in green is the coronary sinus (CS) which is enveloped by muscular fibers which have connections to the atria (green lines). Also shown in green is the vein and ligament of Marshall, which travels from the CS toward the region between the left upper PV and the LA appendage (LAA). IVC, inferior vena cava; LIPV, left inferior pulmonary vein; LSPV, left superior pulmonary vein; RAA, right atrial appendage; RIPV, right inferior pulmonary vein; RSPV, right superior pulmonary vein; SVC, superior vena cava.

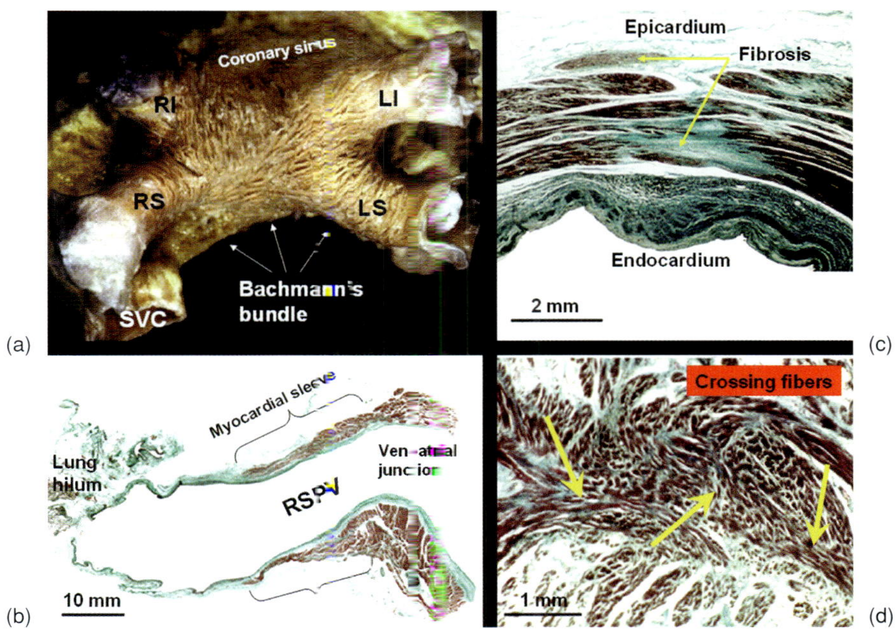

Figure 11.36 (a) Dissection of the left atrium viewed from above shows the entrances and myocardial sleeves of the four pulmonary veins and the anterior interatrial Bachmann bundle. Note the relation of the superior vena cava (SVC) to the right superior (RS) pulmonary vein. (b) Longitudinal sections through three sets of right superior pulmonary veins (RSPV). Note the myocardial sleeve completely surrounding the superior vein and extending from the venoatrial junction. (c) The myocardial sleeve of a left superior PV shows extensive fibrotic replacement. (d) Longitudinal sections of the myocardial sleeve of the right superior pulmonary vein showing a complex arrangement of circular and longitudinal bundles of myocytes. LI, left inferior pulmonary vein; LS, left superior pulmonary vein; RI, right inferior pulmonary vein.

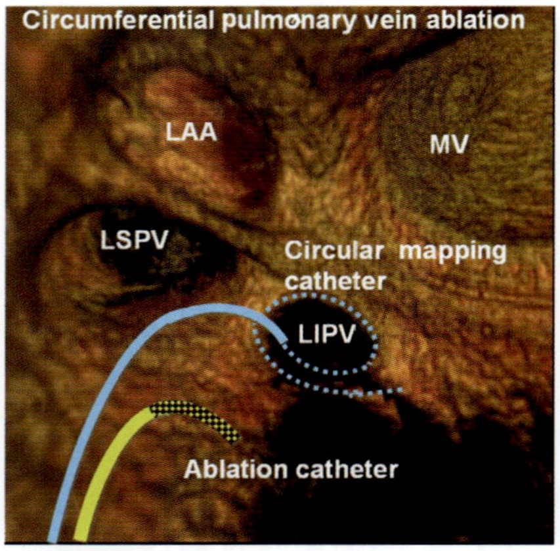

(a)

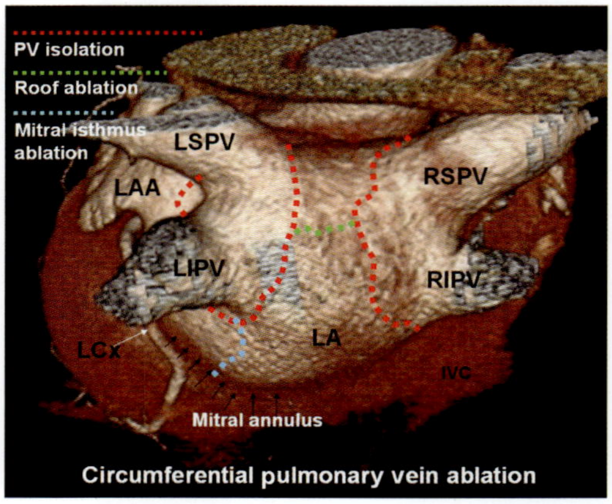

(b)

Figure 11.37 Ablation of atrial fibrillation. (a) Endoscopic view of the left atrium. Two catheters will be introduced into the left atrium through the transseptal puncture. These include a deflectable, circular mapping catheter, and a deflectable ablation catheter. (b) Circumferential pulmonary vein ablation. Posterior three-dimensional view of the left atrium and the pulmonary veins is shown. The two encircling pulmonary vein lesions are connected with an ablation line in the roof. Another ablation line was created along the mitral isthmus between the left inferior pulmonary vein (LIPV) and the lateral mitral annulus. IVC, inferior vena cava; LA, left atrium; LAA, left atrial appendage; LCx, left circumflex artery; LSPV, left superior pulmonary vein; MV, mitral valve; RIPV, right inferior pulmonary vein; RSPV, right superior pulmonary vein. (Reprinted with permission from Saremi and Krishnan [7].)

The left superior PV is in close vicinity to LAA and the left inferior PV courses near the descending aorta. Veins are larger in AF versus non-AF patients, men versus women, and persistent versus paroxysmal patterns.

The PV trunk is defined as the distance from the ostium to the first order branch. The superior PV ostia are larger (19–20 mm) than the inferior PV ostia (16–17 mm) [76,77]. The superior PVs tend to have a longer trunk (21.6 $\pm$ 7.5 mm) than the inferior PVs (14.0 $\pm$ 6.2 mm) [76,77]. It is important to report the ostial diameters of each vein and the length to the first-order branch (Figure 11.40). These diameters influence the selection of circular catheter size used.

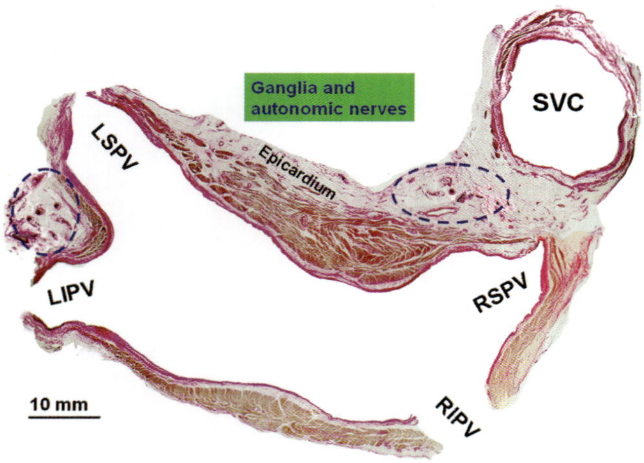

Figure 11.38 Cross histological section stained with elastic van Gieson of the left atrium, pulmonary veins, and superior vena cava. Note the ganglia and autonomic nervous system at the level of epicardium between superior vena cava (SVC) and right superior pulmonary vein (RSPV) (dashed circle) and between the superior and inferior left pulmonary vein (LSPV and LIPV) (dashed circle). RIPV, right inferior pulmonary vein.

Common anomalies include a conjoined (common) left or right PV in 25% of individuals [76,77]. Conjoined PV is more frequently seen on the left than the right [6]. In a recent study comparing MDCT and ICE, conjoined left PV ostia were observed in 79% patients with MDCT and 74% patients with ICE. Conjoined right ostia were observed in 31 and 38% patients, respectively [78]. Compared to ICE, the sensitivity for detection of additional branches was higher for MDCT [78]. Supernumerary veins are also frequently seen (Figure 11.28). The most common is a separate right middle PV, which drains the middle lobe of the lung [79]. One or two separate middle lobe vein ostia can be seen in 26% of patients [6]. The ostial diameter of the right middle PV is smaller than other veins (mean, 9.9 $\pm$ 1.9 mm). The ectopic focus originating from the right middle PV could initiate AF, which is cured by catheter ablation of right middle PV. In some patients, a supernumerary PV exists which shows an aberrant insertion with a perpendicular position in relation to the LA posterior wall. Supernumerary branch usually drains the upper lobe of the right lung and characteristically passes behind the bronchus intermedius (Figure 11.41).

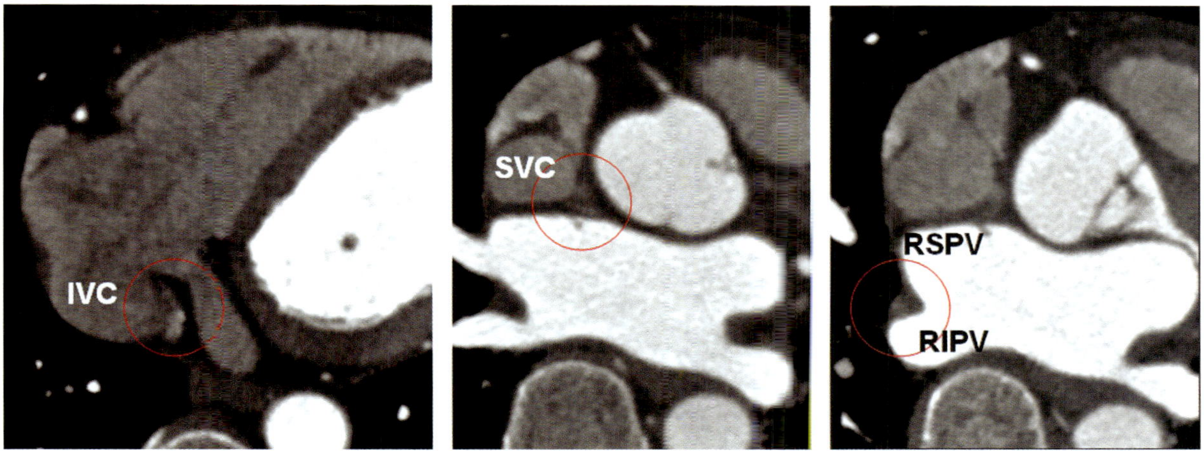

(a), (b) (c)

Figure 11.39 Parasympathetic ganglionic plexi of the heart (within the circles). It is difficult to image vagus plexi of the heart. However, those can indirectly be localized by enhancement of their rich vascular supply. Multiple ganglia exist. The largest collection of ganglia is located in the fad pad of superior and inferior cavoatrial junctions (a and b). Part (c) shows a smaller enhancing LA plexus between the right superior (RS) and right inferior (RI) pulmonary veins. Surgical or catheter ablation of these structures has been used for successful ablation of atrial fibrillation. IVC, inferior vena cava; LA, left atrium; RIPV, right inferior pulmonary vein; RSPV, right superior pulmonary vein; SVC, superior vena cava.

Finally, "early branching" of the PVs is also frequently observed. In this variant, the PV branches in close proximity to the ostium (Figure 11.40). Absence of one PV requires careful examination of all intrathoracic venous system, as it can be associated with partial anomalous venous return (Figure 11.42).

The caliber of the PVs gradually increased as they approached the LA. However, the caliber of the left inferior PV may decrease as it enters the LA and should not be mistaken for stenosis [80] (Figure 11.43). The size of the PV ostia is variable during the cardiac cycle. Therefore, any measurement of the PVs should take place in the same

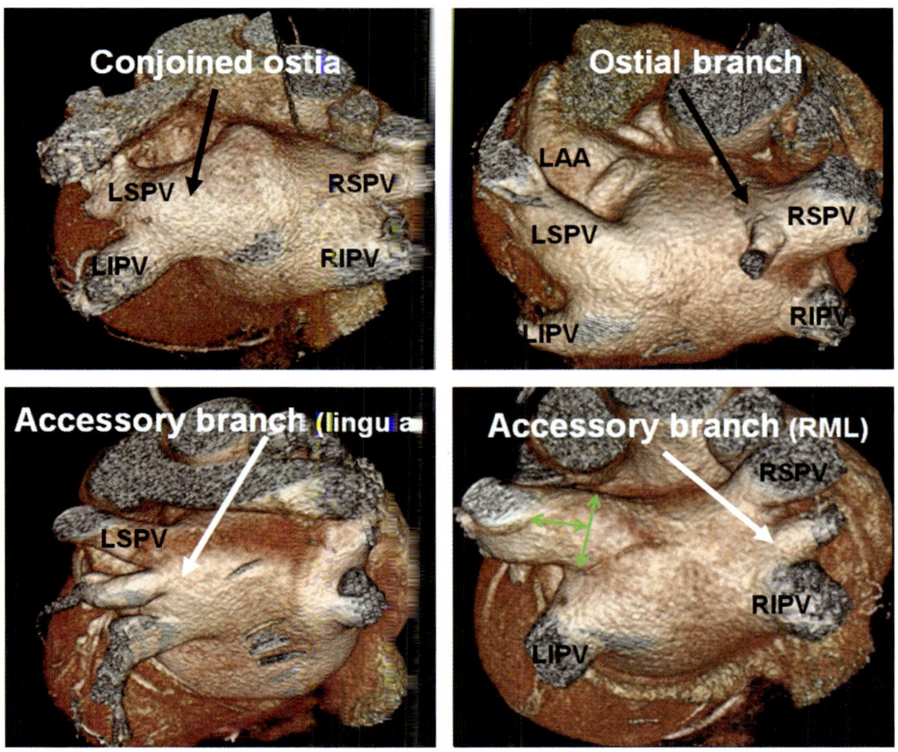

Figure 11.40 Anatomic variants of the pulmonary veins. Three-dimensional images show conjoined ostia, a common variant seen in up to 25% of cases; "early branching" of the pulmonary veins (ostial branch, which is also common; left accessory PV draining the lingual; and a small right middle lobe accessory pulmonary vein draining the right middle lobe (RML), which represents the most common variant. It is important to measure the ostial cross-sectional diameters and the trunk length (the distance from the ostium to the first-order branch) (green double-headed arrows). The superior pulmonary veins have a larger ostium and a longer trunk than do the inferior pulmonary veins. LAA, left atrial appendage; LIPV, left inferior pulmonary vein; LSPV, left superior pulmonary vein; RIPV, right inferior pulmonary vein; RSPV, right superior pulmonary vein.

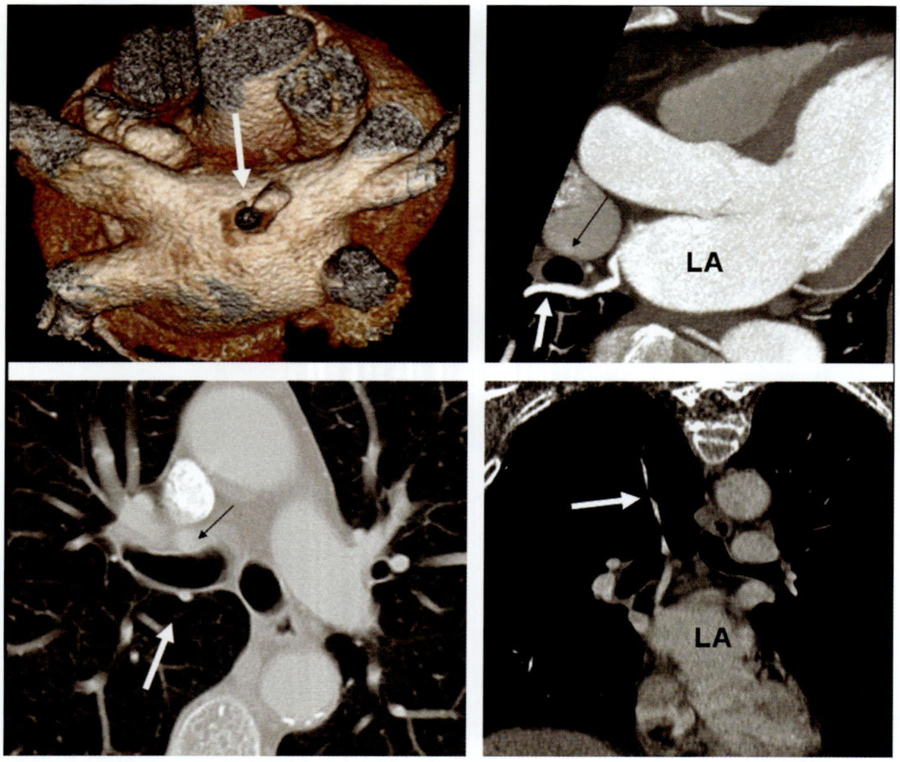

Figure 11.41 Supernumerary pulmonary vein (white arrows) shows an aberrant insertion with a perpendicular position in relation to the posterior wall of left atrium (LA). It usually drains the upper lobe of the right lung and characteristically passes behind the bronchus intermedius (black arrows).

phase of the cardiac cycle during the follow-up studies of patients. In a recent study, the measurement of ostial areas showed that the ostia enlarged at the end of ventricular systole when compared with those at the end of ventricular diastole, by the factors of 1.25–1.44 [81].

Left Atrial Isthmus and AF

In patients with AF, the success rate of catheter ablation depends on adequate electrical isolation by performing linear ablation lesions (Figure 11.37b). However, recurrence

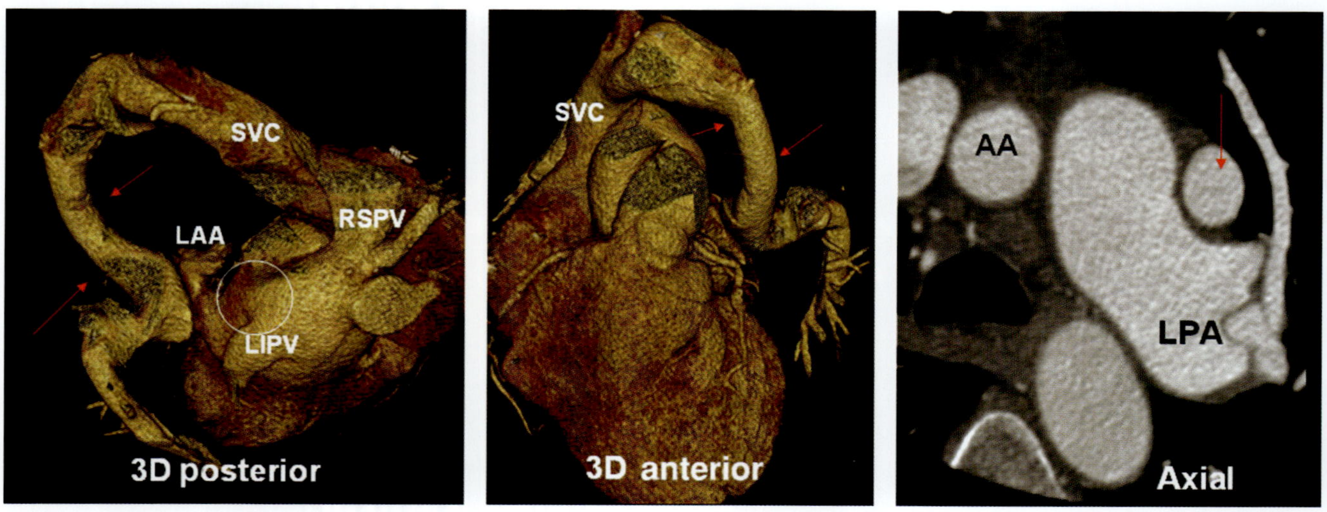

Figure 11.42 Absence of left superior pulmonary vein (circle) with anomalous venous return of the left upper lobe to SVC (red arrows). AA, ascending aorta; LAA, left atrial appendage; LIPV, left inferior pulmonary vein; LPA, left pulmonary artery; RSPV, right superior pulmonary vein; SVC, superior vena cava.

of atrial arrhythmias is not uncommon, particularly in left atrial isthmus, the area between the orifice of the left inferior PV and the posteroinferior mitral annulus (Figure 11.44) [82]. The left atrial isthmus may have a variable length, running from 17 to 51 mm [83]. CT can accurately demonstrate the boundaries of this area including exact location of mitral valve, CS, circumflex artery (Figure 11.44), and great cardiac vein (GCV) and their anatomic variants [7,84] (Chapter 1, Figure 11.19).

Oblique Vein of Marshall and Persistent Left SVC

Non-PV triggers initiating AF can be identified in up to one third of unselected patients referred for catheter ablation for paroxysmal AF [4,85]. The sites of origin for non-PV atrial triggers include the posterior wall of LA, SVC, crista terminalis, fossa ovalis, CS, behind the Eustachian ridge, along the ligament of Marshall, and adjacent to the atrioventricular valve annuli (Figure 11.35).

The oblique vein of Marshall (Figure 11.45), located between the LAA and the left upper and lower PVs, runs inferiorly along the inferior atrial wall to join the CS approximately 3 cm from its ostium. In most hearts (70%), the oblique vein or ligament of Marshall is <3 mm from the endocardium of the left lateral ridge and has muscular connections to the left PVs [86]. The remnant of oblique vein can be detected on coronary CT studies (Figure 11.46, upper row images). It remains patent as an isolated malformation, the persistent left SVC draining into the CS in 0.3% of the normal population and can be the source of AF [87] (Figure 11.46, lower row images).

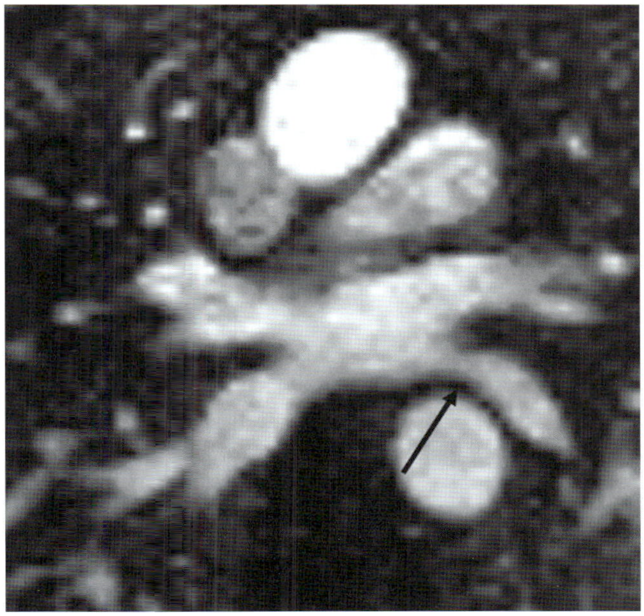

Figure 11.43 MR angiography for anatomic study of the left atrium (LA) and pulmonary veins (PVs). The caliber of the PVs gradually increased as they approached the left atrium. However, the caliber of the inferior pulmonary veins especially left side (arrow) may decrease as it enters the LA. This should not be mistaken with real stenosis.

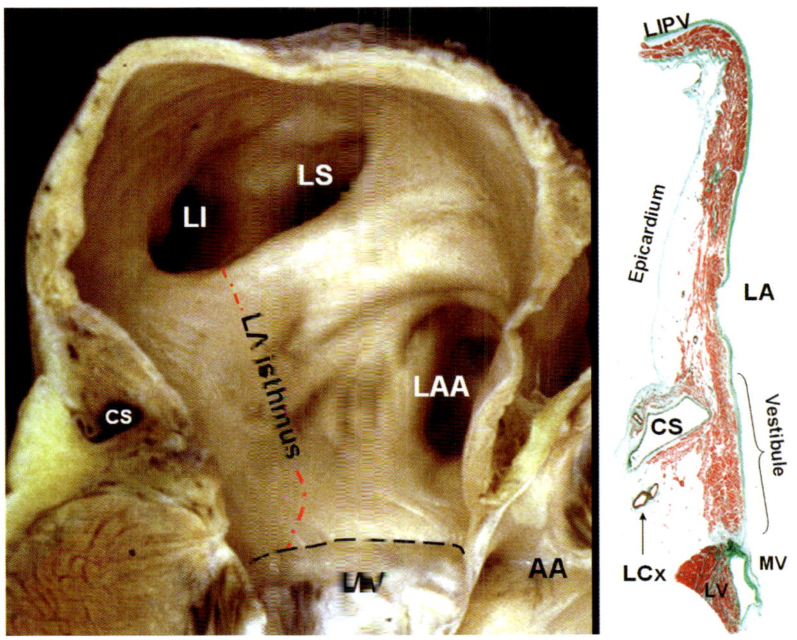

(a) (b)

Figure 11.44 (a) Sagittal section of the heart shows a common vestibule for both left pulmonary veins (PVs). Note the line connecting the inferior margin of the ostium of the left inferior PV to the mitral annulus named left atrial (LA) isthmus. (b) Sagittal sections at the LA isthmus stained with Masson's trichrome illustrate its anatomic relations with the coronary sinus (CS) and circumflex artery (LCx). Note the distance of the CS to the hingeline of the mitral valve (dotted line). AA, ascending aorta; LAA, left atrial appendage; LI, left inferior PV; LIPV, left inferior pulmonary vein; LS, left superior PV; MV, mitral valve.

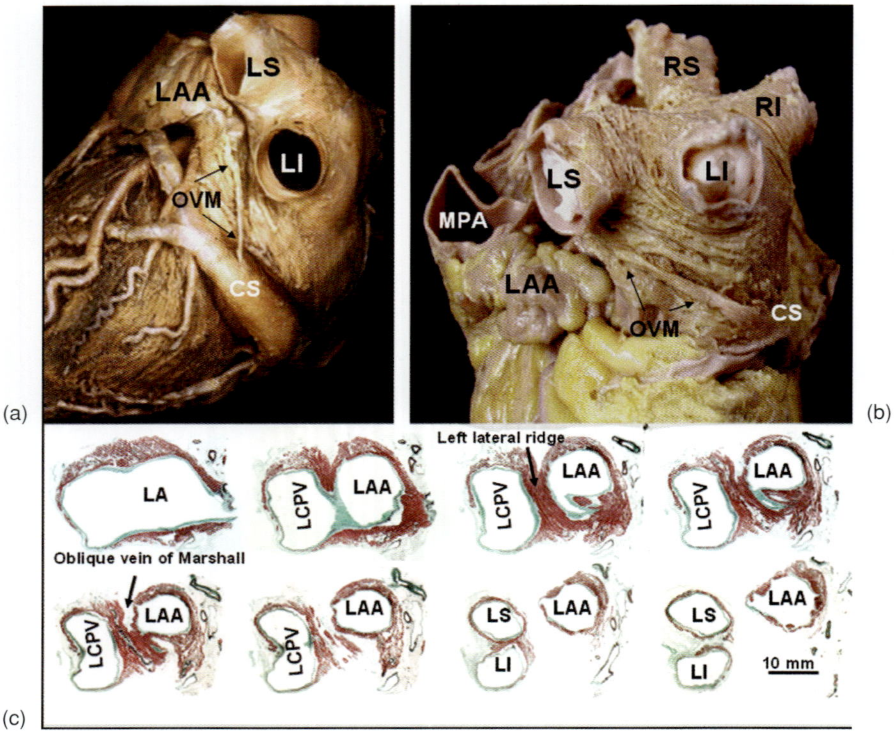

Figure 11.45 Parts (a) and (b) are dissections to show the myofiber arrangement in the subepicardium of the lateral ridge and the trajectory of the oblique vein of Marshall (OVM). (c) Sagittal sections stained with Masson's trichrome showing different levels of the left atrium (LA), common vestibule for both left PVs, left lateral ridge (LLR), left atrial appendage (LAA), and myocardial sleeve of the LS and LI pulmonary veins. Note the vein of Marshall is in direct contact with the myocardium of the left lateral ridge. CS, coronary sinus; LCPV, left common pulmonary vein; LI, left inferior; LS, left superior; MPA, main pulmonary artery; RI, right inferior pulmonary vein; RS, right superior pulmonary vein.

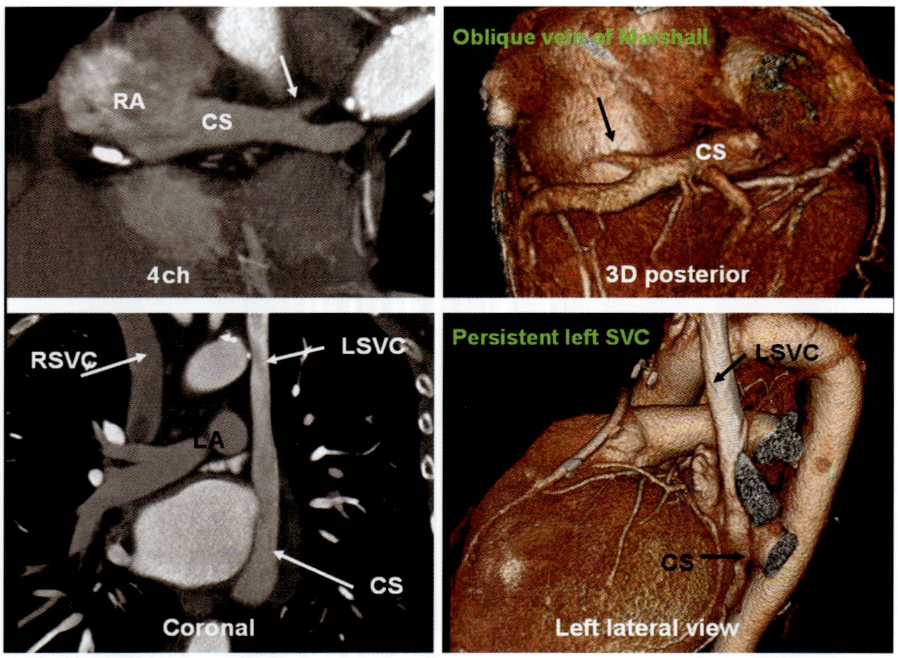

Figure 11.46 The non-PV ectopic beats may arise from the vein of Marshall (upper row) and a persistent left SVC (lower row). It is important to look for these incidental findings. Upper row demonstrates an oblique Vein of Marshall (arrows), which is nicely shown on both four-chamber (4ch) [through the coronary sinus (CS)] and posterior three-dimensional views of the heart. Lower images show a persistent left SVC: Coronal and left lateral three-dimensional views show preferential flow of high density contrast (injected in the left arm) in the left SVC (LSVC) and into the CS. Right SVC (RSVC) is less enhanced. LA, left atrium; LSVC, left SVC; RA, right atrium; SVC, superior vena cava.

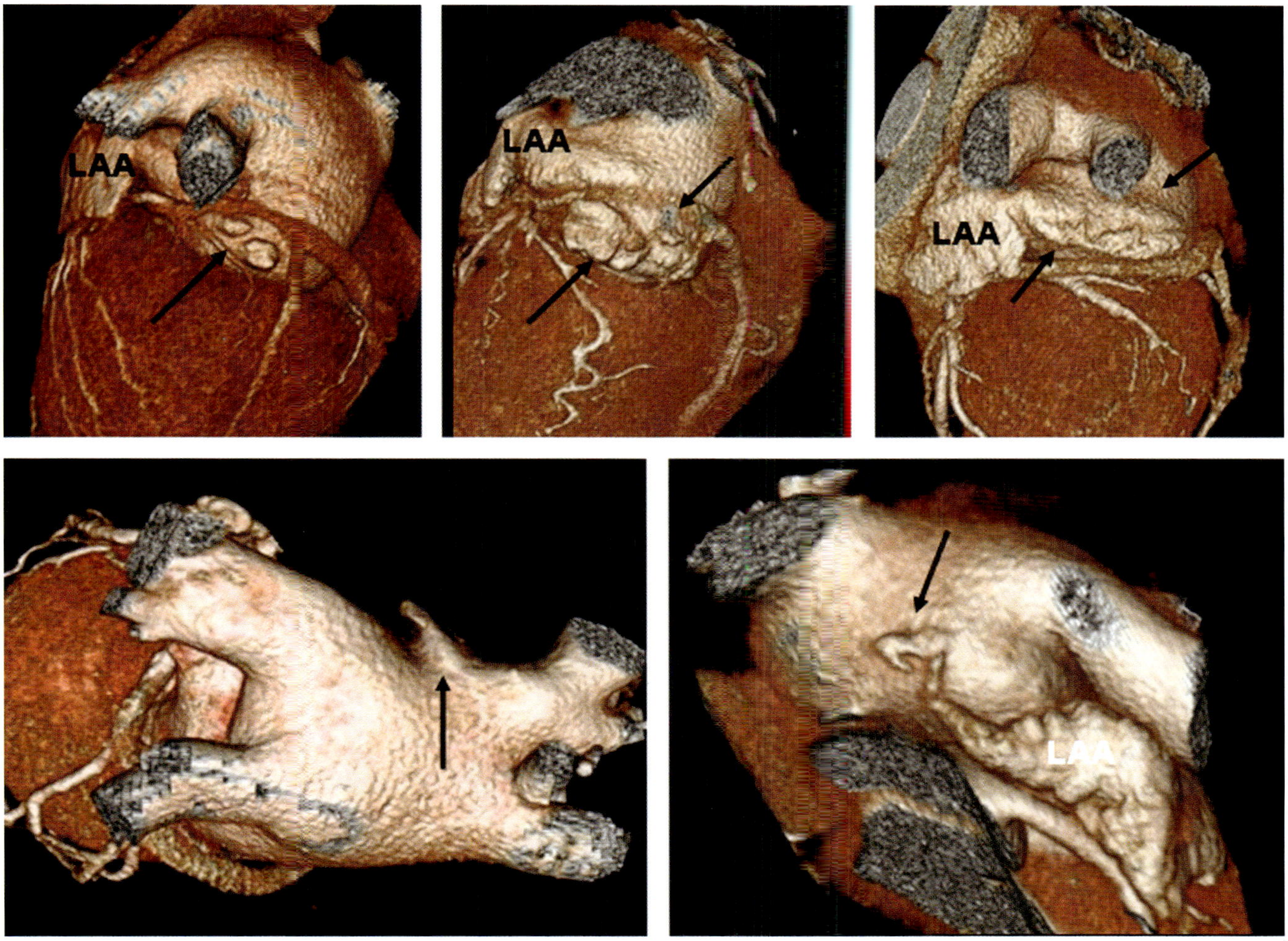

Figure 11.47 Accessory left atrial appendage. This anatomic variant is common. Two common locations are left atrial isthmus (upper row, three different patients) and anterior wall of the LA (lower row, two different patients). LAA, left atrial appendage.

Important Related Structures of the LA

Accessory Left Atrial Appendages

Accessory LAA is a common anatomic variant [88,89] and can be seen in two anatomic locations: the anterior wall of the LA (projects into the transverse sinus) and the left atrial isthmus (Figure 11.47). Description of this anatomic variant is required in radiology reports, as they may be a potential cause of thrombus formation or interfere with ablation procedures.

Intraatrial Membrane: Cor Triatriatum Sinister

Incidental discovery of a nonobstructive membrane within the LA should raise the possibility of cor triatriatum sinister. This congenital anomaly is rare but surgically correctable. Incidental finding of a small incomplete membrane is not rare (Figure 11.48). Cardiac MDCT provides excellent anatomic detail to detect and evaluate this anomaly [90].

S-shaped SAN Artery

S-shaped SAN artery is an anatomic variant of SAN artery originating from the posterolateral part of the LCx artery [91,92] (Figure 11.49). It is common to find it in 14% of coronary CT angiographies [91]. The S-shaped SAN artery has a predictable proximal course in the groove between the orifices of the left superior PV and the LAA close to the left atrial wall (2.43 ± 0.992 mm). MDCT can be used

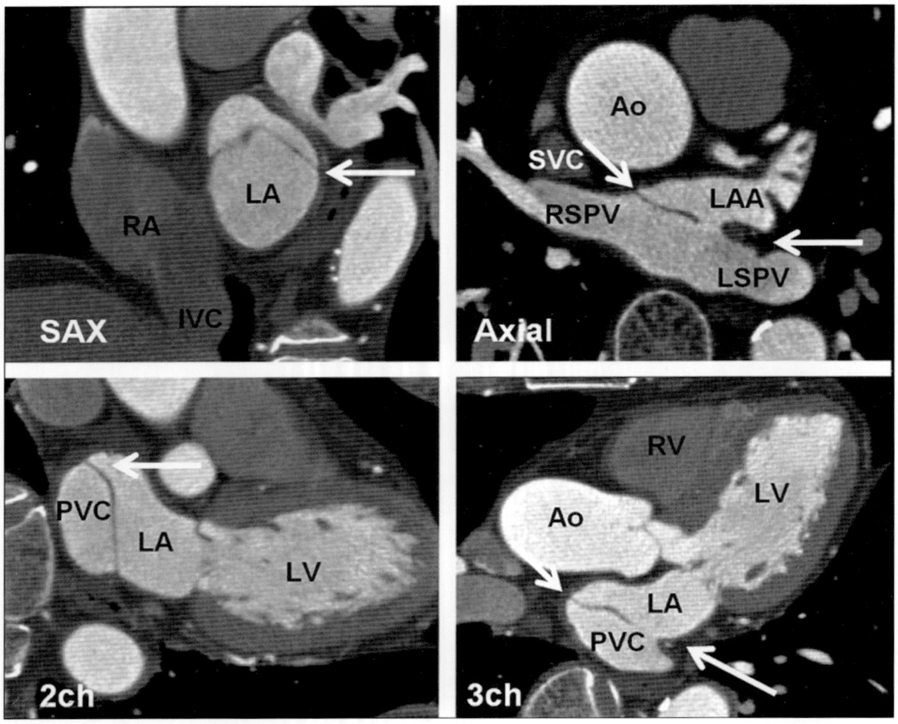

Figure 11.48 Cor triatriatum sinister [90]. Forty-eight-year-old man with incidental discovery of a nonobstructive membrane in the LA. Mid-diastolic images of coronary CT angiography in different views, including short axis (SAX), axial, two chamber (2ch), and four chamber (4ch) show a membranous diaphragm in the left atrium (LA) extending from the anterior wall of the LA near the orifice of the right superior pulmonary vein (RSPV) to the junction of the left atrial appendage (LAA) and the left superior pulmonary vein (LSPV). This membrane with a 2 cm central perforation separates the pulmonary venous compartment (PVC) of the left atrium from the main body of the left atrium. No hemodynamic effect was shown on Doppler examination (not shown). 3ch, three chamber; Ao, aorta; CT, crista terminalis; IVC, inferior vena cava; LV, left ventricle; RA, right atrium; RV, right ventricle; SVC, superior vena cava.

to plan surgical and catheter-based LA interventions in which this artery is at risk of injury.

Large Thebesian (Atrial) Veins

Thebesian veins are small and situated deep in the myocardium. However, various forms and courses of the intramural venous tunnel, sinus, or channel of the atria have been described [93]. Large transmural veins should not be confused with pathologies (Figure 11.50).

Relationship of the Esophagus and LA

Because of the close proximity of the esophagus to the posterior wall of the LA (Figure 11.51) [94], ablation procedures involving this region of the LA may cause esophageal damage and result in formation of an atrial esophageal fistula [95]. MDCT is a valuable tool to show the relation of the atrial wall to the esophagus and the descending aorta prior to the ablation procedure [96] (Figure 11.52). However, peristalsis and dynamic movement of the esophagus during the procedure can result in discordance between the preprocedure and intraprocedure anatomy [96].

Phrenic Nerve

The phrenic nerves lie along the lateral mediastinum and run from the thoracic inlet to the diaphragm [97]. Phrenic nerve injury results from direct thermal injury, usually to the right phrenic nerve, which is located near the right superior PV and the SVC (Figure 11.53) [98]. Less frequently, ablation within the LA appendage can result in left phrenic nerve damage. MDCT coronary angiography can demonstrate the left phrenic neurovascular bundle as it passes over the LV pericardium in 74% of the studies [99] (Figure 11.54). However, it is difficult to image the right phrenic nerve. In some high-quality images, the right phrenic nerve can be seen as a mildly enhancing extrapericardial structure lateral to the SVC and anterior to the right superior PV (Figure 11.54).

Acute Occlusion of the LCx Artery

Acute occlusion of the LCx artery during catheter ablation within the CS to complete the line of block of mitral isthmus has been reported [100]. A more posterior mitral isthmus line may avoid this complication but may increase the risk of injury to the esophagus. CT has the potential of showing the relation of the CS, LCX artery, and left atrial

(a)

(b)

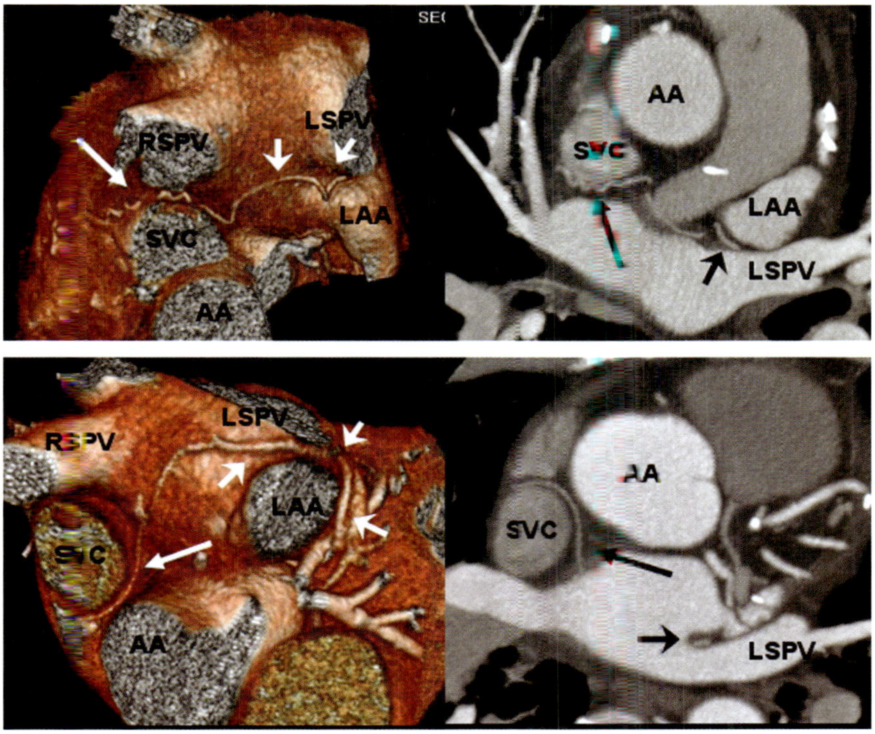

Figure 11.49 Anatomic course of the S-shaped SAN artery. (a) Retrocaval and (b) Precaval modes of termination are shown. The left images are sculptured three-dimensional views showing the S-shaped SAN arteries (short arrows) in two different cases. Corresponding axial images at the level of the superior cavoatrial junction are shown on the right side. The proximal course of the artery is similar in most cases. Arising from the proximal left circumflex (LCx) artery, it turns posteriorly and moves in the groove between the left atrial appendage (LAA) and the left superior pulmonary vein (LSPV) orifices (short arrows). We found that in most cases the distal artery traveled very close to the interatrial groove, penetrated the interatrial muscle bundle, and then followed its course behind the SVC (retrocaval) to reach the SAN area on the lateral aspect of the cavoatrial junction [long arrows in (a)]. This variant is prone to injury in the superior septal approach for mitral valve repair. In the precaval mode of termination [long arrows in (b)], the artery traveled away from the interatrial groove to reach the anterior margin of the superior cavoatrial junction and would be less susceptible to injury. AA, ascending aorta; RSPV, right superior pulmonary vein; SVC, superior vena cava. (Reprinted with permission from Saremi *et al.* [92].)

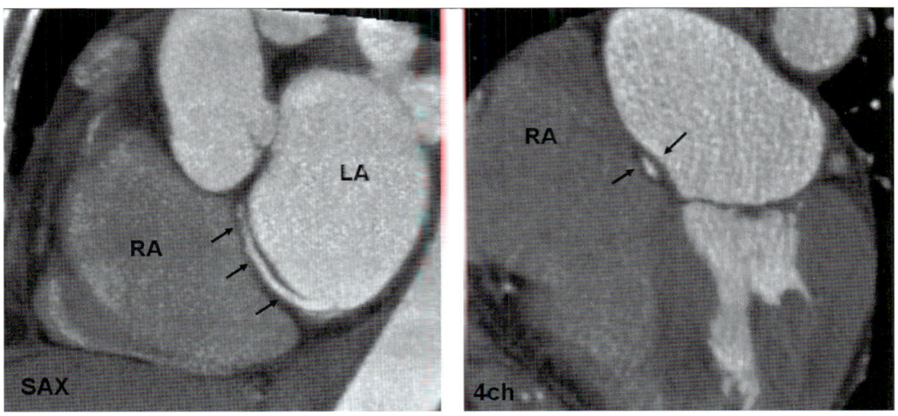

Figure 11.50 Short-axis (SAX) and four-chamber (4ch) images demonstrate a large draining vein in the interatrial septum draining the left atrial (LA) wall. This large Thebesian vein entered into the right atrium near the superior vena cava (not shown). RA, right atrium.

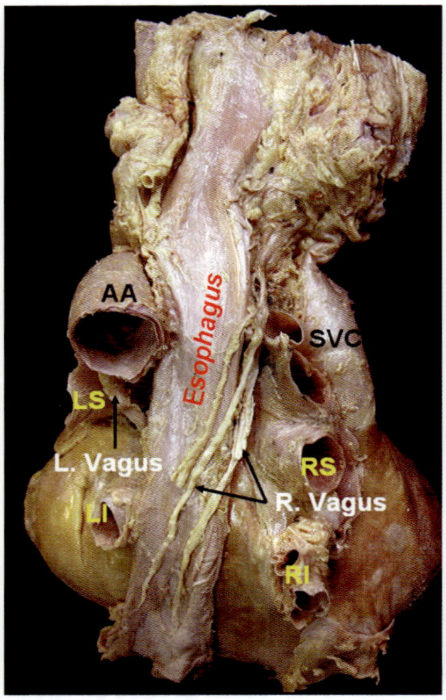

(a)

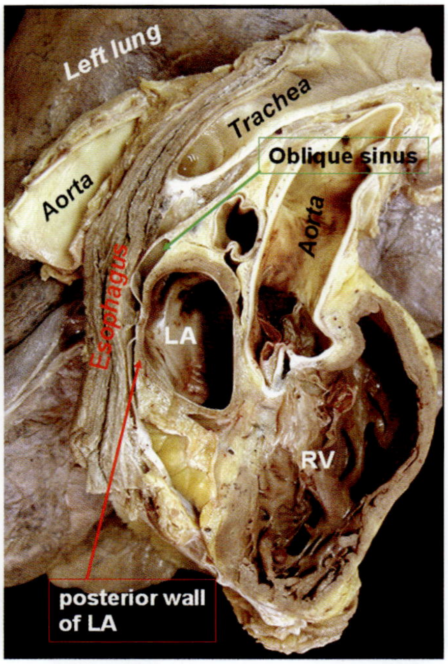

(b)

Figure 11.51 (a) Thoracic organs viewed from the back after removal of the descending thoracic aorta to show the course of the esophagus in situ and its relationship to the right (R) and left (L) vagus nerves, posterior wall of the left atrium, and the left inferior (LI) pulmonary vein. (b) Sagittal section through the heart and esophagus showing a middle section between the left and right PVs. AA, ascending aorta; LA, left atrium; LI, left inferior pulmonary vein; LS, left superior pulmonary vein; PVs, pulmonary veins; RI, right inferior pulmonary vein; RS, right superior pulmonary vein; RV, right ventricle; SVC, superior vena cava.

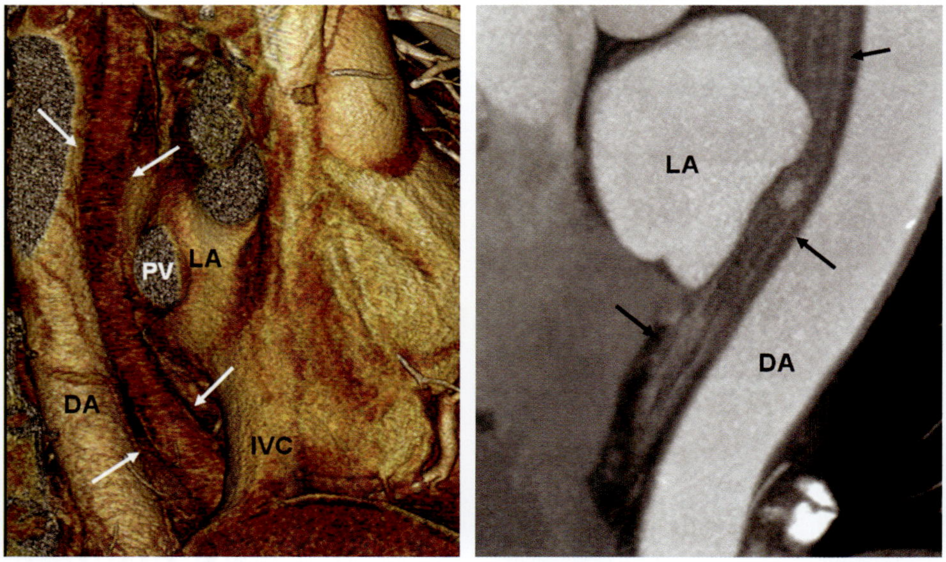

Figure 11.52 Relationship of the esophagus and left atrium (LA). Right lateral three-dimensional image and sagittal view of the heart demonstrate anatomic course of the esophagus (between arrows) along the posterior wall of LA. Note close proximity of the esophagus to the inferior pulmonary vein. DA, descending aorta; IVC, inferior vena cava; PV, pulmonary vein.

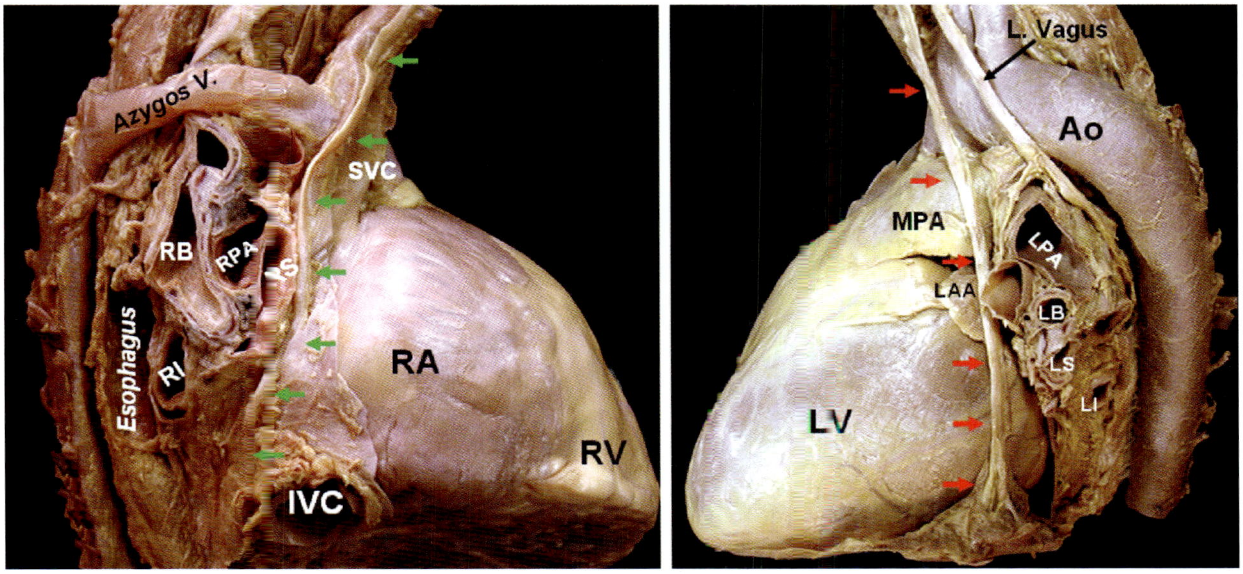

Figure 11.53 (a) Dissection after removal the fibrous pericardium showing the course of the right phrenic nerve indicated by green arrows is closely related to the superior cava vena (SVC) and right superior (RS) pulmonary vein to the undersurface of the diaphragm at the level of the inferior vena cava (IVC). (b) Dissection of the left phrenic nerve (red arrows) that descends on the fibrous pericardium anterior and lateral to the aortic arch (Ao), alongside the distal part of main pulmonary artery (MPA), left atrial appendage (LAA), and the lateral wall of the left ventricle to penetrate the left part of the diaphragm. LB, left bronchus; LI, left inferior pulmonary vein; LPA, left pulmonary artery; LS, left superior pulmonary vein; LV, left ventricle; RA, right atrium; RB, Right bronchus; RI, Right inferior pulmonary vein; RPA, right pulmonary artery; RV, right ventricle.

wall for a safer approach in this type of ablations (Figure 11.55).

Excess Fat Around the RA and within the IAG

The relative thickness of septum secundum and the prominence of fossa ovale margins may vary greatly (Figure 11.56). The thickness is directly proportional to the amount of fat in the IAG. Thickness greater than 2 cm is defined as lipomatose hypertrophy of the septum (LHS) [101]. Although, LHS remains asymptomatic in most people, cardiac arrhythmias including AF are common, especially with increase in thickness of fat in the interatrial septum [102]. CT is an accurate method to study anatomy of the interatrial septum and adjacent structures [58, 103].

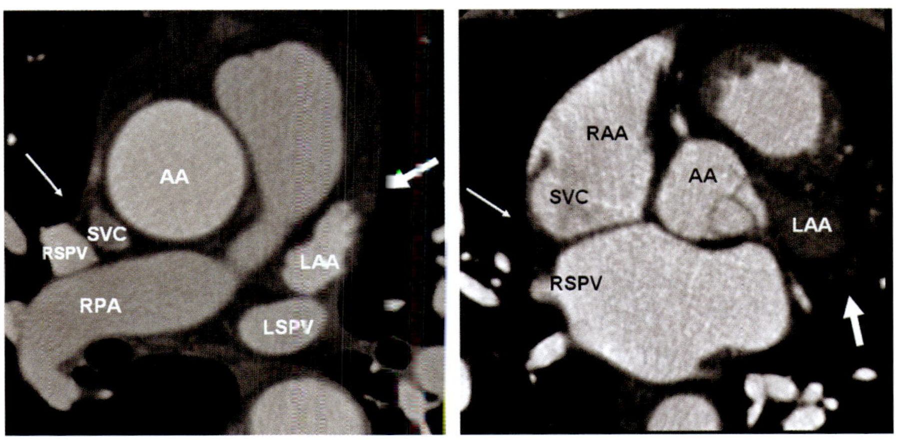

Figure 11.54 Axial images of the heart at the level of the left atrial appendage (LAA) show the anatomic relation of the left phrenic neurovascular bundle with the LAA (thick arrow). Also shown is the right phrenic nerve as it passes between the superior vena cava (SVC) and the right superior pulmonary vein (RSPV). AA, ascending aorta; LSPV, left superior pulmonary vein; RAA, right atrial appendage; RPA, right pulmonary artery.

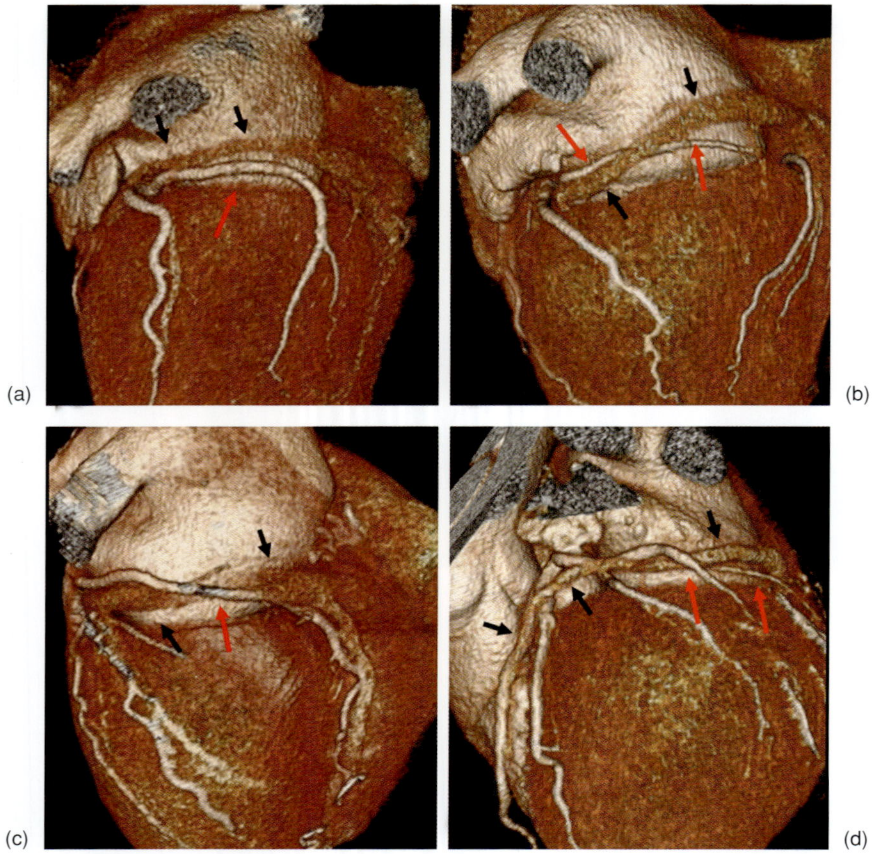

Figure 11.55 Multidetector CT (MDCT) can demonstrate the spatial relationship of the coronary sinus (CS) (black arrows), mitral annulus, and left circumflex (LCx) artery branches (red arrows), important considerations in preprocedure imaging for percutaneous trans-CS interventions. The CS may travel close or at a distance from the mitral ring. The LCx artery move parallel (a), under (b), or above (c) the CS, or encircle it (d).

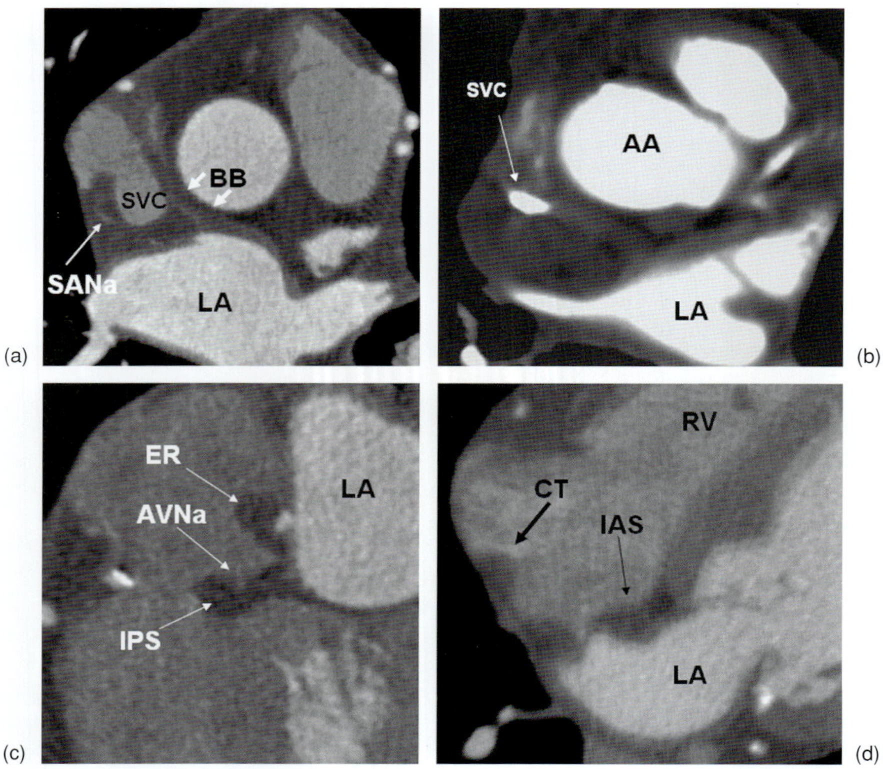

Figure 11.56 Critical places where fat infiltration may interfere with normal conduction include the SAN, Bachmann bundle (BB), interatrial septum (IAS), crista terminalis (CT), and inferior pyramidal space (IPS) where AV node artery (AVNa) is located. (a) Axial CT shows fatty infiltration of BB (small arrows) and SAN. SAN artery (SANa) is shown as it approaches SAN. (b) Axial image. Fatty infiltration around the superior vena cava (SVC) can cause obstruction and difficulty in passing the catheters. (c) Four-chamber view. Fatty infiltration and thickening of the Eustachian ridge (ER) may cause problem in ablation of paraseptal isthmus for atrial flutter. Fatty IPS is also shown. Also note the close proximity of the AVNa to the wall of coronary sinus (CS) as it travels in the inferior pyramidal space. (d) Axial CT shows enlarged CT and IAS due to fatty infiltration. AA, ascending aorta; AV, atrioventricular; LA, left atrium; LV, left ventricle; RV, right ventricle; SAN, sinoatrial node.

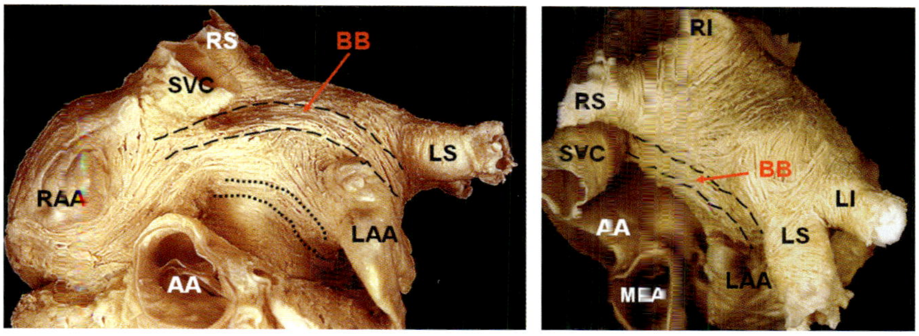

Figure 11.57 Dissections of the subepicardial fibres viewed from the anterior (a) and superior (b) aspects. Bachmann bundle (BB, black broken lines) crosses the anterior interatrial groove, blends into the circumferential fibers of the anterior wall (dotted lines), to pass to either side of the neck of the left atrial appendage (LAA). AA, ascending aorta; LI, left inferior pulmonary vein; LS, left superior pulmonary vein; MPA, main pulmonary artery; RAA, right atrial appendage; RI, right inferior pulmonary vein; RS, right superior pulmonary vein; SVC, superior vena cava.

Imaging of Bachmann Bundle

On the anterior subepicardial aspect of the LA, the most muscular bridge is Bachmann bundle (BB). This broad band of circumferential interatrial myofibers can be traced rightward to the junction between the RA and the superior caval vein, and leftward to either side of the neck of the LAA reuniting posteriorly to run on the epicardial aspect of the lateral wall (Figure 11.57) [86, 104]. On the right, it extends into the anteromedial wall of the RA, anterior to the SVC, where its fibers intermingle with those of the precaval bundle, the superior extension of the crista terminalis. On the left, it blends in with the LAA musculature (Figure 11.58). This interatrial band ensures rapid interatrial conduction, leading to physiological biatrial contraction. Changes in the musculature of BB could block or prolong interatrial conduction, resulting in abnormal atrial excitability, atrial dysfunction, AF, and other arrhythmias [105].

The principal vascular supply of BB is believed to stem from the SAN artery and its branches [88, 106] (Figure 11.59). Anatomic variants of this region are common (Figure 11.60).

In a recent anatomic study of BB and its vascular supply by 64 MDCT in normal and abnormal patients (severe coronary artery disease and interatrial block or AF), the investigators were able to detect detailed anatomy of BB by MDCT [88]. The study showed that BB was less visible in the abnormal groups, as it was replaced with fat (Figure 11.61).

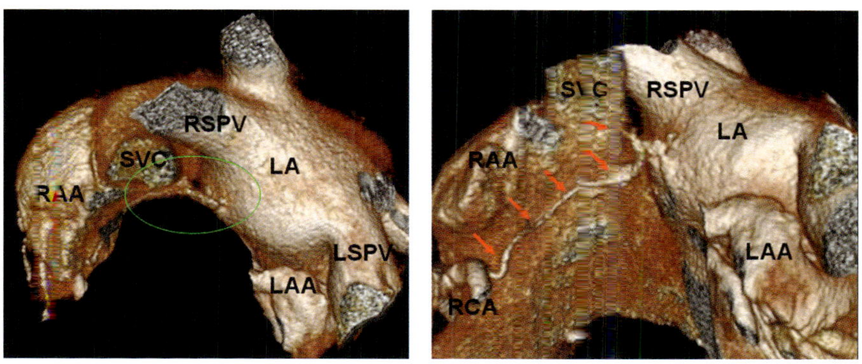

Figure 11.58 Sculptured three-dimensional superior and anterosuperior images of the atria. (a) BB is shown (green circle) connecting the two atria anteriorly up to the junction of the superior vena cava (SVC) in the right atrium (RA) and extending to the left atrial appendage (LAA) in the left atrium (LA). In (b), the SAN artery is shown arising from the right coronary artery (RCA), passing through BB, and ending retrocavally. BB, Bachmann bundle; LIPV, left inferior pulmonary vein; LSPV, left superior pulmonary vein; RAA, right atrial appendage; RSPV, right superior pulmonary vein. (Reprinted with permission from Saremi *et al.* [88].)

(a), (b)

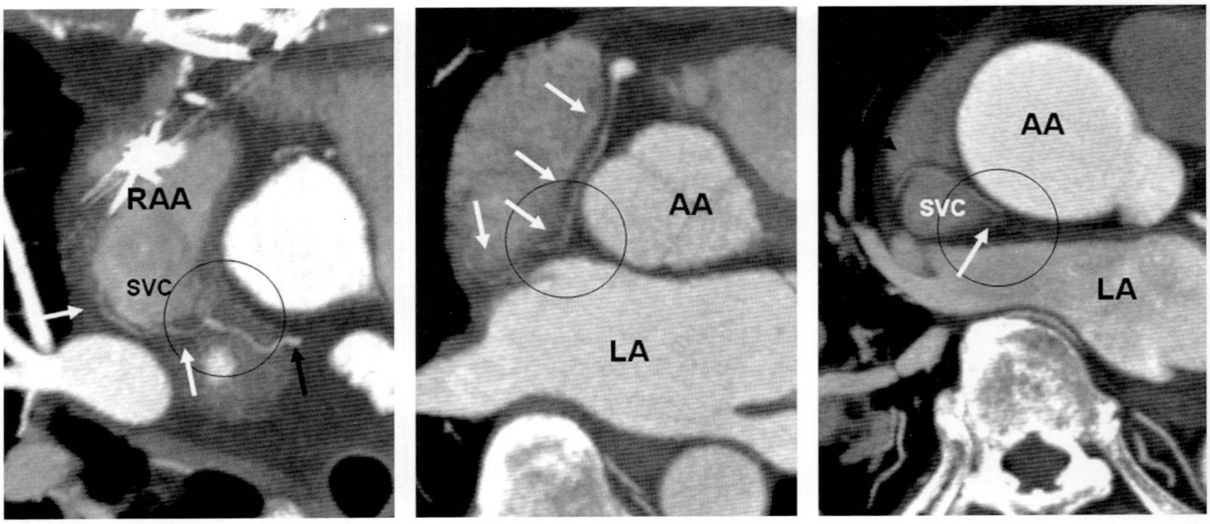

(c)

Figure 11.59 Vascular supply of BB (circles). BB is invariably supplied by the SAN artery (arrows). Part (a) demonstrates the left SAN artery arising from the left circumflex (LCx, not shown), ending retrocavally. Part (b) shows the right SAN artery arising from the RCA, ending retrocavally (arrows). Part (c) demonstrates the left SAN artery ending precavally (arrow). The relation of the artery to BB depends on the mode of termination of the SAN artery in relation to the SVC. In the retrocaval course (a and b), the SAN artery either penetrates BB or passes above BB while giving off small branches to it. In this course, the SAN artery is very close to the interatrial groove. In the precaval version of SAN artery termination (c), the artery approaches BB and gives off branches to supply the region, and then continues its course toward the SAN on the lateral aspect of the superior cavoatrial junction. AA, ascending aorta; BB, Bachmann bundle; LA, left atrium; RAA, right atrial appendage; SVC, superior vena cava.

Anomalous Pulmonary and Systemic Connections

Premature atresia of the right or left portion of the primordial PV while primitive pulmonary–systemic connections are still present results in a partial anomalous pulmonary venous (PAPV) connection [107]. Unlike a total anomalous pulmonary venous connection, a PAPV connection is an acyanotic lesion and may incidentally be detected on imaging studies [108] (Figure 11.42). Classically, a PAPV connection has been described as presenting in childhood, most frequently on the right side and associated with a sinus venosus atrial septal defect [109, 110]. In a PAPV connection of the left upper lobe, intraparenchymal left upper lobe PVs join to form an anomalous vein described as the vertical vein draining into the left brachiocephalic vein (Figures 11.42 and 11.62). The prevalence of a PAPV connection is different in adults [111]. In one recent review of 1825 chest CT reports, the prevalence of PAPV connection was 0.2%. Seventy-nine percent of patients had an anomalous left upper lobe vein connecting to a persistent left vertical vein, and 17% had an anomalous right upper lobe vein draining into the SVC [111]. Three percent had an anomalous right lower lobe vein draining into the suprahepatic IVC (Figure 11.62).

Cardiac Venous System

Implications for Cardiac Resynchronization Therapy

In approximately 30% of patients with chronic heart failure, the disease process affects the conduction pathways by causing a delay in the onset of right or left ventricular systole because of bundle branch block [112]. Intraventricular conduction delay may further impair the ability of the failing heart to eject blood. Cardiac resynchronization therapy (CRT) with biventricular pacing can improve synchrony of contractions of both ventricles, leading to improved hemodynamics and ejection fraction. Pacing the LV is accomplished via the CS. Crucial, however, for positioning the LV lead via transvenous approach is the presence of a suitable branch of the CS. CT has been used to evaluate the CS and coronary veins prior to lead placement [113–115].

Major components of the cardiac venous system include the CS, the GCV, the anterior interventricular vein (AIV), and the posterior interventricular vein (PIV). The GCV courses along with the LCx artery, and subsequently, drains into the CS [116]. It receives two main branches, namely, left marginal vein (LMV), along the lateral border of LV, and posterior (PV) or posterolateral (PLV) veins.

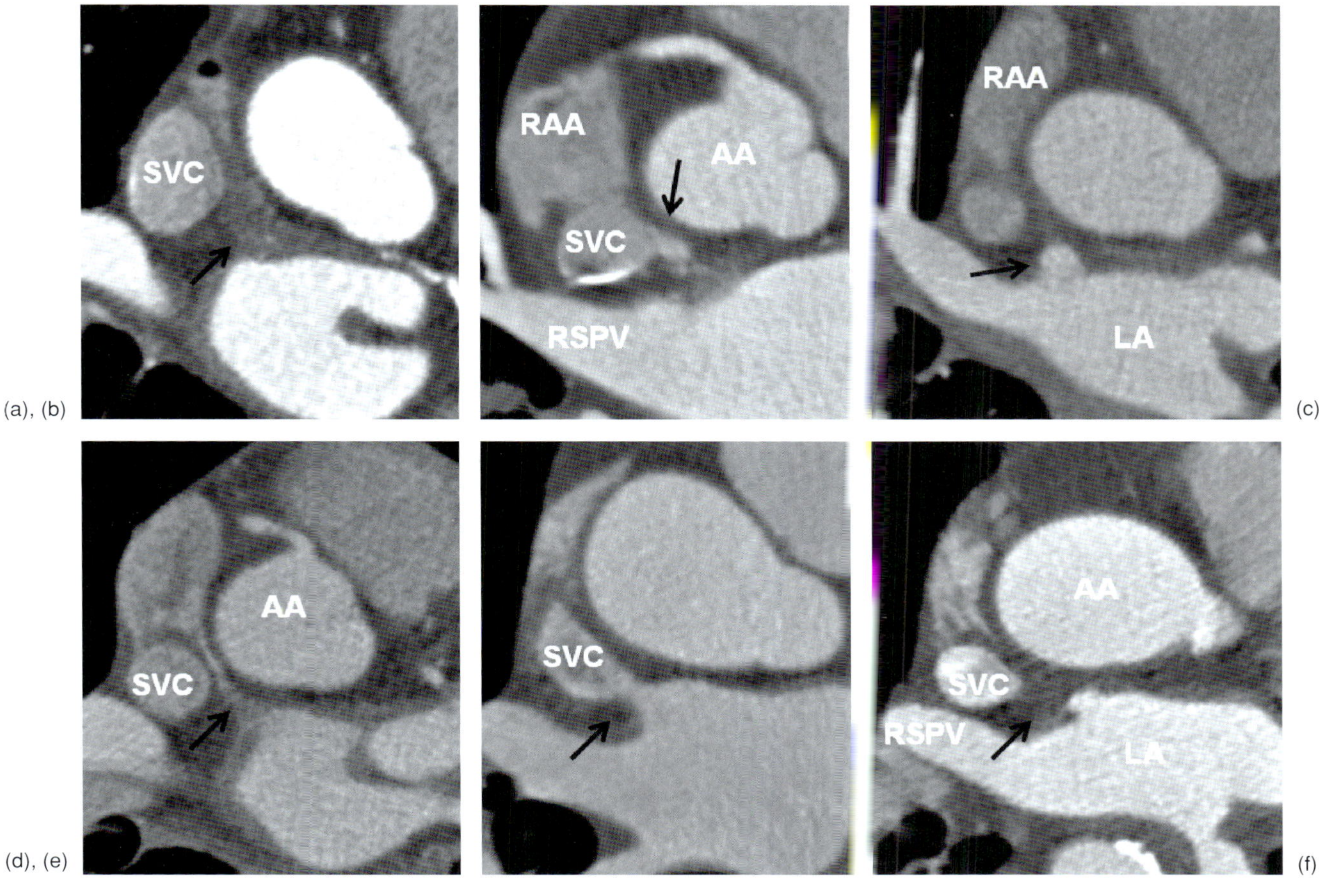

Figure 11.60 Axial views of the heart in different patients showing anatomic variations of the Bachmann bundle (BB) are the following: parts (a) and (b) show thickened BB and BB with contrast filled protrusion on its right atrial side, respectively. Part (c) shows BB with contrast filled protrusion on its left atrial side. Part (d)shows BB filled with contrast. This variation was seen in 0.8% of the normal group. Part (e) shows sinus venosus defect (arrow). BB could not be identified. Part (f) shows fatty replacement of BB. AA, ascending aorta; LA, left atrium; RAA, right atrial appendage; RSPV, right superior pulmonary vein; SVC, superior vena cava.

LMV and PLV are often the target veins for the LV lead in CRT (Figure 11.63).

Coronary Sinus (CS) and Its Anatomic Variants

The CS is described usually as beginning proximally at the right atrial orifice and ending distally at the site of origin of the valve of Vieussens or the GCV, albeit that the direction of flow is from distal to proximal (Figure 11.64). The CS is approximately 45 mm long and 10–12 mm in diameter and highly variable in morphology [117–119]. The beginning of the CS is marked either by an outer constriction, the opening of the oblique vein of Marshall, or by the Vieussens valve internally [118] (Figures 11.46 and 11.65).

The CS ostium is guarded by the Thebesian valve (Figure 11.66). The oval-shaped CS ostium (7 × 9 mm) marks the base of Koch's triangle. The CS opens in the wall of the RA posteroinferior to the commissure between the septal and the posterior leaflets of the TV (Figure 11.15).

From the perspective of ablationists, the CS is an important channel for mapping and for reaching accessory atrioventricular pathways around the mitral valve and those traversing the inferior pyramidal space, the inferior paraseptal pathways. The orifice of the CS may be accessed also for ablating the slow pathway in patients with atrioventricular nodal reentrant tachycardia. The CS is used as a conduit for catheter treatment of arrhythmias as well as LV pacing [120–122]. To obtain recordings of the LA and LV, a catheter is guided into the CS. Because of the sharp angle of the CS with the LA, catheterization of this structure is easier via the SVC (Figure 11.67).

The CS morphology is highly variable (Figure 11.68). Careful evaluation of anatomic barriers is important for treatment success [122]. It is shown that the proximal CS in patients with AV junctional reentry tachycardia is

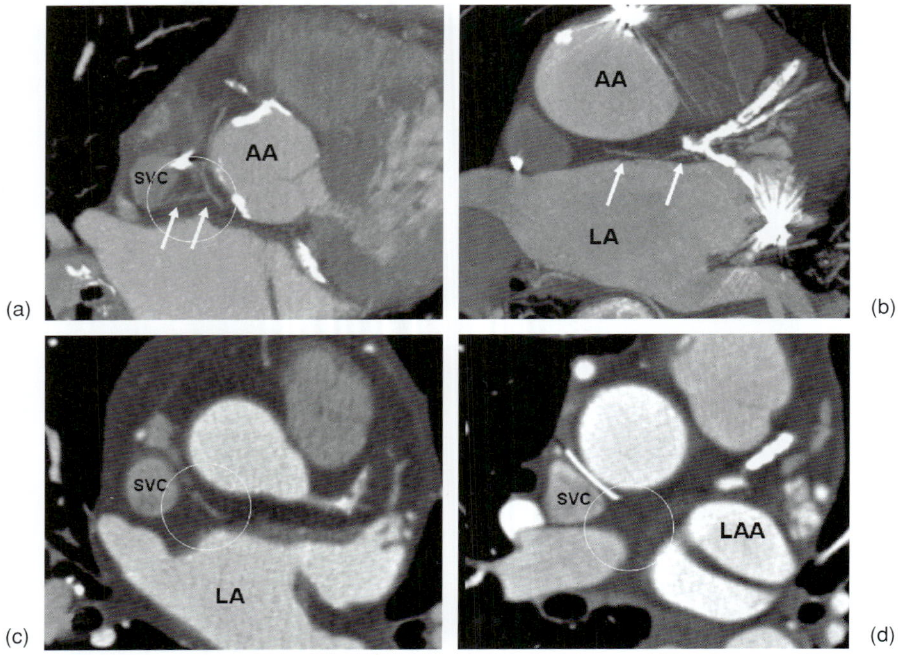

Figure 11.61 Fatty replacement of the anatomic region of BB in four different patients with severe CAD. In spite of severe CAD, the SAN arteries are well opacified in (a) and (b) (arrows). In (a), the SAN artery was arising from a diseased RCA with severe CAD. The SAN artery gives off the BB branch and ends retrocavally (arrows). (b) Status post-CABG patient. The SAN artery, which is arising from a heavily calcified left circumflex artery, shows normal flow and terminates precavally. (c) BB shows a central enhancement with fatty infiltration around it. No muscle bundle is seen. (d) Status post-CABG with a SA nodal lead in place. No SAN artery was visualized in this patient. AA, ascending aorta; BB, Bachmann bundle; CABG, coronary artery bypass grafts; CAD, coronary artery disease; LA, left atrium; LAA, left atrial appendage; RCA, right coronary artery; SAN, sinoatrial node; SVC, superior vena cava. (Reprinted with permission from Saremi *et al.* [88].)

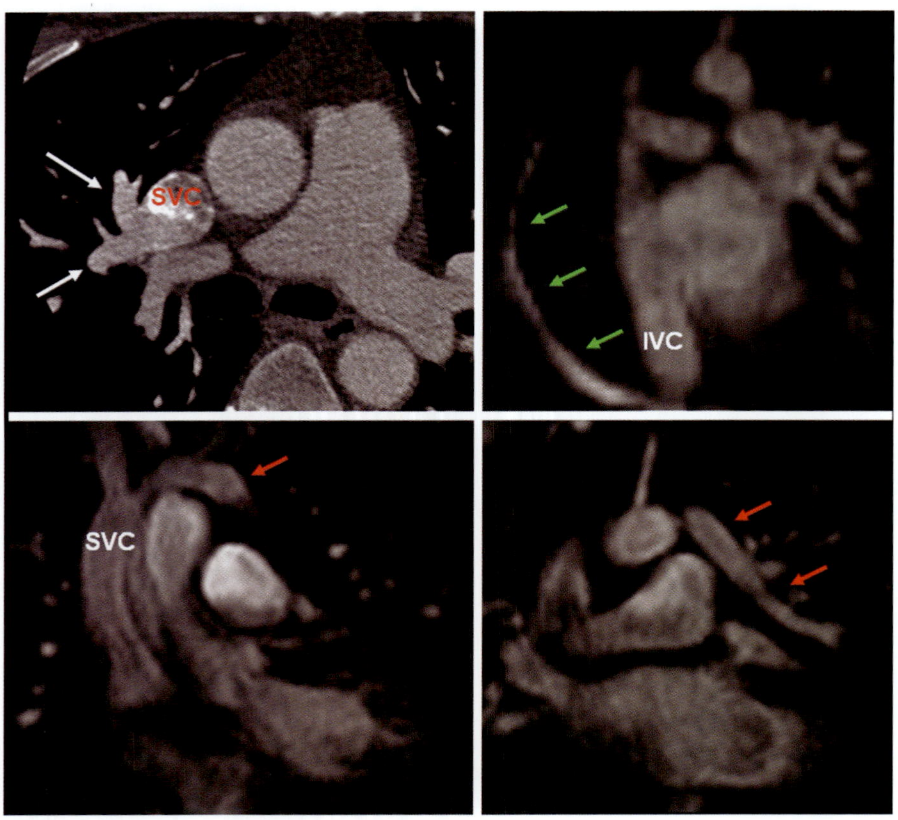

Figure 11.62 Partial anomalous pulmonary venous (PAPV) connections, incidental findings in three different patients. The left upper axial crista terminalis (CT) shows abnormal drainage of right upper lobe pulmonary vein branches directly into the superior vena cava (SVC). Right upper image from a coronal MR angiography show anomalous drainage of right inferior pulmonary vein (green arrows) into the suprahepatic segment of inferior vena cava (IVC) below the diaphragm (scimitar). Lower images from coronal MR angiography show anomalous drainage of left superior pulmonary vein into left brachiocephalic vein via the vertical vein (red arrows).

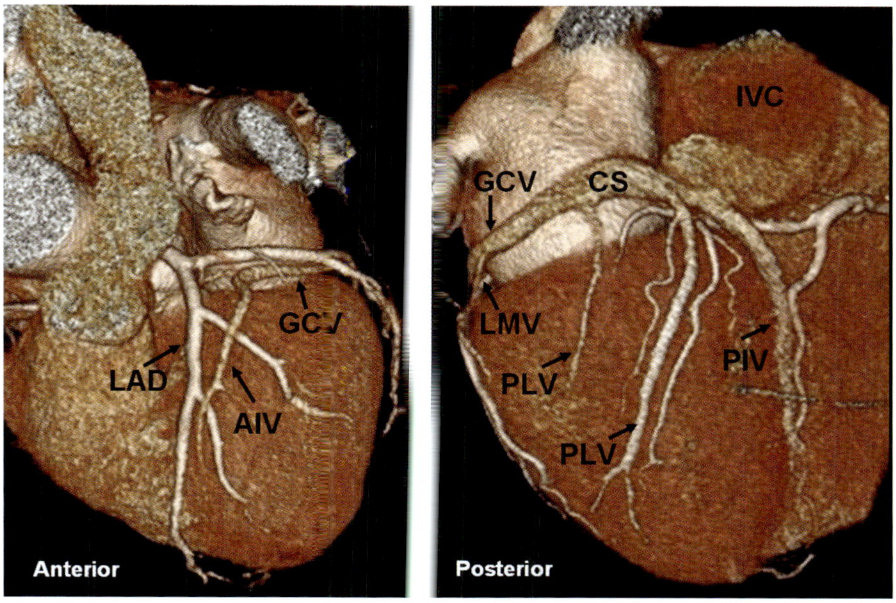

Figure 11.63 Cardiac venous anatomy. The anterior interventricular vein (AIV) forms great cardiac vein (GCV) in left atrioventricular groove. The GCV receives two main branches, lateral marginal vein (LMV), along the lateral border of LV, and posterior (PV) or posterolateral (PLV) veins. Implantation of CS lead usually involves the lateral and posterior (LMV, PV, PLV) branches, which are quite variable in their number, tortuosity, dimensions, and angulation with GCV. The catheter will usually be placed in the periphery of LMV. CS, coronary sinus; IVC, inferior vena cava; LAD, left anterior descending artery; PIV, posterior interventricular vein.

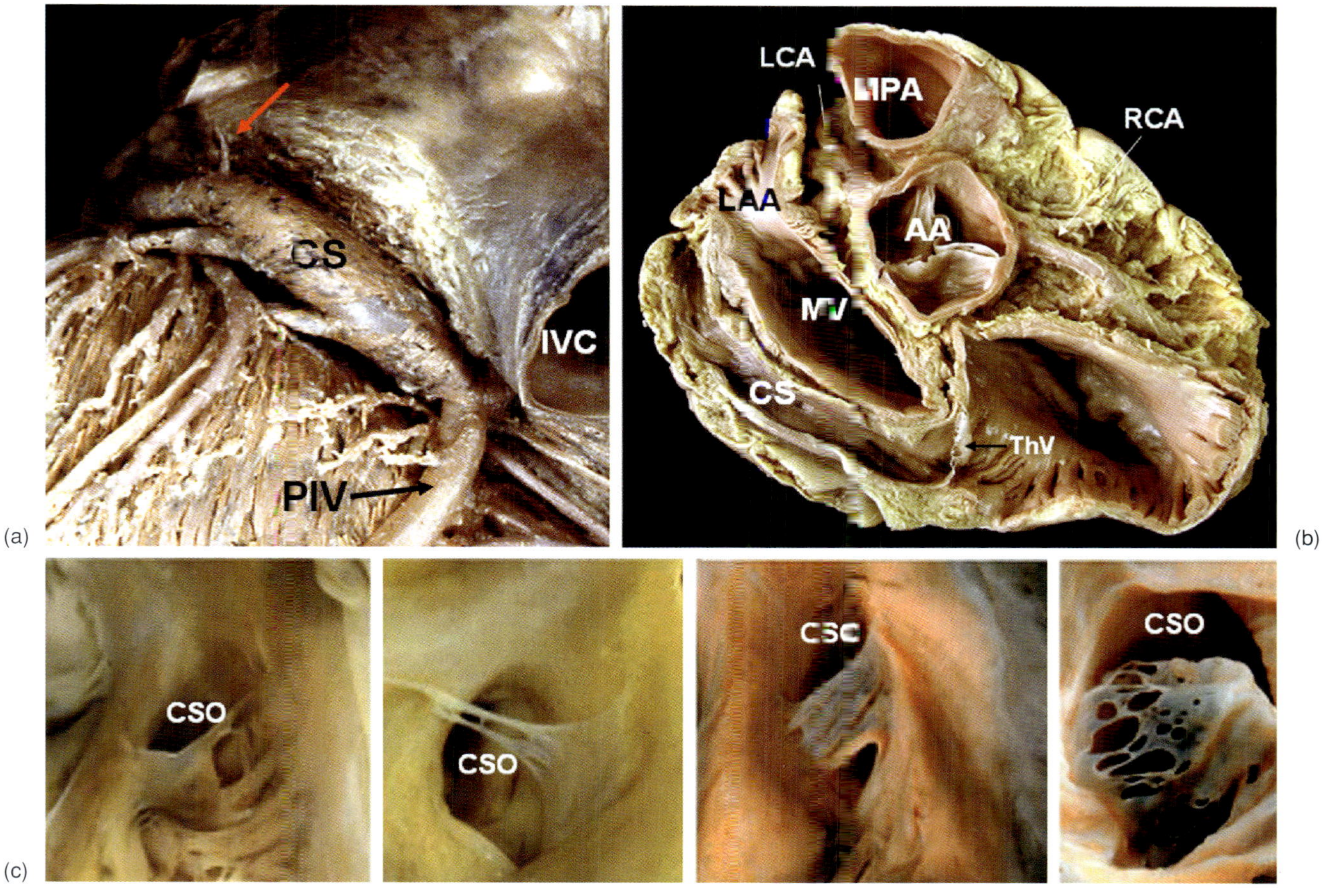

Figure 11.64 (a) Posteroinferior view of a dissection showing the coronary sinus (CS), posterior interventricular vein (PIV) in the inferior aspect of the heart. The remnant of the vein of Marshall (VM) is a short stump (red arrow). (b) Basal view showing the course of the CS across the posterior left atrial wall. At the level of the right atrium note the mouth of the CS that is guarded by the Thebesian valve (ThV) in the base of the triangle of Koch. (c) Variations in morphology of the ThV and CS orifice (CSO) [118]. Ao, aorta; AA, ascending aorta; IVC, inferior vena cava; LAA, left atrial appendage; LCA, left coronary artery; LI, left inferior pulmonary vein; MPA, main pulmonary artery; MV, mitral valve; RCA, right coronary artery.

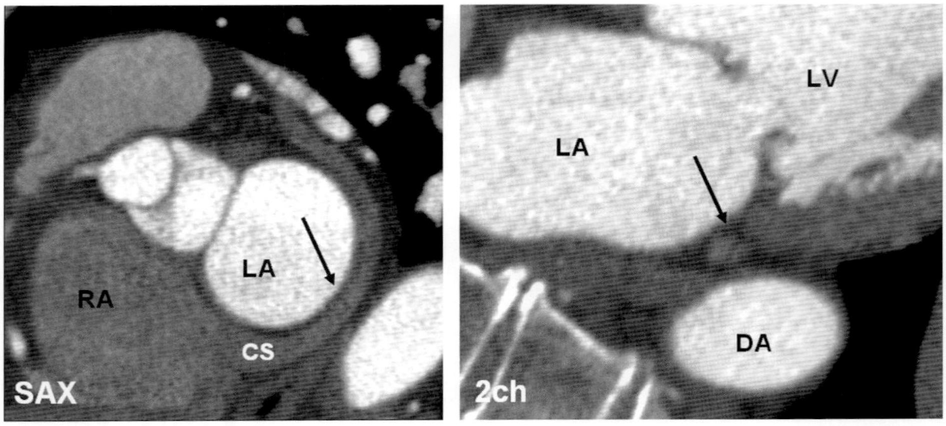

Figure 11.65 Short-axis (SAX) and two-chamber (2ch) views of the heart show the coronary sinus (CS) and the valve of Vieussens (arrows). This valve is usually rudimentary and too small to be resolved by CT, but with careful attention to the images of coronary sinus, it may be seen as a dark line. It can also be marked by relative constriction of the coronary sinus or by the opening of oblique vein of Marshall. CT, crista terminalis; DA, descending aorta; LA, left atrium; LV, left ventricle; RA, right atrium.

significantly larger than the control patients and appears like a windsock [123]. However, this morphology can be seen in normal individuals (Figure 11.68). Excess epicardial fat around the CS may narrow its lumen.

Coronary sinus catheterization procedures are well known for their technical limitations due to the variability of the CS course, valves, and its relationship to adjacent structures. The valve of Vieussens is usually rudimentary and incomplete, but it may be a major source of difficulty in cannulation of CS [124]. The GCV may kink at the level of being crossed by the deeply seated muscular LCx artery, resulting in luminal obstruction [118] (Figure 11.69).

Congenital anomalies of the CS and veins do exist, e.g., diverticulum, stenosis, ectasia, unroofed sinus, ostial atresia, agenesis, or duplication [125] (Figures 11.68–11.70). The majority of the CS diverticula are located along the inferior aspect of the sinus, usually at the junction of the middle cardiac vein with the CS [122] (Figure 11.70). The CS diverticulum is different from the STR, which is an outpouching of the RA wall at the level of the CTI extending below the orifice of the CS (Figure 11.27). CS diverticulum may form the anatomic basis of posteroseptal or left posterior accessory pathways. In such cases, ablation within the diverticulum is necessary [121,126].

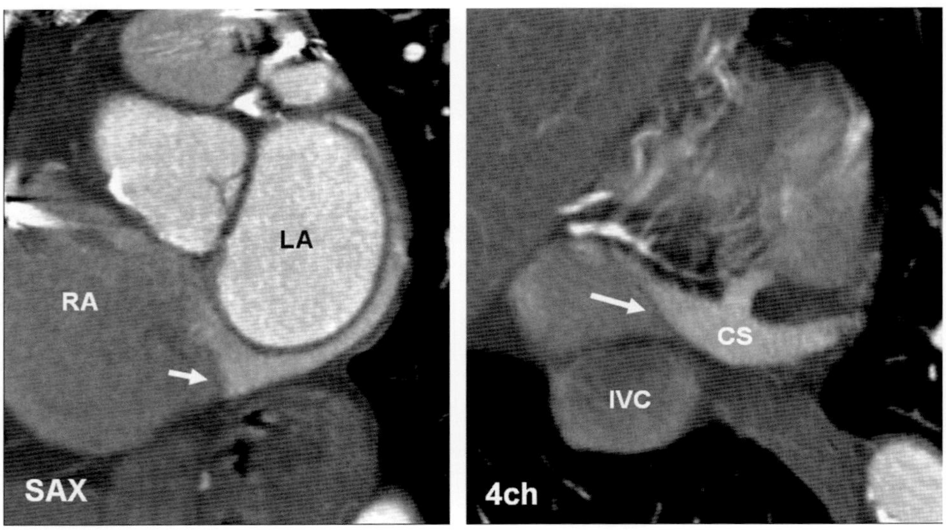

Figure 11.66 Short-axis (SAX) and four-chamber (4ch) views of the heart show the Thebesian valve at the ostium of the coronary sinus. The valve is usually a thin semilunar fold in anteroinferior rim of the ostium. However, its appearance is quite variable. It can be seen in 50% of the good-quality coronary CT studies. CS, coronary sinus; CT, crista terminalis; IVC, inferior vena cava; LA, left atrium; RA, right atrium.

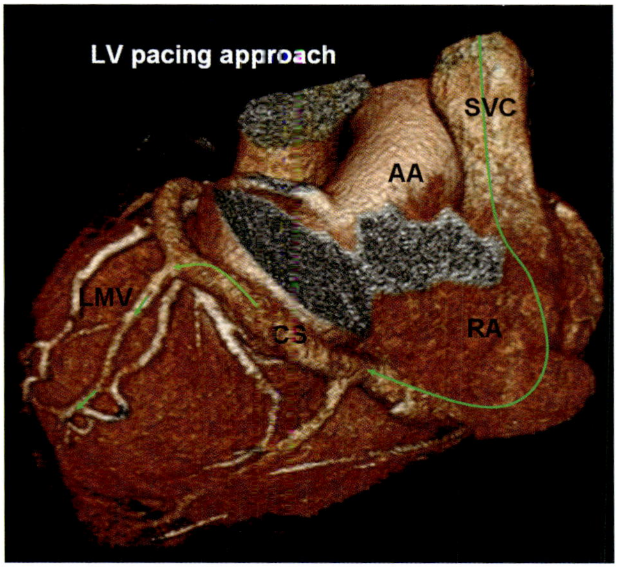

Figure 11.67 Three-dimensional image shows how left ventricular pacing for CRT involves cannulation of the coronary sinus (CS), which is easier to perform via the superior vena cava (SVC). Green arrows indicate the path of the catheter, which is usually placed in the periphery of the lateral marginal vein (LMV). AA, ascending aorta; RA, right atrium.

Left Phrenic Nerve and Its Relation with the Coronary Veins Targeted for LV Pacing

The left phrenic nerve stimulation after CRT is a well-recognized complication [127,128]. The left phrenic nerve passes at a distance of <3 mm of LMV in 43% of cadaveric heart specimens (Figure 11.71) [97]. Given the anatomical variability of the target coronary veins for CRT, and close proximity of the left phrenic nerve to these structures, it is important to show their relationship to stay away from phrenic nerve during LV lead placement. MDCT coronary angiography has the potential to detect the left phrenic nerve in its neurovascular bundle, as it passes over the LV pericardium [99] (Figures 11.71 and 11.72).

Relationship of the Coronary Sinus with LCx Artery

Percutaneous mitral annuloplasty methods exploit the anatomic proximity of the CS to the mitral annulus to deliver an annuloplasty device into the CS to shrink the annulus, thus reducing mitral regurgitation with no need for open cardiac surgery. Some authors have suggested that CS devices may potentially impinge on the LCx artery during annuloplasty via the CS [129]. The LCx artery crosses under the CS the majority of times, but with a significant variability in the location where it crosses the CS (Figure 11.55). These anatomical features should be taken into consideration while selecting percutaneous treatment strategies for mitral valve repair.

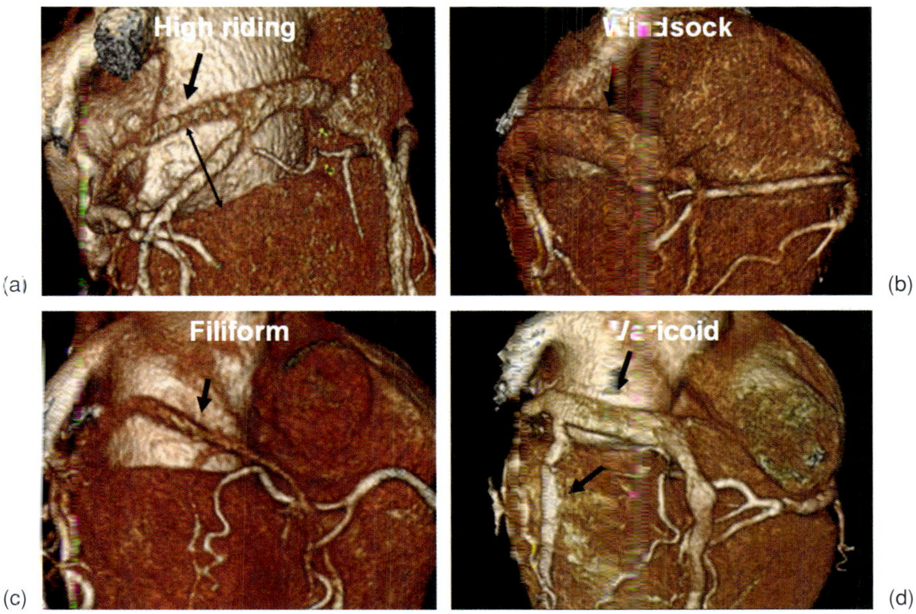

Figure 11.68 Normal anatomic variants of the coronary sinus. Part (a) shows a high-riding coronary sinus (arrow) approximately 3 cm above the atrioventricular groove. Coronary sinus usually travels at the level or up to 10 mm above atrioventricular junction. (b) A dilated coronary sinus is shown giving the appearance of a wind sock (arrow). Part (c) shows a filiform coronary sinus (arrow) because of excessive fat deposition around the coronary sinus. Part (d) shows varicoid appearance of the coronary sinus and veins (arrows).

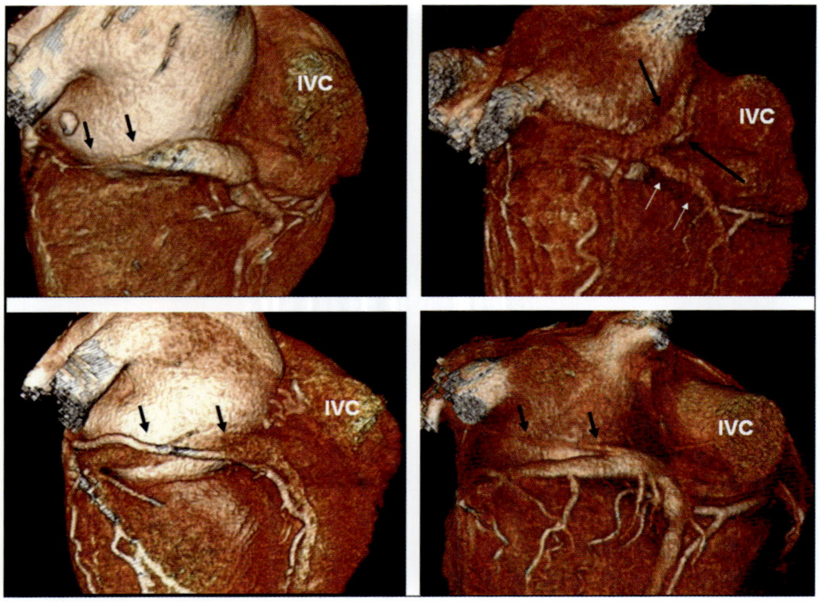

Figure 11.69 Parts (a) to (d) are posterior views of three-dimensional reconstructed cardiac CT images in four different patients showing anatomic barriers that may interfere with cannulation of the coronary sinus. Part (a) demonstrates an atretic coronary sinus at the junction with great cardiac vein. Part (b) is an example of aberrant drainage of the coronary sinus high in the right atrium (black arrows). Note medial insertion of the posterior interventricular vein (white arrows), giving a bifid appearance to the coronary sinus. Part (c) shows compression of the coronary sinus at the level of being crossed by a deeply seated left circumflex artery (arrows). Part (d) shows the oblique vein of Marshall at the origin of the coronary sinus. This vestigial structure may impede further advancement of the catheter into the coronary sinus. IVC, inferior vena cava.

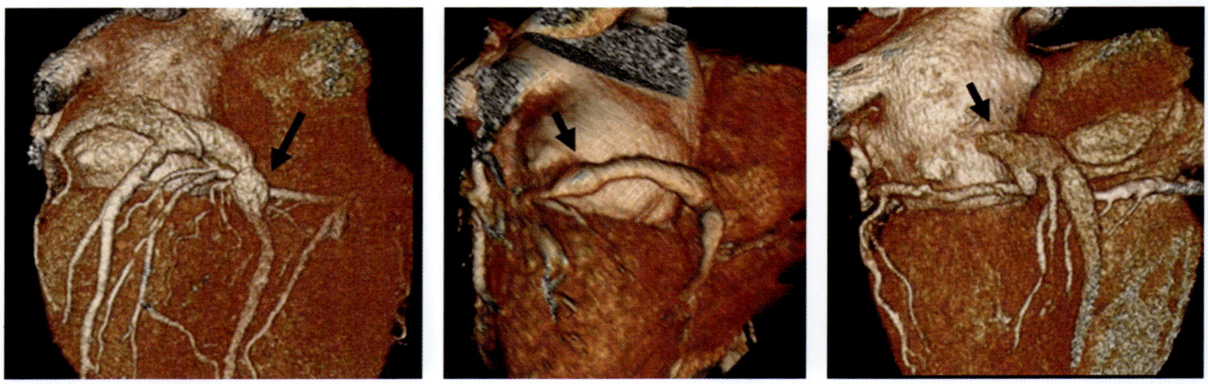

Figure 11.70 Focal dilatation (diverticulum) of the coronary venous system. This anatomic variant is commonly seen at the junction of the posterior interventricular vein with the coronary sinus (arrow in a). The second most common location of this anatomic variant is at the junction of the great cardiac vein with the coronary sinus (arrow in b). Part (c) shows aneurysmal dilatation of the coronary sinus at the origin of the oblique vein of Marshall (arrow).

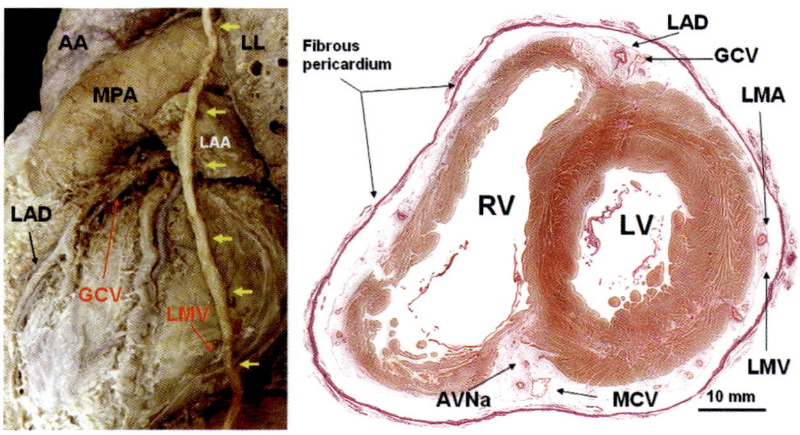

Figure 11.71 (a) The left lateral view after removal the fibrous pericardium and part of the left lung (LL) shows the course of the left phrenic nerve (yellow arrows) running over the tip of the left atrial appendage (LAA) and close to the left marginal vein (LMV). (b) Cross-histological section stained with elastic van Gieson of the right ventricle (RV) and left ventricle (LV) near the leaflets attachment. Note close proximity of the phrenic nerve (black arrow) with the left lateral marginal vein (LMV). AVNa, AV nodal artery; GCV, Great cardiac vein; LAD, left anterior descending artery; LMA, Left marginal artery; MCV, Middle cardiac vein; MPA, main pulmonary artery.

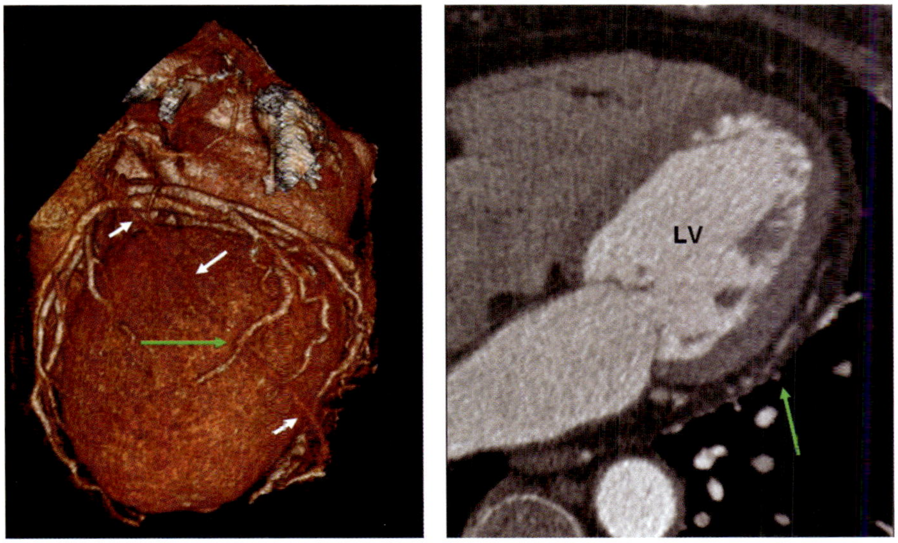

Figure 11.72 Anatomic course of the left phrenic neurovascular bundle. The left lateral view of three-dimensional MDCT and axial image of the heart show the left phrenic nerve running outside pericardium over the coronary vessels toward the diaphragm (white arrows). Note close proximity of the phrenic nerve with the left lateral marginal vein where they cross (green arrows). LV, left ventricle; MDCT, multidetector CT.

References

1. Morady F. (1999) Radio-frequency ablation as treatment for cardiac arrhythmias. *N Engl J Med* 340:534–544.
2. Scheinman MM, Huang S. (2000) The 1998 NASPE prospective catheter ablation registry. *Pacing Clin Electrophysiol* 23:1020–1028.
3. Cazeau S, Leclercq C, Lavergne T *et al.* (2001) Effects of multisite biventricular pacing in patients with heart failure and intraventricular conduction delay. *N Engl J Med* 344:873–880.
4. Haissaguerre M, Shah DC, Jais P *et al.* (2000) Electrophysiological breakthroughs from the left atrium to the pulmonary veins. *Circulation* 102:2463–2465.
5. Marrouche NF, Martin DO, Wazni O *et al.* (2003) Phased-array intracardiac echocardiography monitoring during pulmonary vein isolation in patients with atrial fibrillation: impact on outcome and complications. *Circulation* 107:2710–2716.
6. Marom EM, Herndon JE, Kim YH *et al.* (2004) Variations in pulmonary venous drainage to the left atrium: implications for radiofrequency ablation. *Radiology* 230:824–829.
7. Saremi F, Krishnan S. (2007) Cardiac conduction system: anatomic landmarks relevant to interventional electrophysiologic techniques demonstrated with 64-detector CT. *Radiographics* 27(6):1539–1565.
8. Yee R, Connolly S, Noorani H. (2003) Clinical review of radiofrequency catheter ablation for cardiac arrhythmias. *Can J Cardiol* 19:1273–1284.
9. Veinot JP, Lemery R. (2005) Innovations in cardiovascular pathology: anatomic and electrophysiologic determinants associated with ablation of atrial arrhythmias. *Cardiovasc Pathol* 14:204–213.
10. Sánchez-Quintana D, Ho SY. (2003) Anatomy of cardiac nodes and atrioventricular specialized conduction system. *Rev Esp Cardiol* 56:1085–1092.
11. Malouf JF, Edwards WD, Tajik AJ, Seward JB. (2004) Functional anatomy of the heart. In Fuster V, Alexander RW, O'Rourke RA *et al.* (eds): *The Heart* (11th edition). McGraw-Hill, New York, pp. 75–83.
12. Ho SY, Anderson RH, Sánchez-Quintana D. (2002) Atrial structure and fibres: morphologic bases of atrial conduction. *Cardiovasc Res* 54:325–336.
13. Anderson RH, Brown NA. (1996) The anatomy of the heart revisited. *Anat Rec* 246:1–7.
14. Edwards WD. (1991) Applied anatomy of the heart. In Giuliani ER, Fuster V, Gersh BJ, McGoon MD, McGoon DC (eds): *Cardiology: Fundamentals and Practice* (2nd edition). Mosby-Year Book, St. Louis, pp. 47–112.
15. Sánchez-Quintana D, Anderson RH, Cabrera JA *et al.* (2002) The terminal crest: morphological features relevant to electrophysiology. *Heart* 88:406–411.
16. Matsuyama TA, Inoue S, Kobayashi Y *et al.* (2004) Anatomical diversity and age-related histological changes in the human right atrial posterolateral wall. *Europace* 6:307–315.
17. Pharr JR, Figueredo VM. (2002) Lipomatus hypertrophy of the atrial septum and prominent crista terminalis appearing as a right atrial mass. *Eur J Echocardiogr* 3:159–161.
18. Bharati S, Lev M. (1996) Cardiac conduction system involvement in sudden death of obese young people. *Am Heart J* 129:273–281.
19. Shirani J, Roberts WC. (1993) Clinical, electrocardiograhic and morphologic features of massive fatty deposits (lipomatous hypertrophy) in the atrial septum. *J Am Coll Cardiol* 22:226–238.
20. Mizumaki K, Fujiki A, Nagasawa H *et al.* (2002) Relation between transverse conduction capability and the anatomy of the crista terminalis in patients with atrial flutter and atrial fibrillation: analysis by intracardiac echocardiography. *Circ J* 66:1113–1118.
21. Kalman JM, Olgin JE, Karch MR, Hamdan M, Lee RJ, Lesh MD. (1998) "Cristal tachycardias": origin of right atrial

tachycardias from the crista terminalis identified by intracardiac echocardiography. *J Am Coll Cardiol* 31:451–459.
22. Anderson KR, Ho SY, Anderson RH. (1979) Location and vascular supply of sinus node in human heart. *Br Heart J* 41:28–32.
23. Chiu I, Hung CR, How SW, Chen MR. (1989) Is the sinus node visible grossly? A histological study of normal hearts. *Int J Cardiol* 22:83–87.
24. Sánchez-Quintana D, Cabrera JA, Farré J, Climent V, Anderson RH, Ho SY. (2005) Sinus node revisited in the era of electroanatomical mapping and catheter ablation. *Heart* 91(2):189–194.
25. Inoue S, Shinohara F, Niitani H, Gotoh K. (1986) A new method for the histological study of aging changes in the sinoatrial node. *Jpn Heart J* 27:653–660.
26. Man KC, Knight B, Tse HF *et al.* (2000) Radiofrequency catheter ablation of inappropriate sinus tachycardia guided by activation mapping. *J Am Coll Cardiol* 35:451–457.
27. Berdajs D, Patonay L, Turina MI. (2003) The clinical anatomy of the sinus node artery. *Ann Thorac Surg* 76:732–735.
28. Sow ML, Ndoye JM, Lo EA. (1996) The artery of the sinuatrial node: anatomic considerations based on 45 injection-dissections of the heart. *Surg Radiol Anat* 18:103–109.
29. Saremi F, Abolhoda A, Ashikyan O *et al.* (2008) Arterial supply to sinuatrial and atrioventricular nodes: imaging with multidetector CT. *Radiology* 246(1):99–107
30. Ho SY, Anderson RH. (2000) How constant anatomically is the tendon of Todaro as a marker for the triangle of Koch? *J Cardiovasc Electrophysiol* 11:83–89.
31. Anderson RH, Ho HY, Becker AE. (2000) Anatomy of the human atrioventricular junctions revisited. *Anat Rec* 260:81–91.
32. Sow ML, Ndoye JM, Lo EA. (2000) The artery of the atrioventricular node: an anatomic study based on 38 injection-dissections. *Surg Radiol Anat* 22:93–96.
33. Anderson KR, Murphy JG. (1983) The atrio-ventricular node artery in the human heart. *Angiology* 34:711–716.
34. Arid JM, Armstrong O, Rogez JM, Robert R, Lardoux MC, Leborgne J. (2000) Arterial vascularisation of the atrioventricular node. *Surg Radiol Anat* 22:93–96.
35. Jazayeri MR, Hempe SL, Sra JS *et al.* (1992) Selective transcatheter ablation of the fast and slow pathways using radiofrequency energy in patients with atrioventricular nodal reentrant tachycardia. *Circulation* 85:1318–1328.
36. Sánchez-Quintana D, Ho SY, Cabrera JA, Farre J, Anderson RH. (2001) Topographic anatomy of the inferior pyramidal space: relevance to radiofrequency catheter ablation. *J Cardiovasc Electrophysiol* 12:210–217.
37. Poty H, Saoudi N, Nair M, Anselme F, Letac B. (1996) Radiofrequency catheter ablation of atrial flutter. Further insights into the various types of isthmus block: application to ablation during sinus rhythm. *Circulation* 94:3204–3213.
38. Cauchemez B, Haïssaguerre M, Fischer B, Thomas O, Clementy J, Coumel P. (1996) Electrophysiological effects of catheter ablation of inferior vena cava-tricuspid annulus isthmus in common atrial flutter. *Circulation* 93:284–294.
39. Cabrera JA, Sánchez-Quintana D, Ho SY *et al.* (1999) Angiographic anatomy of the inferior right atrial isthmus in patients with and without history of common atrial flutter. *Circulation* 99:3017–3023.
40. Cabrera JA, Sánchez-Quintana D, Farre J, Rubio JM, Ho SY. (2005) The inferior right atrial isthmus: Further architectural insights for current and coming ablation technologies. *J Cardiovasc Electrophysiol* 16(4):409–410.
41. Heidbuchel H, Willems R, van Rensburg H, Adams J, Ector H, Van de Werf F. (2000) Right atrial angiographic evaluation of the posterior isthmus: relevance for ablation of typical atrial flutter. *Circulation* 101:2178–2184.
42. Da Costa A, Faure E, Thevenin J *et al.* (2004) Effect of isthmus anatomy and ablation catheter on radiofrequency catheter ablation of the cavotricuspid isthmus. *Circulation* 110(9):1030–1035.
43. Nakagawa H, Lazzara R, Khastgir T *et al.* (1996) Role of the tricuspid annulus and the Eustachian valve/ridge on atrial flutter: relevance to catheter ablation of the septal isthmus and a new technique for rapid identification of ablation success. *Circulation* 94:407–424.
44. Da Costa A, Mourot S, Romeyer-Bouchard C *et al.* (2004) Anatomic and electrophysiological differences between chronic and paroxysmal forms of common atrial flutter and comparison with controls. *Pacing Clin Electrophysiol* 27(9):1202–1211.
45. Saremi F, Pourzand L, Krishnan S *et al.* (2008) Right atrial cavotricuspid isthmus: anatomic characterization with multi-detector row CT. *Radiology* 247(3):658–668.
46. Olgin JE, Kalman JM, Fitzpatrick AP, Lesh MD. (1995) Role of right atrial endocardial structures as barriers to conduction during human type I atrial flutter: activation and entrainment mapping guided by intracardiac echocardiography. *Circulation* 92:1839–1848.
47. Chang SL, Tai CT, Lin YJ *et al.* (2007) The electroanatomic characteristics of the cavotricuspid isthmus: implications for the catheter ablation of atrial flutter. *J Cardiovasc Electrophysiol* 18(1):18–22.
48. Anderson RH, Brown NA, Webb S. (2002) Development and structure of the atrial septum. *Heart* 88:104–110.
49. Hagen PT, Scholz DG, Edwards WD. (1984) Incidence and size of patent foramen ovale during the first 10 decades of life: an autopsy study of 965 normal hearts. *Mayo Clin Proc* 59:17–20.
50. Lechat PH, Mas JL, Lascault G *et al.* (1988) Prevalence of patent foramen ovale in patients with stroke. *N Engl J Med* 318:1148–1152.
51. Webster MWI, Smith HJ, Sharpe DN *et al.* (1988) Patent foramen ovale in young stroke patients. *Lancet* 2(8601):11–12.
52. Rome JJ, Keane JF, Perry SB *et al.* (1990) Double-umbrella closure of atrial defects: initial clinical applications. *Circulation* 82:751–758.
53. Divekar A, Gaamangwe T, Shaikh N, Raabe M, Ducas J. (2005) Cardiac perforation after device closure of atrial septal defects with the Amplatzer septal occluder. *J Am Coll Cardiol* 45(8):1213–1218.
54. Schwinger ME, Gindea AJ, Freedberg RS, Kronzon I. (1990) The anatomy of the interatrial septum: a

transesophageal echocardiographic study. *Am Heart J* 119:1401–1405.
55. Ho SY, McCarthy KP, Rigby ML. (2003) Morphological features pertinent to interventional closure of patent oval foramen. *J Interv Cardiol* 16(1):33–38.
56. Mattioli AV, Aquilina M, Oldani A, Longhini C, Mattioli G. (2001) Atrial septal aneurysm as a cardioembolic source in adult patients with stroke and normal carotid arteries. A multicentre study. *Eur Heart J* 22(3):261–268.
57. Saremi F, Channual S, Raney A *et al.* (2008) Imaging of patent foramen ovale with 64-section multidetector CT. *Radiology* 249(2):483–492.
58. Saremi F, Attai SF, Narula J. (2007) 64 multidetector CT in patent foramen ovale. *Heart* 93(4):505.
59. Mugge WG, Daniel C, Angermann C *et al.* (1995) Atrial septal aneurysm in adult patients. A multicenter study using transthoracic and transesophageal echocardiography. *Circulation* 91:2785–2792.
60. Schneider B, Hofmann T, Justen MH, Meinertz T. (1995) Chiari's network: normal anatomic variant or risk factor for arterial embolic events? *J Am Coll Cardiol* 26:203–210.
61. Cooke JC, Gelman JS, Harper RW. (1999) Chiari network entanglement and herniation into the left atrium by an atrial septal defect occluder device. *J Am Soc Echocardiogr* 12:601–603.
62. Solomon SB. (2004) The future of interventional cardiology lies in the left atrium. *Int J Cardiovasc Intervent* 6:101–106.
63. Ho SY, Sánchez-Quintana D, Cabrera JA *et al.* (1999) Anatomy of the left atrium: implications for radiofrequency ablation of atrial fibrillation. *J Cardiovasc Electrophysiol* 10:1525–1533.
64. Nathan H, Eliakim M. (1996) The junction between the left atrium and the pulmonary veins. An anatomic study of human hearts. *Circulation* 34:412–422.
65. Haissaguerre M, Jais P, Shah DC *et al.* (1998) Spontaneous initiation of AF by ectopic beats originating in the pulmonary veins. *N Engl J Med* 339:659–666.
66. Pappone C, Oreto G, Rosanio S *et al.* (2001) Atrial electroanatomic remodeling after circumferential radiofrequency pulmonary vein ablation: efficacy of an anatomic approach in a large cohort of patients with atrial fibrillation. *Circulation* 104:2539–2544.
67. Takahashi A, Iesaka Y, Takahashi Y *et al.* (2002) Electrical connections between pulmonary veins: implication for ostial ablation of pulmonary veins in patients with paroxysmal atrial fibrillation. *Circulation* 105:2998–3003.
68. Ouyang F, Bansch D, Ernst S *et al.* (2004) Complete isolation of left atrium surrounding the pulmonary veins: new insights from the double-Lasso technique in paroxysmal atrial fibrillation. *Circulation* 110:2090–2096.
69. Ernst S, Ouyang F, Lober F *et al.* (2003) Catheter-induced linear lesions in the left atrium in patients with atrial fibrillation: an electroanatomic study. *J Am Coll Cardiol* 42:1271–1282.
70. Nademanee K, Mckenzie J, Kosar E *et al.* (2004) A new approach for catheter ablation of atrial fibrillation: mapping of the electrophysiologic substrate. *J Am Coll Cardiol* 43:2044–2053.
71. Haissaguerre M, Hocini M, Sanders P *et al.* (2005) Catheter ablation of long-lasting persistent atrial fibrillation: clinical outcome and mechanisms of subsequent arrhythmias. *J Cardiovasc Electrophysiol* 16:1138–1147.
72. Singh S, Johnson PI, Lee RE *et al.* (1996) Topography of cardiac ganglia in the adult human heart. *J Thorac Cardiovasc Surg* 112:943–995.
73. Pappone C, Santinelli V, Manguso F *et al.* (2004) Pulmonary vein denervation enhances long-term benefit after circumferential ablation for paroxysmal atrial fibrillation. *Circulation* 109:327–334.
74. Schwartzman D, Lacomis J, Wigginton WG. (2003) Characterization of left atrium and distal pulmonary vein morphology using multidimensional computed tomography. *J Am Coll Cardiol* 41:1349–1357.
75. Wittkampf FH, Vonken EJ, Derksen R *et al.* (2003) Pulmonary vein ostium geometry: analysis by magnetic resonance angiography. *Circulation* 107:21–23.
76. Scharf C, Sneider M, Case I *et al.* (2003) Anatomy of the pulmonary veins in patients with atrial fibrillation and effects of segmental ostial ablation analyzed by computed tomography. *J Cardiovasc Electrophysiol* 14:150–155.
77. Cronin P, Sneider MB, Kazerooni EA *et al.* (2004) MDCT of the left atrium and pulmonary veins in planning radiofrequency ablation for atrial fibrillation: a how-to guide. *AJR Am J Roentgenol* 183:767–778.
78. Jongbloed MR, Bax JJ, Lamb HJ *et al.* (2005) Multislice computed tomography versus intracardiac echocardiography to evaluate the pulmonary veins before radiofrequency catheter ablation of atrial fibrillation: a head-to-head comparison. *J Am Coll Cardiol* 45(3):343–350.
79. Tsao HM, Wu MH, Yu WC *et al.* (2001) Role of right middle pulmonary vein in patients with paroxysmal atrial fibrillation. *J Cardiovasc Electrophysiol* 12:1353–1357.
80. Kim YH, Marom EM, Herndon JE II *et al.* (2005) Pulmonary vein diameter, cross-sectional area, and shape: CT analysis. *Radiology* 235(1):43–49.
81. Choi SI, Seo JB, Choi SH *et al.* (2005) Variation of the size of pulmonary venous ostia during the cardiac cycle: optimal reconstruction window at ECG-gated multi-detector row CT. *Eur Radiol* 15(7):1441–1445.
82. Jais P, Hocini M, Hsu LF *et al.* (2004) Technique and results of linear ablation at the mitral isthmus. *Circulation* 110:2996–3002.
83. Becker AE (2004) Left atrial isthmus. Anatomic aspects relevant for linear catheter ablation procedures in humans. *J Cardiovasc Electrophysiol* 15:809–812.
84. Chiang SJ, Tsao HM, Wu MH *et al.* (2006) Anatomic characteristics of the left atrial isthmus in patients with atrial fibrillation, lessons from computed tomographic images. *J Cardiovasc Electrophysiol* 17(12):1274–1278.
85. Shah D, Haissaguerre M, Jais P, Hocini M. (2003) Nonpulmonary vein foci: do they exist? *Pacing Clin Electrophysiol* 26(7 Pt 2):1631–1635.
86. Cabrera JA, Ho SY, Climent V, Sánchez-Quintana D. (2008) The architecture of the left lateral atrial wall: a particular anatomic region with implications for ablation of atrial fibrillation. *Eur Heart J* 29:356–362.

87. Hsu LF, Jais P, Keane D *et al.* (2004) Atrial fibrillation originating from persistent left superior vena cava. *Circulation* 109:828–832.
88. Saremi F, Channual S, Krishnan S *et al.* (2008) Bachmann bundle and its arterial supply: imaging with multidetector CT-implications for interatrial conduction abnormalities and arrhythmias. *Radiology* 248(2):447–457.
89. Duerinckx AJ, Vanovermeire O. (2008) Accessory appendages of the left atrium as seen during 64-slice coronary CT angiography. *Int J Cardiovasc Imaging* 24(2):215–221.
90. Saremi F, Gurudevan SV, Narula J *et al.* (2007) Multidetector computed tomography (MDCT) in diagnosis of "cor triatriatum sinister". *J Cardiovasc Comput Tomogr* 1(3):172–174.
91. Nerantzis C, Avgoustakis D. (1998) An S-shaped atrial artery supplying the sinus node area: an anatomic study. *Chest* 78:274–278.
92. Saremi F, Channual S, Abolhoda A *et al.* (2008) MDCT of the S-shaped sinoatrial node artery. *AJR Am J Roentgenol* 190(6):1569–1575.
93. Von Ludinghausen M, Ohmachi N, Besch S *et al.* (1995) Atrial veins of the human heart. *Clin Anat* 8(3):169–189.
94. Sánchez-Quintana D, Cabrera JA, Climent V *et al.* (2005) Anatomic relations between the esophagus and left atrium and relevance for ablation of atrial fibrillation. *Circulation* 112:1400–1405.
95. Cummings JE, Schweikert RA, Saliba WI *et al.* (2006) Brief communication: atrial-esophageal fistulas after radiofrequency ablation. *Ann Intern Med* 144:572–574.
96. Lemola K, Sneider M, Desjardins B *et al.* (2004) Computed tomographic analysis of the anatomy of the left atrium and the esophagus: implications for left atrial catheter ablation. *Circulation* 110:3655–3660.
97. Sánchez-Quintana D, Cabrera JA, Climent V *et al.* (2005) How close are the phrenic nerves to cardiac structures? Implications for cardiac interventionalists. *J Cardiovasc Electrophysiol* 16:309–313.
98. Sacher F, Monahan KH, Thomas SP *et al.* (2006) Phrenic nerve injury after atrial fibrillation catheter ablation: characterization and outcome in a multicenter study. *J Am Coll Cardiol* 47:2498–2503.
99. Matsumoto Y, Krishnan S, Fowler SJ *et al.* (2007) Detection of phrenic nerves and their relation to cardiac anatomy using 64-slice multidetector computed tomography. *Am J Cardiol* 100(1):133–137.
100. Takahashi Y, Jais P, Hocini M *et al.* (2005) Acute occlusion of the left circumflex coronary artery during mitral isthmus linear ablation. *J Cardiovasc Electrophysiol* 16:1104–1107.
101. Reyes CV, Jablokow VR. (1979) Lipomatous hypertrophy of the cardiac interatrial septum. A report of 38 cases and review of the literature. *Am J Clin Pathol* 72:785–788.
102. Heyer CM, Kagel T, Lemburg SP *et al.* (2003) Lipomatous hypertrophy of the interatrial septum: a prospective study of incidence, imaging findings, and clinical symptoms. *Chest* 124:2068–2073.
103. Meaney JF, Kazerooni EA, Jamadar DA *et al.* (1997) CT appearance of lipomatous hypertrophy of the interatrial septum. *AJR Am J Roentgenol* 168(4):1081–1084.
104. Lemery R, Guiraudon G, Veinot JP. (2003) Anatomic description of the Bachmann bundle and its relation to the atrial septum. *Am J Cardiol* 91:1482–1485.
105. Leier C, Meacham J, Shaal S. (1978) Prolonged atrial conduction. A major predisposing factor for the development of atrial flutter. *Circulation* 57:213–216.
106. Ariyarajah V, Fernandes J, Apiyasawat S *et al.* (2007) Angiographic localization of potential culprit coronary arteries in patients with interatrial block following a positive exercise tolerance test. *Am J Cardiol* 99(1):58–61.
107. Herlong JR, Jaggers JJ, Ungerleider RM. (2000) Congenital heart surgery nomenclature and database project: pulmonary venous anomalies. *Ann Thorac Surg* 69:56–69.
108. Van Meter Jr, C, LeBlanc JG, Culpepper III, WS *et al.* (1990) Partial anomalous pulmonary venous return. *Circulation* 82:IV195–IV198.
109. Ferrari VA, Scott CH, Holland GA *et al.* (2001) Ultrafast three-dimensional contrast-enhanced magnetic resonance angiography and imaging in the diagnosis of partial anomalous pulmonary venous drainage. *J Am Coll Cardiol* 37:1120–1128.
110. Ammash N, Seward J, Warnes C *et al.* (1997) Partial anomalous pulmonary venous connection: diagnosis by transesophageal echocardiography. *J Am Coll Cardiol* 29:1351–1358.
111. Haramati LB, Moche IE, Rivera VT *et al.* (2003) Computed tomography of partial anomalous pulmonary venous connection in adults. *J Comput Assist Tomogr* 27:743–749.
112. Willerson JT, Kereiakes DJ. (2004) Cardiac resynchronization therapy. Helpful now in selected patients with CHF. *Circulation* 109:308–309.
113. Lemola K, Mueller G, Desjardins B *et al.* (2005) Topographic analysis of the coronary sinus and major cardiac veins by computed tomography. *Heart Rhythm* 2:694–699.
114. Mao S, Shinbane JS, Girsky MJ *et al.* (2005) Coronary venous imaging with electron beam computed tomographic angiography: three-dimensional mapping and relationship with coronary arteries. *Am Heart J* 150:315–322.
115. Jongbloed MRM, Lamb HJ, Bax JJ *et al.* (2005) Noninvasive visualization of the cardiac venous system using multislice computed tomography. *J Am Coll Cardiol* 45:749–753.
116. Meisel E, Pfeiffer D, Engelmann L *et al.* (2001) Investigation of coronary venous anatomy by retrograde venography in patients with malignant ventricular tachycardia. *Circulation* 104:442–447.
117. Silver MA, Rowley NE. (1988) The functional anatomy of the human coronary sinus. *Am Heart J* 115:1080–1084.
118. Ho SY, Sánchez-Quintana D, Becker AE. (2004) A review of the coronary venous system: a road less travelled. *Heart Rhythm* 1(1):107–112.
119. Katritsis DG. (2004) The coronary sinus: passive bystander or source of arrhythmia? *Heart Rhythm* 1:113–116.
120. Giorgberidze I, Saksena A, Kroll RB *et al.* (1995) Efficacy and safety of radiofrequency catheter ablation of left-sided accessory pathways through the coronary sinus. *Am J Cardiol* 76:359–365.
121. Sun Y, Arruda M, Otomo K *et al.* (2002) Coronary sinus ventricular accessory connections producing posteroseptal

and left posterior accessory pathways: incidence and electrophysiological identification. *Circulation* 106:1362–1367.

122. Karaca M, Bilge O, Hakan Dinckal M, Ucerler H. (2005) The anatomic barriers in the coronary sinus: implications for clinical procedures. *J Interv Card Electrophysiol* 14:89–94.
123. Ong MG, Lee PC, Tai CT *et al.* (2006) Coronary sinus morphology in different types of supraventricular tachycardias. *J Interv Card Electrophysiol* 15:21–26.
124. Corcoran SJ, Lawrence C, McGuire MA. (1999) The valve of Vieussens: an important cause of difficulty in advancing catheters into the cardiac veins. *J Cardiovasc Electrophysiol* 10:804–808.
125. Binder TM, Rosenhek R, Frank H *et al.* (2000) Congenital malformations of the right atrium and the coronary sinus: an analysis based on 103 cases reported in the literature and two additional cases. *Chest* 117:1740–1748.
126. Guiraudon GM, Guiraudon CM, Klein GJ *et al.* (1988) The coronary sinus diverticulum: a pathologic entity associated with the Wolff-Parkinson-White syndrome. *Am J Cardiol* 62:733–735.
127. Alonso C, Leclercq C, Revaul d'Allonnes F *et al.* (2001) Six year experience of transvenous left ventricular lead implantation for permanent biventricular pacing in patients with advance heart failure: technical aspects. *Heart* 86:405–410.
128. Albertsen AE, Nielsen JC, Pedersen AK *et al.* (2005) Left ventricular lead performance in cardiac resynchronization therapy: impact of lead localization and complications. *Pacing Clin Electrophysiol* 28:483–488.
129. Block PV. (2005) Percutaneous mitral valve repair: are they changing the guard? *Circulation* 111:2154–2156.

12 Coronary Atherosclerosis: CT Imaging for the Preventive Cardiologist

Stephan Achenbach[1] & Jagat Narula[2]

[1]*University of Erlangen, Erlangen, Germany*
[2]*University of California, Irvine, CA, USA*

Histopathology of Acute Coronary Syndromes

"Acute coronary syndromes" comprise ST-elevation myocardial infarction (STEMI), non-ST elevation myocardial infarction (NSTEMI), and unstable angina. More than one million Americans experience an acute coronary syndrome every year, and acute coronary syndromes contribute significantly to the overall mortality of coronary artery disease, which costs more than 400,000 lives each year in the United States alone [1]. Acute coronary syndromes have a common pathomechanism. In most cases, they are caused by acute rupture or erosion of atherosclerotic plaque in the coronary arteries (Figure 12.1). Erosions are responsible for approximately 20–30% of acute coronary syndromes and are found most frequently in women and younger individuals [2]. Very infrequently, "calcified nodules" are the pathologic substrate underlying acute coronary syndromes [2]. When plaque rupture or erosion occurs, the resulting rough surface is suddenly exposed to the blood stream. Thrombus formation occurs instantaneously and is further accelerated by thrombogenic substances liberated from the ruptured plaque. Depending on the degree of luminal obstruction caused by the thrombus, symptoms vary: Complete or subtotal obstruction of the coronary artery lumen results in myocardial ischemia and potentially necrosis, typically accompanied by severe symptoms and clinically becoming manifest as STEMI, NSTEMI, or unstable angina. However, plaque rupture and erosion can also occur silently, without symptoms. Indeed, repeated rupture and healing is one mechanism of plaque growth and the development of coronary artery stenoses [3].

Plaques that cause acute coronary syndromes are, in most cases, not associated with "significant" (usually assumed above a threshold of 50% diameter stenosis) narrowing of the coronary artery lumen (Figure 12.2). Retrospective analyses have shown that coronary atherosclerotic lesions that cause acute myocardial infarction are associated with a luminal stenosis below 50% in 48% of cases. Plaques that lead to unstable angina have a luminal stenosis of <50% in 72% of cases before the acute onset of symptoms [4,5]. This explains why many individuals are asymptomatic until an acute coronary syndrome occurs. In fact, patients who experience acute myocardial infarction had no prior symptoms of coronary artery disease in approximately 50% of cases. Unfortunately, sudden cardiac death, often without any preceding symptoms, can be the first and only manifestation of coronary artery disease [6].

The underlying histology of *plaque erosion* is typically intimal thickening or fibroatheroma; calcification is rare. The typical atherosclerotic lesion that is associated with *plaque rupture* is the "thin cap fibroatheroma" (TCFA; Figure 12.3); TCFAs are considered to be precursors of plaque rupture [2]. While plaques that rupture or plaques prone to rupture are not necessarily associated with significant luminal stenosis, overall plaque size and volume is typically large (Figure 12.3). Substantial "positive remodeling" [7] is typically found and allows for a preserved coronary artery lumen size in spite of the presence of large plaque volumes.

Typical morphologic characteristics include a thin fibrous cap (<65 μm in thickness), infiltration with macrophages, and a relatively large necrotic core, both in relative and absolute terms. Typically, >10% of the plaque volume are occupied by the necrotic core (Figure 12.3).

Revisiting Cardiac Anatomy: A Computed-Tomography-Based Atlas and Reference, 1st edition. Edited by Farhood Saremi, Eloisa Arbustini, Stephen Achenbach and Jagat Narula.

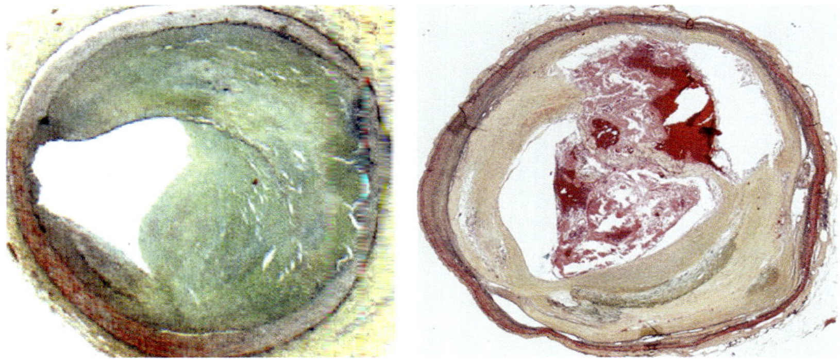

Figure 12.1 Histology of a stable plaque (a) and a ruptured plaque (b). The stable plaque (a) contains mostly collagen and smooth muscle cells; lipid content is minimal. The ruptured plaque is made up mostly of a "necrotic core" (NC), which is acellular, has a high lipid content and semisolid consistency. The NC is covered by a thin fibrous cap. At the site of rupture, material from the NC is exposed to the blood stream and causes thrombosis. (a) (b)

On average, 23% of the plaque volume are occupied by the necrotic core in TCFAs and in plaques that have ruptures; the necrotic core accounts for 34% of the plaque volume [2]. The average length of necrotic cores in TCFAs is 8 mm. Finally, vascularization of the plaque may play a role in plaque instability and the likelihood for rupture. Intraplaque hemorrhage is frequently seen, but it can both be a promoter or a consequence of plaque instability [8,9].

Most plaque ruptures are located in the proximal segments of the coronary arteries. Clinically, the majority of acute coronary syndromes occur in the proximal vessel segments. Similarly, in pathology, 95% of all plaques prone to rupture or erosion are located in the proximal or mid-segments of the major coronary arteries [10–12].

CT Imaging of Plaque

The fact that acute coronary syndromes are difficult to predict, that traditional risk factors only incompletely identify individuals at increased risk, and that a well-known substrate for acute coronary syndromes exists—the coronary atherosclerotic plaque—makes the use of imaging techniques for detecting and characterizing coronary atherosclerotic plaque attractive. The concept is that imaging of plaque may contribute to identifying high-risk individuals, which may benefit from intensive risk factor modification. Demonstrating the *absence* of plaque may, in turn, allow to safely withhold treatment from individuals who may have risk factors, but no detectable coronary atherosclerosis. Much research remains to be done before such concepts can be widely incorporated into clinical practice, but cardiac computed tomography has demonstrated that imaging of coronary atherosclerotic plaque is possible and that it can contribute toward identifying individuals at high and low risk for future coronary artery disease events. By nature of the underlying pathology, sites of future plaque erosion will be more difficult to detect than the often large plaques associated with plaque rupture.

Coronary Calcium

In the coronary arteries, calcifications occur almost exclusively in the context of atherosclerotic plaque [13, 14]. The only exception are patients in renal failure in whom medial (nonatherosclerotic) calcification of the coronary artery wall may occur. Not every atherosclerotic coronary plaque is calcified, but the amount of coronary calcium roughly correlates to the extent of atherosclerotic plaque

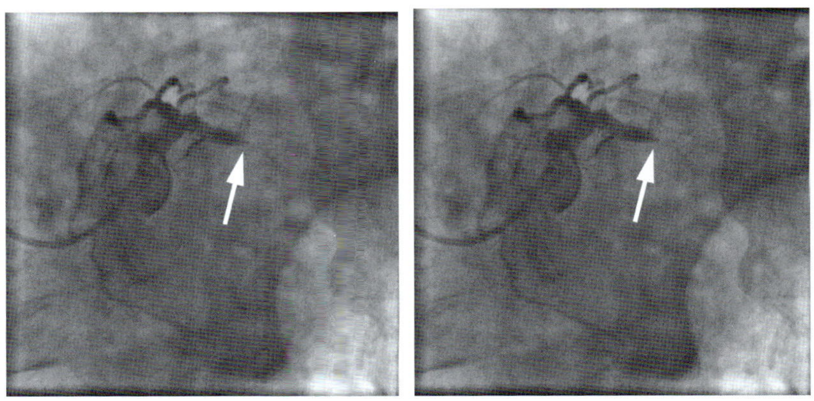

Figure 12.2 Invasive coronary angiogram performed in a 78-year-old male within an interval of 6 days. (a) Invasive angiography in LAO caudal projection ("spider view") shows the left circumflex coronary artery without any significant luminal narrowing (arrow). (b) Six-day slater, the patient developed ST-elevation myocardial infarction. Invasive angiography shows thrombotic occlusion of the proximal left circumflex coronary artery (arrow). LAO, left anterior oblique. (a) (b)

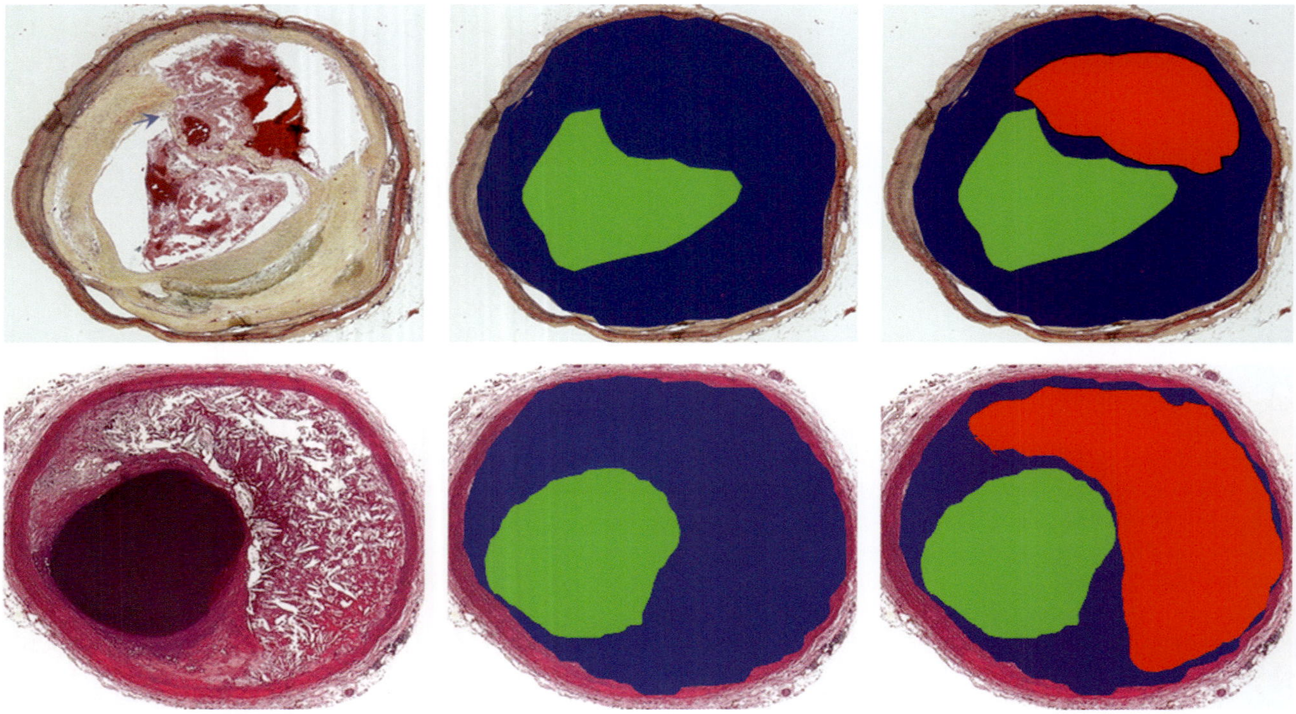

Figure 12.3 Histologic images show very comparable features of a "ruptured plaque" (top panel) and a "thin cap fibroatheroma" (bottom panel). Both lesions have a large necrotic core (NC) that is covered by a thin fibrous cap. The cap is disrupted in the ruptured plaque with necrotic core material in contact with the blood stream. In the "thin cap fibroatheroma," the fibrous cap is intact. Plaques that are vulnerable to rupture are typically large. Corresponding color-coded images show the vessel lumen coded in green and the plaque area coded in blue. The majority of the cross-sectional vessel area is covered by the plaque. This, however, does not mean that luminal stenosis is present, since extensive vessel remodeling often completely compensates for the plaque material and the lumen is not significantly encroached. Large necrotic cores are one of the most prominent features of plaques that are prone to rupture. The necrotic core is coded in red. In both cases, it makes up a substantial proportion of the plaque volume.

burden [13, 14]. Calcification is neither a sign of stability nor instability of an individual plaque, and its presence or absence is not closely associated with the likelihood of an individual lesion to rupture and cause an event [15]. Some research suggests that calcium may be a sign of previous plaque hemorrhage [15]. Plaques with healed ruptures usually contain calcium, whereas plaques with erosions are often not calcified. Coronary calcium is easy to detect by CT and the correlation of calcium with the presence and amount of coronary atherosclerotic plaque makes coronary calcium an interesting target for risk stratification purposes (see Figures 12.4 and 12.5). In the vast majority of

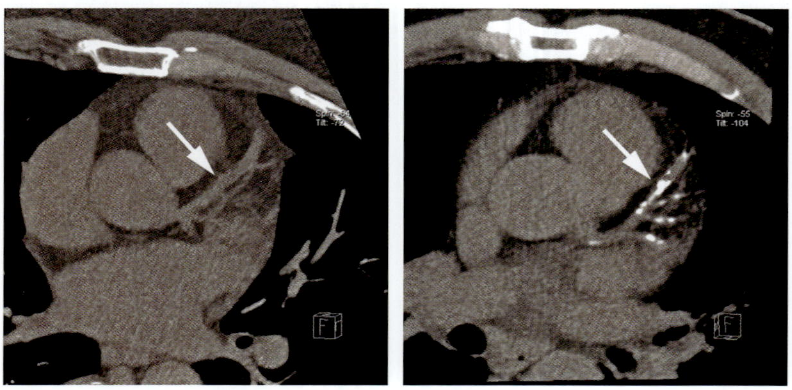

(a) (b)

Figure 12.4 Detection of coronary calcification by computed tomography. (a) Non-contrast-enhanced CT image that shows the left main and proximal left anterior descending coronary artery (arrow) without calcification. (b) Nonenhanced image in a patient with calcification of the proximal left anterior descending coronary artery (arrow). Such calcifications are invariably a sign of coronary atherosclerosis.

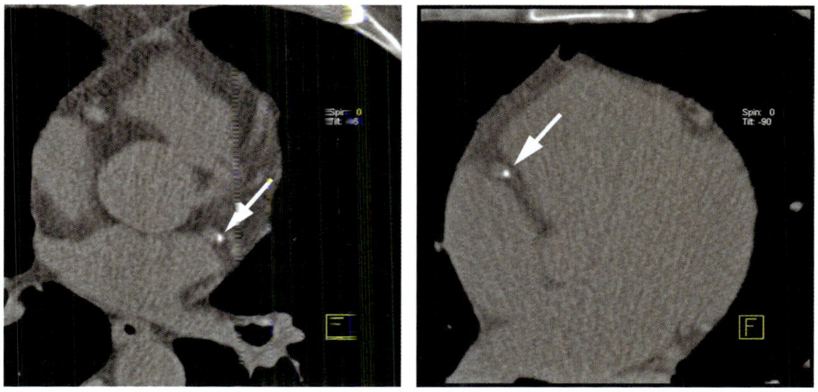

Figure 12.5 Coronary artery calcification. (a) Calcification in the left circumflex coronary artery. (b) Calcification in the right coronary artery. By convention, the presence of calcium is assumed if the CT attenuation—in non-contrast-enhanced images—measures more than 130 Hounsfield Units (HU).

patients with acute coronary syndromes, some coronary calcium can be detected, and the amount of calcium in these patients is substantially greater than in matched control subjects without coronary artery disease. However, calcium is not necessarily present at the site of the culprit lesion [16–18].

Detection and Quantification of Coronary Calcium

Cardiac computed tomography with ECG gating allows for accurate detection and for the quantification of coronary artery calcium. Images are acquired without contrast enhancement, and the radiation dose is relatively low radiation dose (about 0.7–3.0 mSv [19]). The calcified volume or, more frequently, the so-called Agatston Score is determined to quantify the amount of calcium (Figure 12.6). Several large reference datasets describe the distribution of "Agatston Scores" found in the population, stratified by age and gender [17,19–22].

Clinical Significance of Coronary Calcium

Several cohort studies have shown that the presence of coronary calcium demonstrated by computed tomography in asymptomatic individuals is a prognostic parameter with high predictive power regarding the development of hard cardiac events during the following 3–5 years [17,23–32]. It has further been demonstrated that a calcium score of 0 is associated with a very low risk of future myocardial infarction or death due to coronary heart disease (0.4% over 3–5 years) [33]. The presence of any calcium increases the risk for future events by a factor of 4. "Agatston Scores" between 1 and 112 increase the risk of myocardial infarction and coronary artery disease death by 1.9, scores between 100 and 400 by a factor of 4.3, scores between 400 and 999 by a factor of 7.2, and scores of >1000 by a factor of 10.8 or myocardial infarction or death [33]. In a study of 25,253 patients observed for a mean period of approximately 7 years, coronary calcium was a better predictor of overall mortality than standard risk factors. The rate of death from any cause, after adjustment for traditional cardiovascular risk factors, was increased by a factor of 3.6 for "Agatston Scores" between 11 and 100, by a factor of 3.8 for calcium scores between 101 and 399, by a factor of 5.8 for scores between 400 and 699, by a factor of 6.5 for scores between 700 and 999, and by a factor of 9.4 for scores of >1000 [34]. Interestingly, there is an influence of ethnicity both on the prevalence of coronary calcification

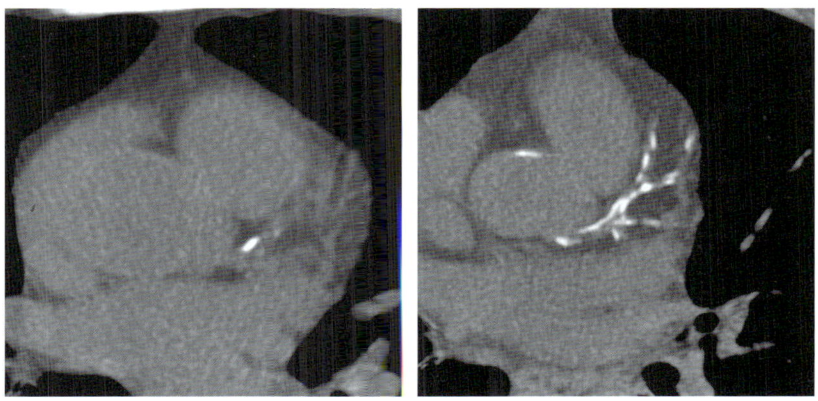

Figure 12.6 Quantification of coronary calcium by the "Agatston Score." The "Agatston Score" is derived from the area and density of calcified coronary artherosclerotic plaques; it has no unit. The sum of the score of all plaques within given vessel provides the "Agatston Score" for that vessel. (a) Moderate amount of calcium in the very proximal left anterior descending coronary artery. The "Agatston Score" is 48. (b) Substantial amount of calcium in the left main and left anterior descending coronary artery. The "Agatston Score" is 665.

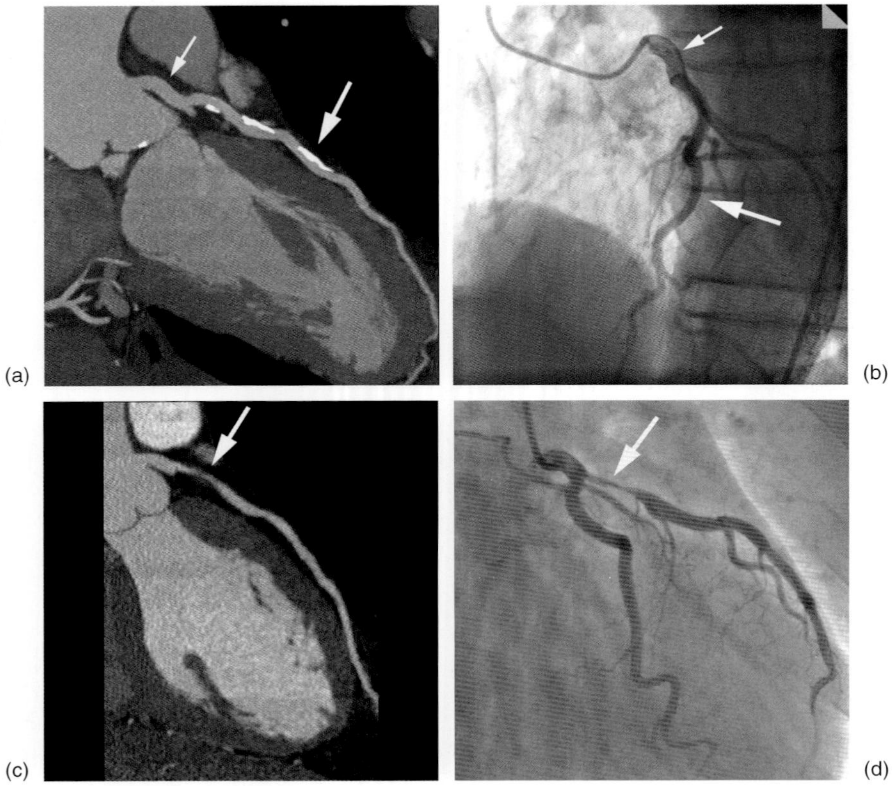

Figure 12.7 The presence and extent of coronary calcium is not necessarily associated with the presence of a significant coronary luminal stenosis. Coronary CT angiogram (a) and invasive coronary angiogram (b) of a patient with substantial coronary artery calcification. Here, the left man (small arrow) and left anterior descending coronary arteries (large arrow) are shown. In spite of the calcification, no stenosis is present. Coronary CT angiogram (c) and invasive coronary angiogram (d) of a patient without detectable coronary artery calcification. The left main and left anterior descending coronary arteries show absence of calcification, but a high-grade proximal stenosis of the left anterior descending coronary artery is present (arrow).

and on the predictive power of coronary calcification, with African Americans being at highest risk when high calcium scores are present [32, 35].

Coronary calcification has been found to be progressive over time [36]. The amount of progression correlates to noncoronary atherosclerosis [37], is related to cardiovascular risk factors [38], and shows a genetic influence [39]. Initial data demonstrated a higher coronary artery disease event rate in individuals who displayed more rapid progression of coronary artery calcium [40].

Clinically, it is currently assumed that individuals at clearly high risk will not profit from coronary calcium imaging, since they need intensive treatment regardless of the result.

> ... the current literature on coronary artery calcium does not provide support for the concept that high-risk asymptomatic individuals can safely be excluded from medical therapy for coronary heart disease even if coronary artery calcium score is 0. [41]

Neither will individuals who have no risk factors and are clearly at low risk profit from "screening" [41]. Individuals who seem to be at intermediate risk for coronary events (10-year event risk between 10 and 20%) based on traditional risk factor analysis will be most likely to profit from coronary calcium imaging in order to determine whether intensive risk modification is necessary.

> ... clinical decision-making could potentially be altered by coronary artery calcium measurement in patients initially judged to be at intermediate risk (10% to 20% in 10 years). The accumulating evidence suggests that asymptomatic individuals with an intermediate Framingham Risk Score may be reasonable candidates for ... testing using coronary artery calcium as a potential means of modifying risk prediction and altering therapy. [41]

Unselected "screening" or patient self-referral is uniformly discouraged [41, 42]. In symptomatic patients, there is no clinical application for coronary calcification measurements, since the presence or absence of coronary calcium, while being correlated to plaque burden, is not closely correlated to the presence or absence of stenosis (Figure 12.7).

Noncalcified Plaque

After intravenous injection of contrast agent, state-of-the-art CT imaging allows visualization of the coronary artery lumen and coronary vessel wall, including imaging of coronary atherosclerotic plaque, both calcified and noncalcified (Figure 12.8). Image acquisition and reconstruction protocols are substantially more elaborate than for coronary calcium measurements, and radiation exposure is also significantly higher. Datasets need to be of high-quality image, with absence of artifacts caused by

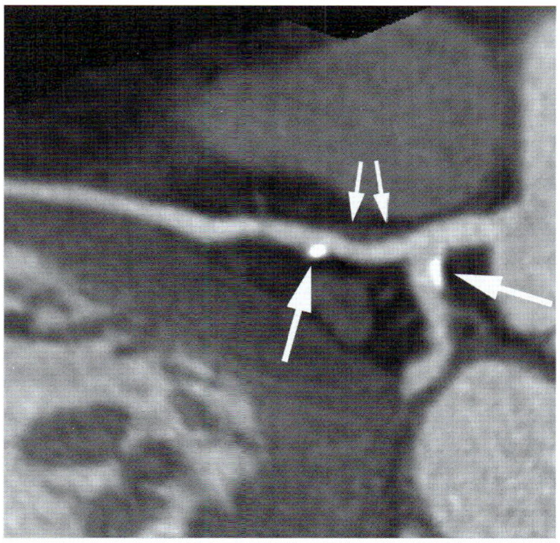

Figure 12.8 Visualization of calcified and noncalcified plaque by contrast-enhanced coronary CT angiography. This image shows the bifurcation of the left main coronary artery into the left anterior descending coronary artery (of which a longer segment is shown) and the left circumflex artery (of which only a short segment is shown before it leaves the imaging plane). Both calcified (large arrows) and noncalcified coronary atherosclerotic plaque (small arrows) is present.

coronary artery motion or high image noise, which cannot be achieved in all cases. Two-dimensional postprocessing techniques are used and permit to display coronary atherosclerotic plaques, with calcified plaque of substantially higher CT attenuation than the contrast-enhanced coronary lumen and noncalcified plaque typically assuming a CT attenuation value that is lower than the contrast-enhanced vessel lumen but higher than the surrounding perivascular tissue (Figure 12.9). Obviously, the ability to not only depict calcium but also to potentially detect, quantify, and characterize noncalcified plaque components is of tremendous interest for risk stratification. Currently, data about the ability of coronary CT angiography to provide this information are limited. In comparison to intravascular ultrasound (IVUS), accuracy for detecting noncalcified plaque has been found to be approximately 80–90% [43–47] (Figure 12.10). To a certain extent, coronary CT angiography allows plaque characterization: On average, the CT attenuation within "fibrous" plaques is higher than within "lipid-rich" plaques (mean attenuation values of 91–116 HU versus 47–71 HU) [48–51]. However, the variability of density measurements within plaque types is large [51], and density measurements within plaque are heavily influenced by the contrast attenuation in the adjacent lumen [52]. While, therefore, accurate classification of plaque composition by measuring the CT attenuation is not always possible, it has been speculated that very low densities (below 30 HU) are associated with a higher predisposition toward rupture [53]. Measurement of plaque dimensions constitutes another possible approach by which CT could identify plaques at a higher risk for rupture. CT has a relatively limited spatial resolution, but it can be used to estimate plaque area and

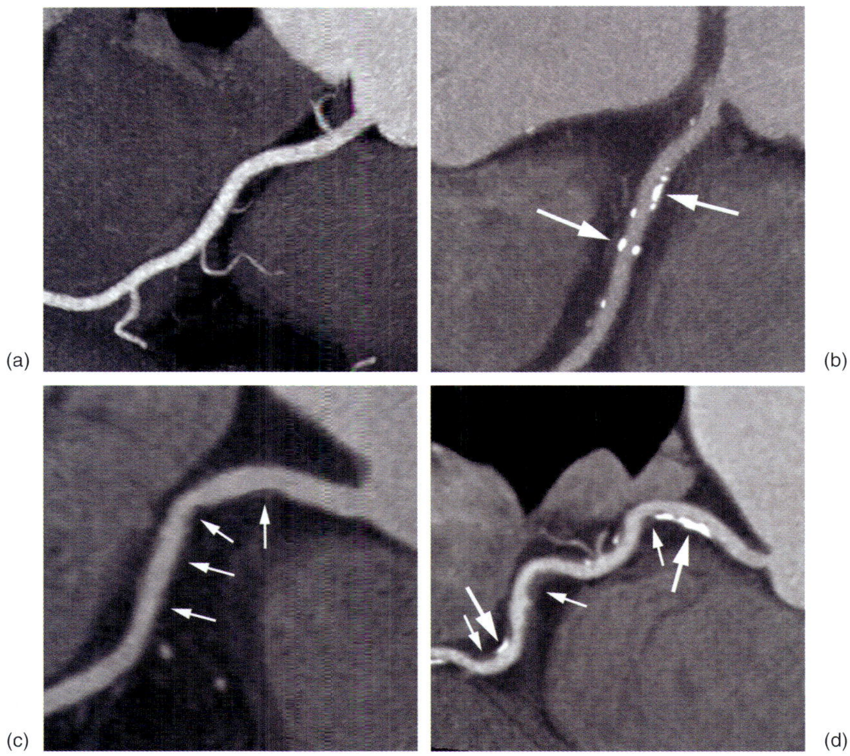

Figure 12.9 Various types of coronary atherosclerotic plaque demonstrated by coronary CT angiography. In all cases, the proximal right coronary artery is shown. (a) Proximal right coronary artery without any detectable plaque. (b) Proximal right coronary artery with calcified plaque (large arrows). Noncalcified plaque is not detectable. (c) Proximal right coronary artery with exclusively noncalcified plaque (small arrows). No calcified plaque is present. (d) Proximal right coronary artery with both calcified and noncalcified plaque (sometimes referred to as "mixed plaque"). Some calcified components are indicated by a large arrow; some noncalcified components are indicated by small arrows.

(a) (b) (c) (d)

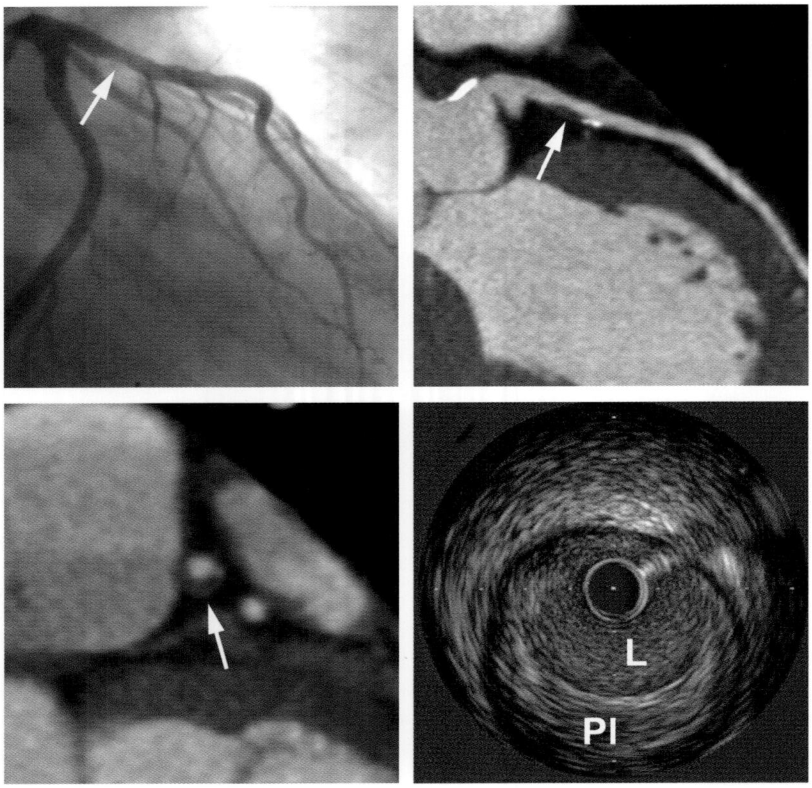

Figure 12.10 Visualization of coronary atherosclerotic plaque in coronary CT angiography as compared to invasive angiography and intravascular ultrasound (IVUS). (a) Invasive coronary angiography shows very mild luminal narrowing of the proximal left anterior descending coronary artery (arrow). (b) Coronary CT angiography, here a longitudinal visualization of the left main and proximal left anterior descending coronary artery, shows a large, partly calcified plaque of the proximal left anterior descending coronary artery (arrow). (c) Cross-sectional visualization of the lesion by CT angiography shows the large dimension of the plaque in comparison to the coronary artery lumen. (d) Cross-sectional imaging by IVUS shows the presence of a large eccentric plaque, which at this level is not calcified (L, Lumen; Pl, Plaque).

volume [43, 47, 54–56]. Since plaques that lead to acute coronary syndromes tend to be large in volume, CT measurement of plaque size and volume may contribute to risk stratification. Similarly, "positive" (outward) remodeling is associated with plaque vulnerability, and the extent of remodeling can be estimated by CT [54] (Figures 12.11 and 12.12).

In a landmark study which comprised 1059 patients who were followed over a mean period of 2.3 years, Motoyama *et al.* could clearly show that plaques with positive

(a) (b)

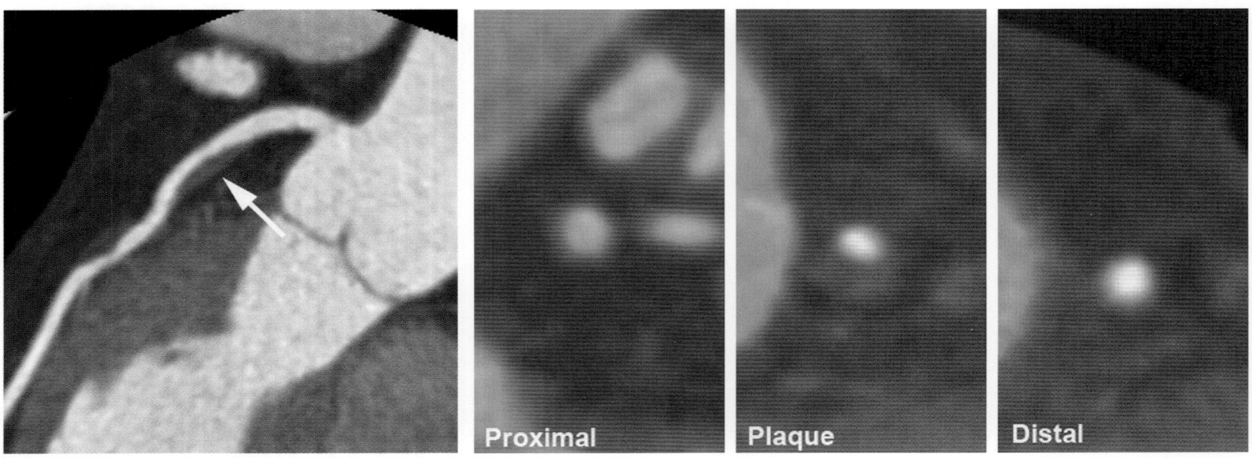

Figure 12.11 Positive remodeling. (a) Longitudinal visualization of a positively remodeled, noncalcified plaque of proximal left anterior descending coronary artery (arrow). (b) Consecutive cross sections of the left anterior descending coronary artery by CT angiography proximal to the plaque, at the level of the plaque, and immediately distal to the plaque. All images are of the same scale. The total vessel cross section at the site of the plaque is larger than proximal or distal to the plaque. This is referred to as "outward," "compensatory," or "positive" remodeling.

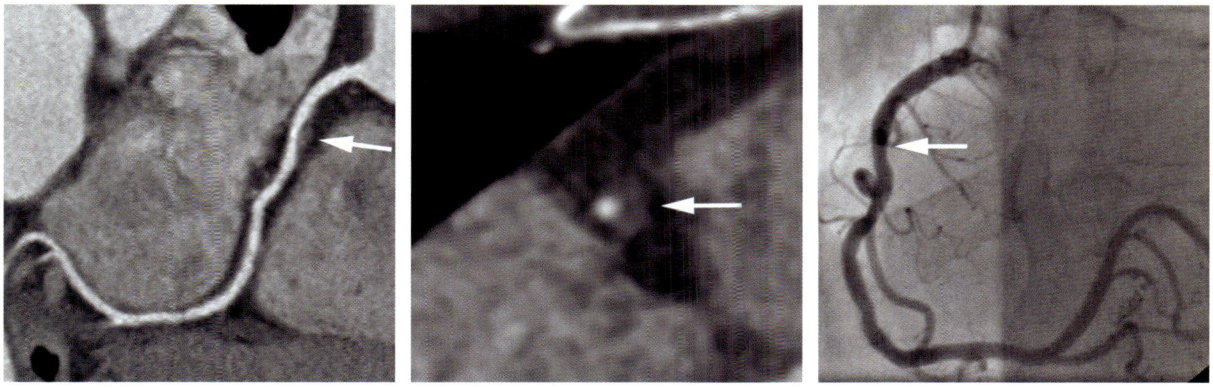

(a), (b) (c)

Figure 12.12 Sometimes, very large plaques can be present with only very mild encroachment of the coronary artery lumen. (a) Coronary CT angiography with a longitudinal visualization of the right coronary artery. (a) large, noncalcified, positively remodeled plaque is present in the proximal right coronary artery (arrow). (b) A cross-sectional view at the level of the plaque confirms the large plaque dimensions. (c) Invasive coronary angiography shows only mild luminal reduction at the site of the atherosclerotic lesion (arrow).

remodeling and low-CT attenuation were at particularly high risk for causing future cardiovascular events [57] (Table 12.1, Figure 12.13). Surrogate markers of plaque burden have been shown to be predictive of overall mortality in two other large trials. Ostrom *et al.* demonstrated that the presence of nonobstructive plaque in all three coronary arteries was associated with increased mortality (risk ratio 1.77 as compared to individuals without any detectable plaque). The presence of nonobstructive plaque in only one or two coronary vessels was not associated with an increased risk [58]. Min *et al.* could demonstrate that the presence of coronary atherosclerotic plaque in at least five coronary artery segments in symptomatic patients was associated with increased mortality as compared with patients with detectable plaque in less than five segments [59].

The actual clinical utility of these observations is uncertain, especially when considering to extend these findings to a "screening" situation. The above named trials were all performed in symptomatic individuals. Because of the lower overall event rates, predicting acute coronary syndromes in *asymptomatic* individuals is more difficult. In fact, a trial of 1000 middle-aged asymptomatic Korean individuals (of which 22% had detectable plaque in CT) was not able to identify any prognostic value of coronary CT angiography over a 17 months follow-up period [60]. Clinically, the use of coronary CT angiography to detect stenoses or plaque in asymptomatic individuals is not currently considered an "appropriate" indication [61].

In patients after acute coronary syndromes, CT can display typical morphologic features of the acute lesion. Typically, acute lesions show pronounced positive remodeling, low-CT attenuation and absence of calcification or small, spotty calcified plaque segments [62–65]. A "rim" of contrast around a central filling defect, a finding know to indicate thrombotic occlusion of a vessel in CT angiography is found in some but not all cases (Figure 12.14). Infrequently, a plaque ulceration as a consequence of old, "healed" plaque rupture can be observed (Figure 12.15).

Table 12.1 Results of a prospective study by Motoyama *et al.* [57].

Finding at baseline	Total number of patients	ACS during follow-up	No ACS during follow-up
Plaques with positive remodeling and CT attenuation <30 HU	45	10	35
Plaques with positive remodeling or CT attenuation <30 HU	27	1	26
Plaques with neither positive remodeling nor CT attenuation <30 HU	822	4	816
No plaque	167	0	167

One thousand and fifty-nine patients were followed for a mean period of 27 months after a clinically indicated coronary CT angiogram. Coronary atherosclerotic plaques were identified and evaluated concerning the presence of positive remodeling and low-CT attenuation (attenuation values <30 HU). It could be demonstrated that the rate of acute coronary syndromes (ACS) during follow-up was substantially higher in patients with plaques that demonstrated positive remodeling and low-CT attenuation as compared to patients with plaque of other type or without plaque.

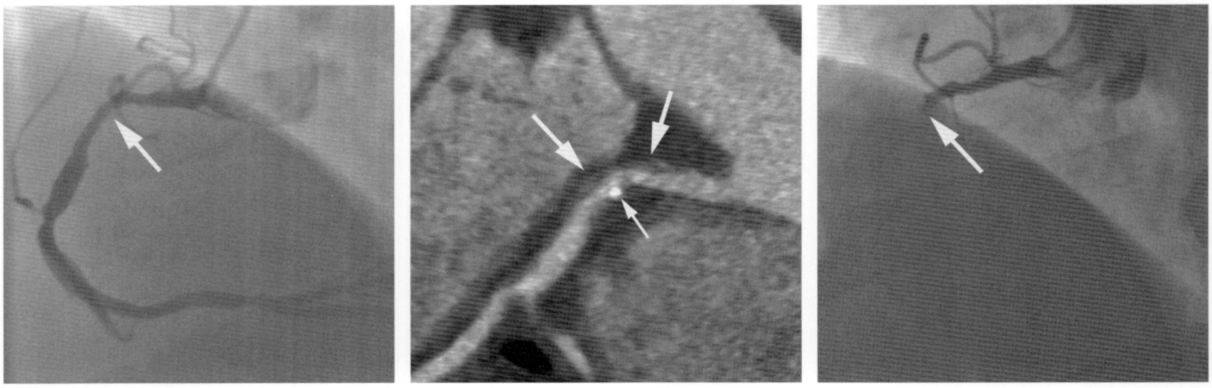

(a), (b) (c)

Figure 12.13 Visualization of a "rupture-prone" plaque in coronary CT angiography. (a) Invasive coronary angiography shows a mid lumen stenosis of the proximal right coronary artery. (b) Coronary CT angiography, performed at the same time as the invasive angiogram in panel A demonstrates a large, mostly noncalcified coronary atherosclerotic plaque of the proximal right coronary artery (large arrows), with positive remodeling, mostly low CT attenuation, and a small "spotty" calcification (small arrow). (c) The same patient, 4 months later, experienced an acute coronary syndrome with ST-elevation myocardial infarction due to sudden occlusion of the right coronary artery at the site of the plaque shown in panel B.

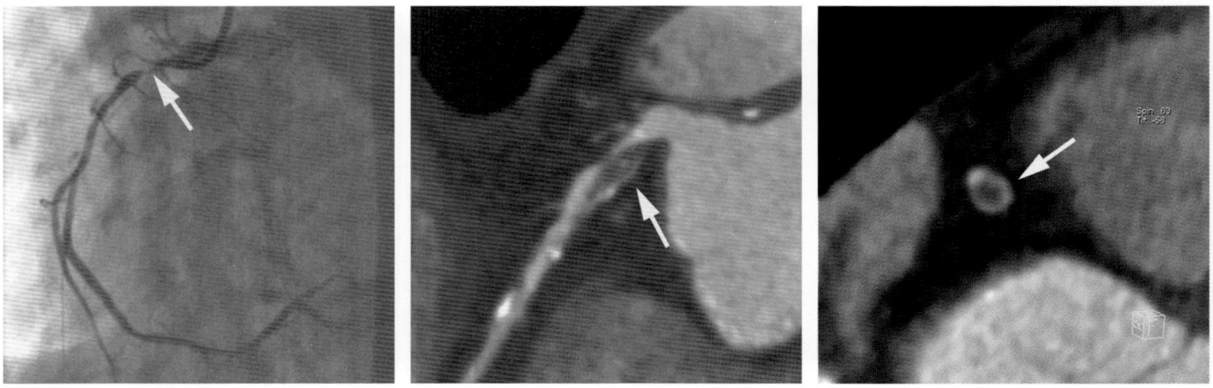

(a), (b) (c)

Figure 12.14 Acute coronary syndrome with plaque rupture visualized in coronary CT angiography. (a) Invasive coronary angiography of a patients with acute non-ST elevation myocardial infarction of the right coronary artery. A high grade stenosis of the very proximal right coronary artery is seen (arrow). (b) CT angiography shows a high grade luminal stenosis and substantial positive remodeling at the site of the lesion (arrow). (c) A cross-sectional view of the right coronary artery obtained by CT angiography at the site of most severe luminal stenosis demonstrates a central filling defect, surrounded by a "rim" of contrast agent (arrow). This finding is observed in approximately one-half of all patients with acute coronary syndromes. The central filling defect is assumed to represent thrombus.

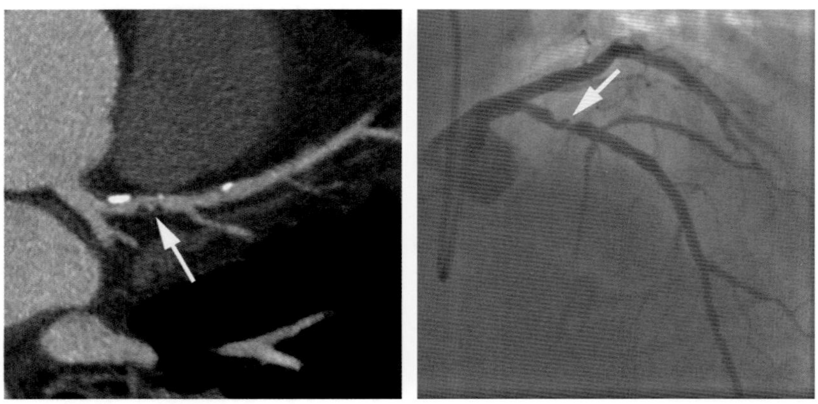

(a) (b)

Figure 12.15 Plaque ulceration seen in invasive coronary angiography and coronary CT angiography. Plaque ulcerations occur as a consequence of "healed" rupture. (a) Invasive coronary angiography (arrow: plaque ulceration in the proximal left anterior descending coronary artery). (b) Coronary CT angiography (arrow: ulcerated plaque).

Summary

In summary, CT imaging of the coronary arteries has tremendous potential to provide uniquely valuable information concerning coronary atherosclerosis. Both for risk stratification of an individual and for obtaining new information on the disease process itself, the ability to directly visualize coronary atherosclerotic lesions as of great potential. As image quality of coronary CT angiography shows continuous improvement, the amount of detailed information that can be obtained from a coronary CT angiogram will undoubtedly increase and even better characterization of coronary atherosclerosis will become possible.

References

1. American Heart Association. (2009) Heart and Stroke Statistics—2009 Update. *Circulation* 119:e21–e181.
2. Virmai R, Burke AP, Farb A, Kolodgie FD. (2006) Pathology of the vulnerable plaque. *J Am Coll Cardiol* 47:C13–C18.
3. Burke AP, Kolodgie FD, Farb A *et al.* (2001) Healed plaque ruptures and sudden coronary death: evidence that subclinical rupture has a role in plaque progression. *Circulation* 103:934–940.
4. Ambrose JA, Winters SL, Stern A *et al.* (1985) Angiographic morphology and the pathogenesis of unstable angina pectoris. *J Am Coll Cardiol* 5:609–616.
5. Ambrose JA, Winters SL, Arora RR *et al.* (1985) Coronary angiographic morphology in myocardial infarction: a link between the pathogenesis of unstable angina and myocardial infarction. *J Am Coll Cardiol* 6:1233–1238.
6. Feinleib M, Simon AB, Gillum RF, Margolis JR. (1975 Dec) Prodromal symptoms and signs of sudden death. *Circulation* 52(6 Suppl):III155–III159.
7. Glagov S, Weisenberg E, Zarins CK, Stankunavicius R, Kolettis GJ. (1987) Compensatory enlargement of human atherosclerotic coronary arteries. *N Engl J Med* 316:1371–1375.
8. Virmani R, Kolodgie FD, Burke AP *et al.* (2005) Atherosclerotic plaque progression and vulnerability to rupture: angiogenesis as a source of intraplaque hemorrhage. *Arterioscler Thromb Vasc Biol* 25:2054–2061.
9. Kolodgie FD, Gold HK, Burke AP *et al.* (2003) Intraplaque hemorrhage and progression of coronary atheroma. *N Engl J Med* 349:2316–2325.
10. Wang JC, Normand SL, Mauri L, Kuntz RE. (2004 Jul 20) Coronary artery spatial distribution of acute myocardial infarction occlusions. *Circulation* 110:278–284.
11. Hong MK, Mintz GS, Lee CW *et al.* (2005) The site of plaque rupture in native coronary arteries: a three-vessel intravascular ultrasound analysis. *J Am Coll Cardiol* 46:261–265.
12. Virmami R, Burke AP, Willerson JT *et al.* (2007) The pathology of the vulnerable plaque. In Virmani R, Narula J, Leon MB, Willerson JT (eds) *The Vulnerable Atherosclerotic Plaques. Strategies for Diagnosis and Management*. Blackwell Futura Publishing, Oxford, UK, pp. 21–36.
13. Burke AP, Virmani R, Galis Z *et al.* (2003) Task Force #2—What is the pathologic basis for new atherosclerosis imaging techniques? *J Am Coll Cardiol* 41:1874.
14. O'Rourke RA, Brundage B, Froelicher VF *et al.* (2000) ACC/AHA Expert Consensus Document on electron-beam computed tomography for the diagnosis and prognosis of coronary artery disease. *Circulation* 102:126.
15. Pham PH, Rao DS, Vasunilashorn F, Fishbein MC, Goldin JG. (2006) Computed tomography calcium quantification as a measure of atherosclerotic plaque morphology and stability. *Invest Radiol* 41:674–680.
16. Pohle K, Ropers D, Mäffert R *et al.* (2003) Coronary calcifications in young patients with first, unheralded myocardial infarction: A risk factor matched analysis by electron beam tomography. *Heart* 89:625.
17. Raggi P, Callister TQ, Cooil B *et al.* (2000) Identification of patients at increased risk of first unheralded acute myocardial infarction by electron-beam computed tomography. *Circulation* 101:850.
18. Schmermund A, Schwartz RS, Adamzik M *et al.* (2001) Coronary atherosclerosis in unheralded sudden coronary death under age fifty: histopathologic comparison with "healthy" subjects dying out of hospital. *Atherosclerosis* 155:499.
19. Gerber TC, Kuzo RS, Morin RL. (2005) Techniques and parameters for estimating radiation exposure and dose in cardiac computed tomography. *Int J Cardiovasc Imaging* 21:165–176.
20. Hoff JA, Chomka EV, Krainik AJ *et al.* (2001) Age and gender distribution of coronary artery calcium detected by electron beam tomography in 35246 adults. *Am J Cardiol* 87:1335.
21. McClelland RL, Chung H, Detrano R *et al.* (2006) Distribution of coronary artery calcium by race, gender, and age. Results from the Multi-Ethnic Study of Atherosclerosis (MESA). *Circulation* 113:30–37.
22. Schmermund A, Mohlenkamp S, Berenbein S *et al.* (2006) Population-based assessment of subclinical coronary atherosclerosis using electro-beam computed tomography. *Atherosclerosis* 185:117–182.
23. Arad Y, Spadaro LA, Goodman K *et al.* (2000) Prediction of coronary events with electron beam computed tomography. *J Am Coll Cardiol* 36:1253.
24. Park R, Detrano R, Xiang M *et al.* (2002) Combined use of computed tomography coronary calcium scores and C-reactive protein levels in predicting cardiovascular events in nondiabetic individuals. *Circulation* 106:2073.
25. Vliegenthart R, Oudkerk M, Song B *et al.* (2002) Coronary calcification detected by electron-beam computed tomography and myocardial infarction. The Rotterdam Coronary Calcification Study. *Eur Heart J* 23:1596.
26. Wong ND, Hsu JC, Detrano RC *et al.* (2000) Coronary artery calcium evaluation by electron beam computed tomography and its relation to new cardiovascular events. *Am J Cardiol* 86:495.
27. Kondos GT, Hoff JA, Sevrukov A *et al.* (2003) Electron-beam tomography coronary artery calcium and coronary events: A 37-month follow-up of 5635 initially asymptomatic low- to intermediate-risk adults. *Circulation* 107:2571.

28. Church TS, Levine BD, McGuire DK *et al.* (2006 Mar 13) Coronary artery calcium score, risk factors, and incident coronary heart disease events. *Atherosclerosis* 190(1):224–231.[Epub ahead of print.]
29. Taylor AJ, Bindeman J, Feuerstein I *et al.* (2005) Coronary calcium independently predicts incident premature coronary heart disease over measured cardiovascular risk factors: mean three-year outcomes in the Prospective Army Coronary Calcium (PACC) project. *J Am Coll Cardiol* 46:807–814.
30. Greenland P, LaBree L, Azen SP *et al.* (2004) Coronary artery calcium score combined with Framingham score for risk prediction in asymptomatic individuals. *JAMA* 291:210–215.
31. Arad Y, Goodman KJ, Roth M *et al.* (2005) Coronary calcification, coronary disease risk factors, C-reactive protein, and atherosclerotic cardiovascular disease events: the St. Francis Heart Study. *J Am Coll Cardiol* 46:158–165.
32. Detrano R, Guerci AD, Carr JJ *et al.* (2008) Coronary calcium as a predictor of coronary events in four racial or ethnic groups. *N Engl J Med* 358:1336–1345.
33. Budoff MJ, Achenbach S, Blumenthal RS *et al.* (2006) Assessment of coronary artery disease by cardiac computed tomography: a scientific statement from the American Heart Association Committee on Cardiovascular Imaging and Intervention, Council on Cardiovascular Radiology and Intervention, and Committee on Cardiac Imaging, Council on Clinical Cardiology. *Circulation* 114:1761–1791.
34. Budoff MJ, Shaw LJ, Liu ST *et al.* (2007) Long-term prognosis associated with coronary calcification: observations from a registry of 25253 patients. *J Am Coll Cardiol* 49:1860–1870.
35. Nasir K, Shaw LJ, Liu ST *et al.* (2007) Ethnic differences in the prognostic value of coronary artery calcification for all-cause mortality. *J Am Coll Cardiol* 50:953–960.
36. Schmermund A, Baumgart D, Möhlenkamp S *et al.* (2001) Natural history and topographic pattern of progression of coronary calcification in symptomatic patients. *Arterioscler Thromb Vasc Biol* 21:421.
37. Taylor AJ, Bindeman J, Le TP *et al.* (2008) Progression of calcified coronary atherosclerosis: relationship to coronary risk factors and carotid intima-media thickness. *Atherosclerosis* 197:339–345.
38. Kronmal RA, McClelland RL, Detrano R *et al.* (2007) Risk factors for the progression of coronary artery calcification in asymptomatic subjects: results from the Multi-Ethnic Study of Atherosclerosis (MESA). *Circulation* 115:2722–2730.
39. Cassidy-Bushrow AE, Bielak LF, Sheedy PF 2nd *et al.* (2007) Coronary artery calcification progression is heritable. *Circulation* 116:25–31.
40. Raggi P, Callister TQ, Shaw LJ. (2004) Progression of coronary artery calcium and risk of first myocardial infarction in patients receiving cholesterol-lowering therapy. *Arterioscler Thromb Vasc Biol* 24:1272–1277.
41. Greenland P, Bonow RO, Brundage BH *et al.* (2007) ACCF/AHA 2007 clinical expert consensus document on coronary artery calcium scoring by computed tomography in global cardiovascular risk assessment and in evaluation of patients with chest pain: a report of the American College of Cardiology Foundation Clinical Expert Consensus Task Force (ACCF/AHA Writing Committee to Update the 2000 Expert Consensus Document on Electron Beam Computed Tomography). *Circulation* 115:402–426.
42. De Backer G, Ambrosioni E, Borch-Johnsen K *et al.* (2003) European guidelines on cardiovascular disease prevention in clinical practice. Third Joint Task Force of European and Other Societies on Cardiovascular Disease Prevention in Clinical Practice. *Eur Heart J* 24:1601–1610.
43. Achenbach S, Moselewski F, Ropers D *et al.* (2004) Detection of calcified and noncalcified coronary atherosclerotic plaque by contrast-enhanced, submillimeter multidetector spiral computed tomography: a segment-based comparison with intravascular ultrasound. *Circulation* 109:14–17.
44. Leber AW, Knez A, Becker A *et al.* (2004) Accuracy of multidetector spiral computed tomography in identifying and differentiating the composition of coronary atherosclerotic plaques: a comparative study with intracoronary ultrasound. *J Am Coll Cardiol* 43:1241–1247.
45. Leber AW, Becker A, Knez A *et al.* (2006) Accuracy of 64-slice computed tomography to classify and quantify plaque volumes in the proximal coronary system: a comparative study using intravascular ultrasound. *J Am Coll Cardiol* 47:672–627.
46. Petranovic M, Soni A, Bezzera H *et al.* (2009) Assessment of nonstenotic coronary lesions by 64-slice multidetector computed tomography in comparison to intravascular ultrasound: evaluation of nonculprit coronary lesions. *J Cardiovasc Comput Tomogr* 3:24–31.
47. Sun J, Zhang Z, Lu B *et al.* (2008 Mar) Identification and quantification of coronary atherosclerotic plaques: a comparison of 64-MDCT and intravascular ultrasound. *AJR Am J Roentgenol* 190:748–754.
48. Schroeder S, Kopp AF, Baumbach A *et al.* (2001) Noninvasive detection and evaluation of atherosclerotic coronary plaques with multislice computed tomography. *J Am Coll Cardiol* 37:1430–1435.
49. Caussin C, Ohanessian A, Ghostine S *et al.* (2004) Characterization of vulnerable nonstenotic plaque with 16-slice computed tomography compared with intravascular ultrasound. *Am J Cardiol* 94:99–100.
50. Carrascosa PM, Capunay CM, Garcia-Merletti P, Carrascosa J, Garcia MF. (2006) Characterization of coronary atherosclerotic plaques by multidetector computed tomography. *Am J Cardiol* 97:598–602.
51. Pohle K, Achenbach S, MacNeill B *et al.* (2007) Characterization of non-calcified coronary atherosclerotic plaque by multi-detector row CT: Comparison to IVUS. *Atherosclerosis* 190:174–180.
52. Cademartiri F, Mollet NR, Runza G *et al.* (2005) Influence of intracoronary attenuation on coronary plaque measurements using multislice computed tomography: observations in an ex vivo model of coronary computed tomography angiography. *Eur Radiol* 15:1426–1431.
53. Motoyama S, Kondo T, Anno H *et al.* (2007) Atherosclerotic plaque characterization by 0.5-mm-slice multislice computed tomographic imaging. *Circ J* 71:363–366.
54. Achenbach S, Ropers D, Hoffmann U *et al.* (2004) Assessment of coronary remodeling in stenotic and nonstenotic coronary atherosclerotic lesions by multidetector spiral computed tomography. *J Am Coll Cardiol* 43:842–847.

55. Moselewski F, Ropers D, Pohle K *et al.* (2004) Comparison of measurement of cross-sectional coronary atherosclerotic plaque and vessel areas by 16-slice multidetector computed tomography versus intravascular ultrasound. *Am J Cardiol* 94:1294–1297.
56. Bruining N, Roelandt JR, Palumbo A *et al.* (2007) Reproducible coronary plaque quantification by multislice computed tomography. *Catheter Cardiovasc Interv* 69:857–865.
57. Motoyama S, Sarai M, Harigaya H *et al.* (2009) Computed tomographic angiography characteristics of atherosclerotic plaques subsequently resulting in acute coronary syndrome. *J Am Coll Cardiol* 54:49–57.
58. Ostrom MP, Gopal A, Ahmadi N *et al.* (2008) Mortality incidence and the severity of coronary atherosclerosis assessed by computed tomography angiography. *J Am Coll Cardiol* 52:1335–1343.
59. Min JK, Shaw LJ, Devereux RB *et al.* (2007) Prognostic value of multidetector coronary computed tomographic angiography for prediction of all-cause mortality. *J Am Coll Cardiol* 50:1161–1170.
60. Choi EK, Choi SI, Rivera JJ *et al.* (2008) Coronary computed tomography angiography as a screening tool for the detection of occult coronary artery disease in asymptomatic individuals. *J Am Coll Cardiol* 52:357–365.
61. Hendel RC, Patel MR, Kramer CM *et al.* (2006) ACCF/ACR/SCCT/SCMR/ASNC/NASCI/SCAI/SIR appropriateness criteria for cardiac computed tomography and cardiac magnetic resonance imaging: a report of the American College of Cardiology Foundation Quality Strategic Directions Committee Appropriateness Criteria Working Group, American College of Radiology, Society of Cardiovascular Computed Tomography, Society for Cardiovascular Magnetic Resonance, American Society of Nuclear Cardiology, North American Society for Cardiac Imaging, Society for Cardiovascular Angiography and Interventions, and Society of Interventional Radiology. *J Am Coll Cardiol* 48:1475–1497.
62. Leber AW, Knez A, White CW *et al.* (2003) Composition of coronary atherosclerotic plaques in patients with acute myocardial infarction and stable angina pectoris determined by contrast-enhanced multislice computed tomography. *Am J Cardiol* 91:714–718.
63. Inoue F, Sato Y, Matsumoto N, Tani S, Uchiyama T. (2004) Evaluation of plaque texture by means of multislice computed tomography in patients with acute coronary syndrome and stable angina. *Circ J* 68:840–844.
64. Hoffmann U, Moselewski F, Nieman K *et al.* (2006) Noninvasive assessment of plaque morphology and composition in culprit and stable lesions in acute coronary syndrome and stable lesions in stable angina by multidetector computed tomography. *J Am Coll Cardiol* 47:1655–1662.
65. Motoyama S, Kondo T, Sarai M *et al.* (2007) Multislice computed tomographic characteristics of coronary lesions in acute coronary syndromes. *J Am Coll Cardiol* 50:319–326.

13 Nomograms for Coronary Computed Tomographic Angiography

Leslee J. Shaw,[1] James K. Min[2] & Daniel S. Berman[3]

[1]*Emory University School of Medicine, Atlanta, GA, USA*
[2]*Weill Medical College of Cornell University, The New York Presbyterian Hospital, New York, NY, USA*
[3]*Cedars-Sinai Medical Center, Los Angeles, CA, USA*

For the current chapter, we plan to focus on two issues: (1) to define the normative standards for coronary computed tomographic angiography (CCTA) measurements of size and volume and (2) to examine the role of CCTA in the estimation of both diagnosis of obstructive coronary artery disease (CAD) and its utility in prognostication. Within this chapter, we focus on normative standards and clinical algorithms of testing that may employ CCTA and integrate systematic or pooled evidence from the peer-reviewed literature to support a given decision tree for selected patient series. Despite the rapid evolution of evidence with CCTA, the breadth and depth of data remains low. and as such, we will also culminate our review by proposing future strategies where CCTA may play a novel role in the detection of at-risk patients.

Normative Values for CT Measurements

Normative values for cardiac dimensions, volumes, function, and mass have recently been devised from a cohort of 103 normotensive, nonobese, and apparently healthy individuals [1]. The normative ranges defined as 95% confidence intervals for the left and right ventricles, and atria are reported in Tables 13.1–13.3. Several notable results may be observed in these tables. In general, these results revealed similar measures for CT to that of cardiovascular magnetic resonance (MR) imaging [2]. Moreover, consistent with prior reports for both CT and MR, there was an underestimation of left atrial end-systolic volume by echocardiography, using several formulas, was observed (i.e., the Simpson's rule and area-length volume formulas) [3]. There may also be a slight underestimation of left ventricular ejection fraction with CT when using 10 phases. Finally and importantly, variability within left ventricular volumes was apparent by age, gender, and body mass index; with slightly increasing values for older, men, and obese patients.

Diagnosis of Obstructive CAD

Although numerous studies have been published in the diagnostic accuracy of CCTA, we will be highlighting several systematic reviews on the subject as well as three controlled clinical trials have recently been published [4–8]. One recent systematic review published a diagnostic sensitivity and specificity for the detection of obstructive CAD of 94 and 85% [5]. For 64-slice CCTA, the numbers improve slightly with a range of sensitivity values from 94 to 98% and a range of specificity values from 89 to 92%. Importantly there have been 3 controlled clinical trials recently published on the diagnostic accuracy of CCTA compared to invasive coronary angiography [9–11]. In each case, the trials included patients clinically referred for invasive angiography, and as such, the ensuing referral bias will lead to greater accuracy statistics than that realized in a noncatheterization cohort. Despite this limitation, the pooled results note a high diagnostic accuracy in 881 patients with sensitivity and specificity measurement of 94 and 80% (Figure 13.1) [6–8]. A diminished specificity was noted in the report by Meijboom and colleagues and may be driven by the higher CAD likelihood population [7]. However, the overestimation of percentage stenosis by CCTA has been noted [12], and in this higher CAD cohort, a greater prevalence of coronary artery calcium could have precipitated this reduced specificity measurement.

Revisiting Cardiac Anatomy: A Computed-Tomography-Based Atlas and Reference, 1st edition. Edited by Farhood Saremi, Eloisa Arbustini, Stephen Achenbach and Jagat Narula.

Table 13.1 Median CT measurements of LV dimensions, function, and mass

LV dimensions and function	95% CI	LV mass	95% CI
1D			
LVIDD, septal-lateral	38.2–56.6	Wall thickness (mm)	4.8–9.8
LVIDD, antero-inferior	46.9–68.5	Relative wall thickness (%)	0.16–0.44
LV apical-annular length, ED	69.4–105.8	ASE estimated LV mass (g)	56.7–207.7
2D		ASE estimated LVMI (g/m^2)	36.6–102.8
LVESV (mL)	24.2–106.2	ASE LVM/Ht$^{2.7}$ (g/m$^{2.7}$)	15.3–45.1
LVEDV (mL)	80.6–220.2	2D LVM ED (g)	47.7–165.7
LVEDVI (mL/m^2)	49.9–109.1	2D LVMI ED (g/m^2)	31.3–81.1
LVEF (%)	43.9–70.5	2D LVM/Ht$^{2.7}$ (g/m$^{2.7}$)	13.3–35.3
3D		2D LVM ED papillary free (g)	54.2–175.4
LVESV (mL)	15.0–90.2		
LVEDV (mL)	72.3–214.9		
LVEDVI (mL/m^2)	46.4–105.2		
LVEF (%)	48.7–78.9		

LVIDD, left ventricular internal diastolic dimension; ED, end diastolic; LVESV, left ventricular end systolic dimension; LVEDV, left ventricular end diastolic dimension; LVEDVI, left ventricular end diastolic volume index; LVEF, left ventricular ejection fraction; ASE, American Society of Echocardiography; ASE LVM, American Society of Echocardiography left ventricular mass; LVM ED left ventricular mass end-diastolic; LVMI ED left ventricular mass index end-diastolic; 2D, two dimensions; 3D, three dimensions; CI, confidence intervals; LV, left ventricle.

The pooling of this data does allow us to propose a work-up algorithm for patients. If you envision that the Assessment by Coronary Computed Tomographic Angiography of Individuals Undergoing Invasive Coronary Angiography (ACCURACY) trial [6] enrolled lower CAD likelihood patients, the resulting high accuracy for CCTA from within the ACCURACY trial may result in this test being favored for similarly lower-risk patients. By comparison, the Meijboom *et al.* [7] series was largely high CAD likelihood patients and the diminished specificity reduces our enthusiasm for this modality in this patient cohort. Within the context of management, given a high likelihood cohort, the wealth of evidence would support an ischemia test, such as stress myocardial perfusion single-photon emission computed tomography (SPECT) or positron emission tomography (PET), rather than CCTA. Given that CAD prevalence is quite high, the need for repeat invasive angiography is elevated and documentation of ischemia is critical to focusing therapeutic decision making in this high likelihood patient. As such, our algorithm in Figure 13.2 supports CCTA in lower likelihood patients and ischemia testing in higher likelihood patients. Randomized clinical trials are now in preparation (e.g., Functional or Anatomic or Both Functional and Anatomic Testing in Symptomatic Individuals Undergoing EvaLuation by MPS or CCTA: Costs and Clinical OUtcomeS) to examine the optimal test of choice for the intermediate CAD likelihood patient.

Table 13.2 Mean RV dimensions, volumes, and function

RV dimensions	End systolic	End diastolic	Other RV measures	
Linear			*Remodeling*	
Mid-cavity, septal-medial (mm)	19.2–40.0	25.8–48.2	RV free wall thickness	1.0–3.8
Mid-cavity, anterior-inferior (mm)	42.2–73.6	55.0–90.2		
Apical-annular length (mm)	44.8–79.2	57.3–98.1		
3D			*Functional measures*	
3D volume (mL)	24.9–139.3	80.8–269.0	Tricuspid annular excursion (mm)	19.2–40.0
3D volume index (mL/m^2)		53.5–133.1	3D RVEF (%)	42.2–73.6

RVEF, right ventricular ejection fraction; 3D, three dimensions; RV, right ventricle.

Table 13.3 LA and RA volumes

	2D LAESV	3D LAESV	3D RAESV
Atrial dimensions	**95% CI**	**95% CI**	**95% CI**
Volume (mL)	29.5–143.5	54.5–150.1	54.9–168.9
Volume index (mL/m^2)	19.0–73.4	31.1–77.7	30.3–89.1

LAESV, left atrial end systolic volume; RAESV, right atrial end systolic volume; RA, right atrium; LA, left atrium; CI, confidence intervals.

Prognostic Accuracy of CCTA

Obstructive CAD

A primary goal of an imaging procedure is to examine more than the probability of an obstructive lesion. Over the past few decades, the aim of a noninvasive procedure has shifted toward a goal of noninvasive-risk stratification for the estimation of near-term risk of a major adverse cardiovascular event (MACE) in patients undergoing stress testing with or without imaging [13–15]. To date, there are a number of studies evaluating the prognostic accuracy of CCTA measurements of the extent and severity of obstructive CAD [16–22]. Although the cohorts evaluated for prognosis with CCTA are small and the follow-up is limited to ~1 year, the data reveal the importance of anatomy in guiding MACE risk. Figure 13.3 reports the relative risk ratios for all of the published series with CCTA examining the presence of significant, obstructive CAD. From this meta-analysis, the cumulative relative risk ratio is elevated 10.6-fold (95% confidence intervals = 4.1–27.5) as compared to a summary risk ratio of 6.0 for stress myocardial perfusion SPECT.

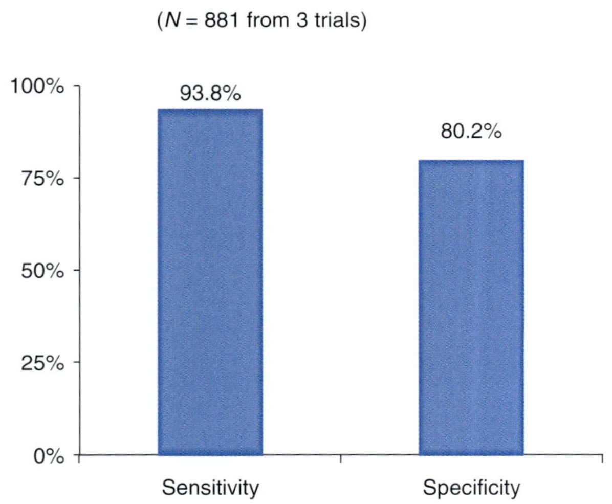

Figure 13.1 Pooled diagnostic accuracy statistics from three controlled clinical trials of CCTA compared to invasive coronary angiography including ACCURACY, CORE-64, and Meijboom *et al.* [10] series.

The rationale for the higher relative risk with CCTA is the relationship between anatomy and MACE risk. If we were able to plot more than the mere presence of obstructive CAD and include more extensive three-vessel CAD, proximal left anterior descending stenosis, or more severe lesions, one would expect that the relative risk ratios would be even higher, as much as 50-fold higher risk ratios [14]. Conversely, the lower risk of ischemia may be explained by presence of technical artifact and ischemia occurring in the setting of endothelial dysfunction but mild CAD. Thus, it appears that as a noninvasive test, CCTA has the potential to provide valuable information as to the underlying burden of obstructive CAD.

A more thorough review of the prognostic literature with CCTA reveals several additional insights into the utility of this modality. In a recent series of 1127 patients, 15-month follow-up for the occurrence of all-cause mortality was ascertained [14]. In this series, we employed the Duke CAD prognostic index to estimate all-cause mortality. The Duke CAD index, initially devised and validated in invasive angiographic population, hierarchically ranks angiographic CAD by both the severity of a lesion, the extent or involvement within the epicardial coronary arteries, and the site of a lesion (i.e., proximal or distal as well as left anterior descending coronary artery involvement). Within the invasive literature, the Duke CAD index is scored from 0 for normal coronary arteries to 100 for left main coronary stenosis with ensuing 5-year cardiovascular mortality corresponding to each score. That is, a score of 0 for normal coronaries would indicate that the expected 5-year cardiovascular mortality of 0%. Importantly, an invasive cohort is decidedly higher risk and we expected that the ranking or scoring from the original Duke CAD prognostic index reports would overestimate mortality for an outpatient population referred for CCTA. However, the *ranking* of mortality should be similar and reveal a graded relationship between the Duke CAD index and mortality risk. This graded relationship is important because it provides enhanced validation of this angiographic index in a lower-risk outpatient cohort. Importantly, all-cause mortality ranged from 0.3% for no CAD stenosis to 12% for patients with left main CAD (≥50% stenosis) (Figure 13.4, $p < 0.0001$) [14]. Figure 13.3 reveals the graded linear relationship between risk and angiographic disease. The low rate of all-cause mortality in patients without epicardial CAD was also recently validated in a large cohort of 2538 patients [18].

The use of the Duke index has important implications for CCTA; in that the wealth of evidence on risk assessment with invasive angiography and the number of

	Accuracy	Meijboom
N =	*230*	*360*
Sensitivity (%)	95	99
Specificity (%)	83	64
PPV (%)	64	86
NPV (%)	99	97
CAD prevalence (%)	**25**	**68**

Low CAD likelihood	**Intermediate CAD likelihood**	**High CAD likelihood**
CCTA favored	Fabulous randomized trial comparing CCTA versus myocardial perfusion SPECT	Ischemia testing favored*

**Consideration of invasive coronary angiography*

Figure 13.2 Diagnostic accuracy trials applied to a given pretest CAD likelihood population. In this example, the ACCURACY trial was more typical of a low CAD likelihood cohort, while the Meijboom report included higher CAD likelihood patients. CAD, coronary artery disease; CCTA, coronary computed tomographic angiography; NPV, negative predictive value; PPV, positive predictive value.

Study name	Cumulative statistics		
	N	**RR (95% CI)**	***p* Value**
Pundziute	100	55.3 (2.9–1042.3)	.01
Min	1127	114.0 (14.2–916.7)	<.001
Gilard	141	24.3 (5.1–116.3)	<.001
Gaemperli	220	22.6 (6.0–84.6)	<.001
Matsumoto	310	13.3 (4.2–42.0)	<.001
Ostrom	2538	10.8 (3.9–30.2)	<.001
Hadamitzky	1667	10.6 (4.1–27.5)	<.001
Summary RR For CCTA	6603	10.6 (4.1–27.5)	<.001
SPECT Meta-analysis	69,655	6.0 (5.4–7.0)	<.0001

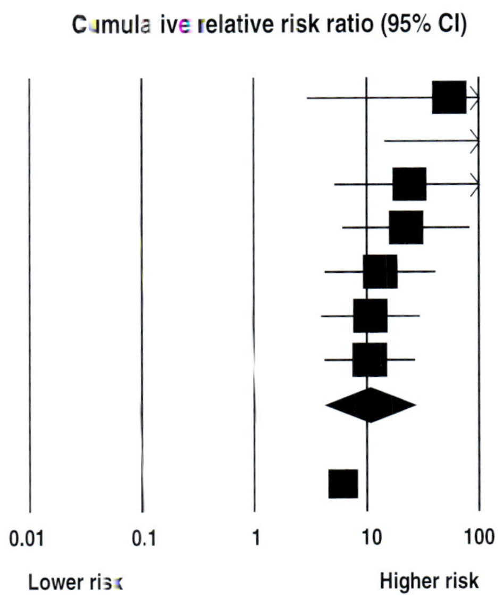

Figure 13.3 Cumulative relative risk (RR) ratio* and 95% confidence intervals (CI) for abnormal or obstructive coronary artery disease (CAD), as compared to no CAD derived from published prognostic series using coronary computed tomographic angiography. Over time, the RR has been refined with more narrow CI around the point estimate of 10.6. In a second analysis, the RR for an abnormal versus normal myocardial perfusion SPECT study (as derived from a meta-analysis of Shaw and Iskandrian [13]) is also listed for comparative purposes. Although the RR will continue to decline with larger patient series (along with the CI), it appears that the RR is higher for CCTA versus SPECT. Note that a combination of events was used for this calculation including all-cause mortality, acute myocardial infarction, late revascularization, and unstable angina. Cumulative relative risk (RR) ratio calculated using a Mantel-Haenszel random effects model. To Calculate a RR for Gilard and Matsumoto, the event data were added solely for no CAD by CCTA. Exclusion of these latter two series does not change the presented results. Note that the heterogeneity statistics for these seven reports was $p < .0001$. An evaluation of publication bias using this meta-analytic data revealed all but two reports were outside the funnel plot (of the standard error by log odds ratio using random effects calculations). CCTA, coronary computed tomographic angiography.

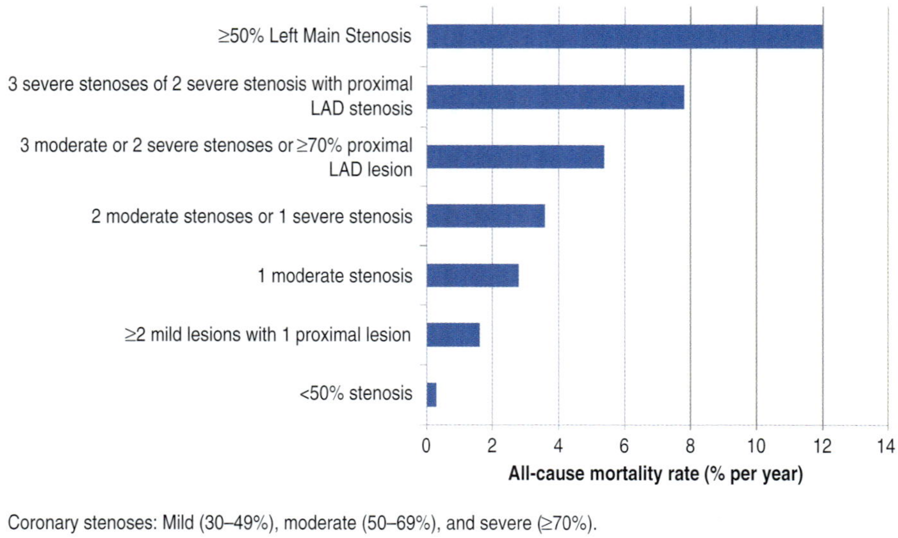

Figure 13.4 Annual mortality by the Duke CAD Prognostic Index derived from a CCTA cohort of 1127 patients. LAD, left anterior descending artery; CCTA, coronary computed tomographic angiography.

clinical risk tools devised over the past several decades can now be validated using CCTA. This would mean that the years of developmental work on stratifying CAD subsets, and importantly, the alteration in risk with surgical intervention or medical management strategies should have applicability for CCTA. Of course, each score requires validation in lower-risk outpatient cohorts. Yet, CCTA has the benefit of this invasive experience in order to "jump start" and focus the risk stratification research. As this evidence starts to unfold, the invasive evidence that has identified CAD subsets that benefit from percutaneous coronary intervention (PCI) or coronary artery bypass surgery (CABS) or medical management may be applied to CCTA strategies. For example, using the Duke CAD index, risk reduction with PCI may be observed in patients with significant CAD, yet the therapeutic benefit may be greater with CABS in patients with more extensive, three-vessel CAD. And, importantly, medical management may result in optimal risk reduction for those with mild CAD. Although this evidence will require validation in outpatient cohorts, one may easily envision how the invasive literature can guide the development of future research in prognostication with CCTA.

Nonobstructive CAD

In a related large series of 2538 patients undergoing electron beam angiography, long-term follow-up data was reported through 6.5 years [18]. This report is similar to the Min series in that higher mortality rates were reported by the number of major epicardial coronary artery vessels with obstructive CAD. In fact, for those with single, double, and triple vessel CAD, the hazard ratios were 1.8, 2.3, and 2.6, respectively ($p < 0.0001$). This larger series with longer-term follow-up also reported on the mortality risk of nonobstructive CAD. And, in this series, the presence of nonobstructive CAD in each of the three major epicardial coronary arteries conferred similar risk to that of patients with single-vessel CAD. This initial report is instrumental, in that it provided insight into novel risk markers that may be uniquely detected with CCTA; that is, nonobstructive CAD including characterization of plaque type (i.e., calcified, noncalcified, or mixed).

As part of this, our knowledge base as to the ensuing risk with coronary artery calcification (CAC) is an important component of risk stratification with plaque and provides us with an understanding of the expected predictive value of nonobstructive plaque. It is important to note that most of the risk information with CAC has been derived in asymptomatic individuals [23]. Several reports derived using electron beam tomography can be helpful in discerning the prognostic potential of CAC as applied in today's CT technology. From a report by Williams *et al.* [24], calcified plaque in the left main and left anterior descending coronary arteries had a high mortality risk similar when compared to what was reported above with obstructive CAD. Importantly, the number of vessels with significant CAC of 100 or 400 and higher reveal a similar ability to risk stratify that is graded from low risk for none to higher and higher risk subsets for those with single and multiple vessels with CAC. Using this report, one can envision in the patient without obstructive CAD that the extent of calcified plaque may provide an estimated MACE risk that is graded. Evidence of calcified plaque within each of the epicardial coronary arteries confers a high-risk status. And, from the Williams series [21], CAC within the left main or left anterior descending coronary arteries connotes higher risk than plaque within

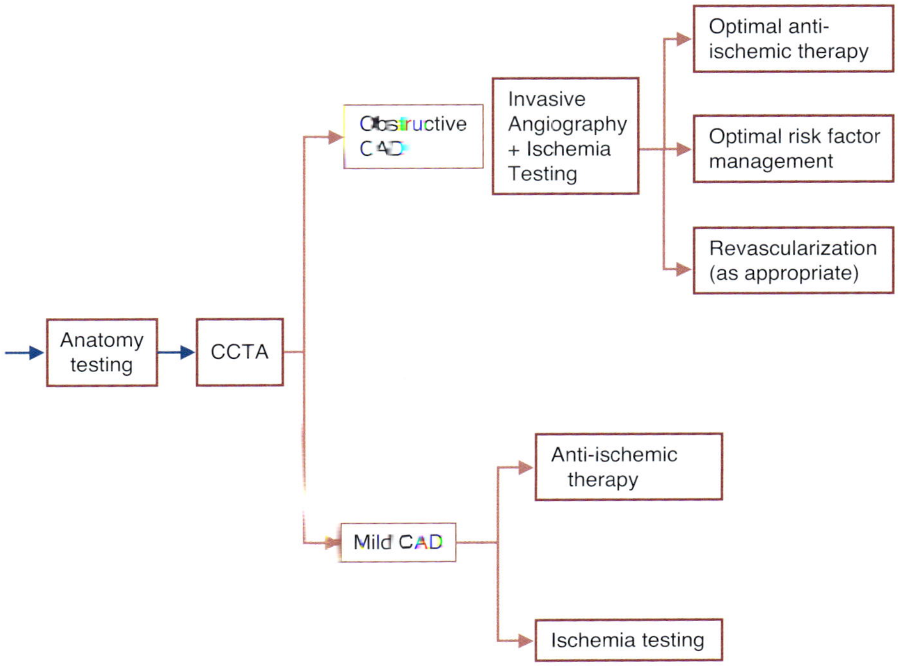

Figure 13.5 Future paradigm for testing intermediate risk, symptomatic women and men. CAD, coronary artery disease; CCTA, coronary computed tomographic angiography.

the right or left circumflex coronary arteries. One or a few larger CAC lesions also confer higher-risk status. Moreover, within this report, frequent CAC lesions (i.e., >20 lesions) were associated with higher mortality.

The data as to the value of CAC in symptomatic patients is, however, sparse. From a systematic review [25], the diagnostic sensitivity and specificity of CAC in symptomatic patients is 85 and 75%. Although data are not available as to the risk of MACE by CAC in symptomatic patients, there are a number of published reports as to the relationship between CAC and myocardial ischemia [26]. From the largest series that include a mixture of symptomatic and asymptomatic patients, the frequency of ischemia increases with more extensive CAC scores. Thus, in the patient with a CAC score ≥1000, one in five will have significant ischemia encumbering at least 5% of the myocardium [27]. At least 5% of the myocardium is considered a moderate-severely abnormal myocardial perfusion SPECT study with ensuing high MACE event rates of 3–5% per year [13, 28]. For this reason, many propose a follow-up ischemia test in patients with a CAC score of 400 or higher. In patients whose clinical risk is elevated (including diabetics, those with the metabolic syndrome or a family history of premature coronary heart disease), ischemia testing is recommended in patients with a CAC score of 100 or higher.

Given the potential for a noninvasive test to discern not only obstructive CAD but also nonobstructive plaque, one can easily envision the role of this modality in lower-risk symptomatic cohorts. Although this data have yet to be published (in particular providing CCTA at a low radiation exposure), we envision a testing algorithm such as that noted in Figure 13.5. In this figure, for patients with nonobstructive CAD or mild coronary stenosis, the ensuing management may either assess the extent and severity of ischemia or the initiation of medical management may prove optimal. The decision to proceed to direct medical management as compared to ischemia testing to further delineate risk should be evaluated in a randomized trial in order to provide definitive guidance to clinicians. Until that time, this strategy should be viewed as opinion based. Yet, the focus of CCTA as the cornerstone of noninvasive management has intuitive appeal. Given that, technical artifact is a challenge for stress myocardial perfusion SPECT, if testing was limited solely to patients with a higher risk of ischemia being related to underlying mild or significant CAD, then the post-test management approaches may be more effectively guided toward targeted anti-ischemic therapy or surgical intervention.

Cost-Efficient Testing Algorithms Using CCTA

Although CCTA is a rather new modality, there are several reports that have examined the economic implications of its use and the potential cost savings that may be achieved with CCTA. One primary role for CCTA is its utility as a gatekeeper to invasive coronary angiography. In one report by Danciu *et al.* [29], selective invasive coronary angiography was performed solely for those with moderate-severe stenosis by CCTA, notably, in a region with a corresponding perfusion abnormality by SPECT. This report presented an interesting management approach. That is, if there was a mismatch between CCTA and myocardial perfusion SPECT where significant nonischemic CAD was documented, then the patient was medically managed. Importantly, in this latter cohort of patients, patients were not referred to invasive coronary angiography with the result being a reduction in invasive procedure use by an estimated 20%. Notably, no MACE, by 1 year, was reported in patients who did not undergo invasive coronary angiography. Thus, this study identified the potential for CCTA to select patients appropriate for the more invasive angiographic procedure. In a larger series, implementation of CCTA within the clinical work-up of patients resulted in a reduction in the normal invasive catheterization rate (32–27%, $p < 0.0001$) [30].

Moreover, several reports have evaluated the cost efficiency of CCTA in stable angina patients [31,32]. In both reports, CCTA provided a lower cost approach to evaluation of stable chest pain while providing equivalent quality in terms of near-term MACE. In one report of 8235 matched low-risk individuals undergoing CCTA or myocardial perfusion SPECT [27], 1-year adjusted CAD costs were reduced 26% for those undergoing CCTA (i.e., an average cost savings of $1075 per patient). From this matched cohort, the major drivers of reduced cost for CCTA were the 24% reduction in likelihood of coronary revascularization ($p < 0.001$). In a related report [28] of 9690 matched intermediate-risk individuals undergoing CCTA or myocardial perfusion SPECT, cost savings with CCTA were similar to the prior report at 33% ($p < 0.001$) with an average cost that reduced by $467 per patient. For CCTA, the major drivers of eliciting cost savings are the lower rates of CAD medications and coronary revascularization as compared to myocardial perfusion SPECT. Importantly for each of these two examples, clinical outcomes were similar, and therefore, no reduction in quality was achieved with CCTA following a more cost-efficient diagnostic strategy.

Future of CCTA

For the majority of this chapter, we have focused on clinical utility of CCTA in the assessment of suspected CAD. The evidence base with CCTA has evolved rapidly, but there are several ongoing clinical trials that have the potential to add considerably to these data. The Study of Myocardial Perfusion and Coronary Anatomy Imaging Roles in Coronary Artery Disease, or SPARC, is an observational registry of >3000 symptomatic patients undergoing CCTA or myocardial perfusion SPECT or PET. The primary aim of this study is to examine costs and clinical outcomes (www.sparctrial.org). This trial is completing follow-up and will add to our knowledge of the comparative effectiveness of CCTA in relation to more conventional ischemia testing. More recently, a pilot phase of the FABULOUS trial was completed with the aim of examining feasibility of this randomized trial of CCTA versus myocardial perfusion SPECT. Within this pilot trial, approximately 200 patients were enrolled, and near-term health status data (i.e., angina) were collected. This data may provide insight into the ability of CCTA or myocardial perfusion SPECT to target therapeutic intervention that will reduce angina stability or frequency. The main trial of FABULOUS has been proposed and is currently under review. As such, in the next few years, we expect an onslaught of high-quality data with CCTA that may drastically change current patient management approaches. Importantly, the goal of all future randomized trials in CCTA would be to establish its ability to improve patient outcomes including life expectancy as well as quality of life.

Recent concerns over radiation exposure have prompted ongoing efforts aimed at providing testing at a minimal burden to the patient. In addition to tube current modulation and lower (i.e., <100 kV) tube voltage as well as other techniques, the goal for CCTA would be to achieve a modest degree of radiation exposure, and therefore, garnering more wide-scale acceptance of this modality in diverse patient populations.

Conclusions

This chapter provides a synopsis of available diagnostic and prognostic data on CCTA. This evidence has been accrued over a very short period of time and reveals a high degree of predictive accuracy. The current evidence base noting a high degree of accuracy for risk detection, and correlation with invasive angiography is reason for enthusiasm with CCTA. The diagnostic accuracy is superbly high and appears to be improved in lower likelihood patients. The prognostic data note a graded relationship between the extent and severity of obstructive CAD and MACE, with limited data known regarding the long-term outcomes of patients undergoing CCTA. Further validations of the invasive jeopardy scores and their application in therapeutic decision making may help to devise CCTA-guided management approaches. In the near future, several large clinical trials will be completed that may further aid in the development of prognostic data with CCTA, in particular, as its effectiveness compares to other modalities such as myocardial perfusion SPECT.

References

1. Lin FY DR, Roman MJ, Meng J, *et al.* (2008) Cardiac chamber volumes, function, and mass as determined by 64-multidetector row computed tomography: mean values among healthy adults free of hypertension and obesity. http://www.ncbi.nlm.nih.gov/pubmed/19356515?ordinalpos=3&itool=EntrezSystem2.PEntrez.Pubmed.Pubmed_ResultsPanel.Pubmed_DefaultReportPanel.Pubmed_RVDocSum. *JACC Cardiovasc Imaging* 1(6):782–786.
2. Rodevan O BR, Ljosland M, Maehle J, Smith HJ, Ihlen H. (1999) Left atrial volumes assessed by three- and two-dimensional echocardiography compared to MRI estimates. *Int J Card Imaging* 15:397–410.
3. Suzuki S, Furui S, Kaminaga T *et al.* (2006) Accuracy and efficiency of left ventricular ejection fraction analysis, using multidetector row computed tomography: effect of image reconstruction window within cardiac phase, slice thickness, and interval of short-axis sections. *Circ J* 70:289–296.
4. Hamon M, Biondi-Zoccai GG, Malagutti P, Agostoni P, Morello R, Valgimigli M. (2006) Diagnostic performance of multislice spiral computed tomography of coronary arteries as compared with conventional invasive coronary angiography: a meta-analysis. *J Am Coll Cardiol* 48(9):1896–1910.
5. Schuijf JD, Bax JJ, Shaw LJ *et al.* (2006) Meta-analysis of comparative diagnostic performance of magnetic resonance imaging and multislice computed tomography for noninvasive coronary angiography. *Am Heart J* 151(2):404–411.
6. Sun Z, Jiang W. (2006) Diagnostic value of multislice computed tomography angiography in coronary artery disease: a meta-analysis. *Eur J Radiol* 60(2):279–286.
7. Stein PD, Beemath A, Kayali F, Skaf E, Sanchez J, Olson RE. (2006) Multidetector computed tomography for the diagnosis of coronary artery disease: a systematic review. *Am J Med* 119(3):203–216.
8. Janne d'Othee B, Siebert U, Cury R, Jadvar H, Dunn EJ, Hoffmann U. (2008) A systematic review on diagnostic accuracy of CT-based detection of significant coronary artery disease. *Eur J Radiol* 65(3):449–461.
9. Budoff MJ, Dowe D, Jollis JG *et al.* (2008) Diagnostic performance of 64-multidetector row coronary computed tomographic angiography for evaluation of coronary artery stenosis in individuals without known coronary artery disease: results from the prospective multicenter ACCURACY (Assessment by Coronary Computed Tomographic Angiography of Individuals Undergoing Invasive Coronary Angiography) trial. *J Am Coll Cardiol* 52(21):1724–1732.
10. Meijboom WB, Van Mieghem CA, van Pelt N *et al.* (2008) Comprehensive assessment of coronary artery stenoses: computed tomography coronary angiography versus conventional coronary angiography and correlation with fractional flow reserve in patients with stable angina. *J Am Coll Cardiol* 52(8):636–643.
11. Miller JM, Rochitte CE, Dewey M *et al.* (2008) Diagnostic performance of coronary angiography by 64-row CT. *N Engl J Med* 359(22):2324–2336.
12. Raff GL, Gallagher MJ, O'Neill WW, Goldstein JA. (2005) Diagnostic accuracy of noninvasive coronary angiography using 64 slice spiral computed tomography. *J Am Coll Cardiol* 46(3):552–557.
13. Shaw LJ Iskandrian AE. (2004) Prognostic value of gated myocardial perfusion SPECT. *J Nucl Cardiol* 11(2):171–185.
14. Shaw LJ, Vasey C, Sawada S, Rimmerman C, Marwick TH. (2005) Impact of gender on risk stratification by exercise and dobutamine stress echocardiography: long-term mortality in 4234 women and 6898 men. *Eur Heart J* 26(5):447–456.
15. Mieres JH, Shaw LJ, Arai A *et al.* (2005) Role of noninvasive testing in the clinical evaluation of women with suspected coronary artery disease: consensus statement from the Cardiac Imaging Committee, Council on Clinical Cardiology, and the Cardiovascular Imaging and Intervention Committee, Council on Cardiovascular Radiology and Intervention, American Heart Association. *Circulation* 111(5):682–696.
16. Pundziute G, Schuijf JD, Jukema JW *et al.* (2007) Prognostic value of multislice computed tomography coronary angiography in patients with known or suspected coronary artery disease. *J Am Coll Cardiol* 49(1):62–70.
17. Min JK, Shaw LJ, Devereux RB *et al.* (2007) Prognostic value of multidetector coronary computed tomographic angiography for prediction of all-cause mortality. *J Am Coll Cardiol* 50(12):1161–1170.
18. Gilard M, Le Gal G, Cornily JC *et al.* (2007) Midterm prognosis of patients with suspected coronary artery disease and normal multislice computed tomographic findings: a prospective management outcome study. *Arch Intern Med* 167(15):1686–1689.
19. Gaemperli O, Valenta I, Schepis T *et al.* (2008) Coronary 64-slice CT angiography predicts outcome in patients with known or suspected coronary artery disease. *Eur Radiol* 18(6):1162–1173.
20. Matsumoto N, Sato Y, Yoda S *et al.* (2007) Prognostic value of non-obstructive CT low-dense coronary artery plaques detected by multislice computed tomography. *Circ J* 71(12):1898–1903.
21. Ostrom MP, Gopal A, Ahmadi N *et al.* (2008) Mortality incidence and the severity of coronary atherosclerosis assessed by computed tomography angiography. *J Am Coll Cardiol* 52(16):1335–1343
22. Hadamitzky M, Freißmuth B, Meyer T *et al.* (2009) Prognostic value of coronary computed tomographic angiography for prediction of cardiac events in patients with suspected coronary artery disease. *J Am Coll Cardiol Img* 2:404–411.
23. Greenland P, Bonow RO, Brundage BH *et al.* (2007) ACCF/AHA 2007 clinical expert consensus document on coronary artery calcium scoring by computed tomography in global cardiovascular risk assessment and in evaluation of patients with chest pain: a report of the American College of Cardiology Foundation Clinical Expert Consensus Task Force (ACCF/AHA Writing Committee to Update the 2000 Expert Consensus Document on Electron Beam Computed

Tomography) developed in collaboration with the Society of Atherosclerosis Imaging and Prevention and the Society of Cardiovascular Computed Tomography. *J Am Coll Cardiol* 49(3):378–402.

24. Williams M, Shaw LJ, Raggi P *et al.* (2008) Prognostic value of number and site of calcified coronary lesions compared with the total score. *JACC Cardiovasc Imaging* 1(1):61–69.
25. Budoff MJ, Cohen MC, Garcia MJ *et al.* (2005) ACCF/AHA clinical competence statement on cardiac imaging with computed tomography and magnetic resonance. *Circulation* 112(4):598–617.
26. Shaw LJ, Heller GV, Casperson P *et al.* (*2006*) Gated myocardial perfusion single photon emission computed tomography in the clinical outcomes utilizing revascularization and aggressive drug evaluation (COURAGE) trial, Veterans Administration Cooperative study no. 424. *J Nucl Cardiol* 13(5):685–698.
27. Berman DS, Wong ND, Gransar H *et al.* (2004) Relationship between stress-induced myocardial ischemia and atherosclerosis measured by coronary calcium tomography. *J Am Coll Cardiol* 44(4):923–930.
28. Berman DS, Kang X, Hayes SW *et al.* (2003) Adenosine myocardial perfusion single-photon emission computed tomography in women compared with men. Impact of diabetes mellitus on incremental prognostic value and effect on patient management. *J Am Coll Cardiol* 41(7):1125–1133.
29. Danciu SC, Herrera CJ, Stecy PJ, Carell E, Saltiel F, Hines JL. (2007) Usefulness of multislice computed tomographic coronary angiography to identify patients with abnormal myocardial perfusion stress in whom diagnostic catheterization may be safely avoided. *Am J Cardiol* 100(11):1605–1608.
30. Chow BJ, Hoffmann U, Nieman K. (2005) Computed tomographic coronary angiography: an alternative to invasive coronary angiography. *Can J Cardiol* 21(11):933–940.
31. Min JK, Kang N, Shaw LJ *et al.* (2008) Costs and clinical outcomes after coronary multidetector CT angiography in patients without known coronary artery disease: comparison to myocardial perfusion SPECT. *Radiology* 249(1):62–70.
32. Min JK, Shaw LJ, Berman DS, Gilmore A, Kang N. (2008) Costs and clinical outcomes in individuals without known coronary artery disease undergoing coronary computed tomographic angiography from an analysis of Medicare category III transaction codes. *Am J Cardiol* 102(6):672–678.

Appendix

Body planes: axial, coronal, sagital

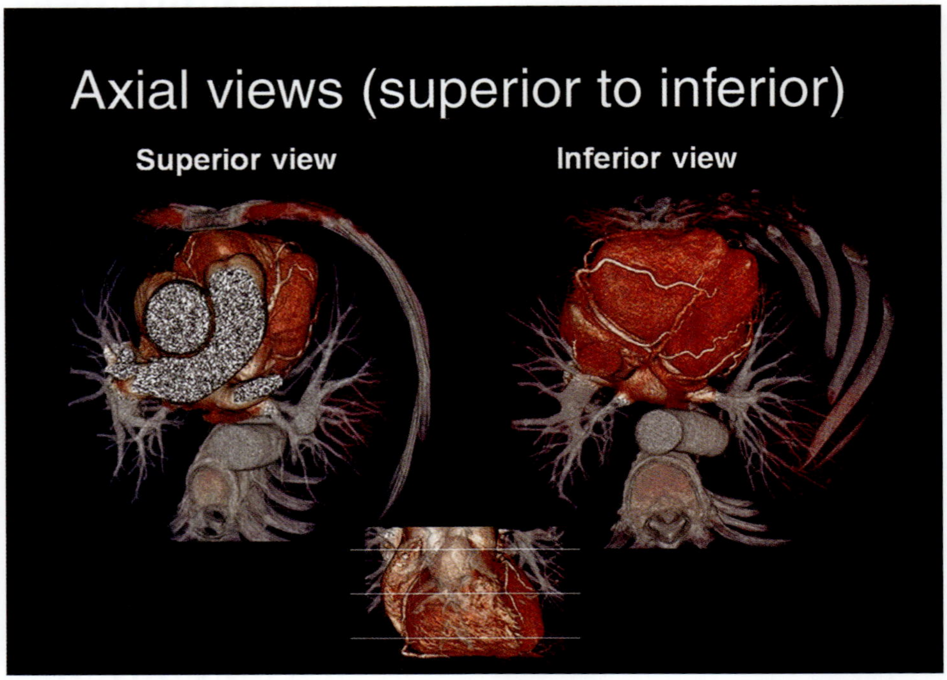

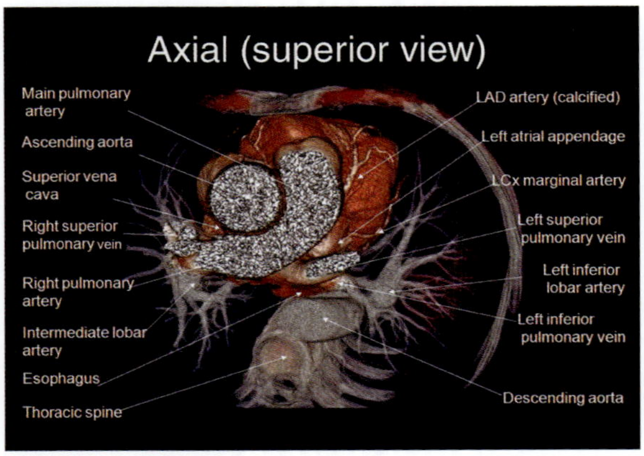

Axial 1

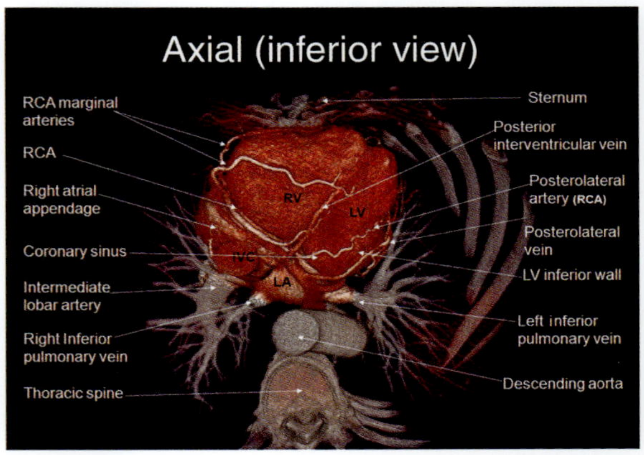

Axial 2

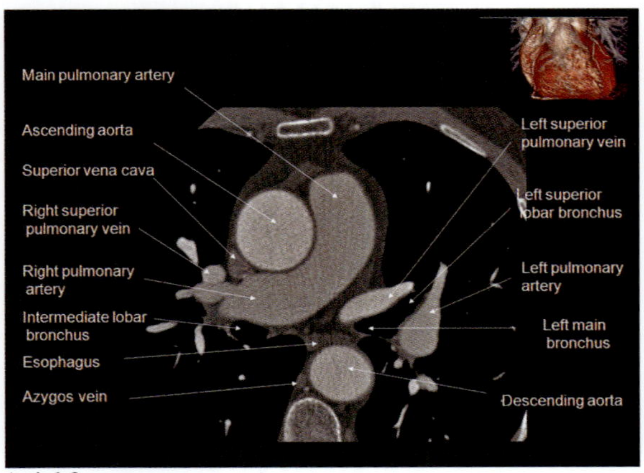

Axial 3

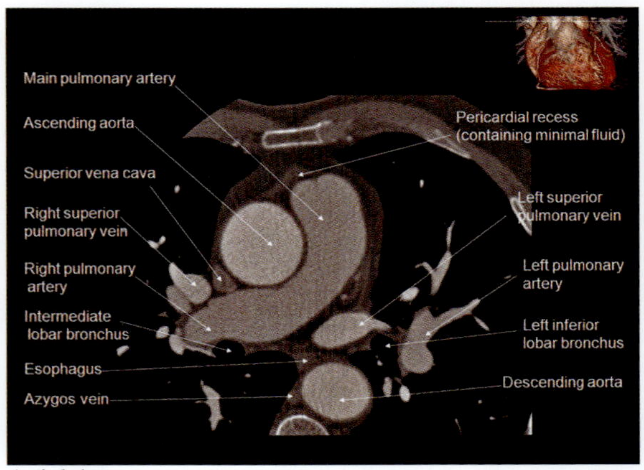

Axial 4

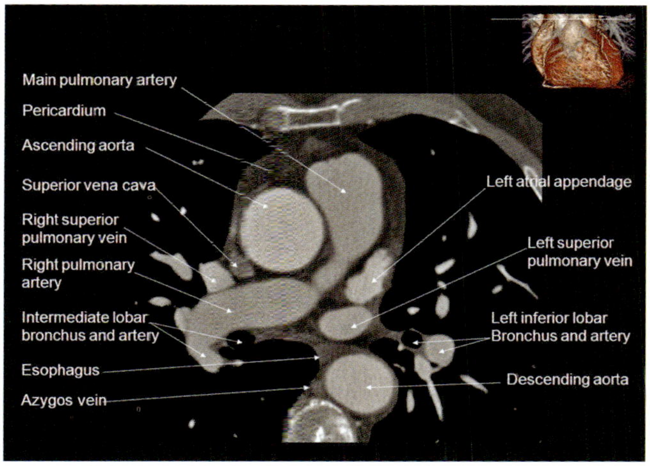

Axial 5

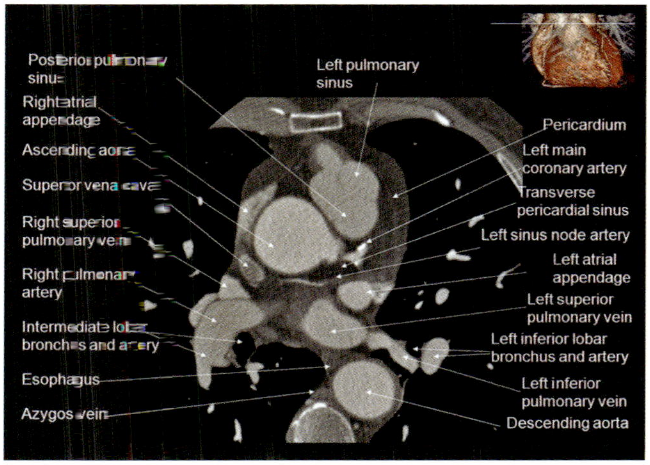

Axial 6

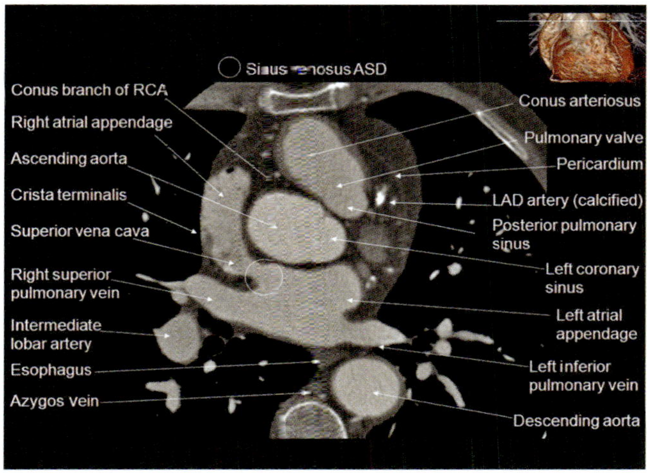

Axial 7

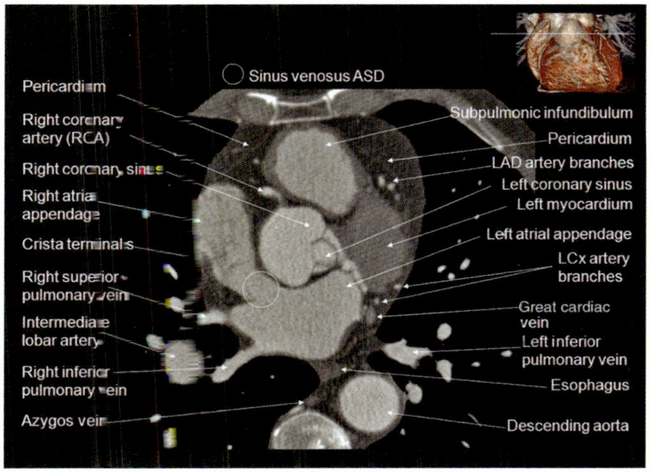

Axial 8

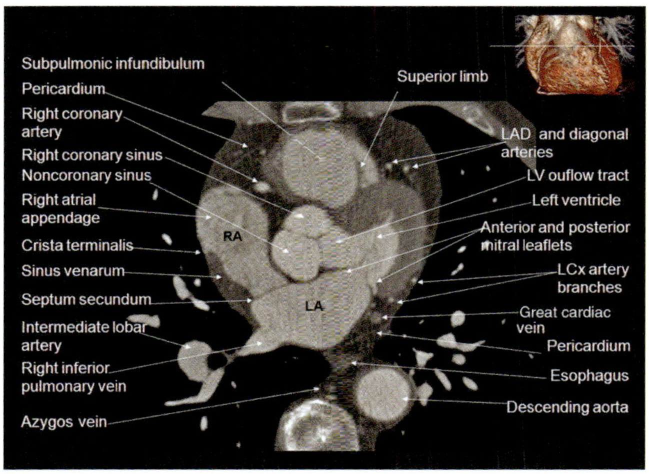

Axial 9

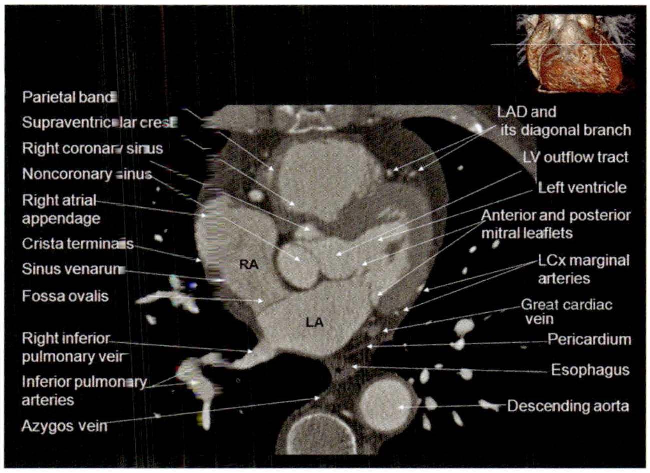

Axial 10

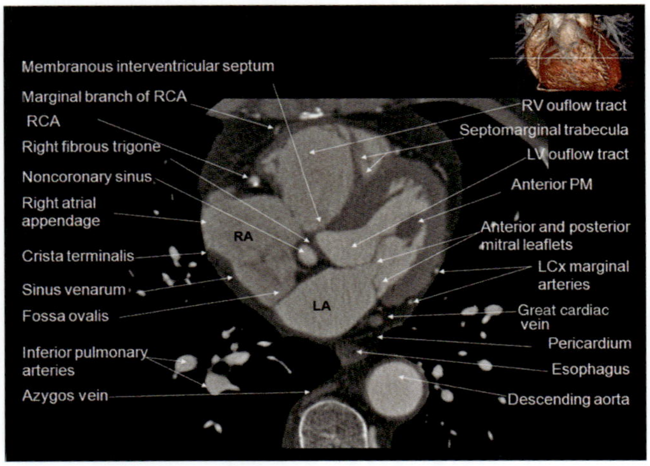

Axial 11

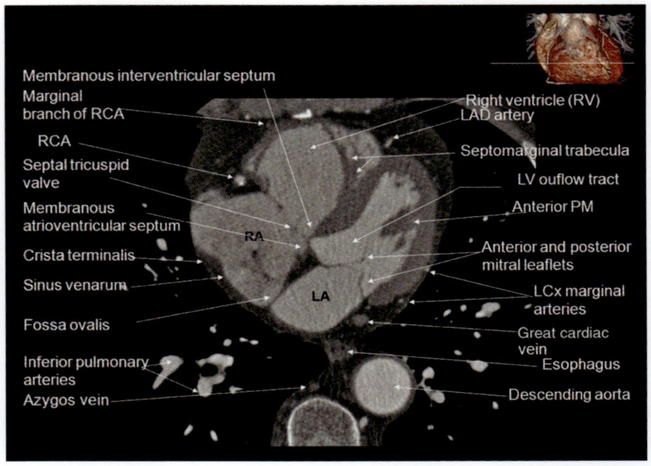

Axial 12

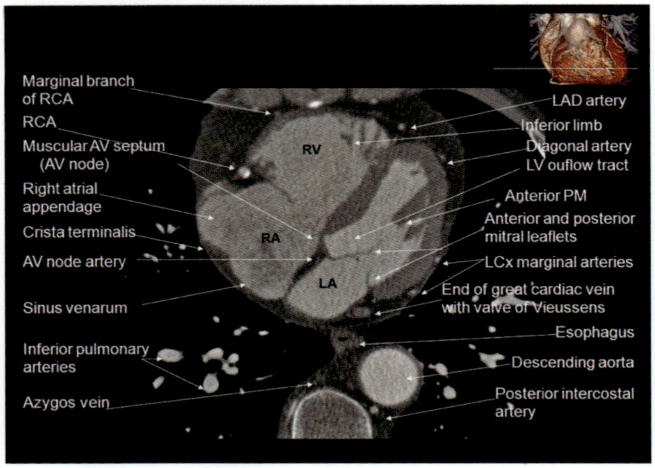

Axial 13

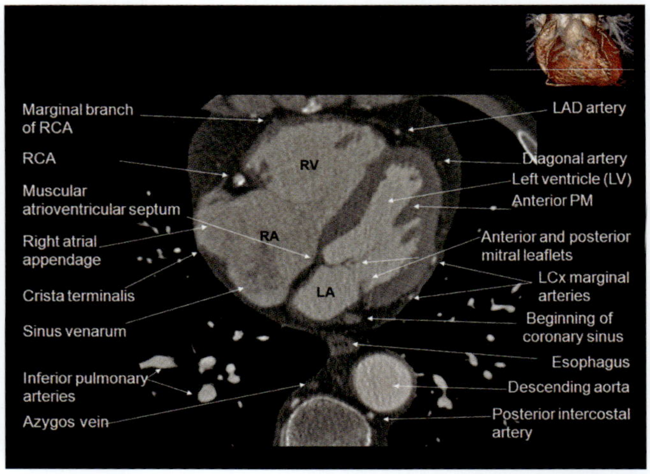

Axial 14

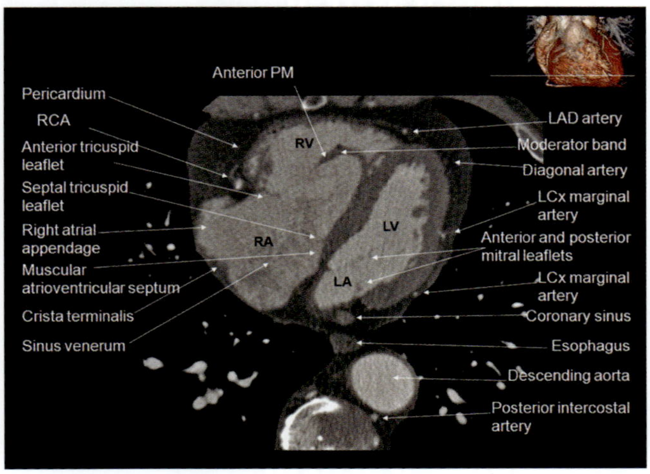

Axial 15

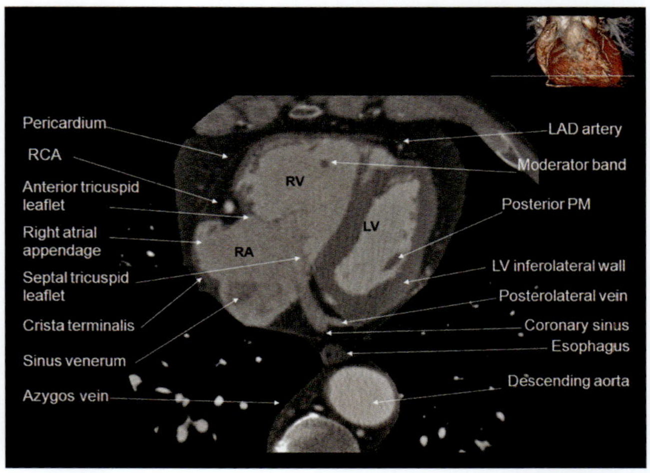

Axial 16

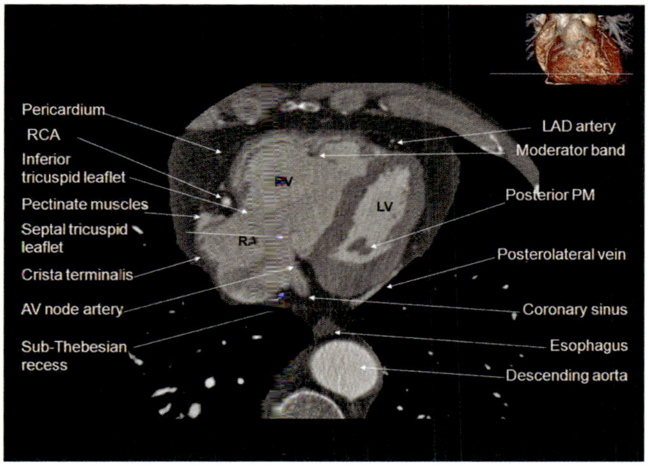

Axial 17

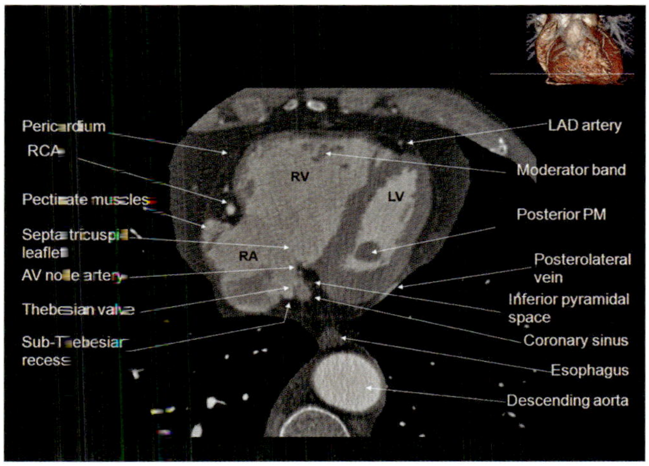

Axial 18

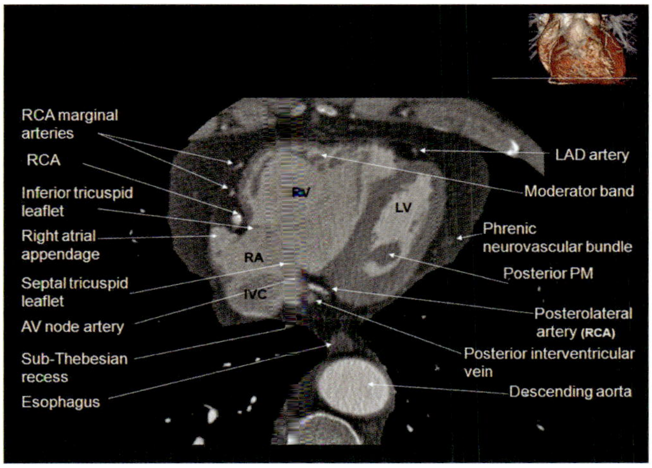

Axial 19

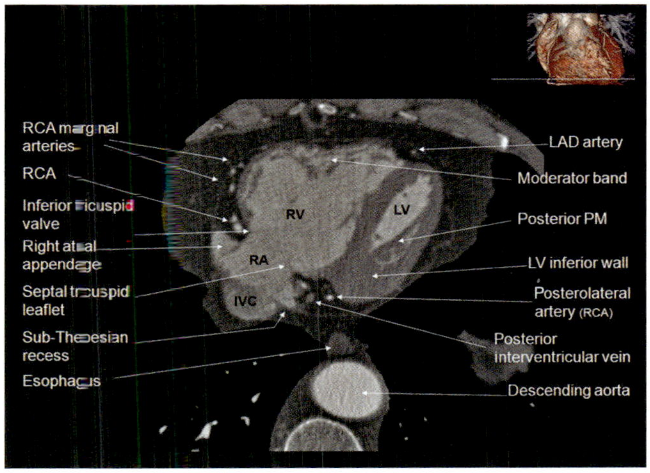

Axial 20

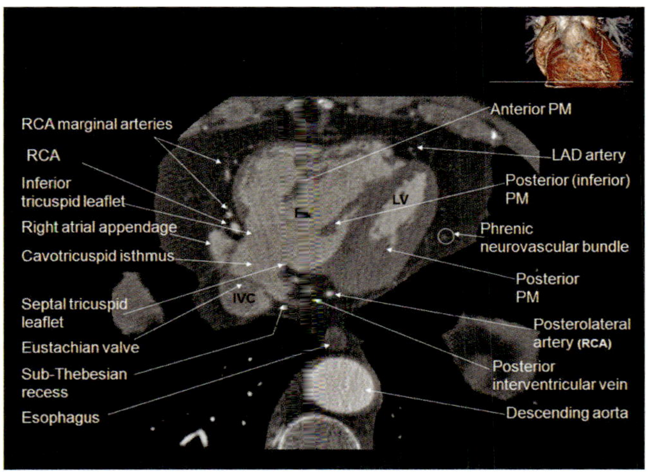

Axial 21

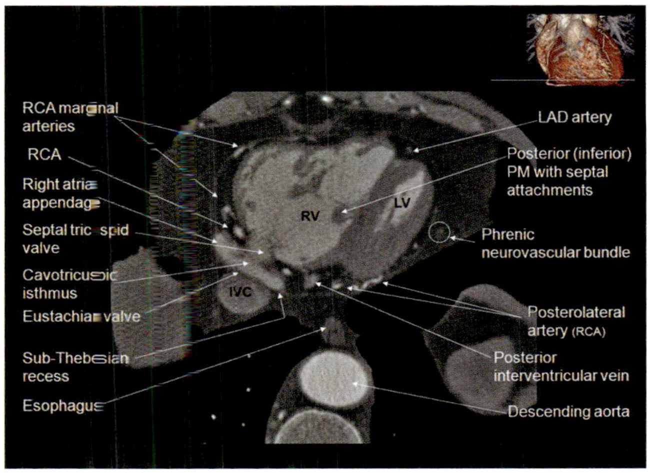

Axial 22

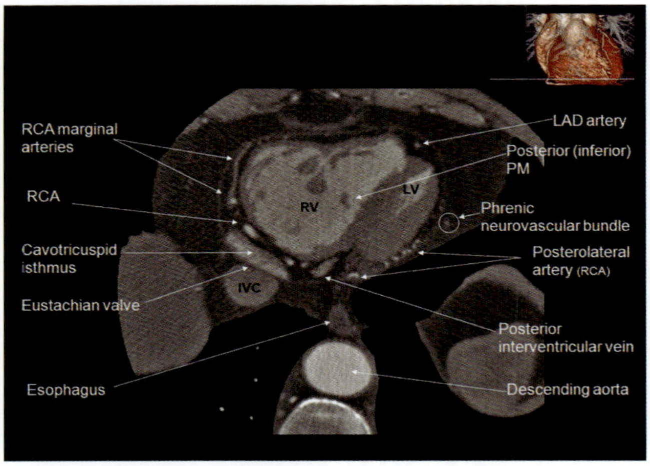

Axial 23

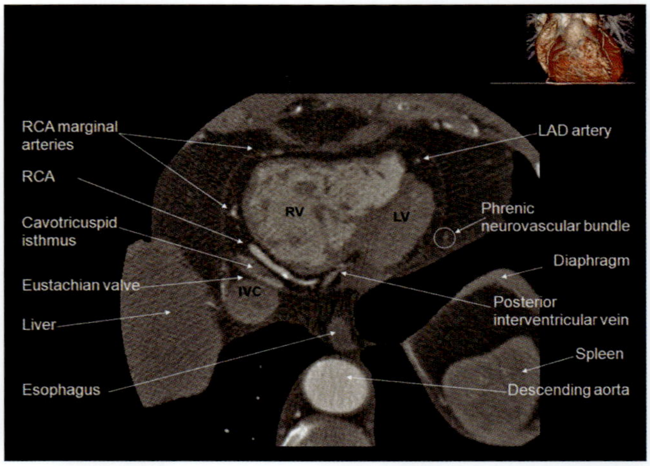

Axial 24

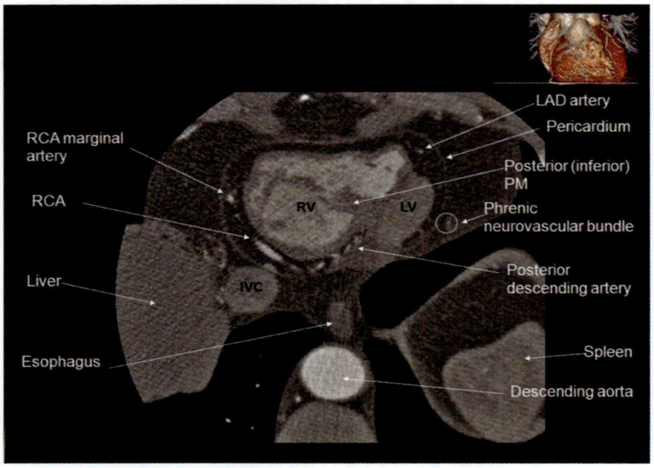

Axial 25

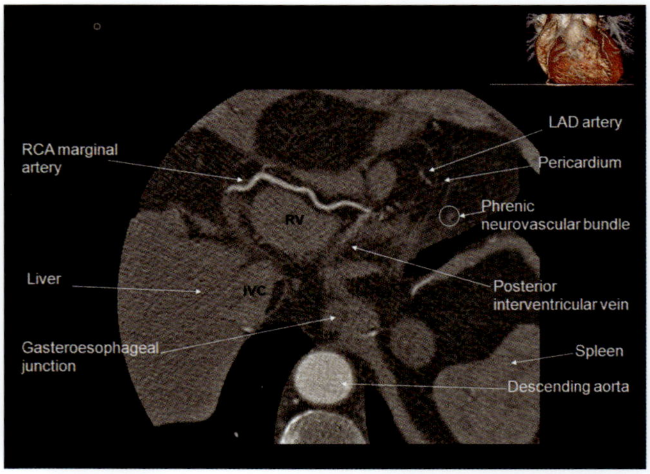

Axial 26

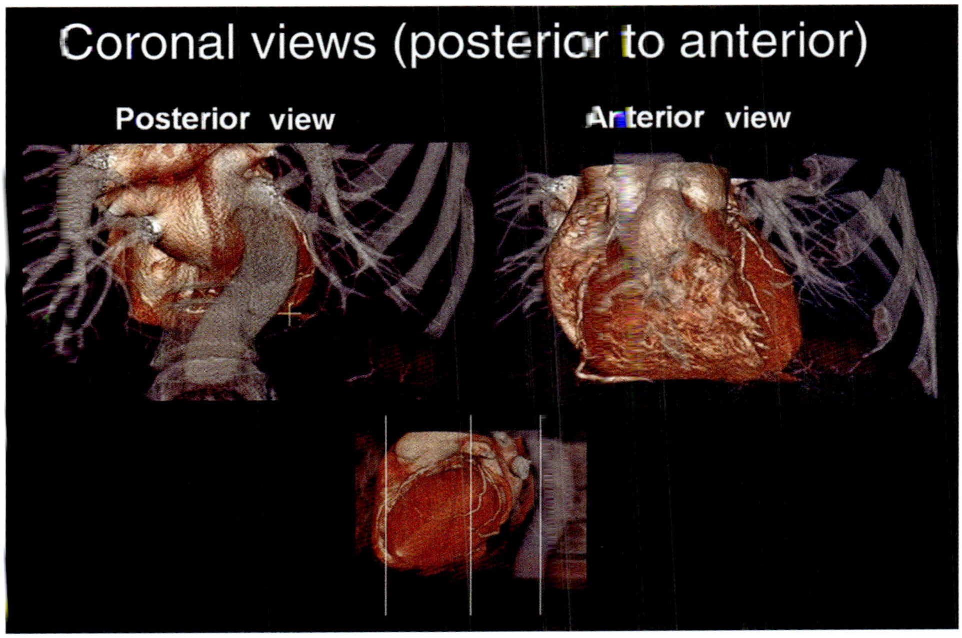

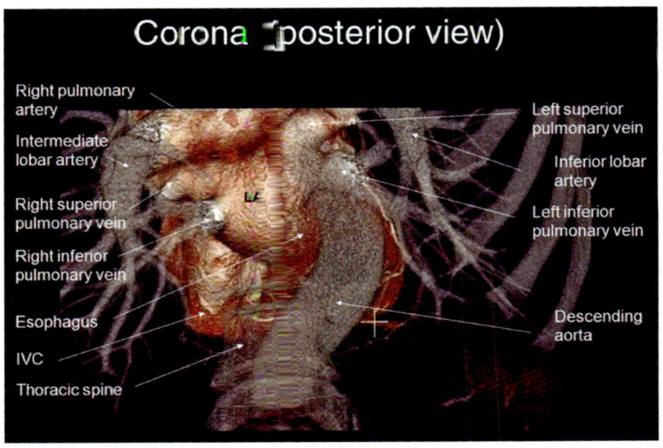

Coronal 1

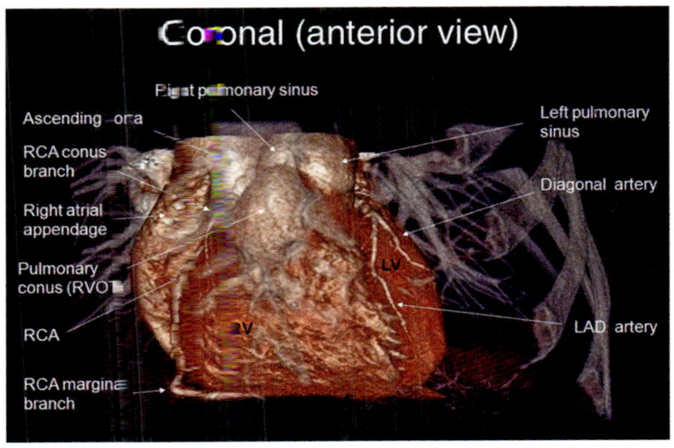

Coronal 2

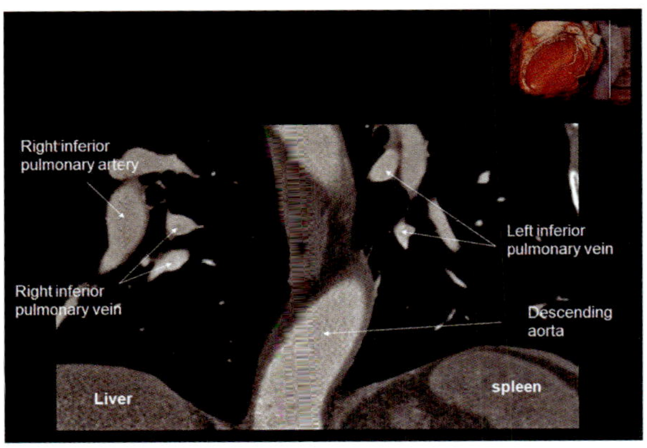

Coronal 3

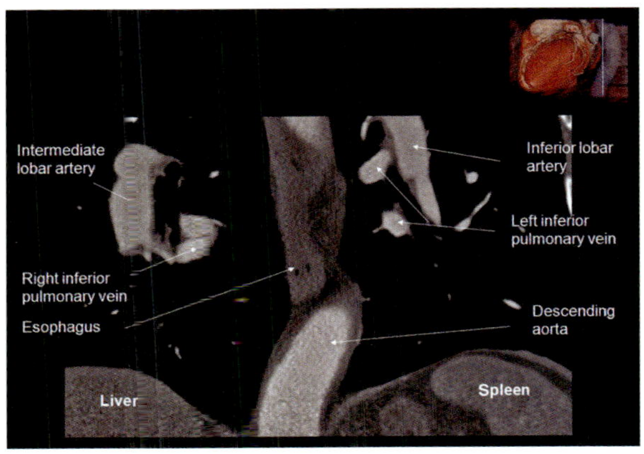

Coronal 4

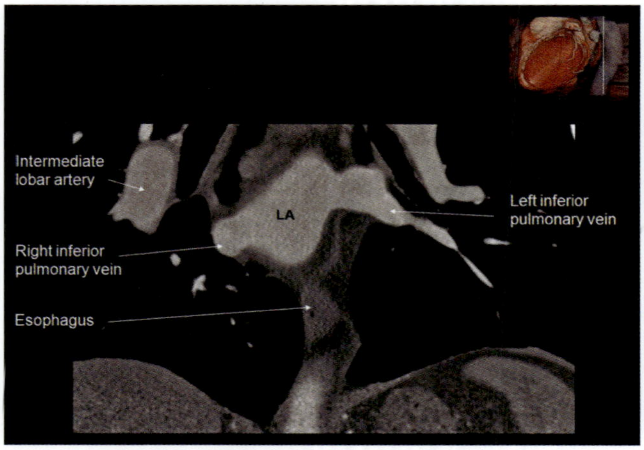

Coronal 5

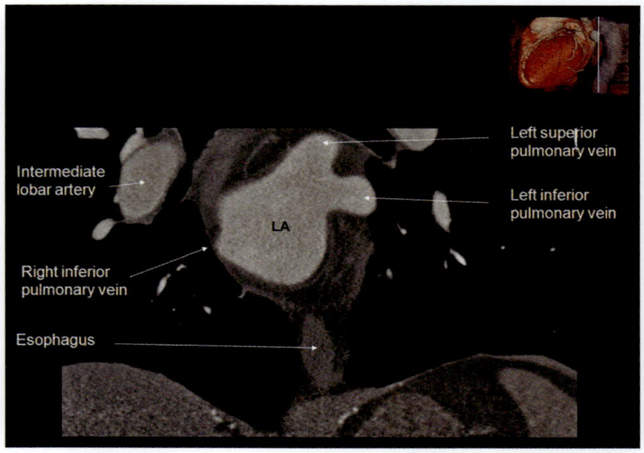

Coronal 6

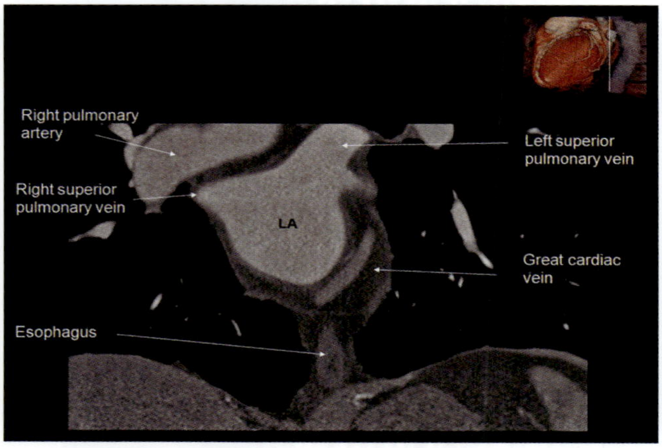

Coronal 7

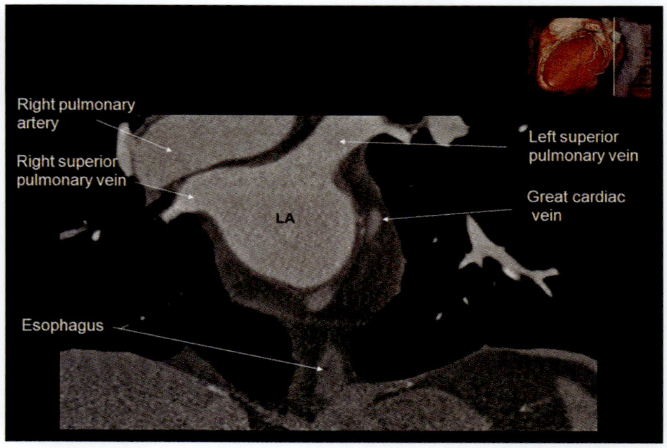

Coronal 8

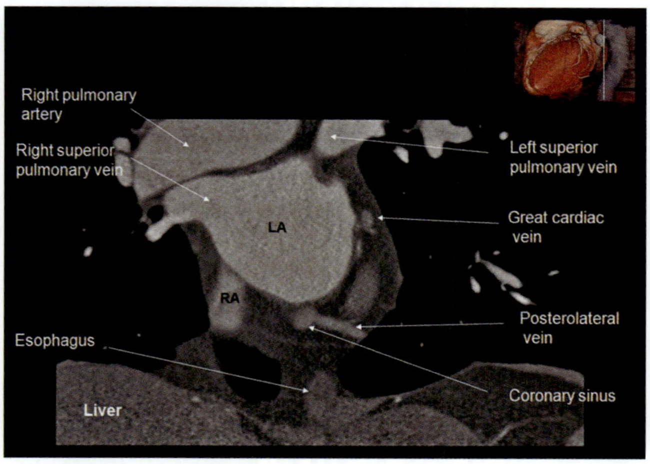

Coronal 9

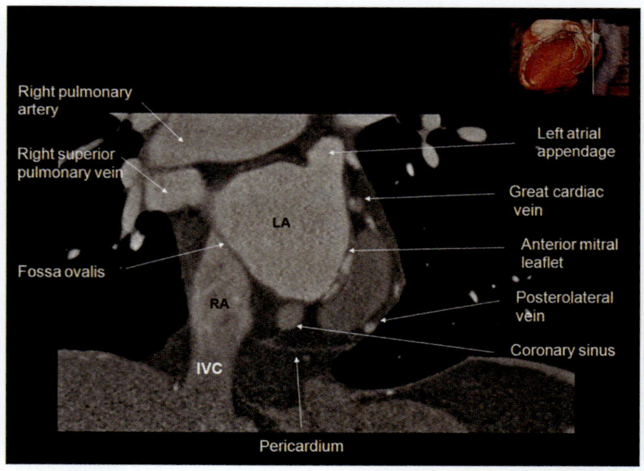

Coronal 10

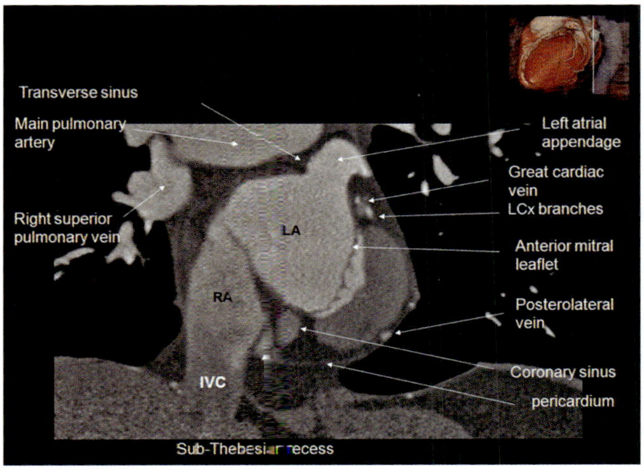

Coronal 11

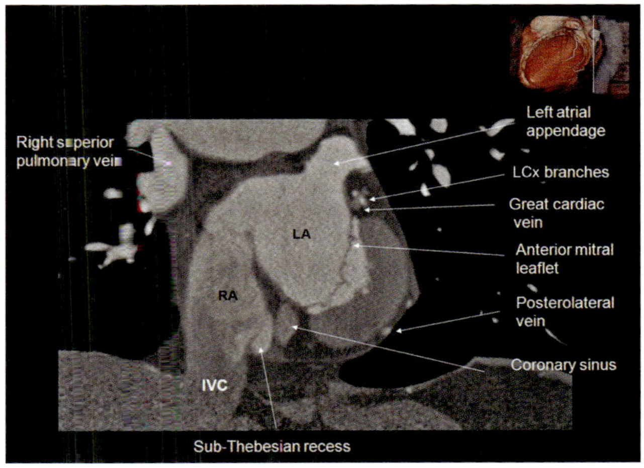

Coronal 12

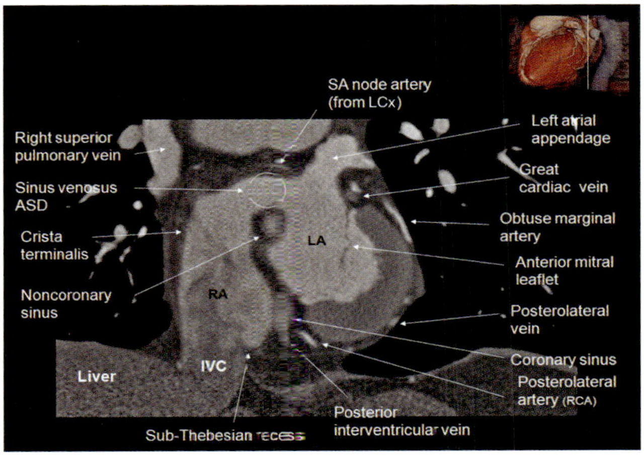

Coronal 13

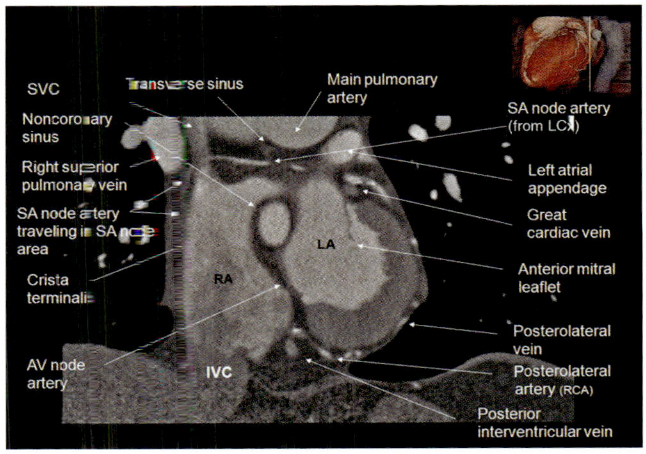

Coronal 14

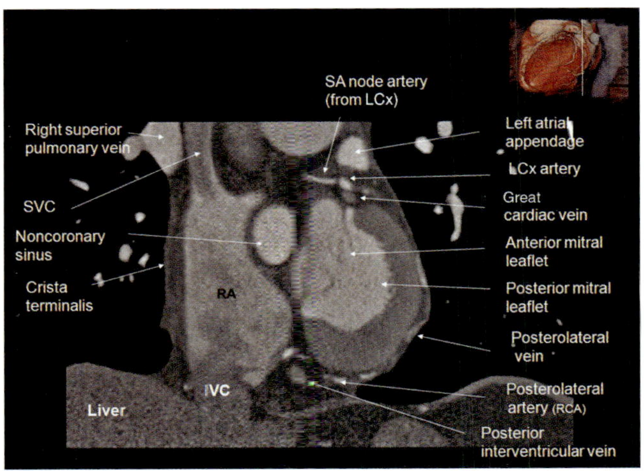

Coronal 15

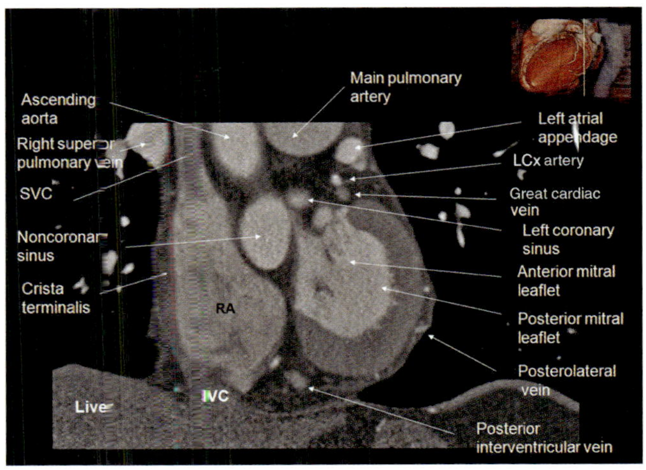

Coronal 16

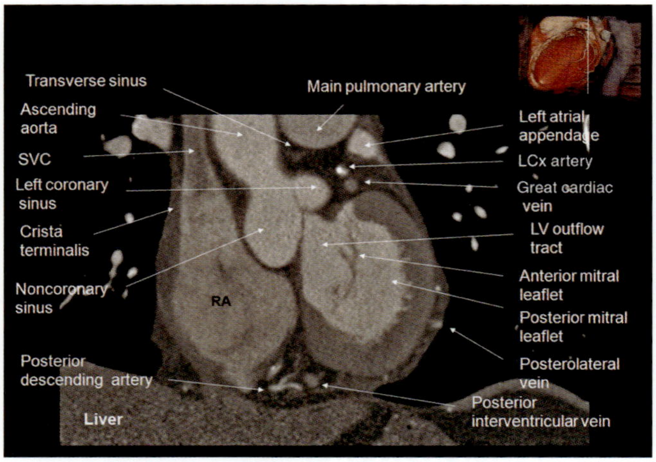

Coronal 17

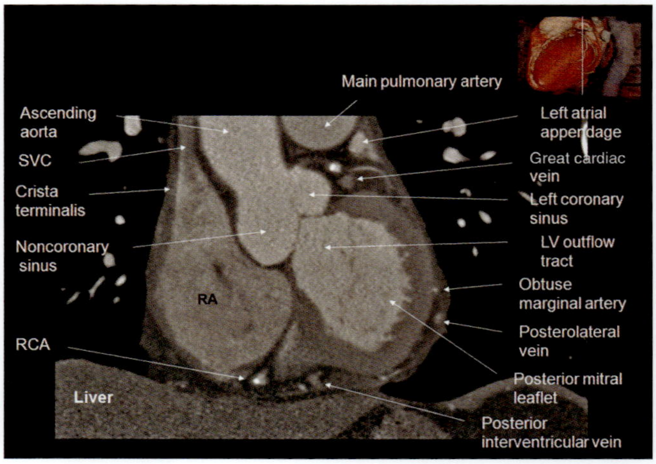

Coronal 18

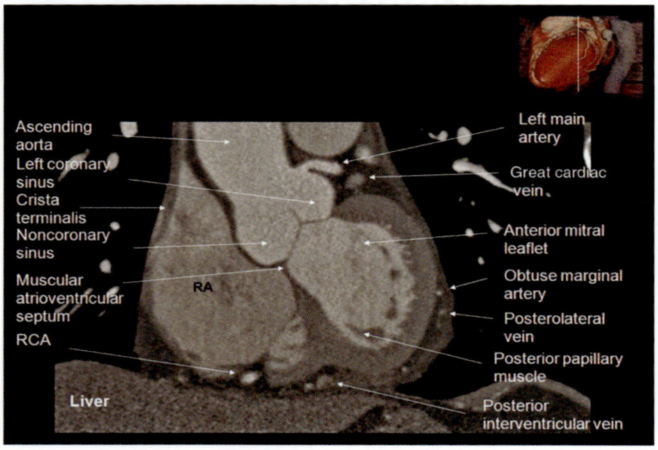

Coronal 19

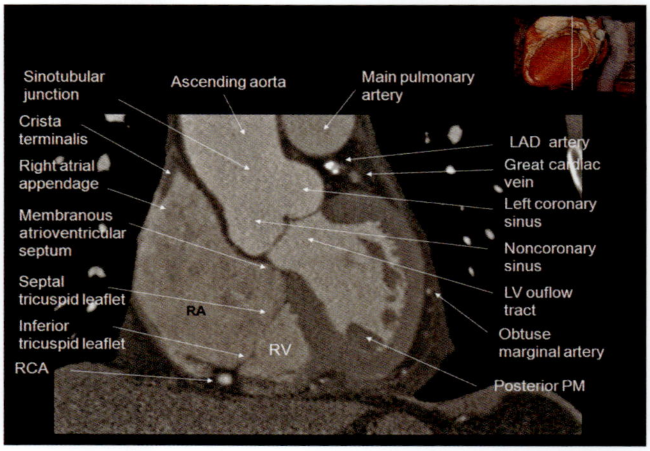

Coronal 20

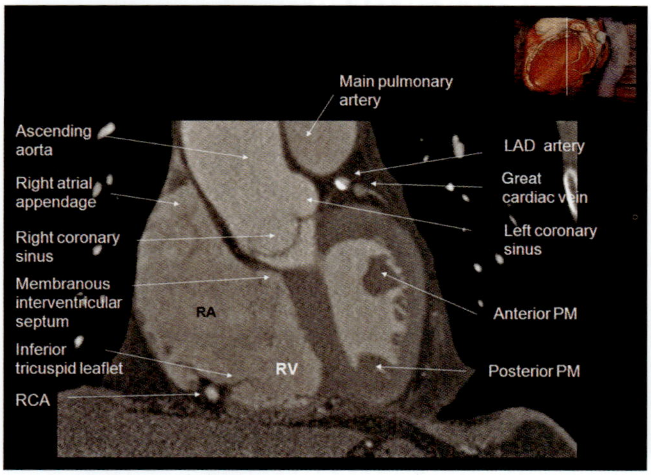

Coronal 21

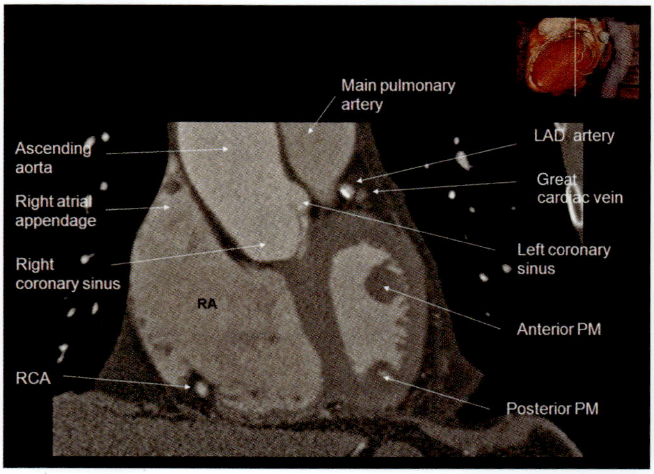

Coronal 22

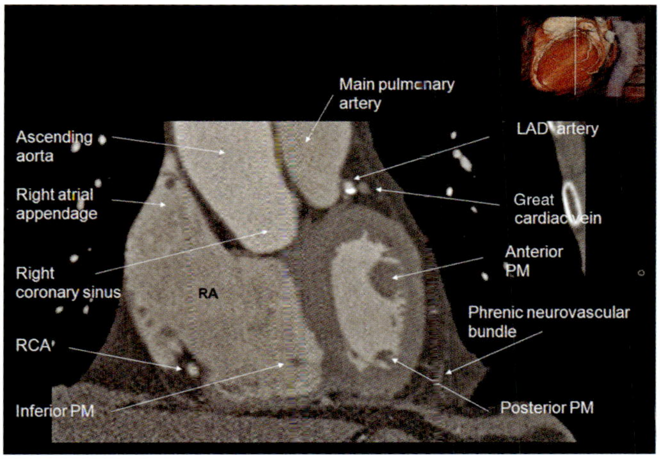

Coronal 23

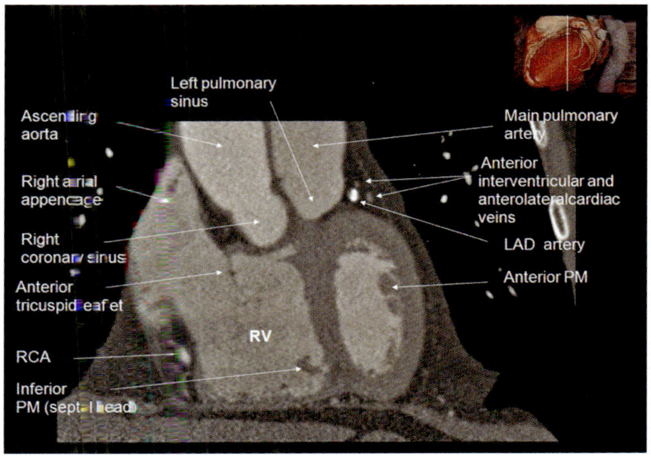

Coronal 24

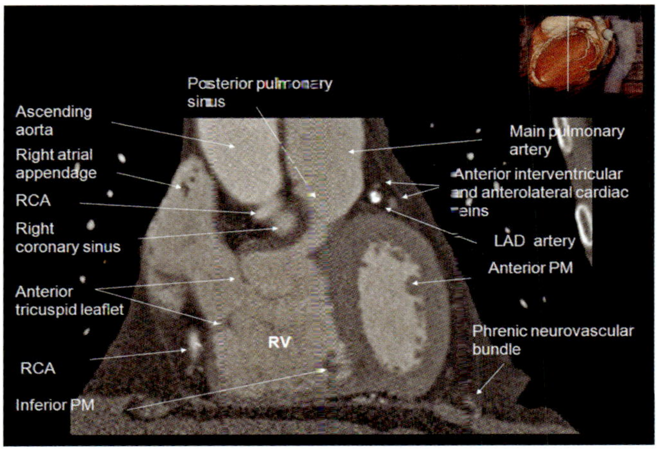

Coronal 25

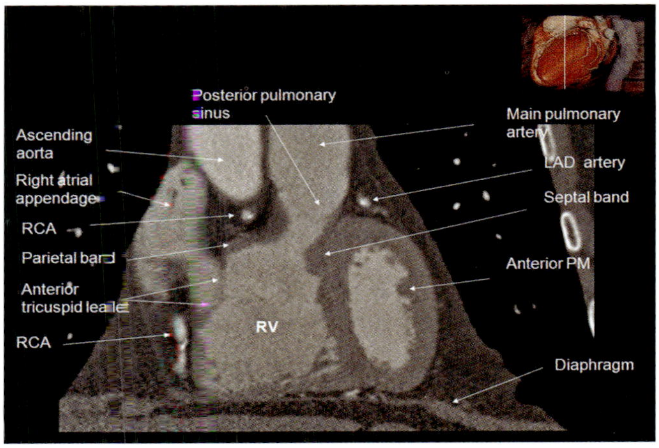

Coronal 26

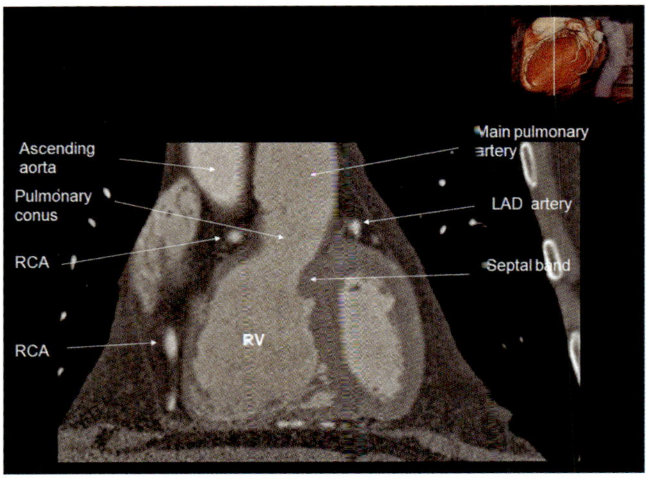

Coronal 27

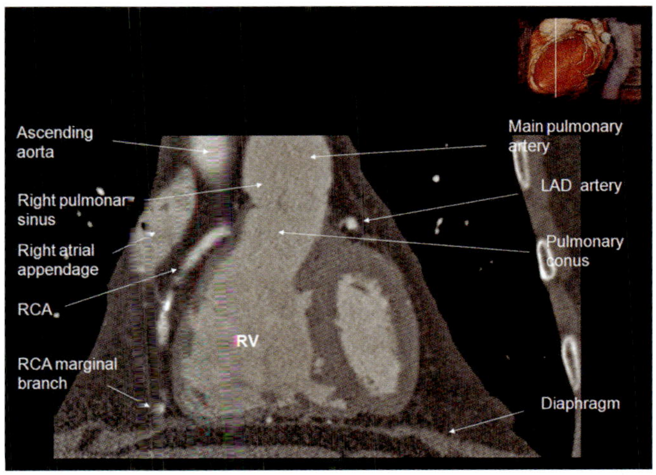

Coronal 28

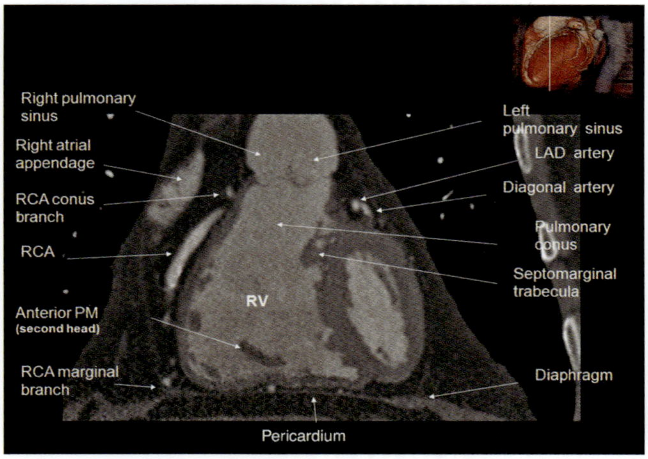

Coronal 29

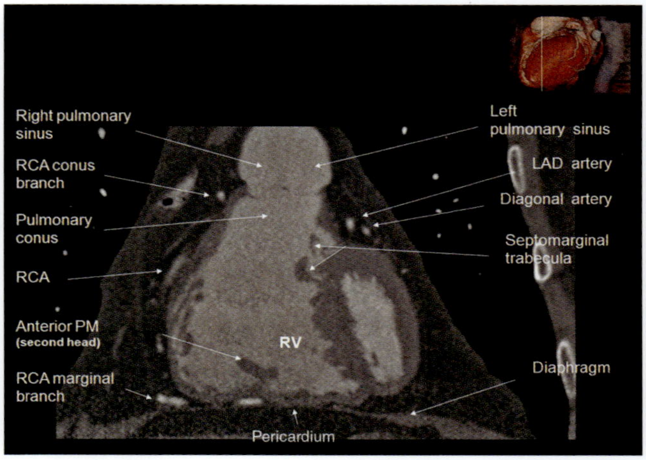

Coronal 30

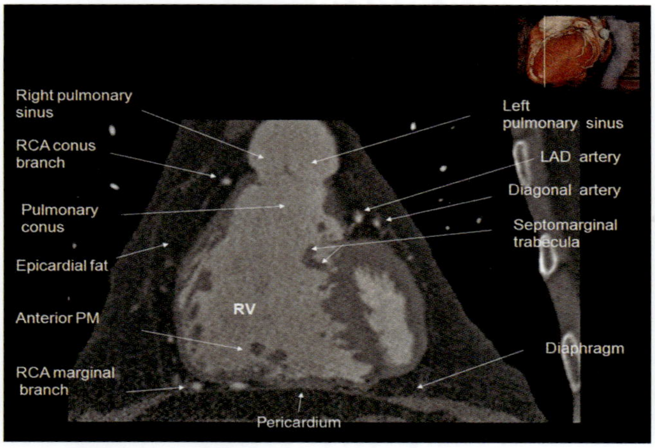

Coronal 31

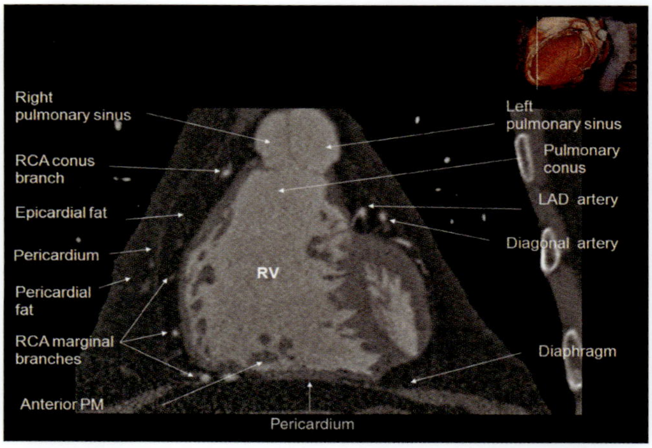

Coronal 32

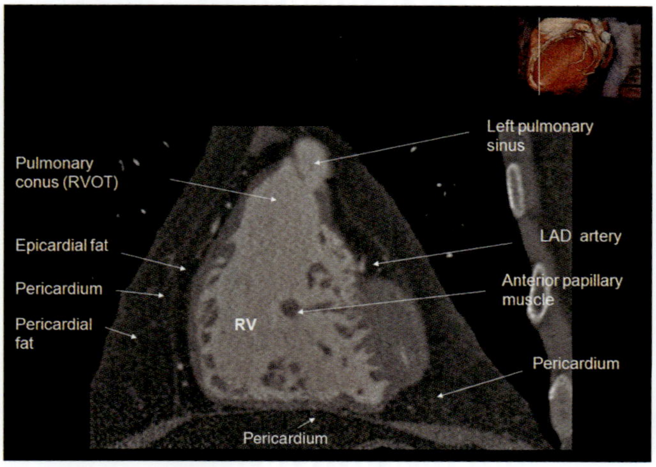

Coronal 33

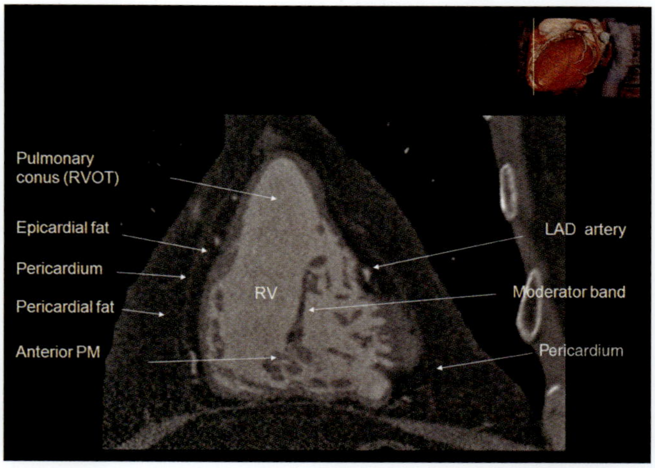

Coronal 34

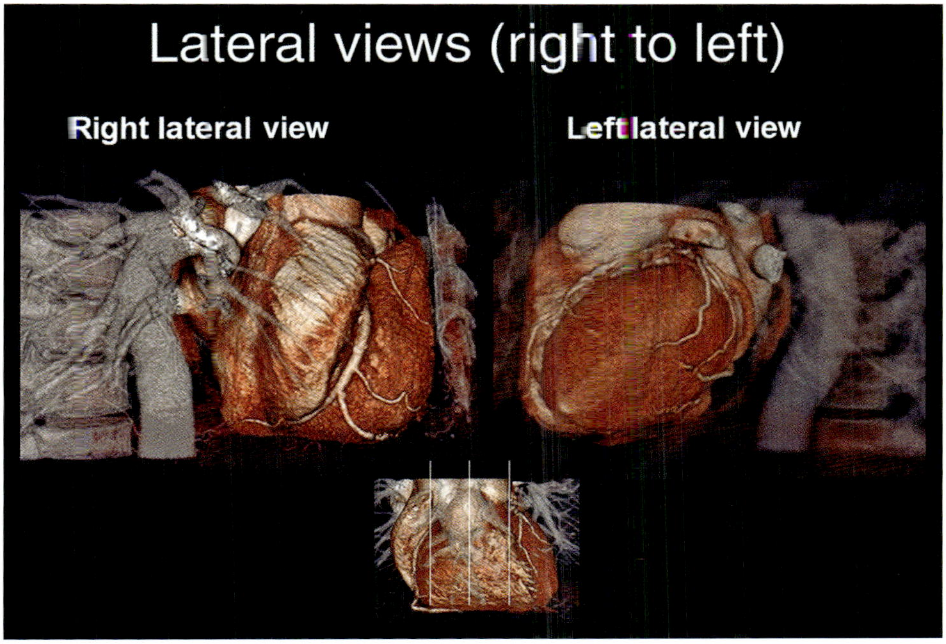

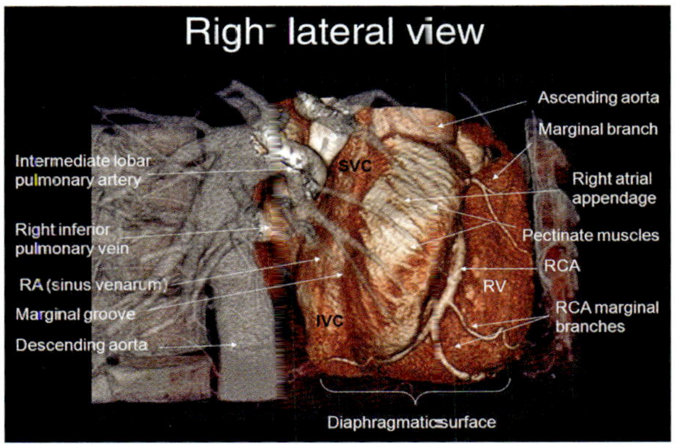

Sagittal 1

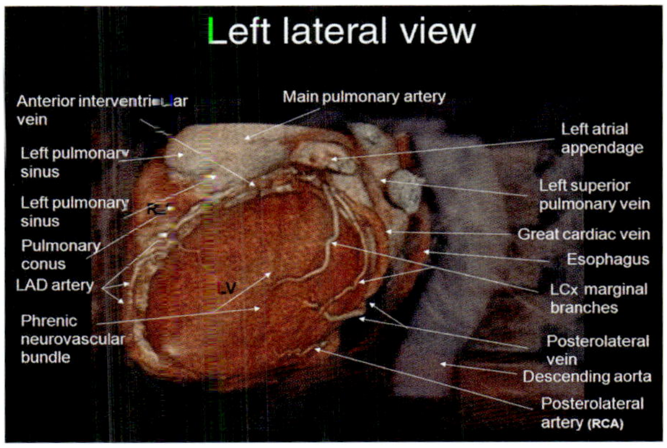

Sagittal 2

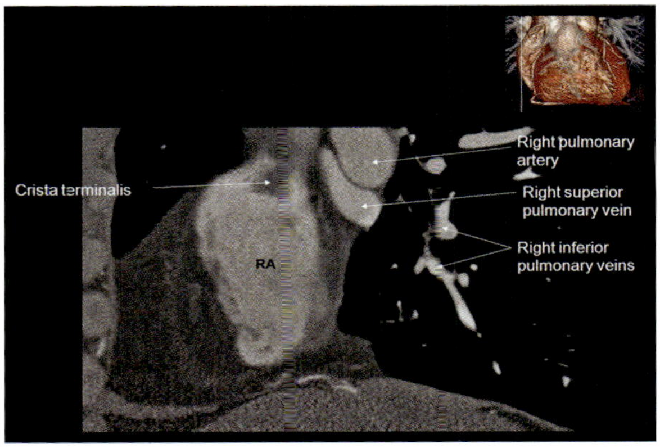

Sagittal 3

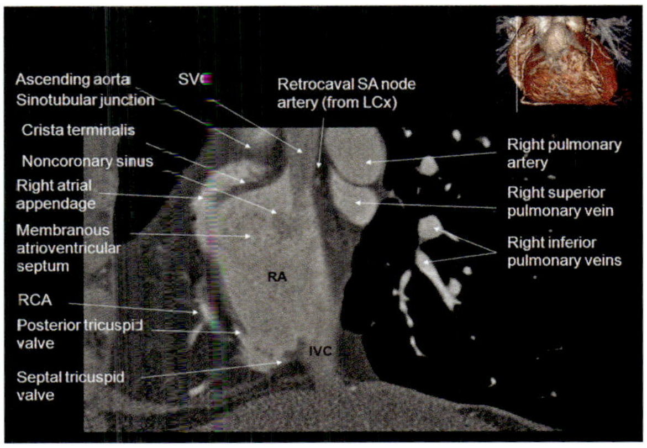

Sagittal 4

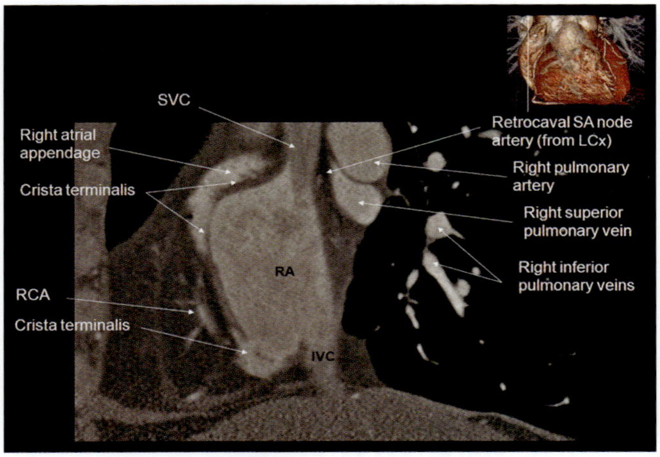

Sagittal 5

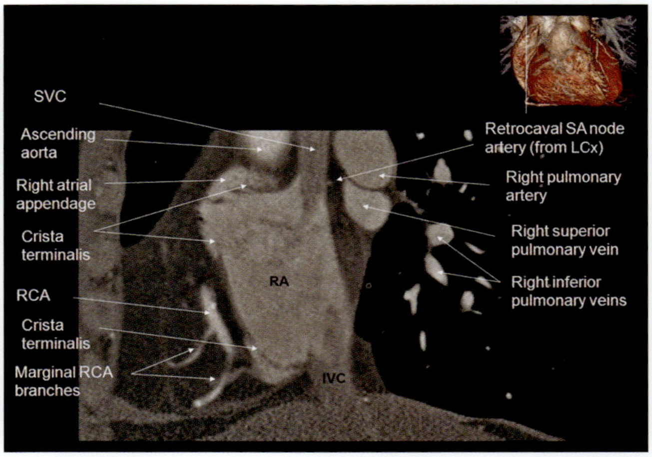

Sagittal 6

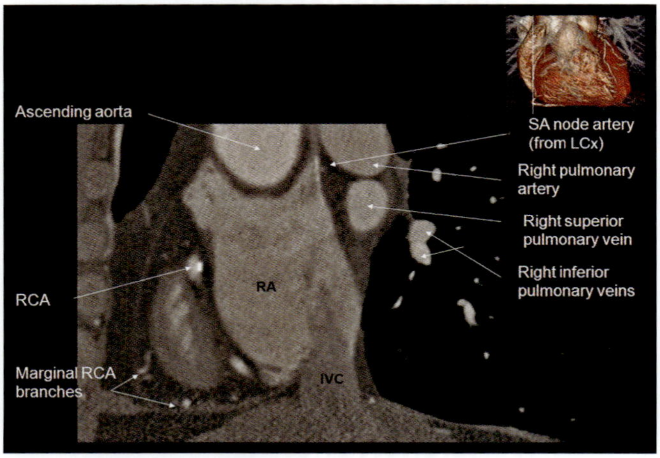

Sagittal 7

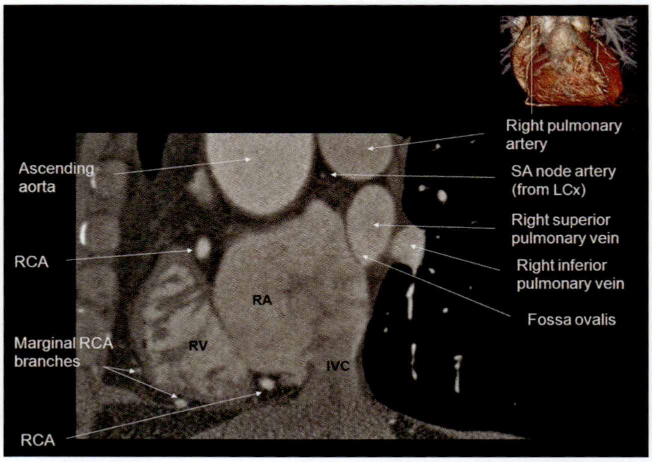

Sagittal 8

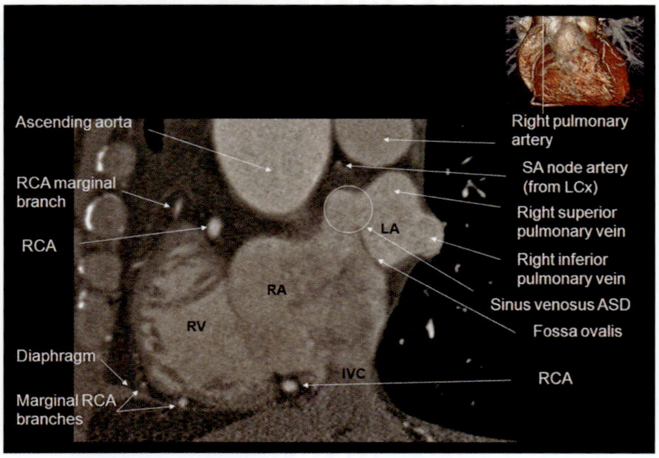

Sagittal 9

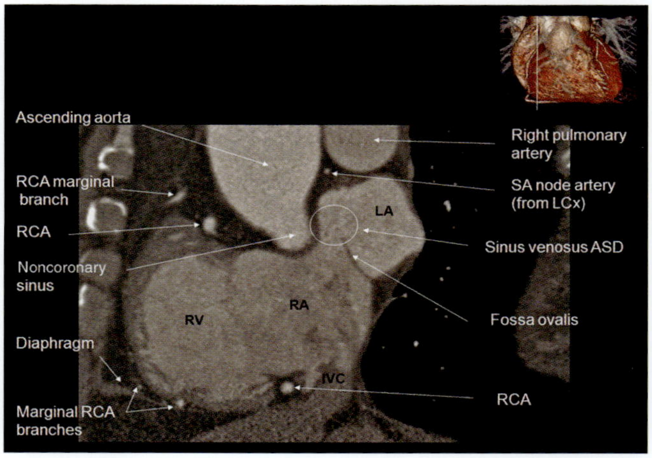

Sagittal 10

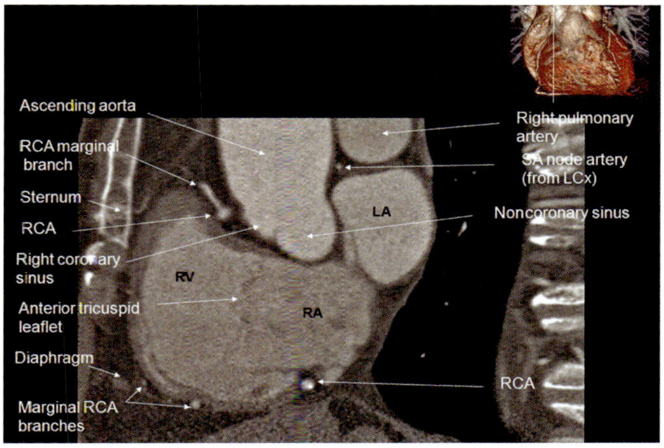

Sagittal 11

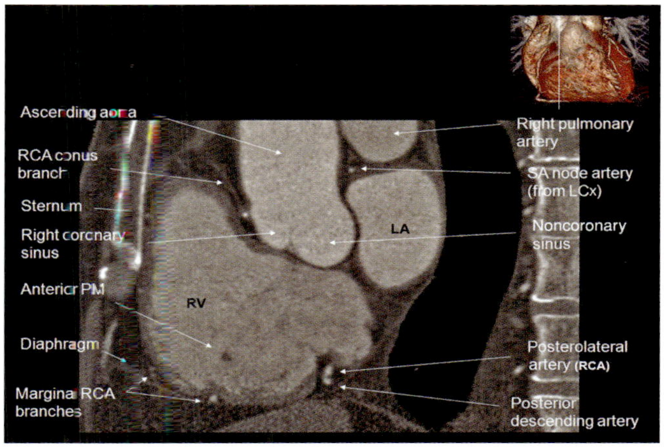

Sagittal 12

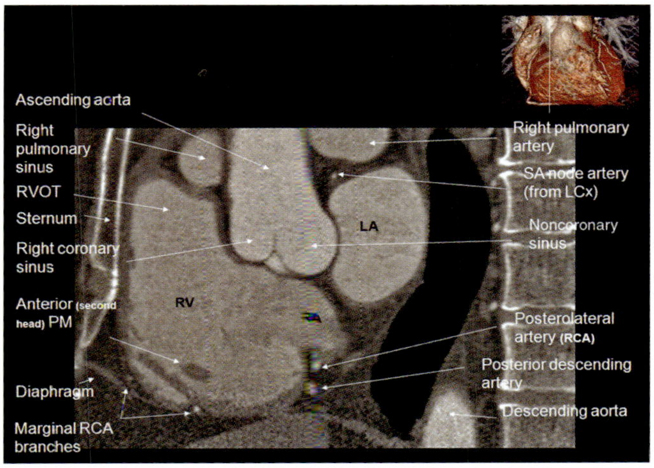

Sagittal 13

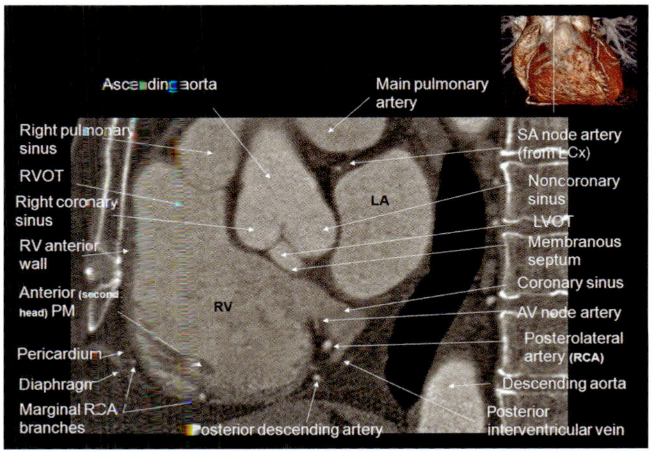

Sagittal 14

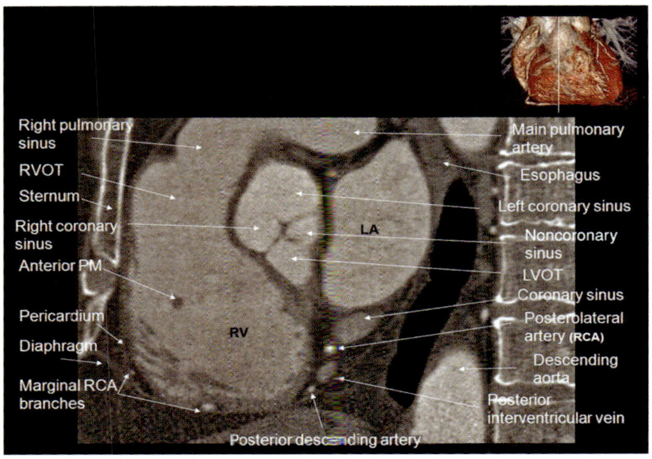

Sagittal 15

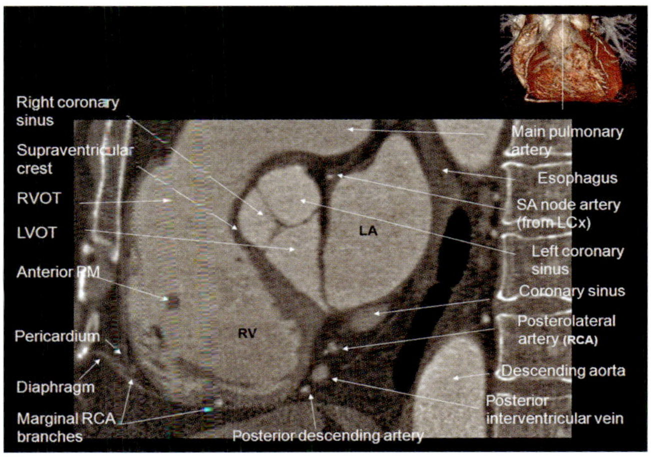

Sagittal 16

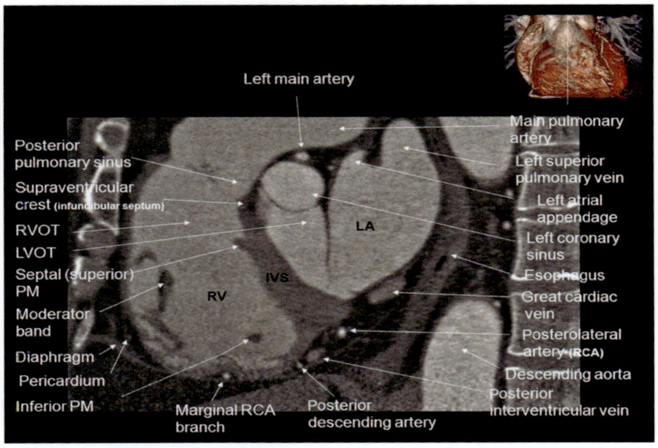

Sagittal 17

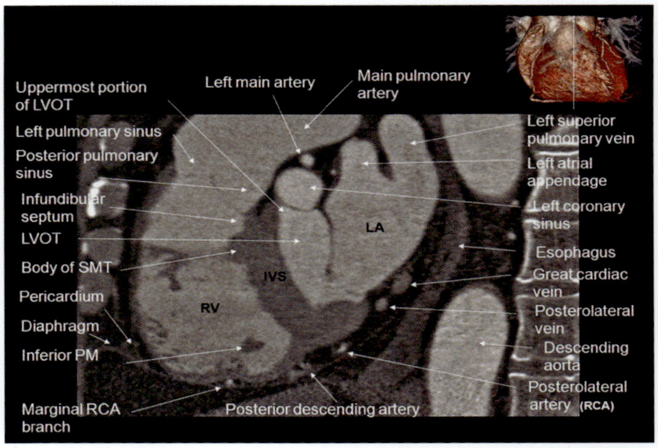

Sagittal 18

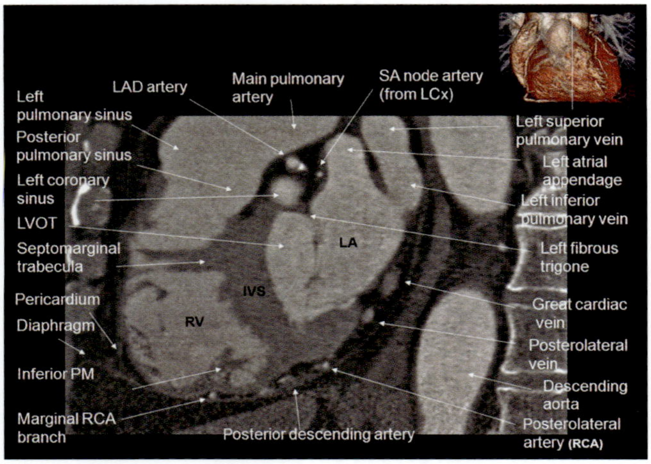

Sagittal 19

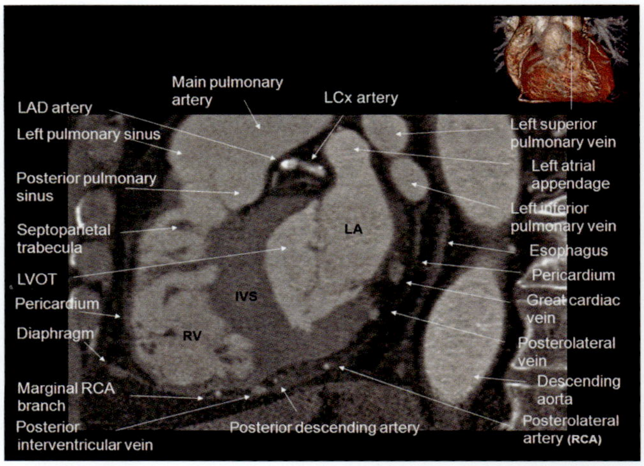

Sagittal 20

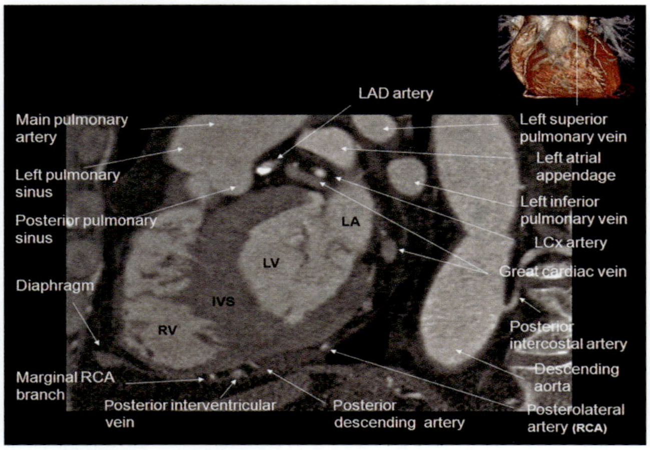

Sagittal 21

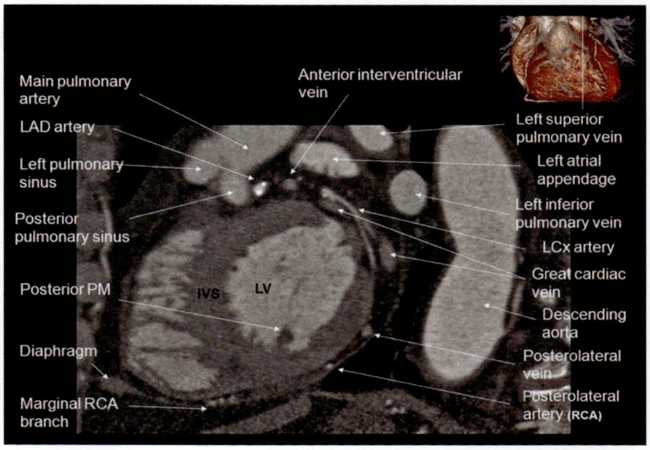

Sagittal 22

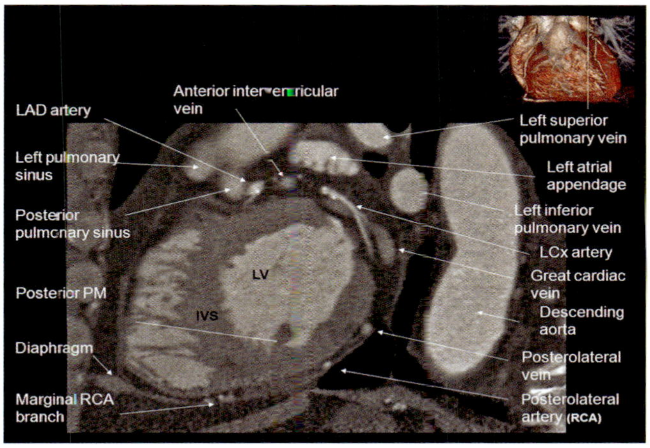

Sagittal 23

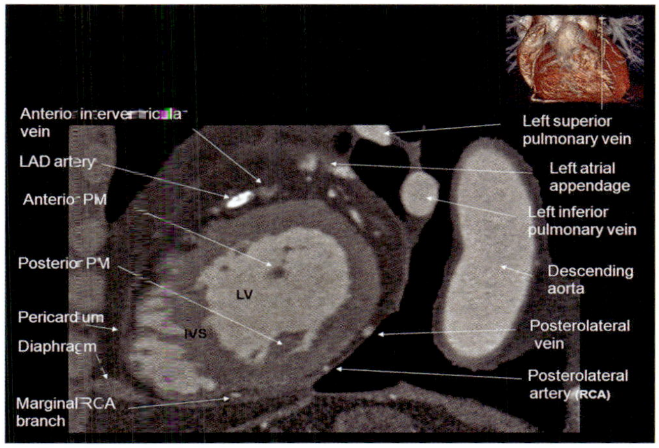

Sagittal 24

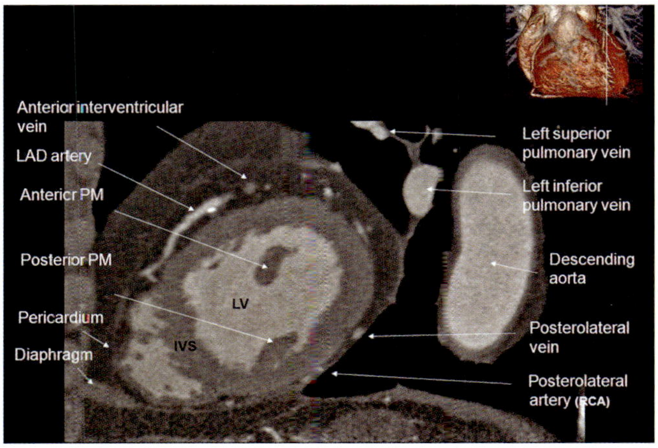

Sagittal 25

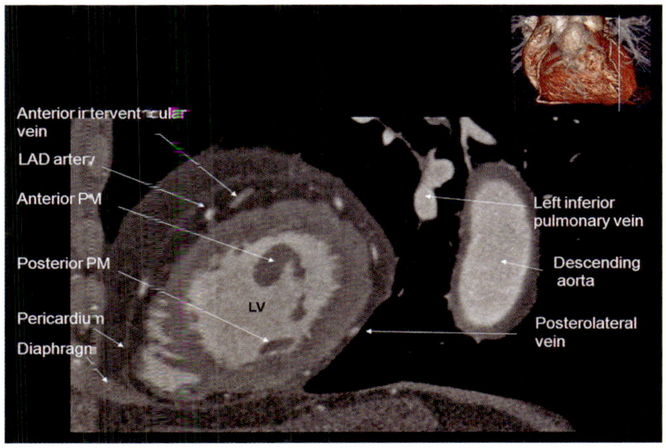

Sagittal 26

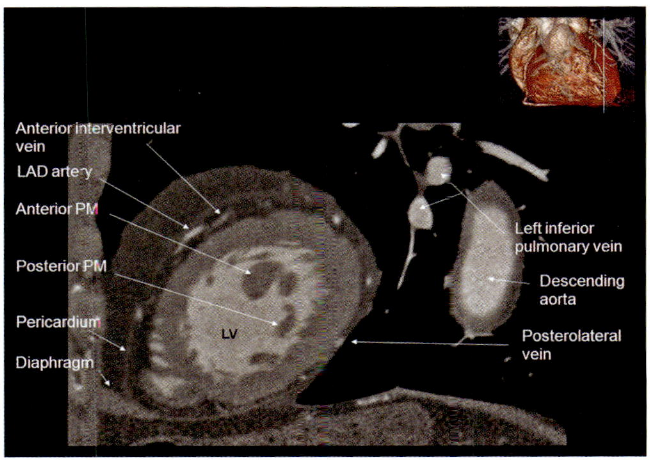

Sagittal 27

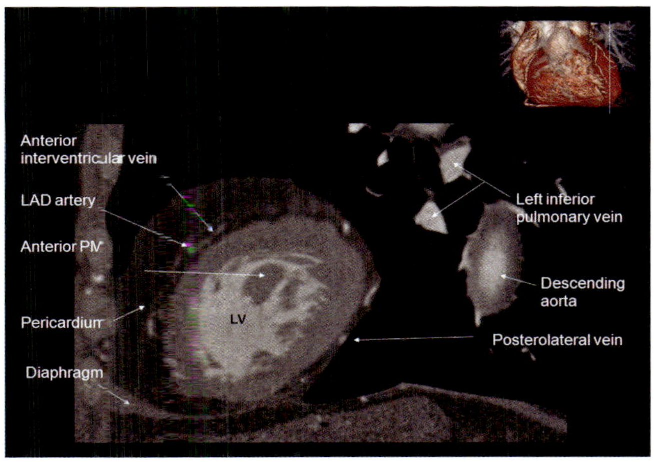

Sagittal 28

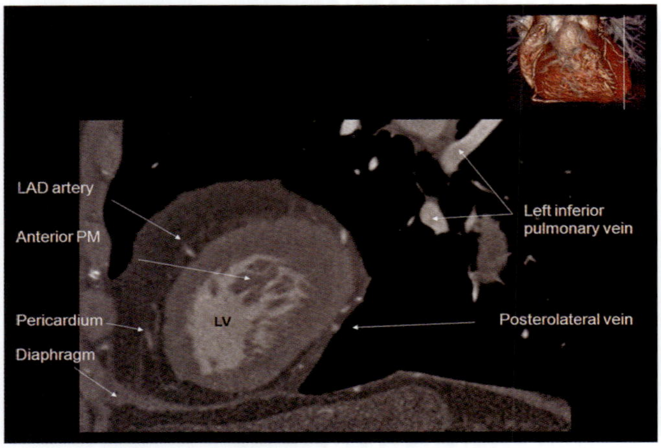

Sagittal 29

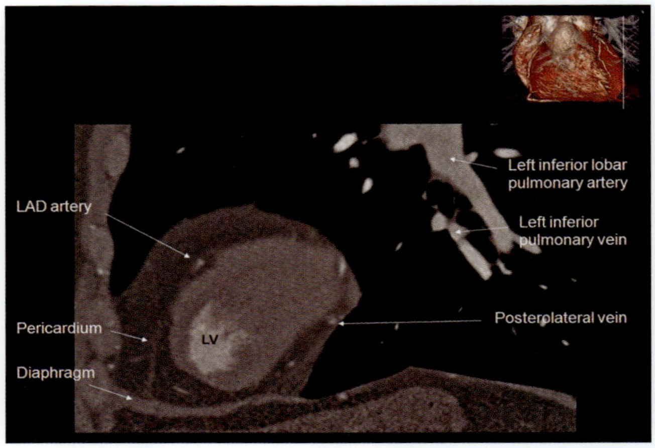

Sagittal 30

Heart planes: short axis, two chamber, four chamber

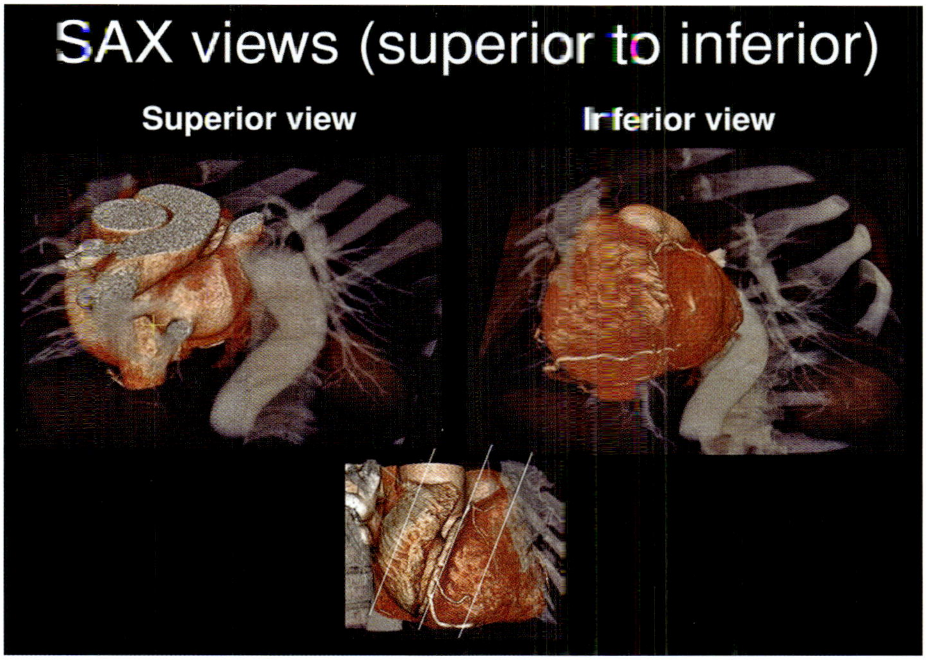

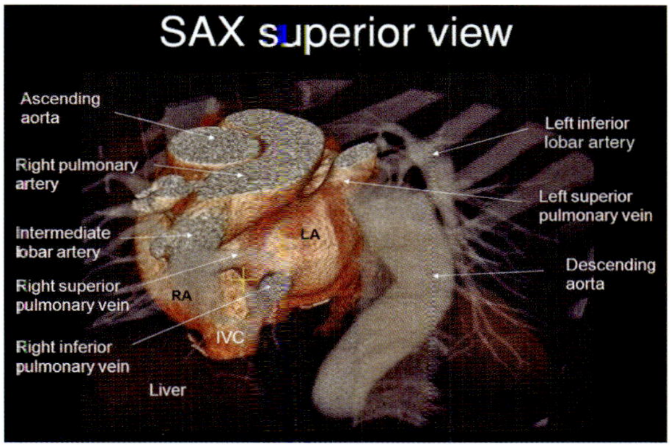

Short axis 1

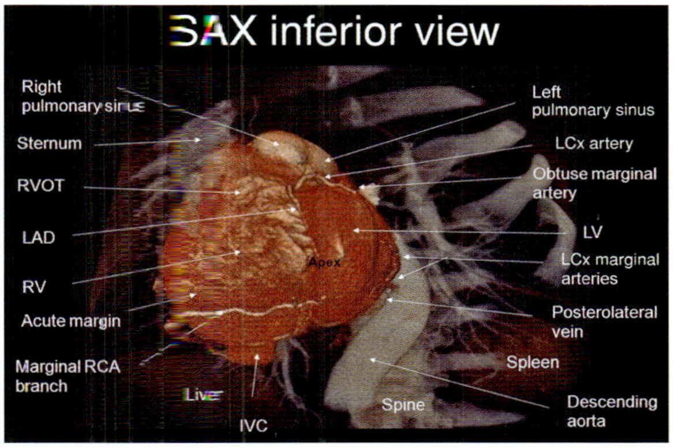

Short axis 2

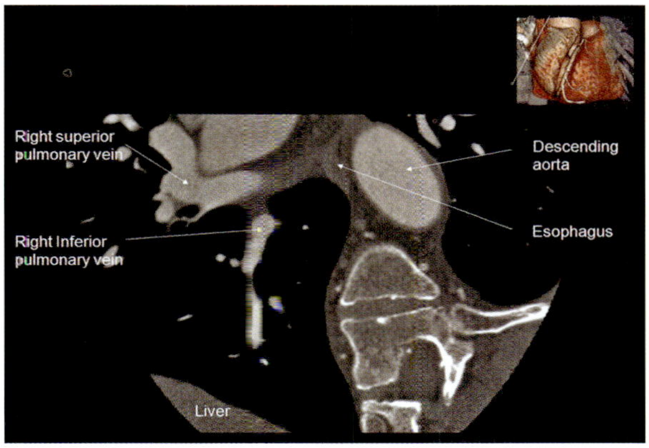

Short axis 3

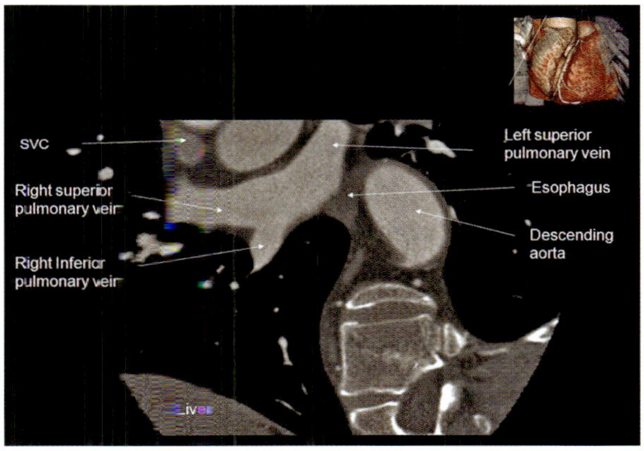

Short axis 4

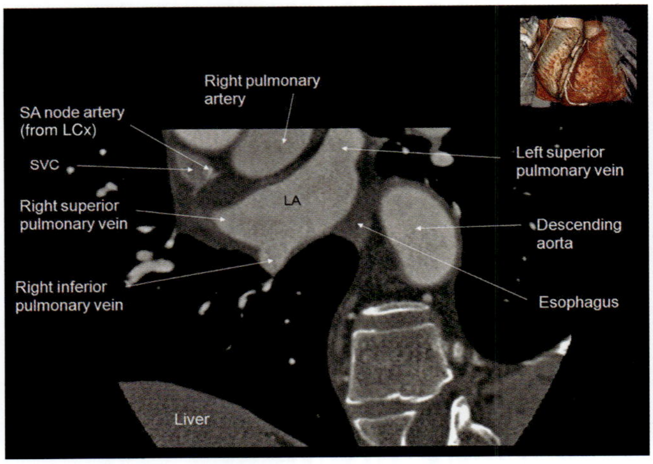

Short axis 5

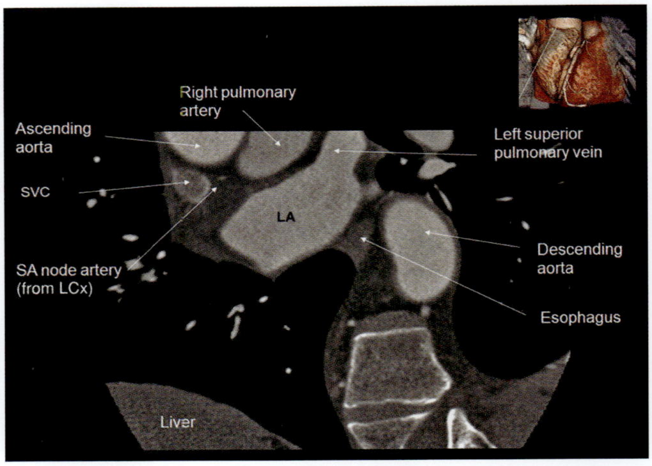

Short axis 6

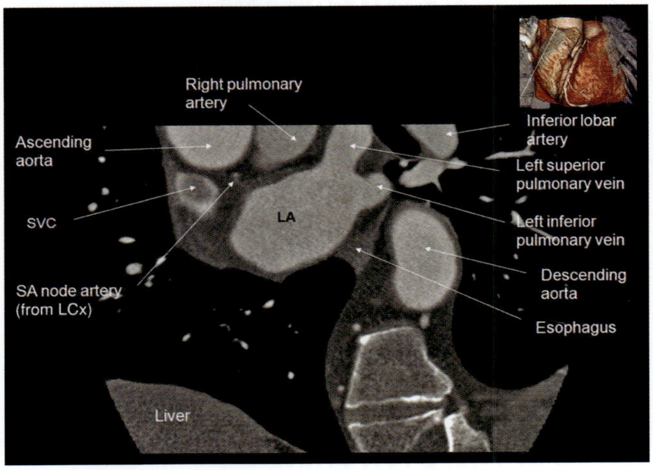

Short axis 7

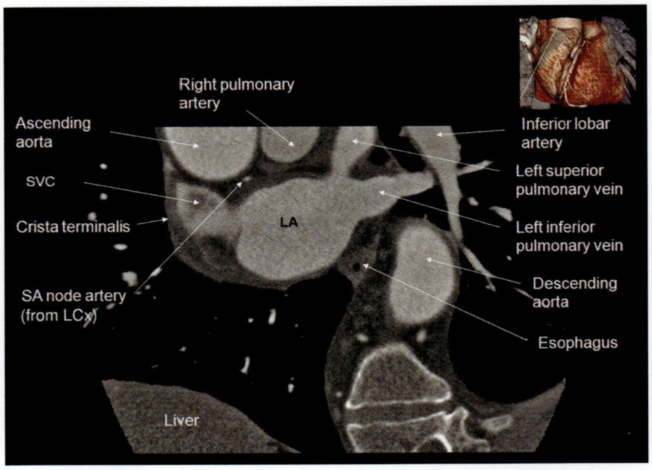

Short axis 8

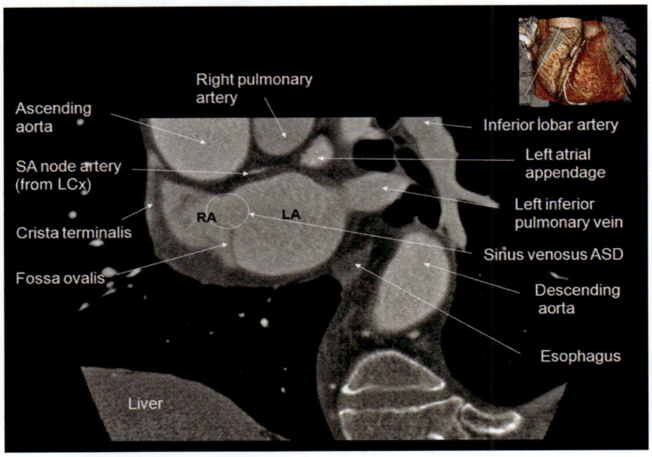

Short axis 9

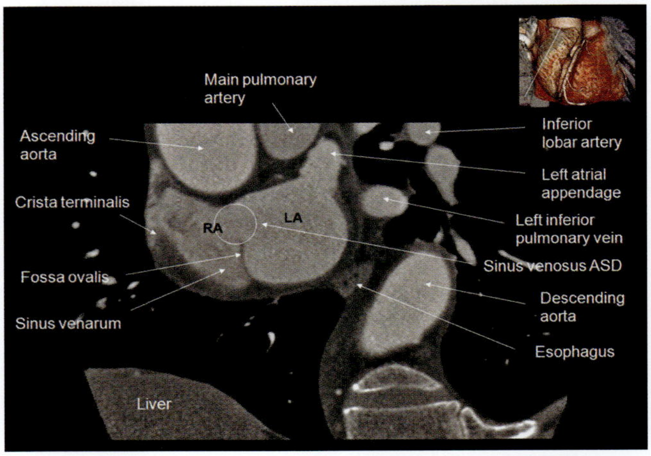

Short axis 10

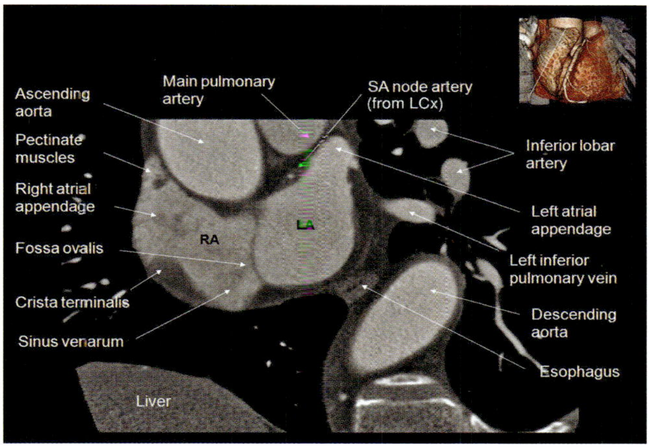

Short axis 11

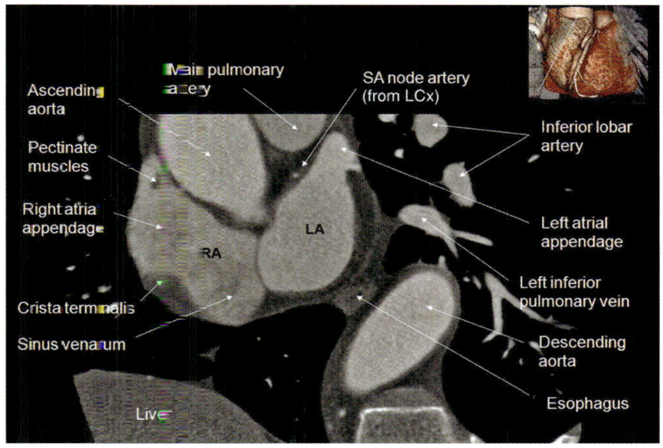

Short axis 12

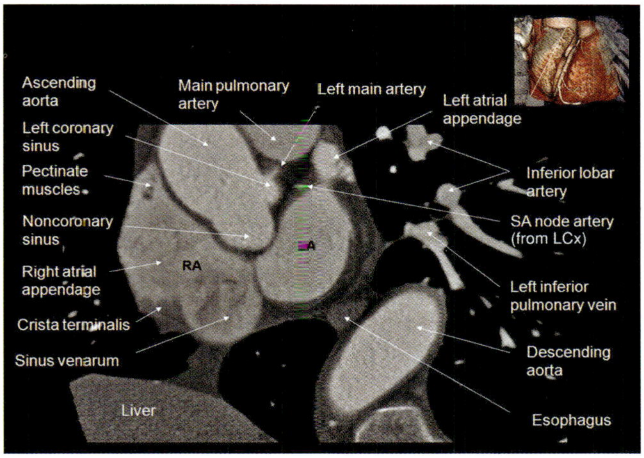

Short axis 13

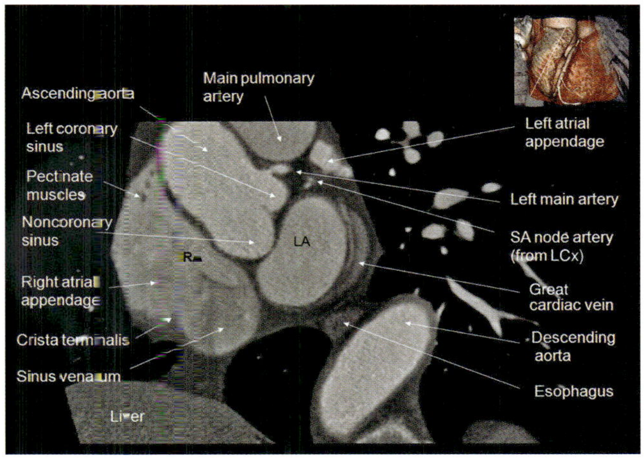

Short axis 14

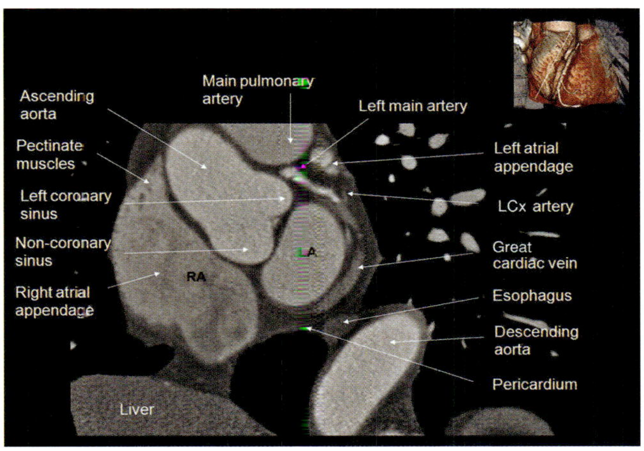

Short axis 15

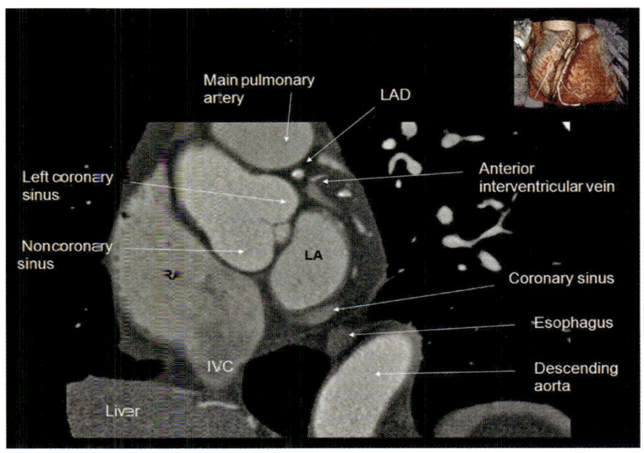

Short axis 16

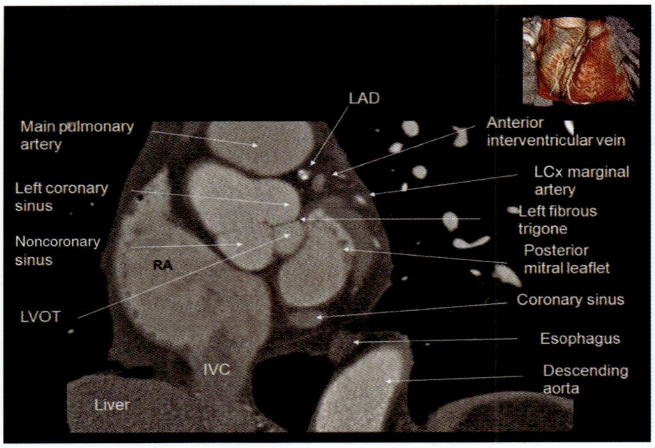

Short axis 17

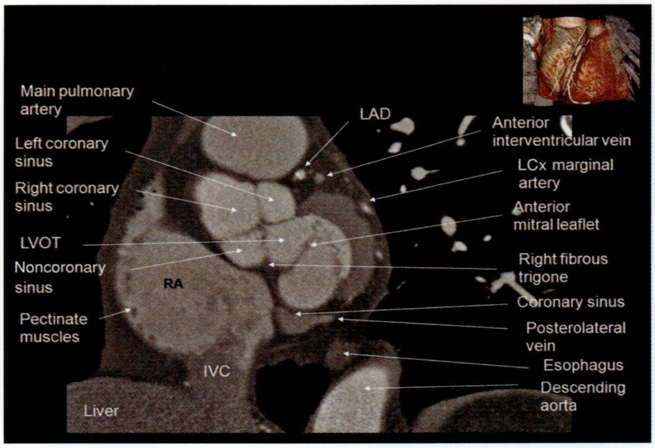

Short axis 18

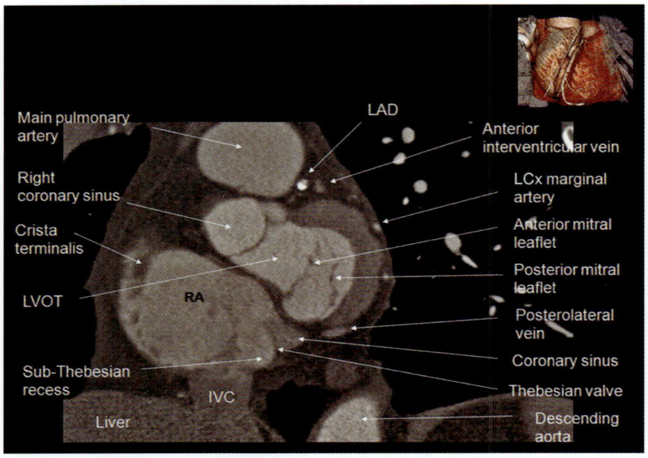

Short axis 19

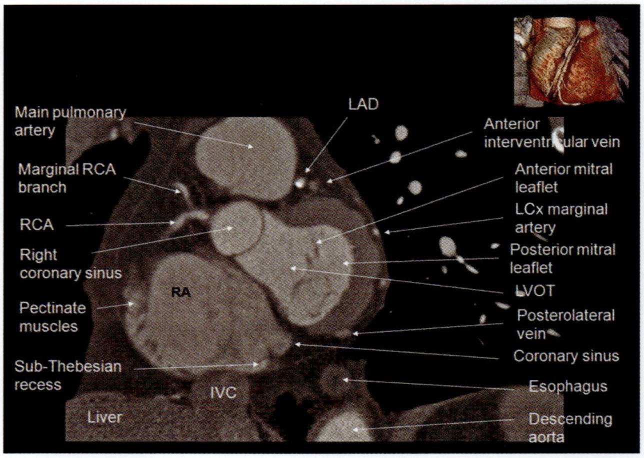

Short axis 20

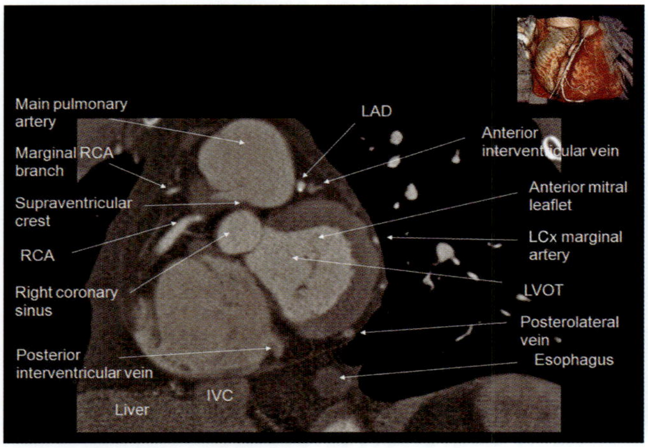

Short axis 21

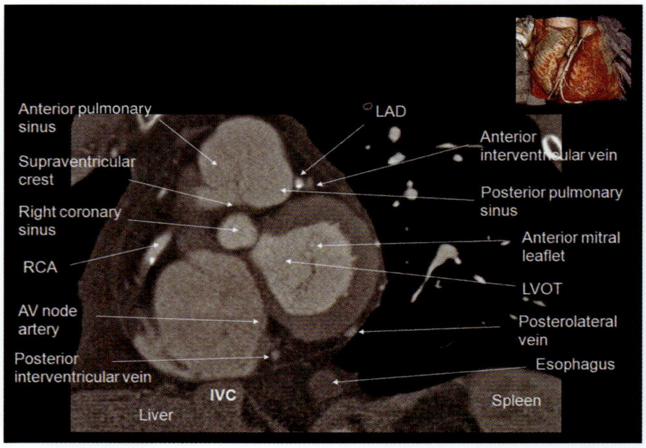

Short axis 22

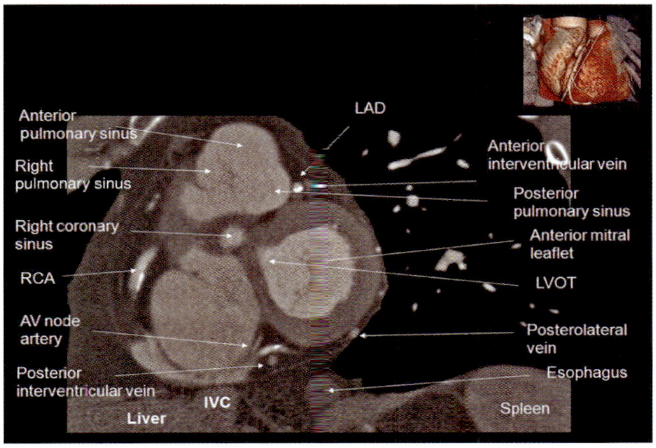

Short axis 23

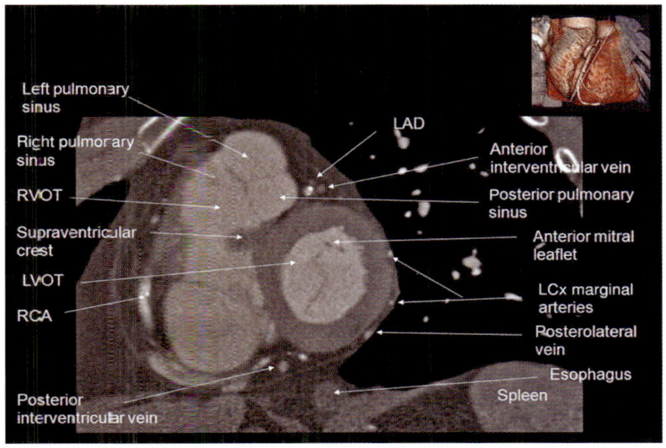

Short axis 24

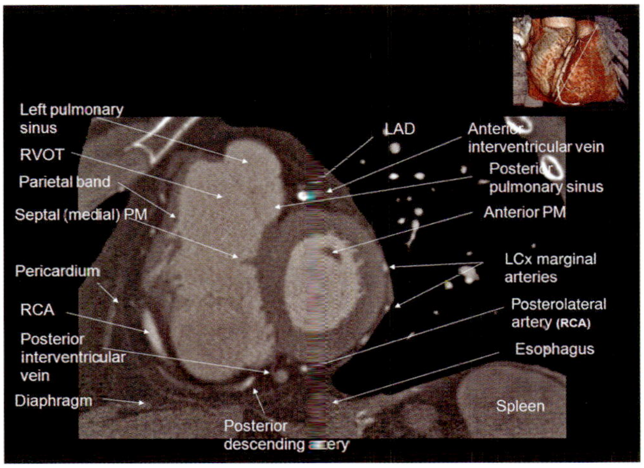

Short axis 25

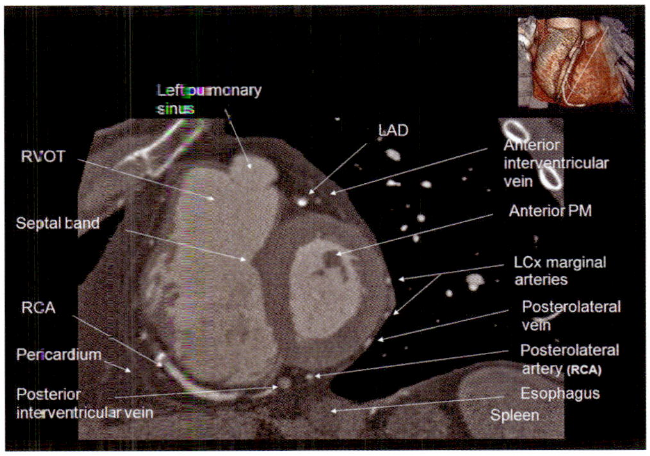

Short axis 26

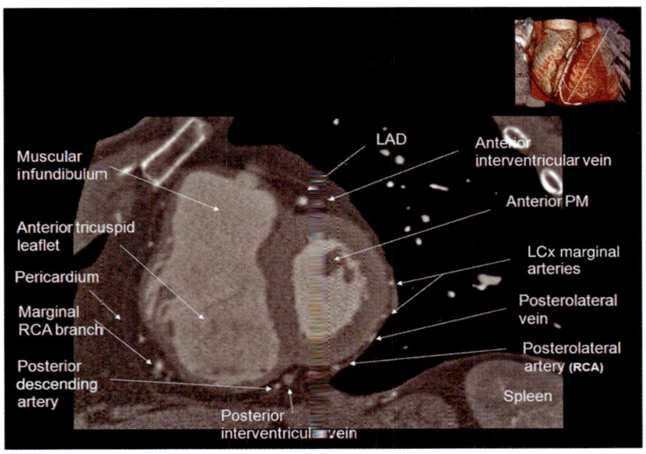

Short axis 27

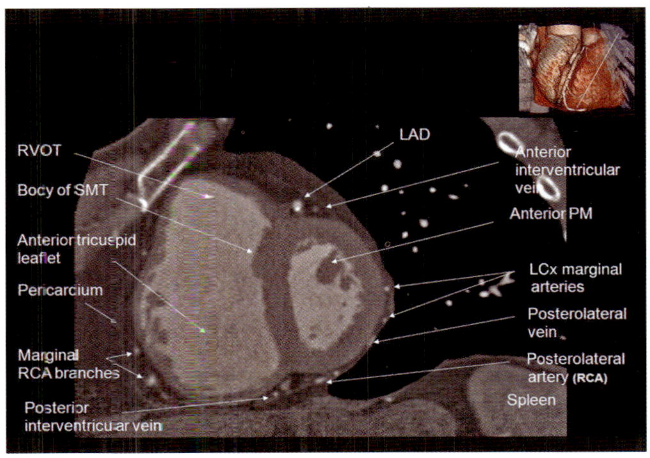

Short axis 28

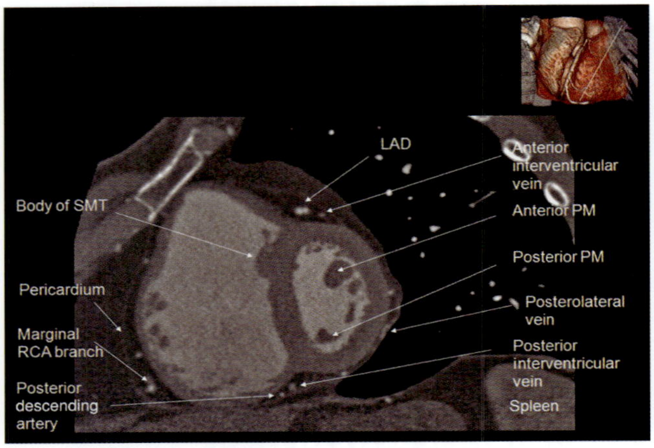

Short axis 29

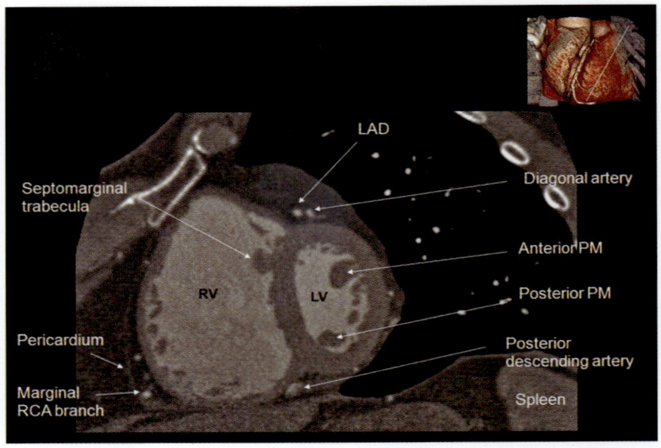

Short axis 30

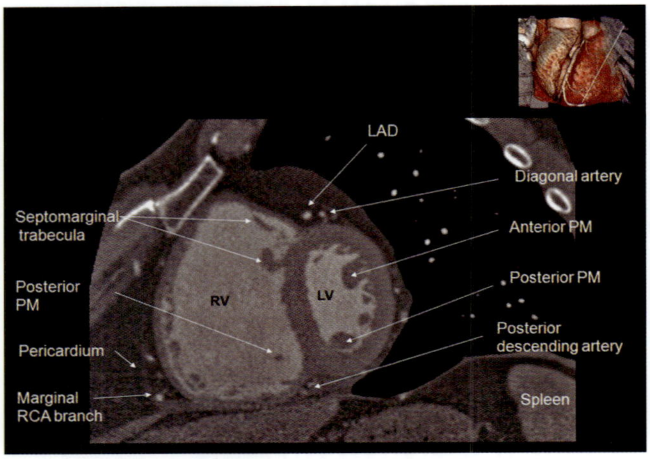

Short axis 31

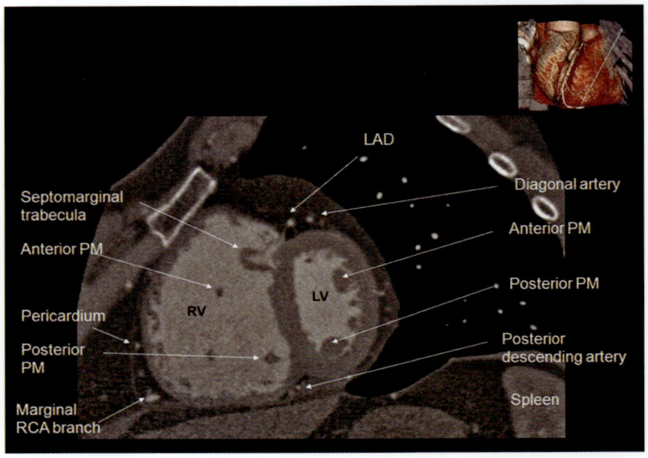

Short axis 32

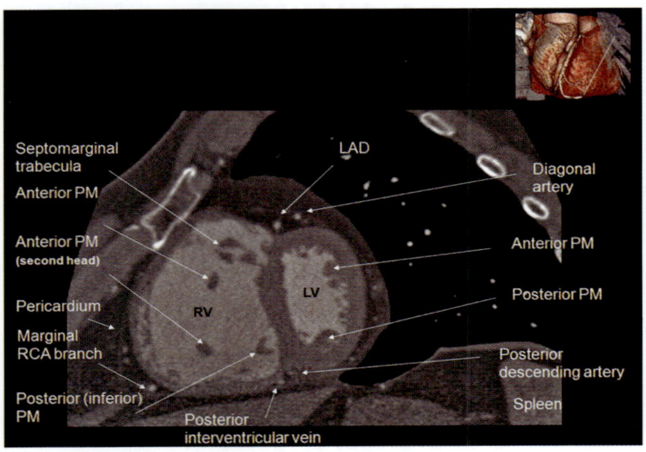

Short axis 33

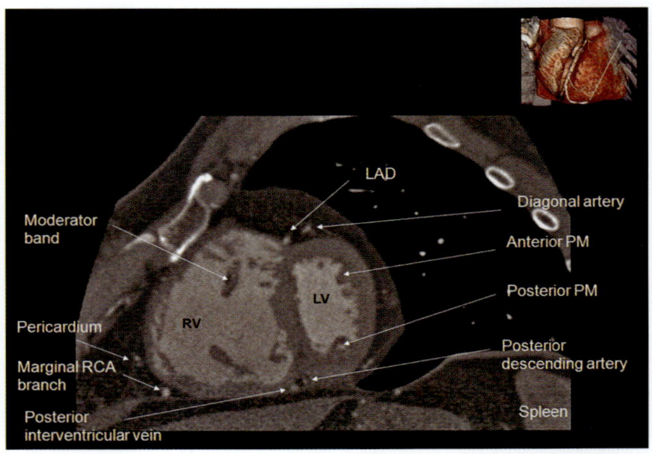

Short axis 34

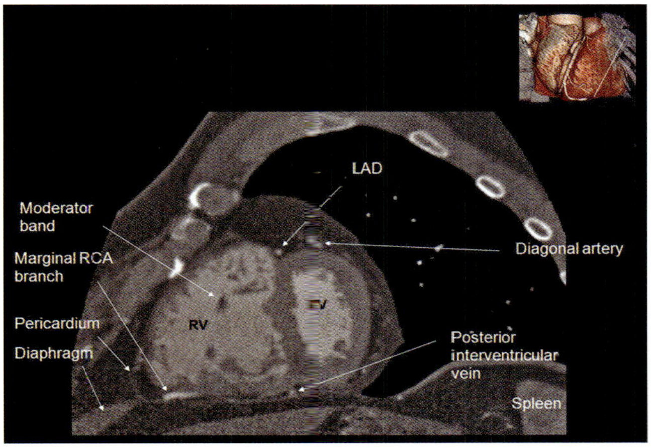

Short axis 35

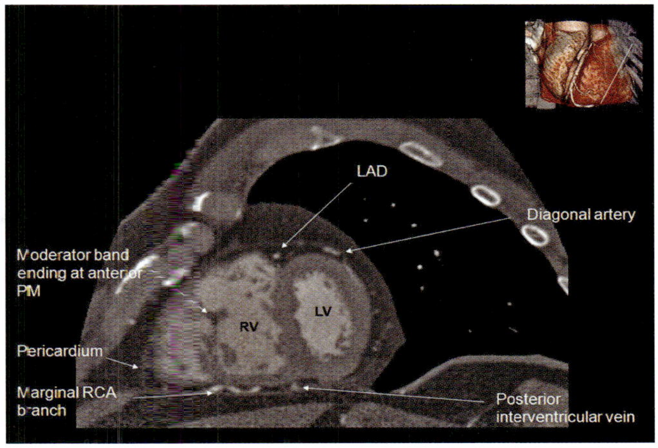

Short axis 36

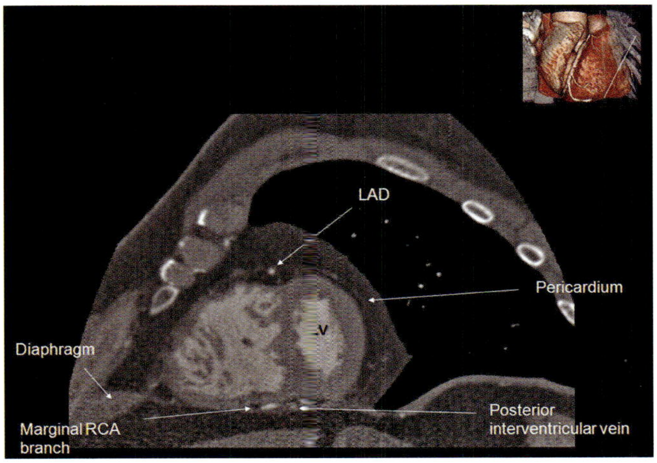

Short axis 37

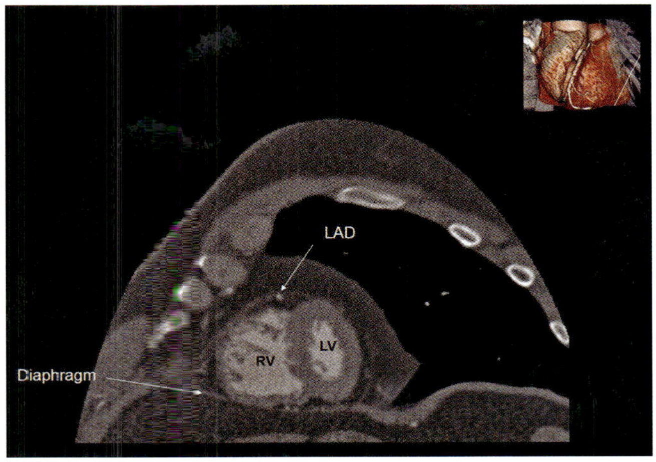

Short axis 38

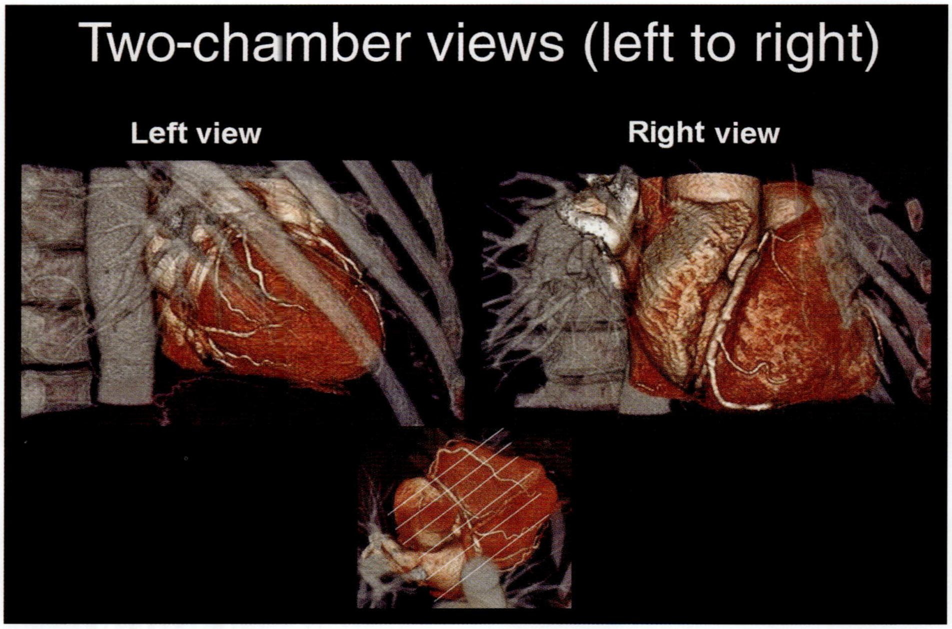

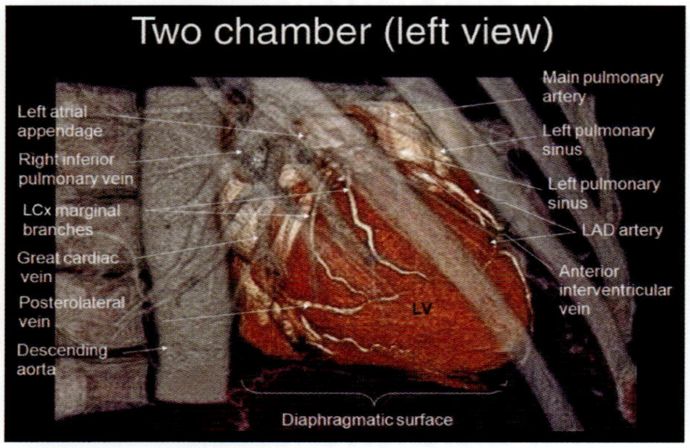

Two chamber 1

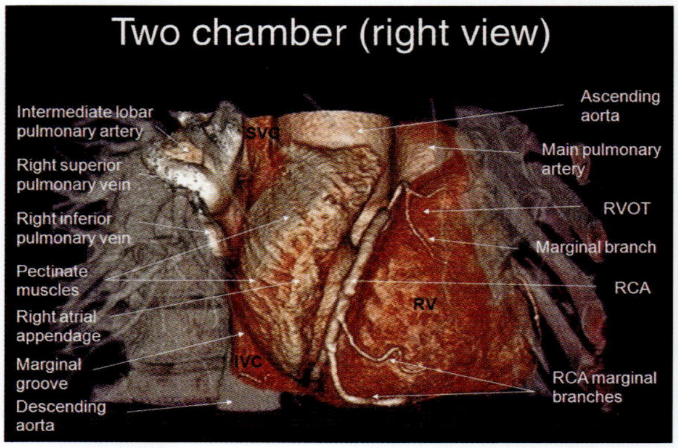

Two chamber 2

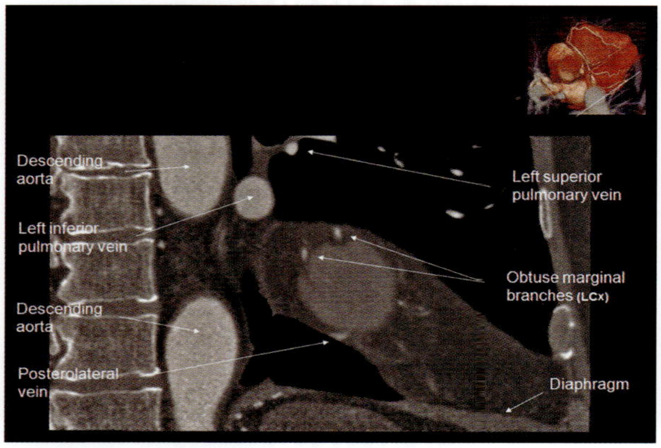

Two chamber 3

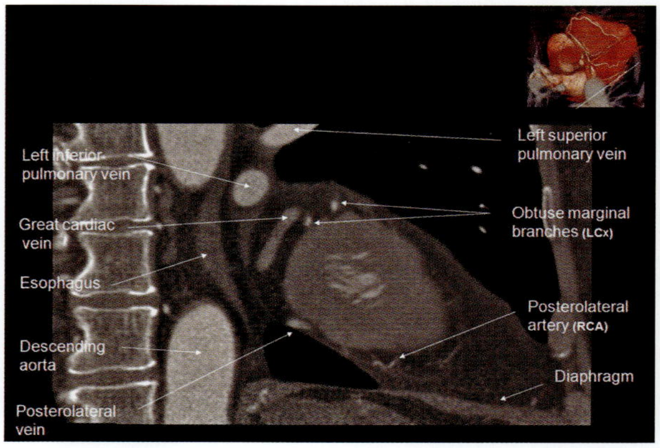

Two chamber 4

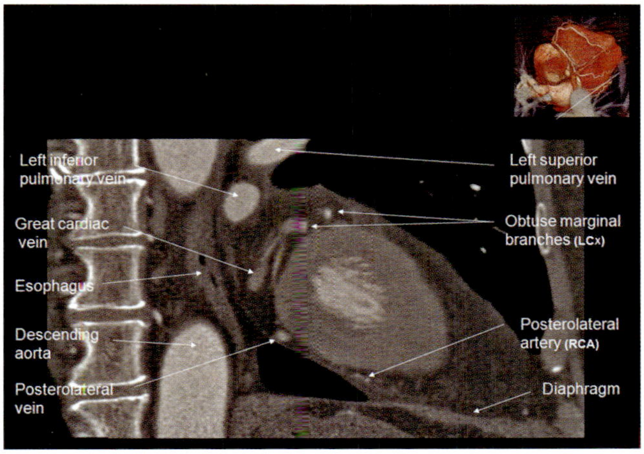

Two chamber 5

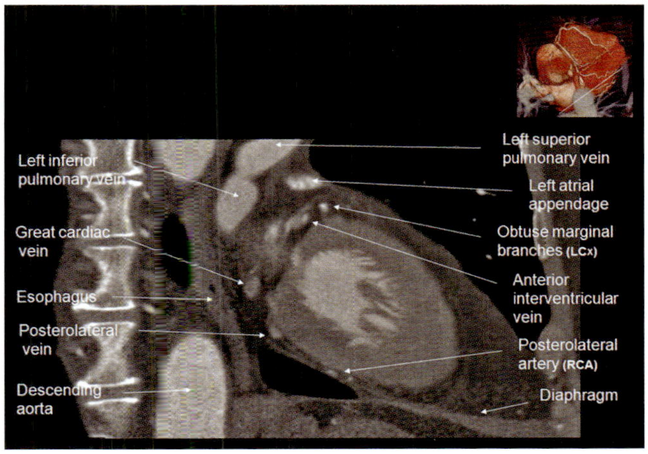

Two chamber 6

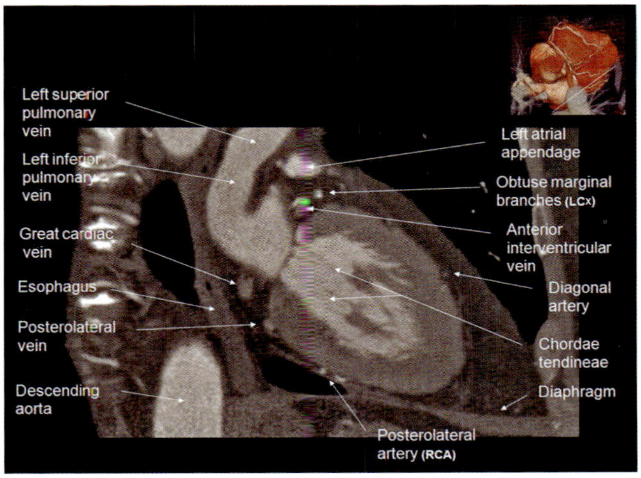

Two chamber 7

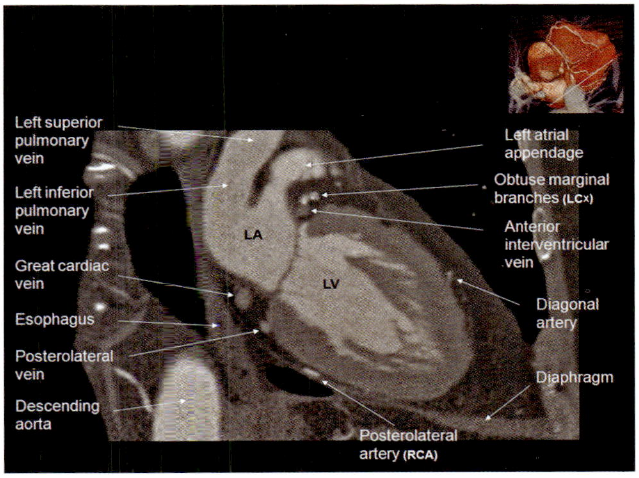

Two chamber 8

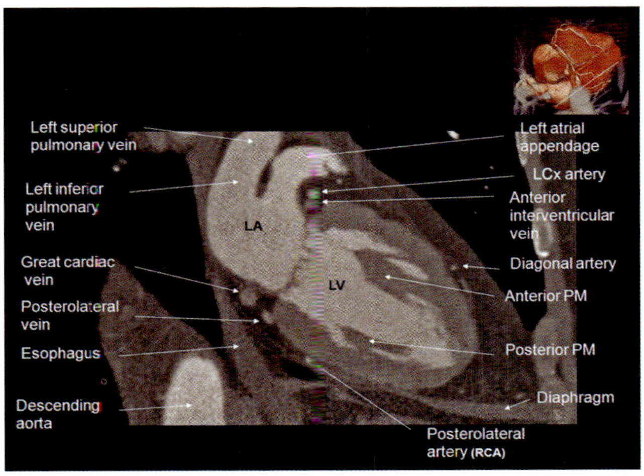

Two chamber 9

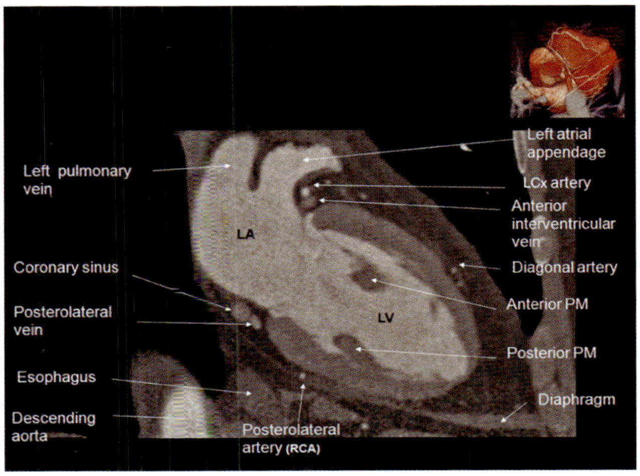

Two chamber 10

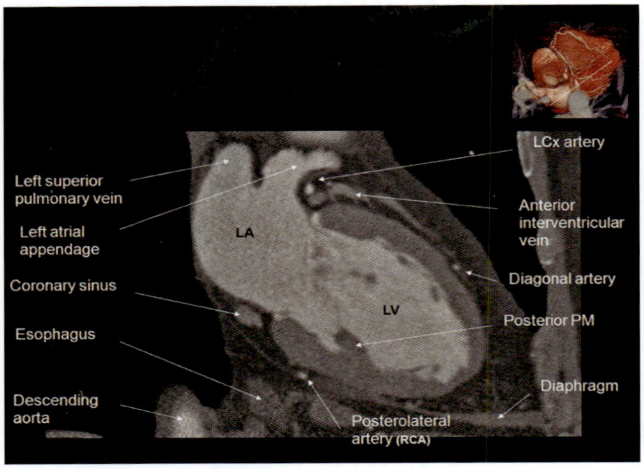

Two chamber 11

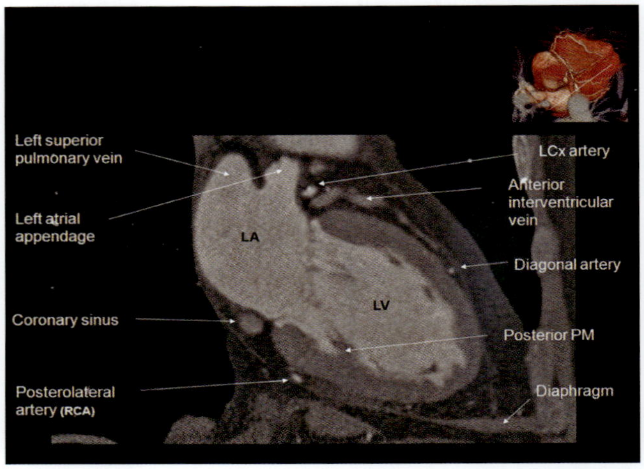

Two chamber 12

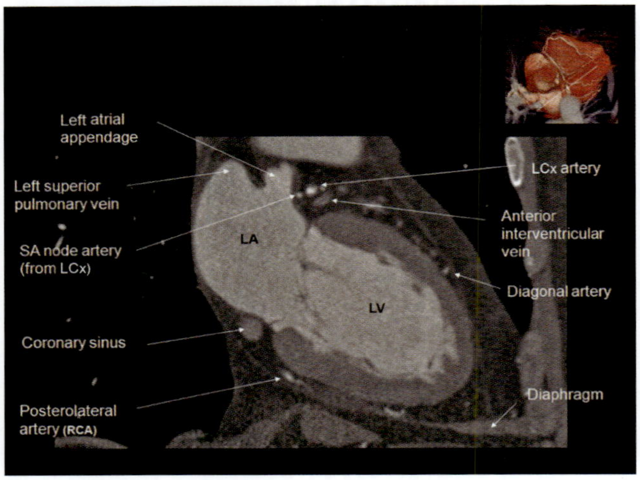

Two chamber 13

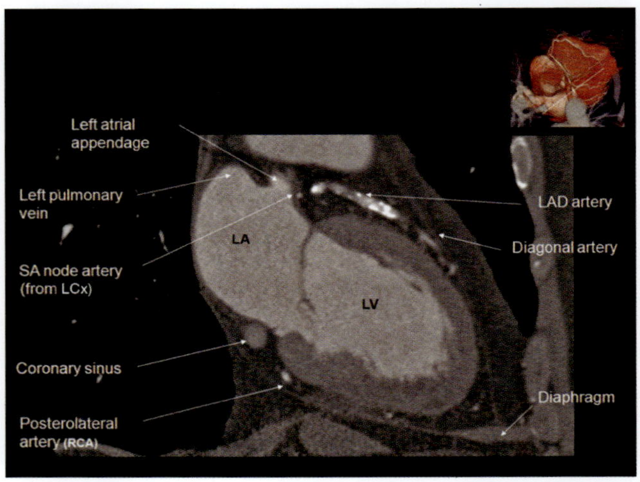

Two chamber 14

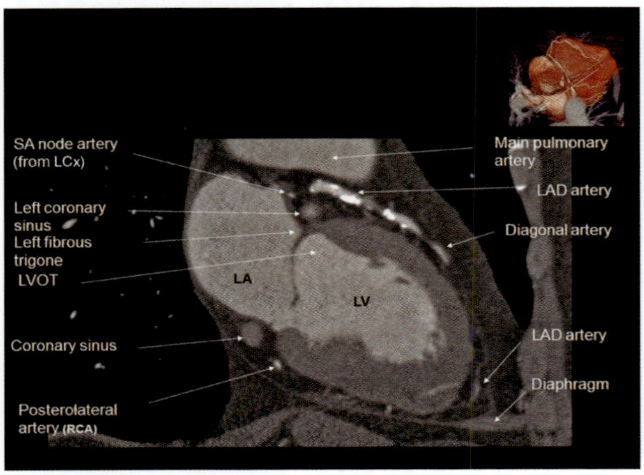

Two chamber 15

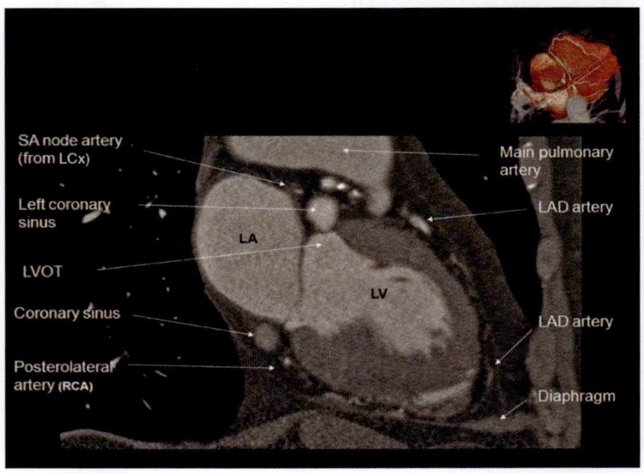

Two chamber 16

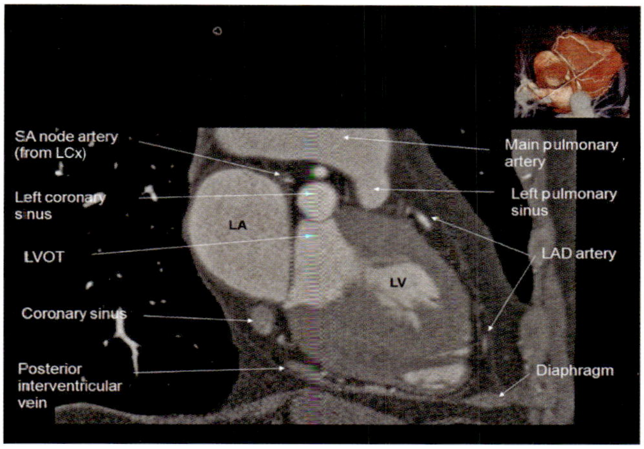

Two chamber 17

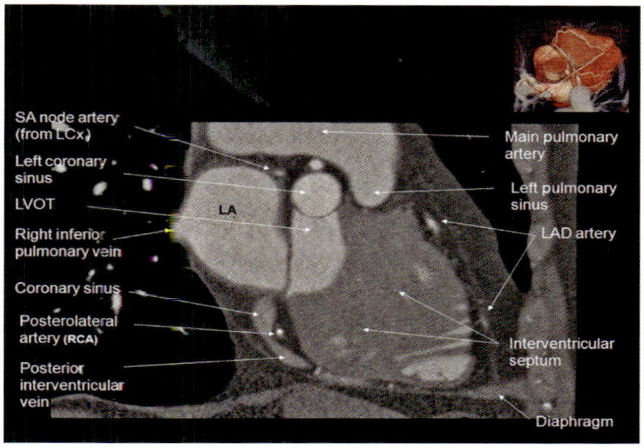

Two chamber 18

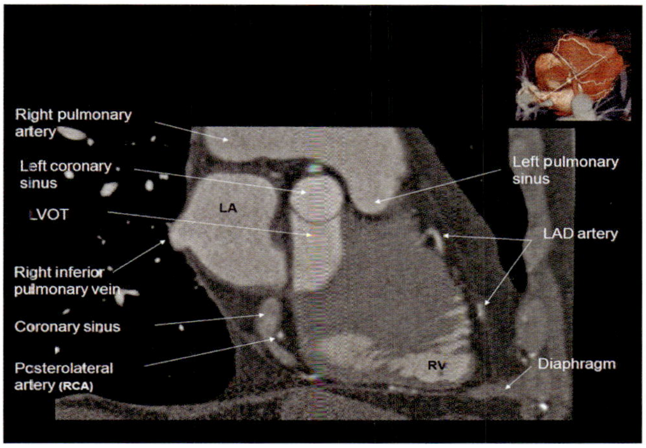

Two chamber 19

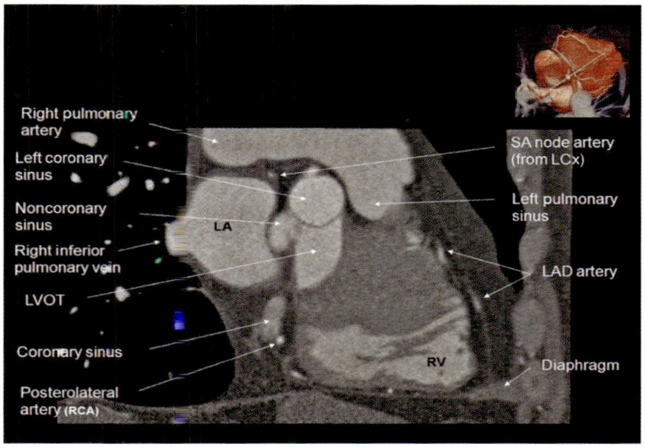

Two chamber 20

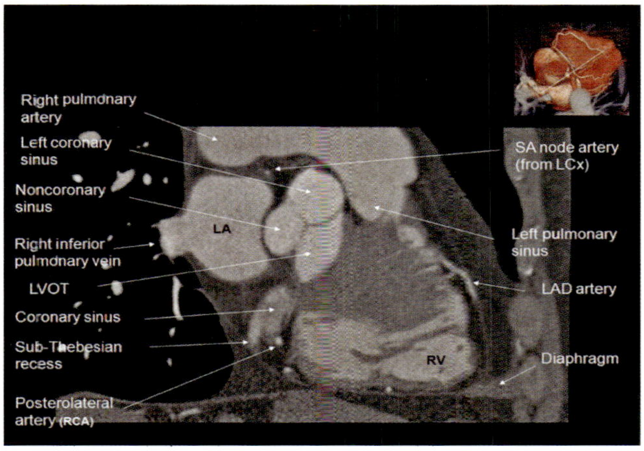

Two chamber 21

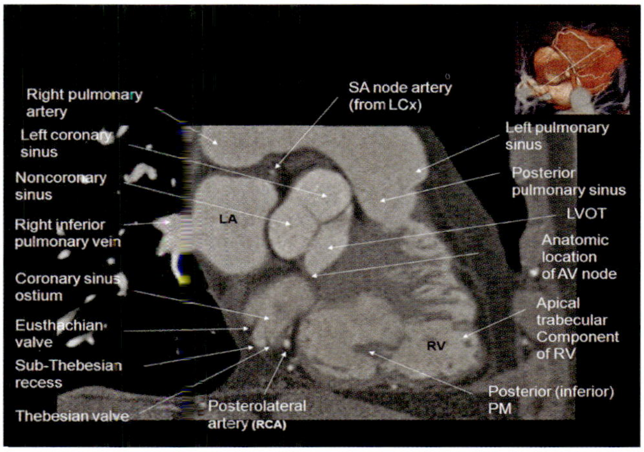

Two chamber 22

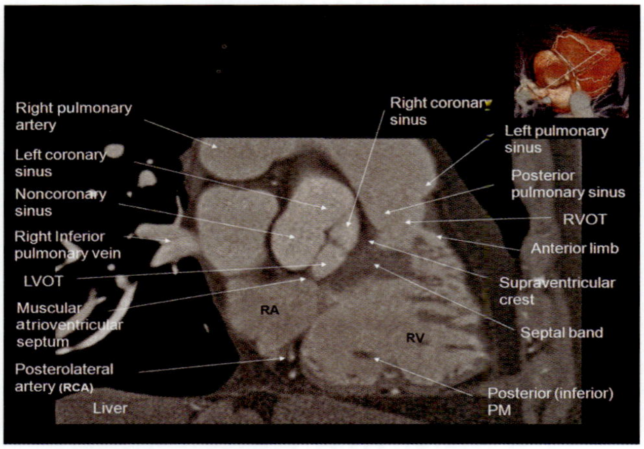

Two chamber 23

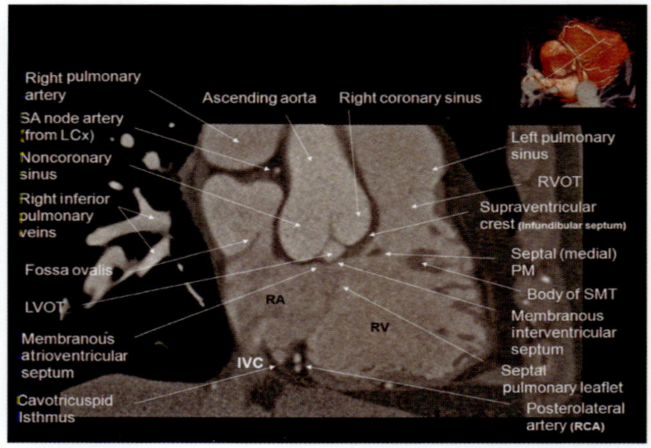

Two chamber 24

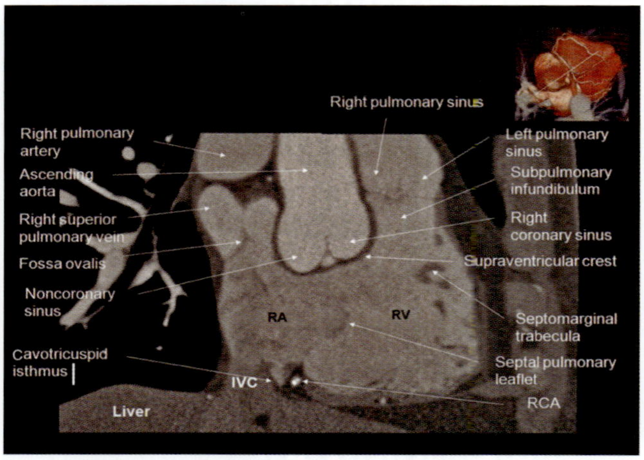

Two chamber 25

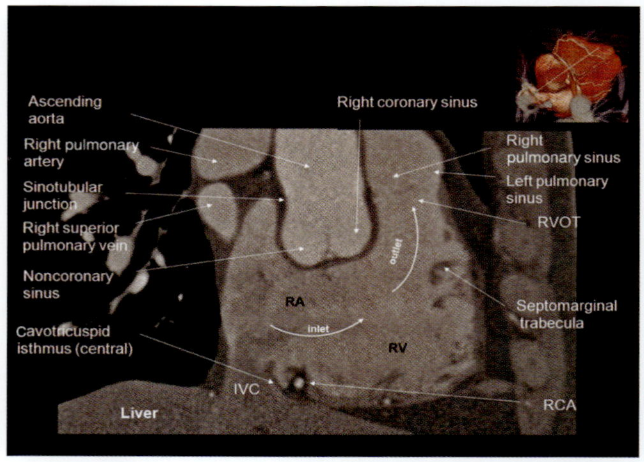

Two chamber 26

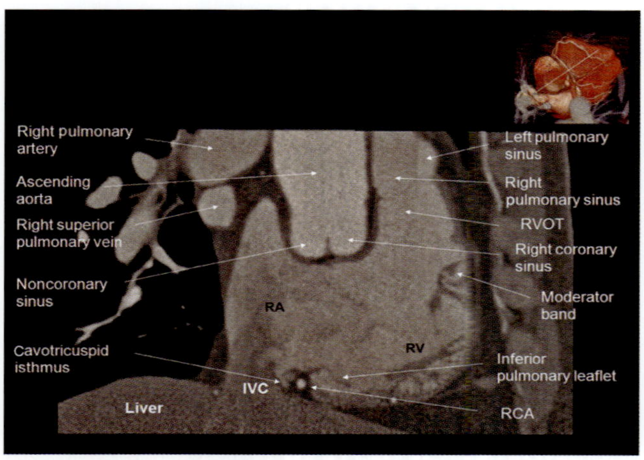

Two chamber 27

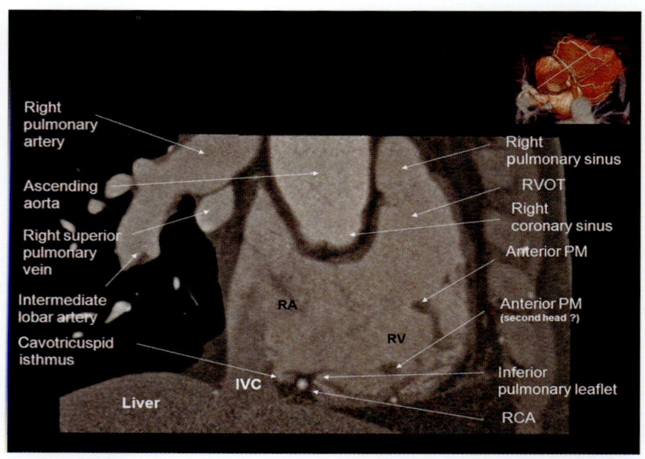

Two chamber 28

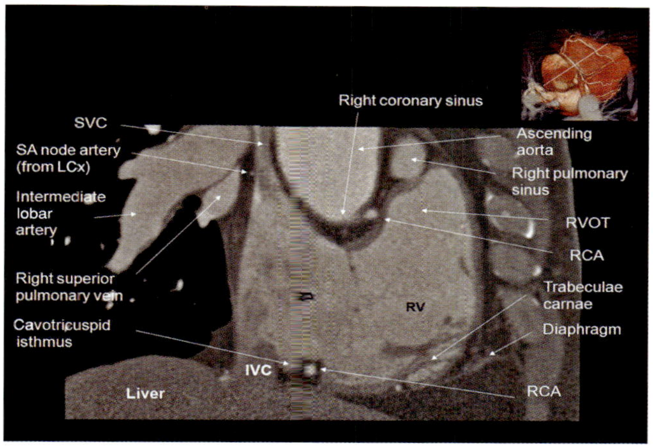

Two chamber 29

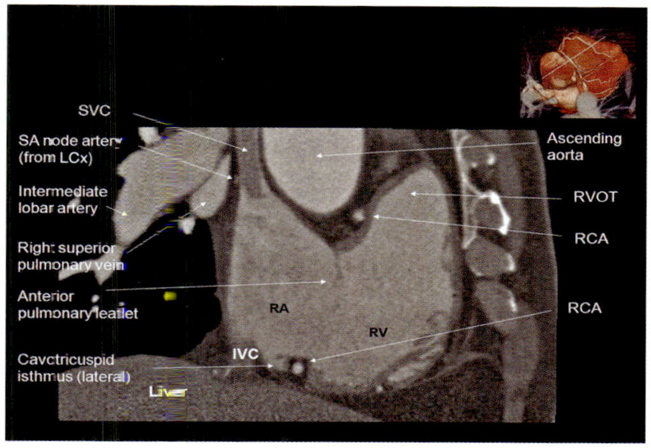

Two chamber 30

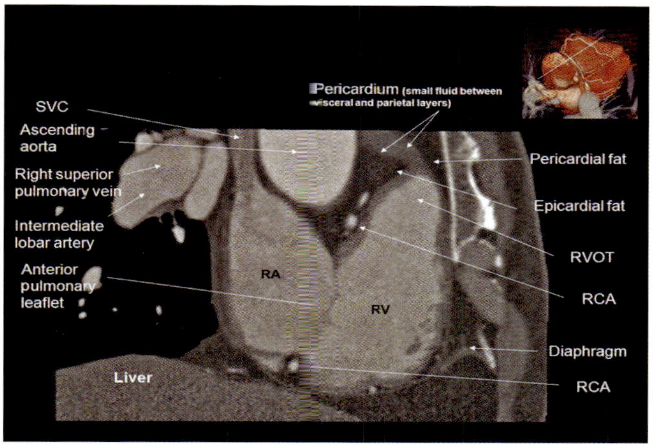

Two chamber 31

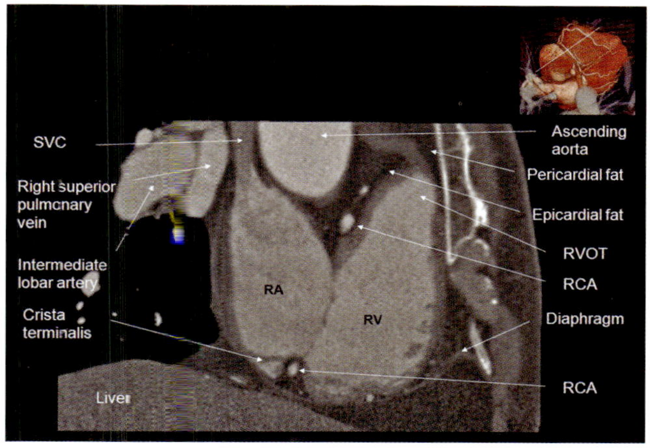

Two chamber 32

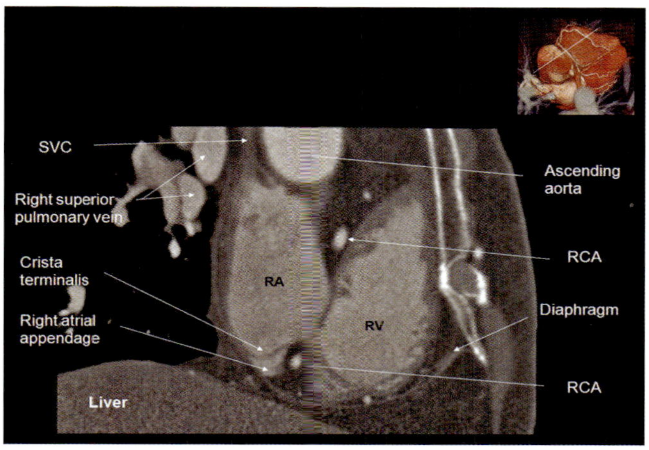

Two chamber 33

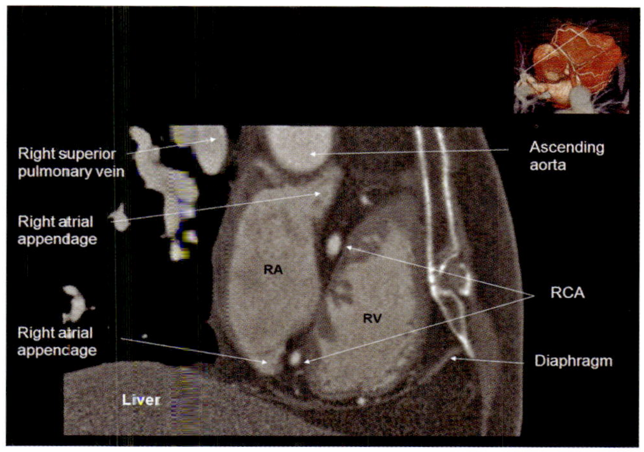

Two chamber 34

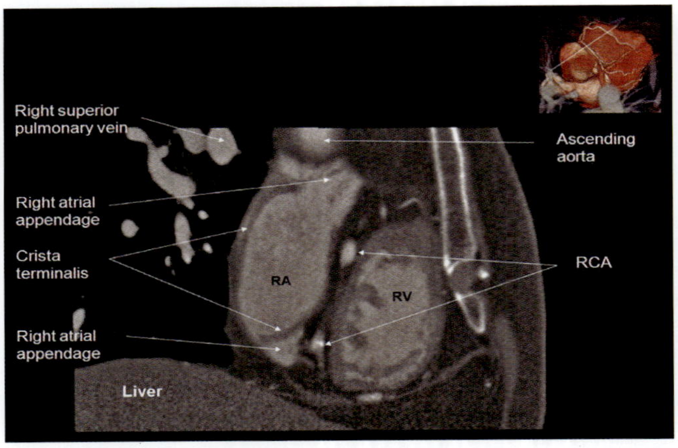

Two chamber 35

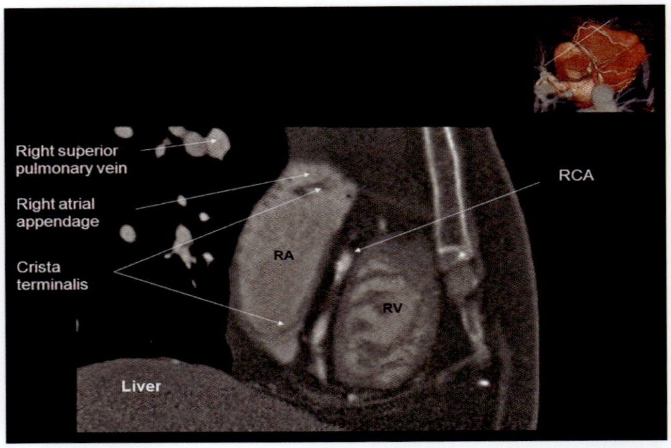

Two chamber 36

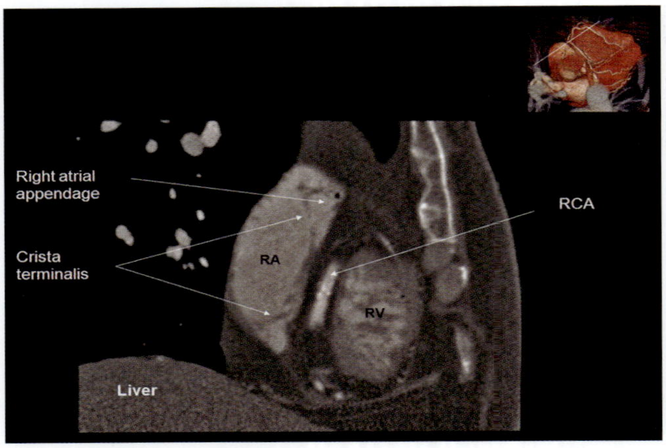

Two chamber 37

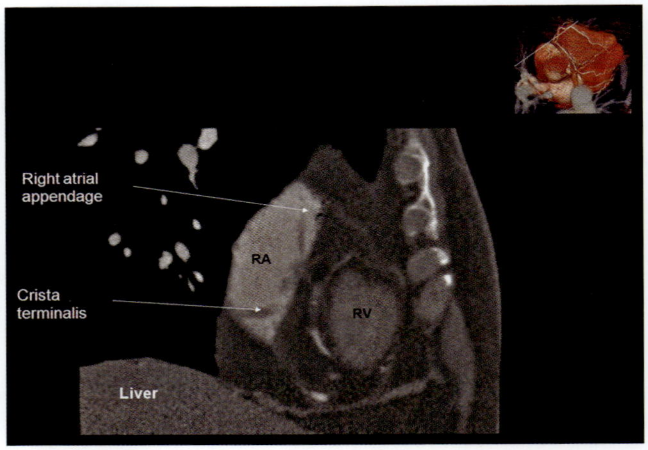

Two chamber 38

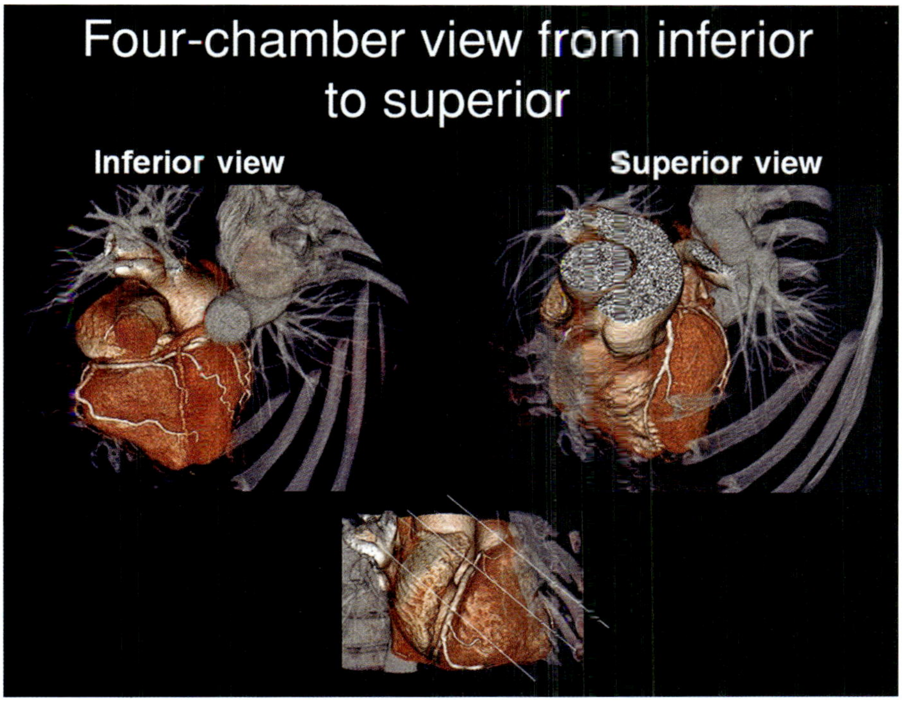

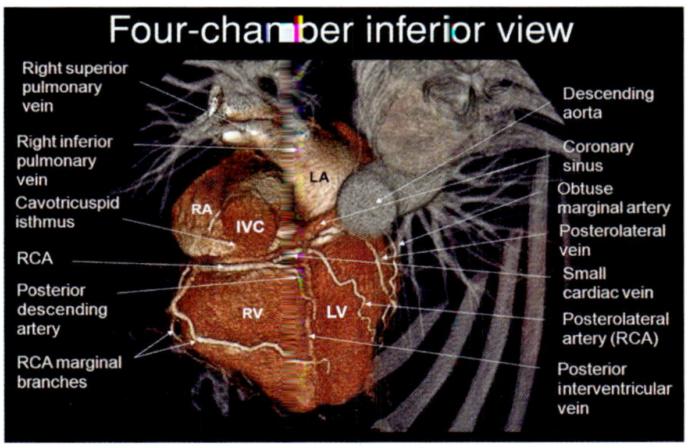

Four chamber 1

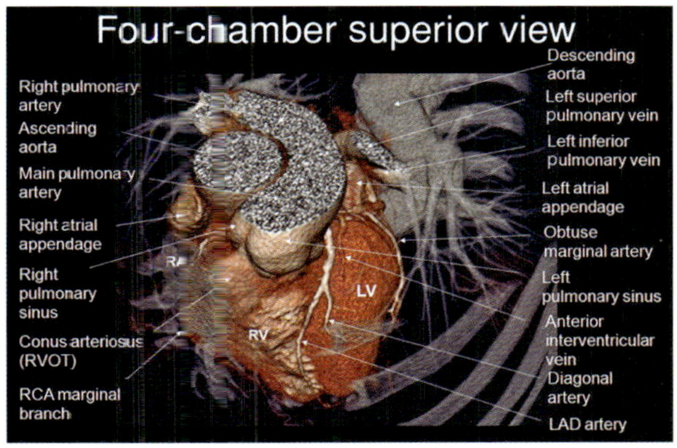

Four chamber 2

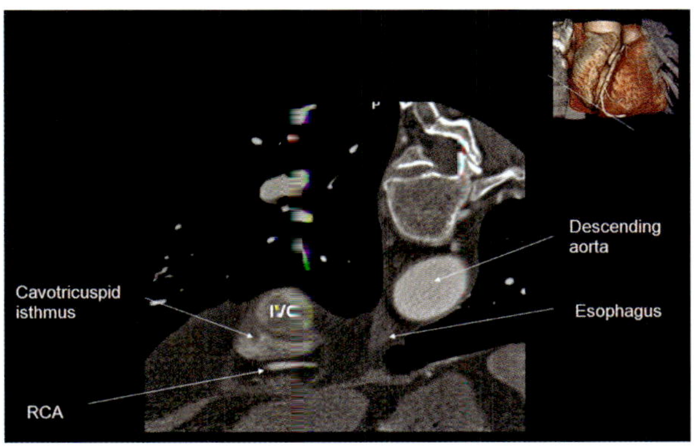

Four chamber 3

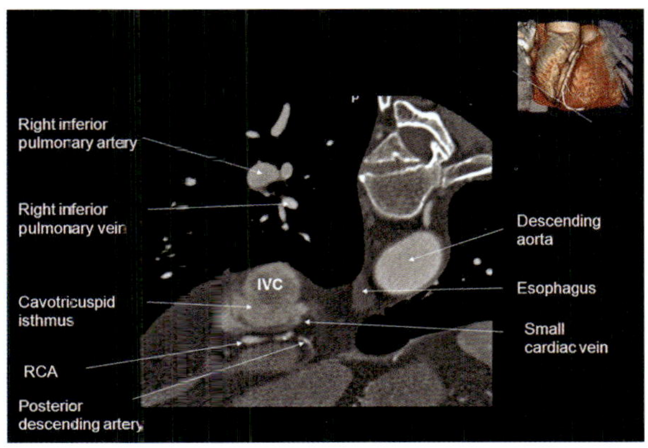

Four chamber 4

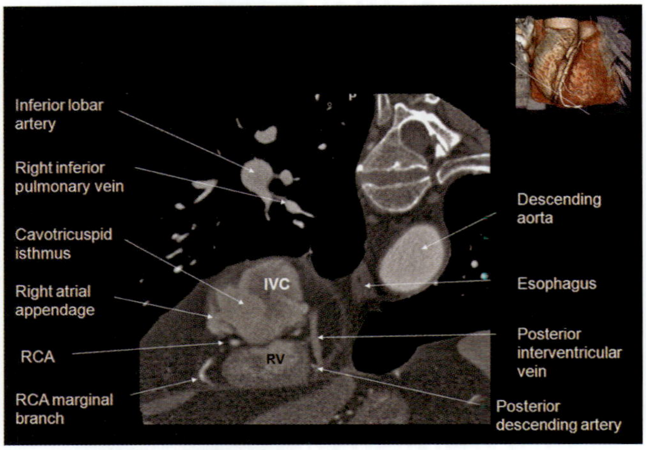

Four chamber 5

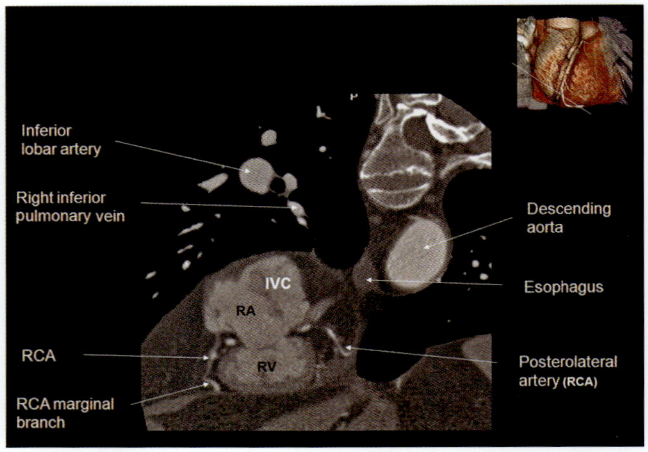

Four chamber 6

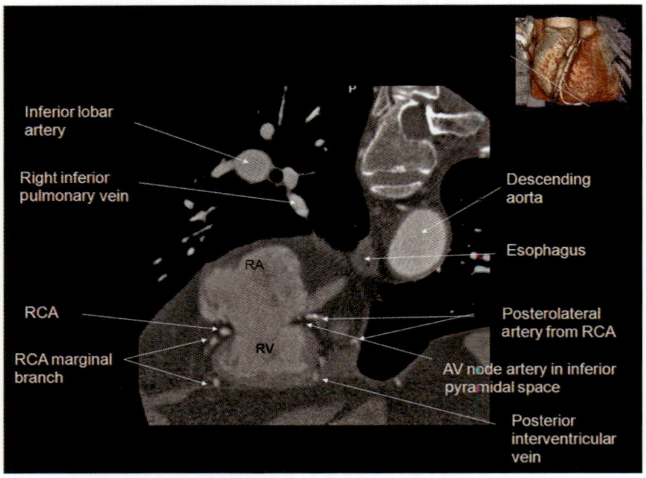

Four chamber 7

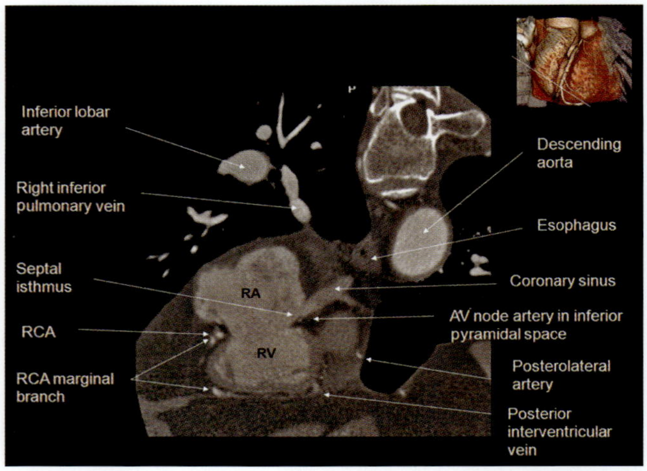

Four chamber 8

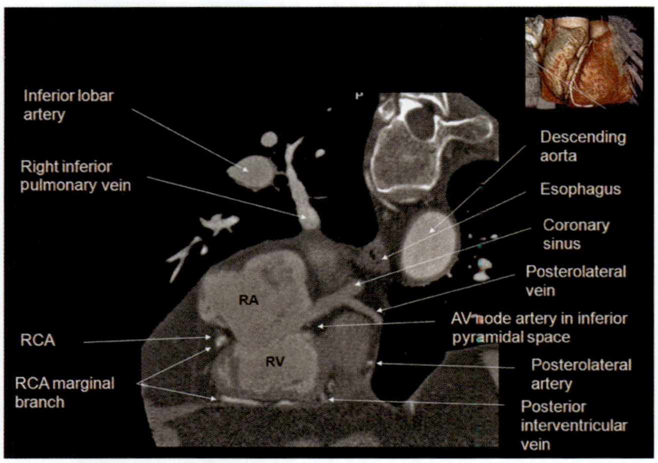

Four chamber 9

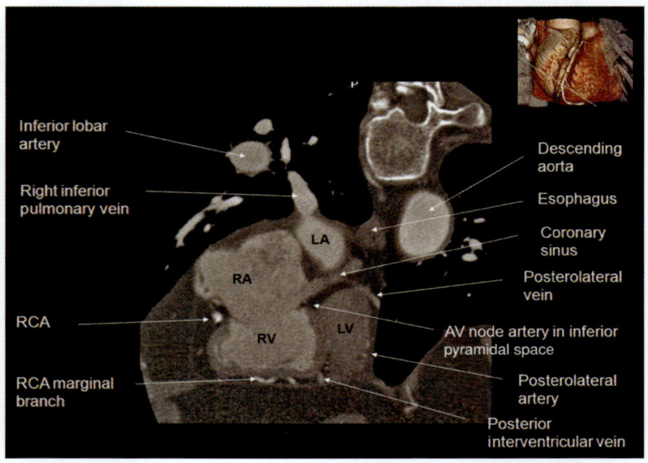

Four chamber 10

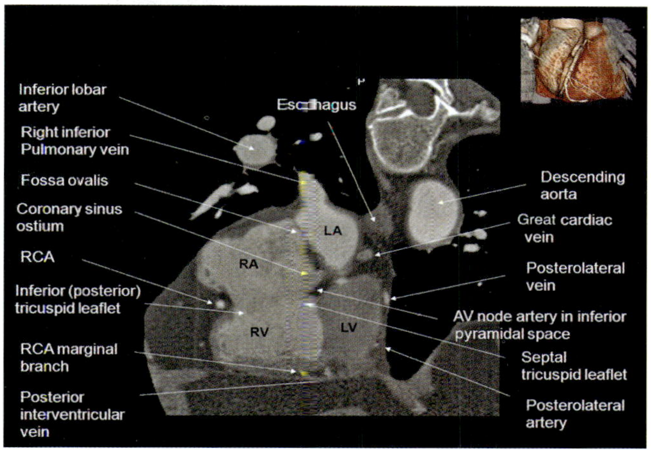

Four chamber 11

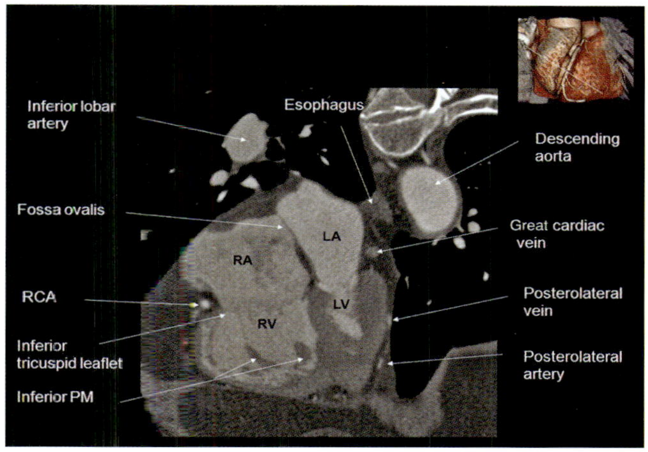

Four chamber 12

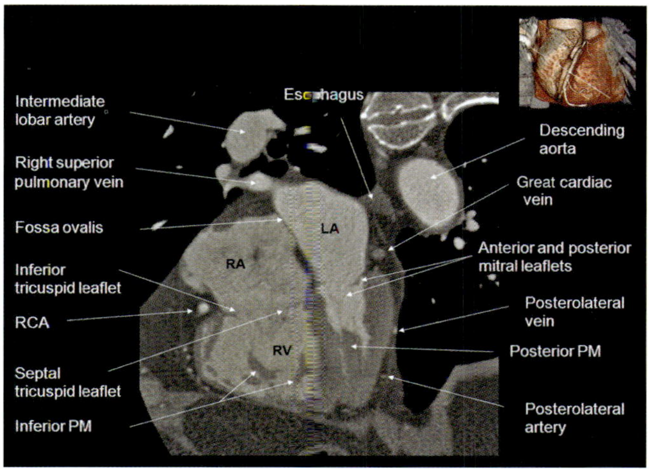

Four chamber 13

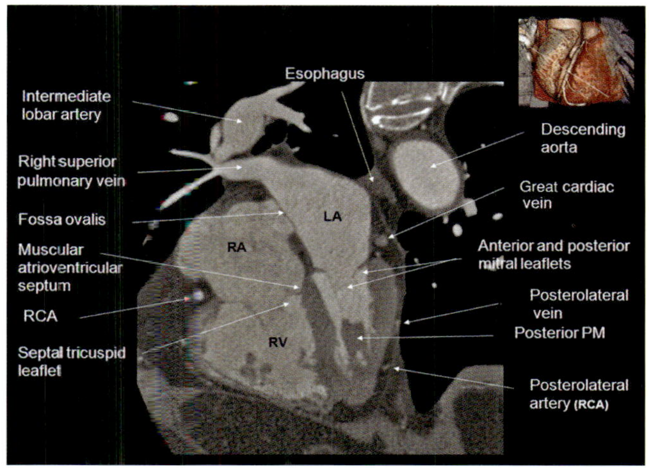

Four chamber 14

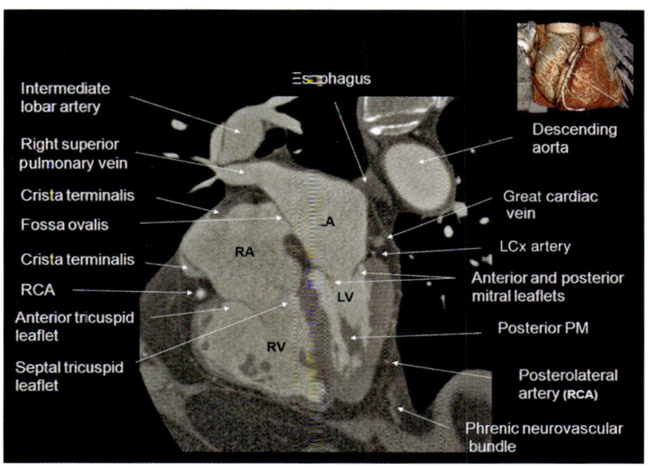

Four chamber 15

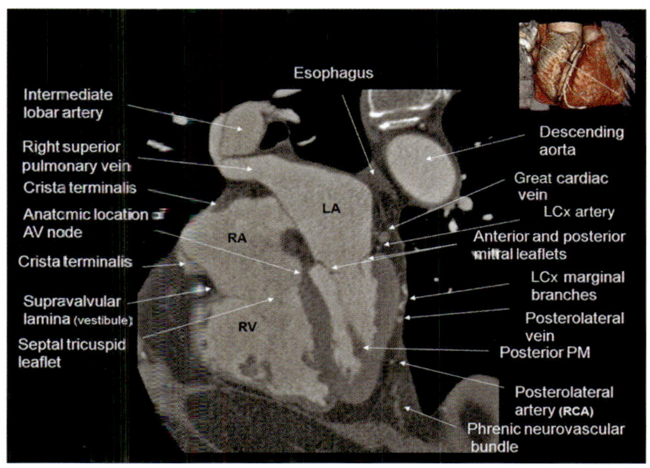

Four chamber 16

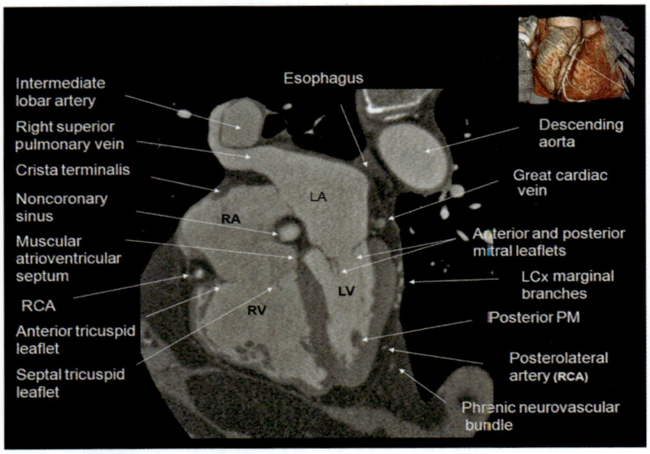

Four chamber 17

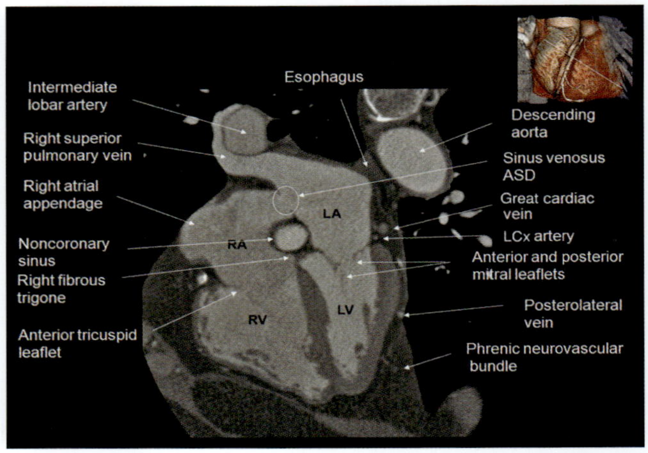

Four chamber 18

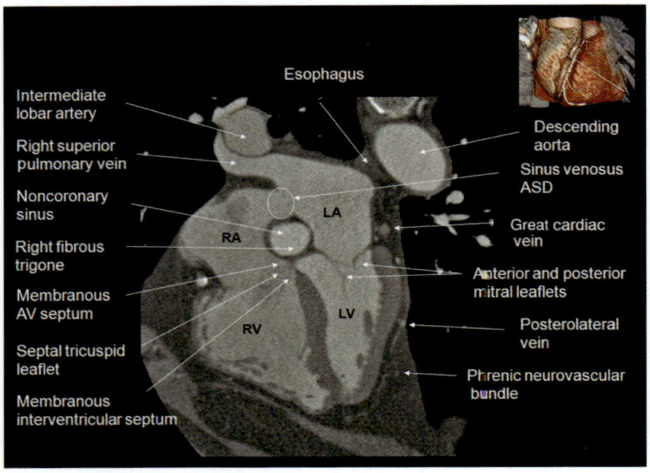

Four chamber 19

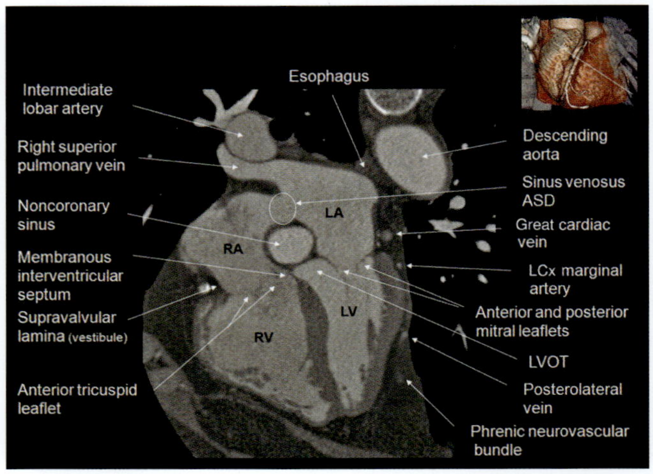

Four chamber 20

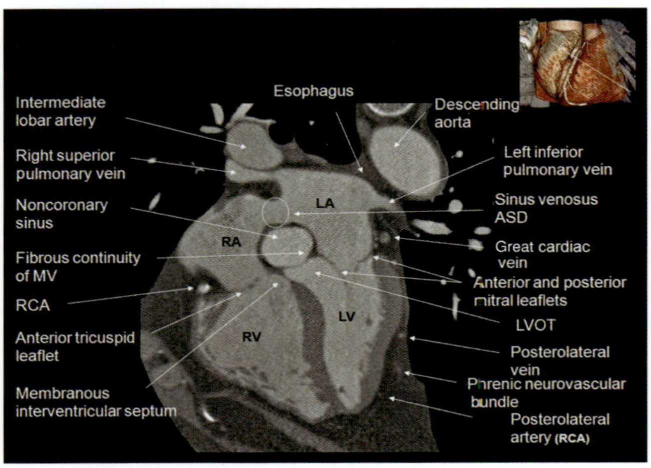

Four chamber 21

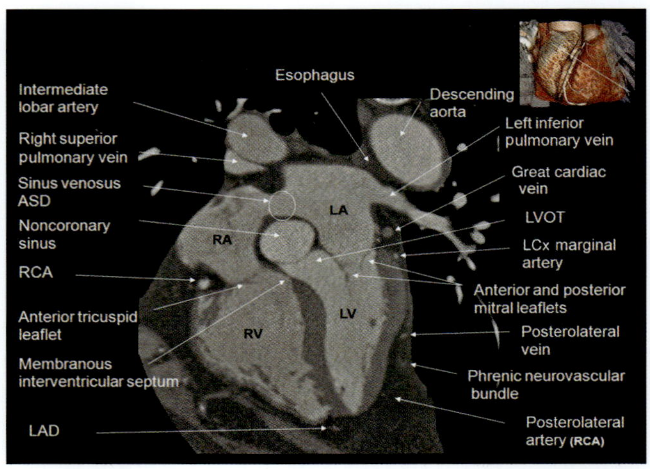

Four chamber 22

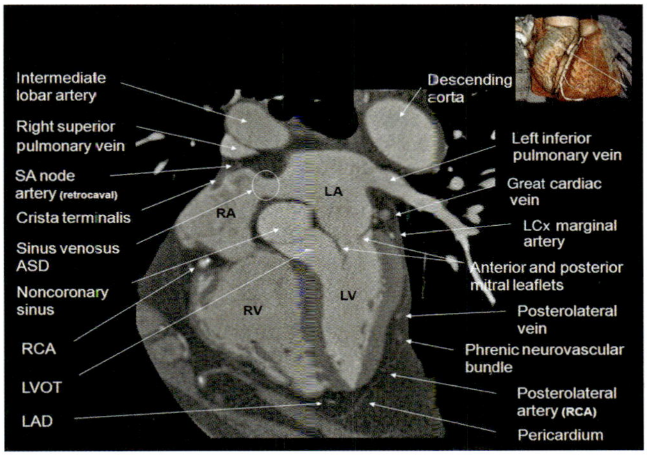

Four chamber 23

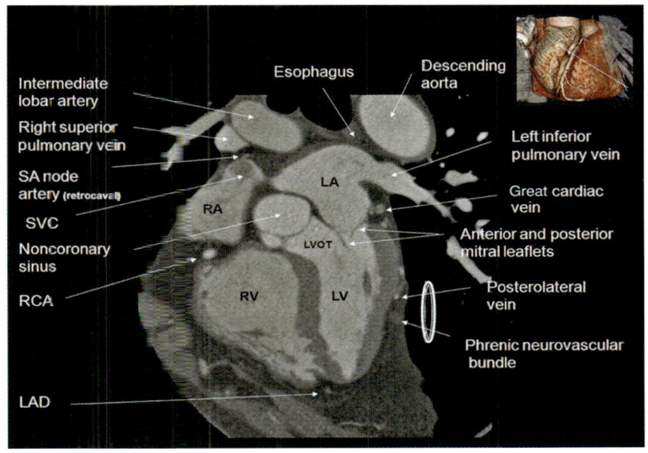

Four chamber 24

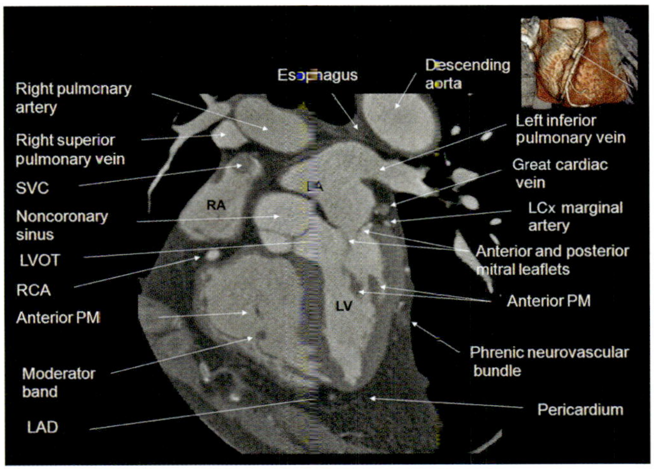

Four chamber 25

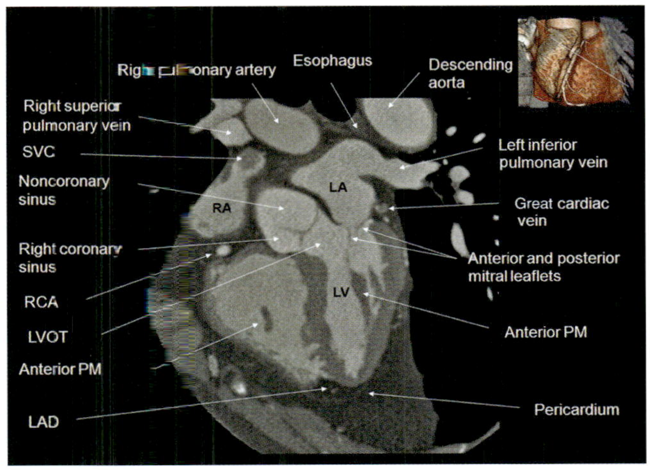

Four chamber 26

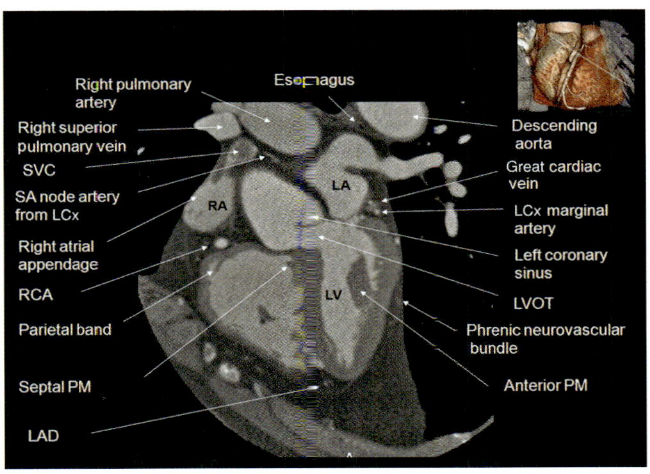

Four chamber 27

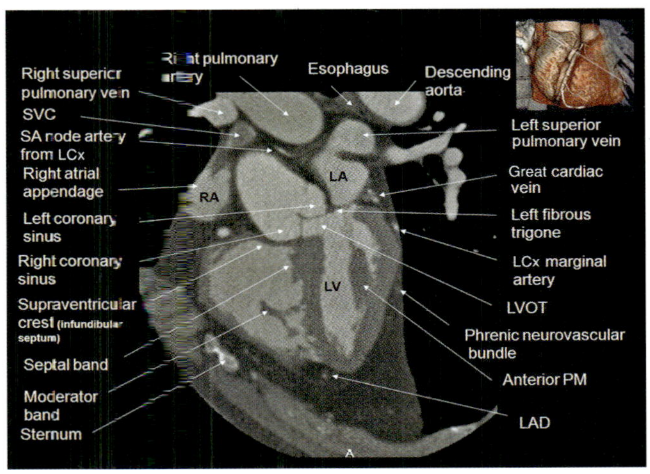

Four chamber 28

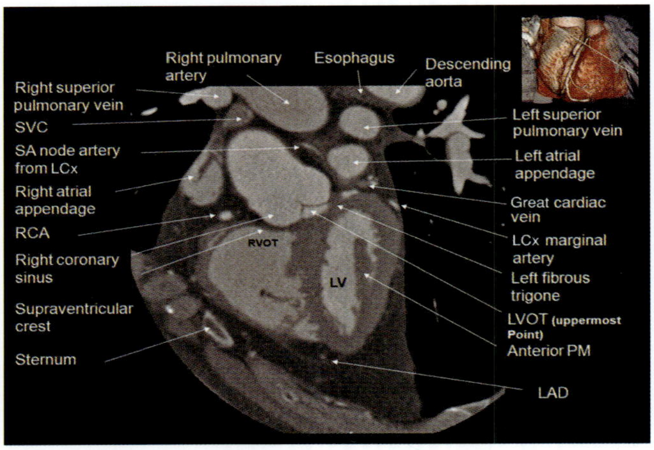

Four chamber 29

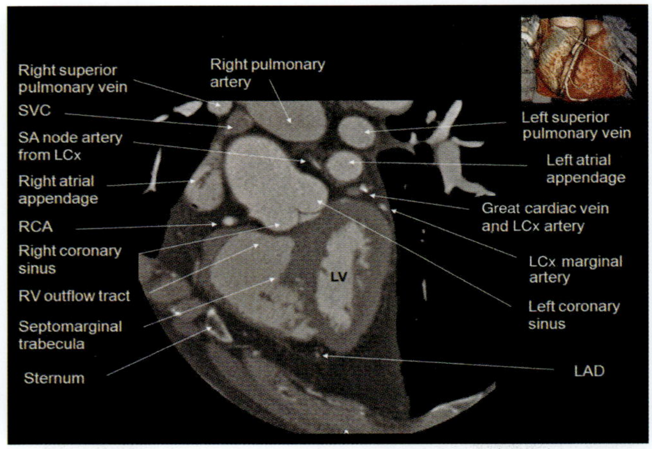

Four chamber 30

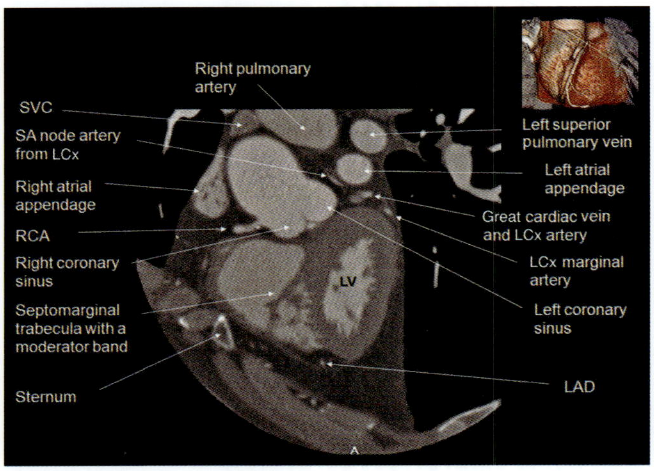

Four chamber 31

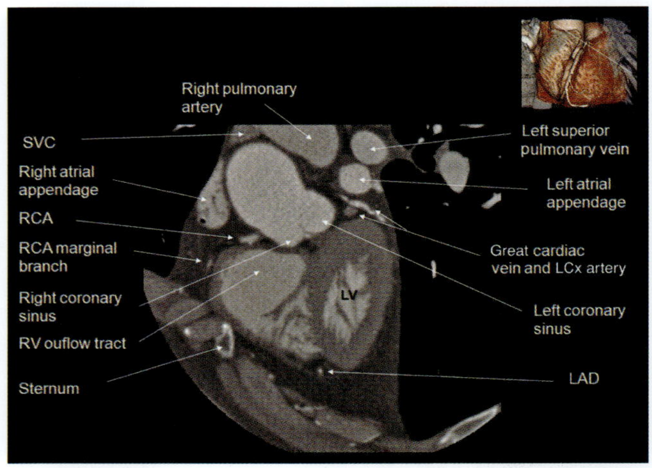

Four chamber 32

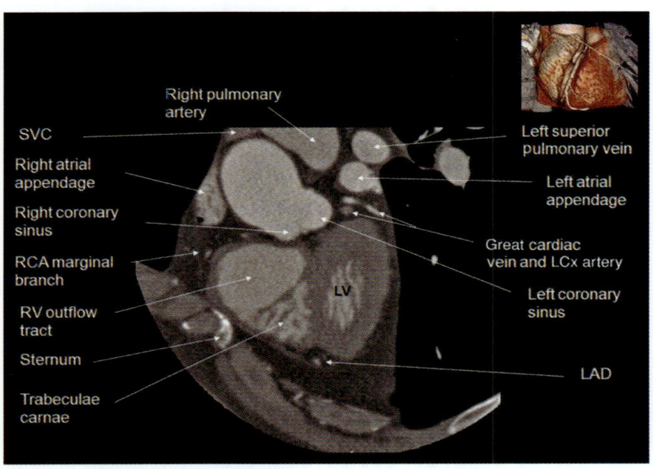

Four chamber 33

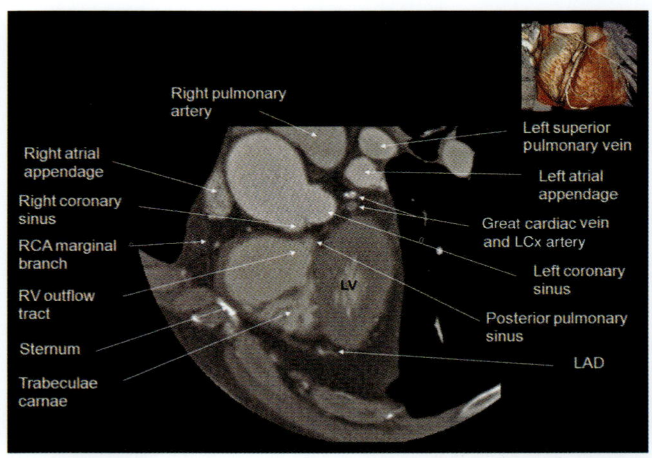

Four chamber 34

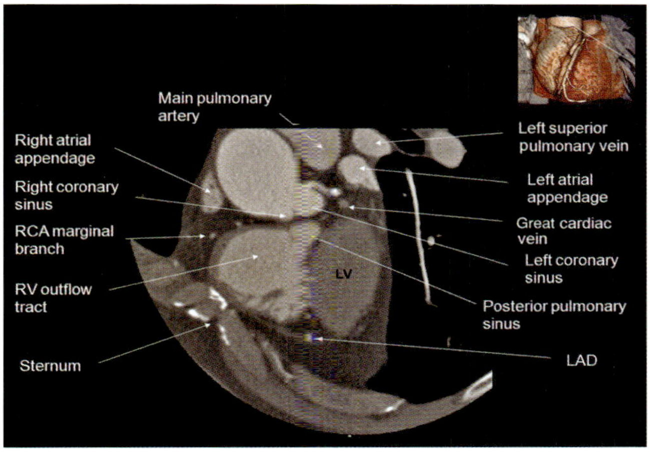

Four chamber 35

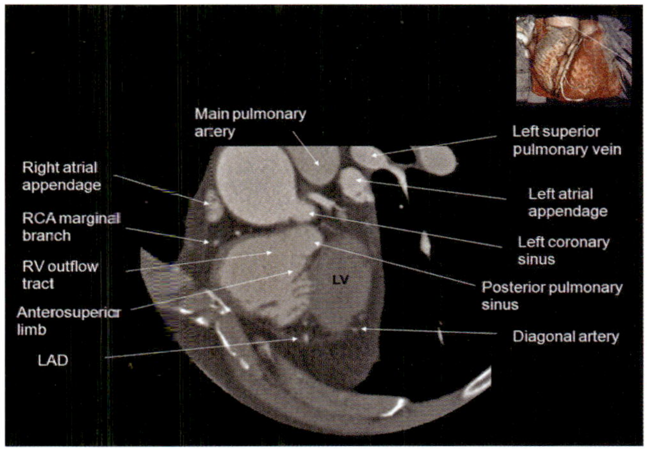

Four chamber 36

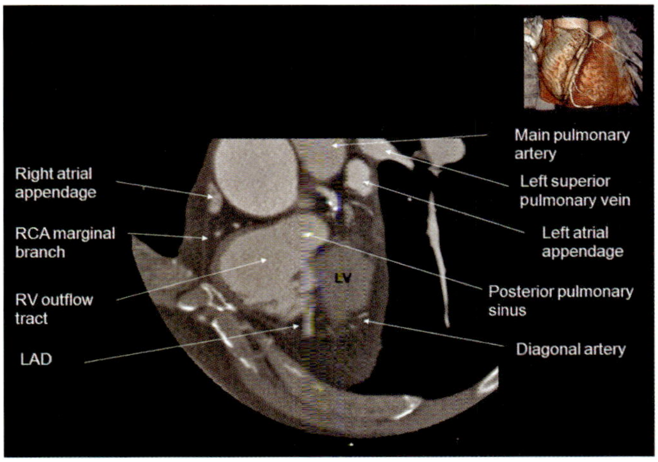

Four chamber 37

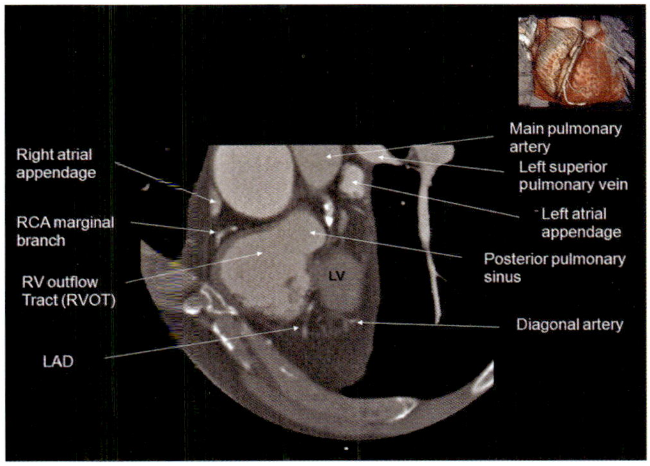

Four chamber 38

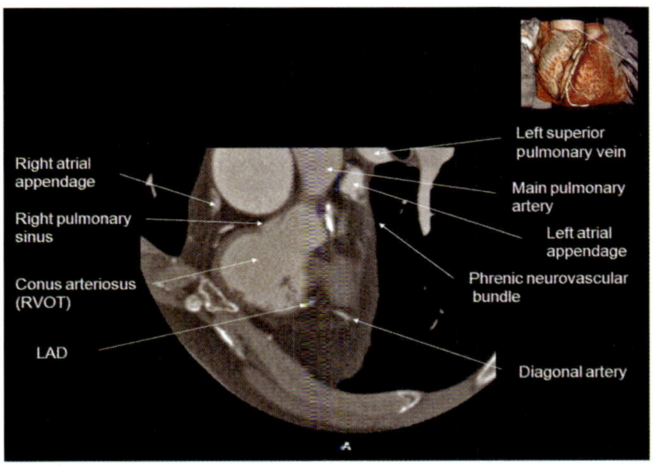

Four chamber 39

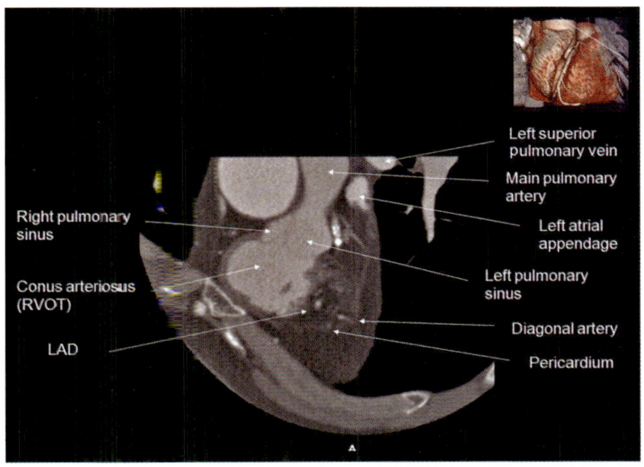

Four chamber 40

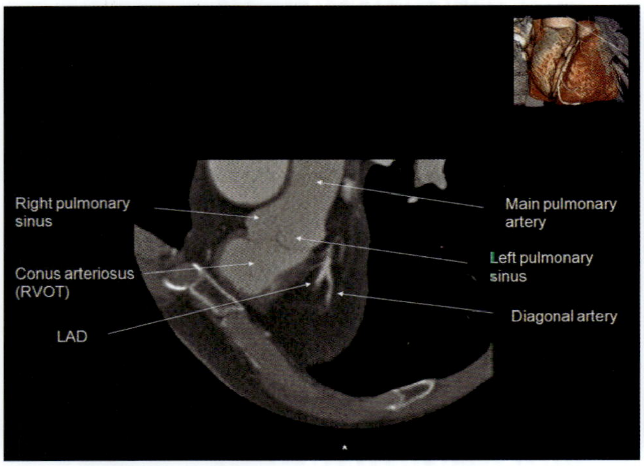

Four chamber 41

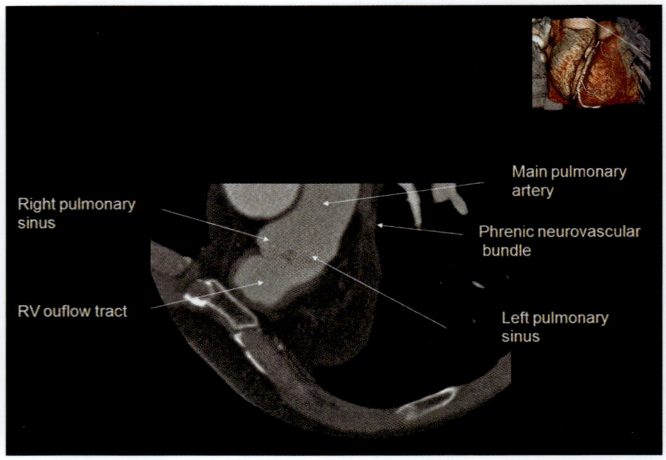

Four chamber 42

Index

Note: Italicized *f* and *t* refer to figures and tables.